Fluid, Electrolyte, and Acid-Base Physiology

THIRD EDITION

Fluid, Electrolyte, and Acid-Base Physiology

A Problem-Based Approach

Mitchell L. Halperin, MD, FRCPC
University of Toronto
Toronto, Ontario

Marc B. Goldstein, MD, FRCPC
University of Toronto
Toronto, Ontario

W.B. SAUNDERS COMPANY
A *Harcourt Health Sciences Company*
Philadelphia   London   New York   St. Louis   Sydney   Toronto

W.B. SAUNDERS COMPANY
A *Harcourt Health Sciences Company*

The Curtis Center
Independence Square West
Philadelphia, Pennsylvania 19106

Library of Congress Cataloging-in-Publication Data

Halperin, M. L. (Mitchell L.)

Fluid, electrolyte, and acid-base physiology: a problem-based approach / Mitchell L. Halperin, Marc B. Goldstein.—3rd ed.

p.   cm.

Includes bibliographical references and index.

ISBN 0–7216–7072–5

1. Water-electrolyte imbalances.   2. Acid-base imbalances.   3. Water-electrolyte imbalances—Case studies.   4. Acid-base imbalances—Case studies.   I. Goldstein, Marc B.   II. Title.   [DNLM: 1. Acid-Base Imbalance—physiopathology.   2. Acid-Base Imbalance—diagnosis. 3. Water-Electrolyte Imbalance—physiopathology.   4. Water-Electrolyte Imbalance—diagnosis.   5. Potassium—metabolism. WD 220 H195f 1999]

RC630.H34 1999   616.3′992—dc21

DNLM/DLC   97-48341

FLUID, ELECTROLYTE, AND ACID-BASE PHYSIOLOGY: ISBN 0–7216–7072–5
A PROBLEM-BASED APPROACH

Last digit is the print number: 9   8   7   6   5   4   3

Special thanks to the following who made excellent suggestions to improve this book:

KAMEL S. KAMEL

JEAN PIERRE MALLIE

JAMES OSTER

BOB RICHARDSON

ADRIENNE SCHEICH

MARTIN SCHREIBER

HARALD SONNENBERG

BOBBY JOE STINEBAUGH

Preparation of this book with great appreciation:

JOLLY MANGAT

□ □ □

BRENDA AND ELLEN. AT LAST!

Preface

There have been many insights gained at the subcellular level on the mechanisms operating in the areas we address as well as the substantial advances in our understanding of many important and common disorders. These have provided the impetus to proceed with this Third Edition, despite the fact that it is only five years since the last edition of *Fluid, Electrolyte, and Acid-Base Physiology*. We have also added many new challenging cases, which we hope will stimulate the reader as much as they have stimulated us. The philosophical priorities of the book remain unchanged.

- Our commitment to "learn by understanding" is further reinforced by the new information from the discipline of cell biology. We also stress the relevant physiology and biochemistry, bringing the basic science to the bedside to explain the disorders and make their therapy obvious. A good example is the pathophysiology of metabolic alkalosis in Chapter 4 and the implications for therapy.

- The book must be useful to readers with different needs:

  In the emergency room, the diagnostic flow charts (identified in their own table of contents) quickly guide one to the appropriate diagnosis. The approach to therapy is then readily available.

  For the reader with little time and looking for a quick overview of a topic, we provide an initial outline of major principles at the beginning of each chapter. Each key point is highlighted in a shadow box, and the reader can pursue these key points of interest by reading the subsequent details.

- Our teaching has always been "problem-based," even prior to it being in vogue, and we continue to add challenging and instructive cases to reinforce the clinical messages. We also have review cases at the end of each chapter, and for those readers who enjoy the clinical challenges, we have a table of contents for the cases.

- In addition to the clinical cases, we pose numerous challenges in the form of questions and provide the answers at the end of the chapter. Additional information is also provided in the margins so as not to distract the reader and disrupt the flow of thought.

HOW TO USE THIS BOOK:

FACED WITH AN EMERGENCY? Go to the Diagnostic Flow Chart Table of Contents, page xv, and find the therapeutic approach in the Table of Contents at the beginning of the relevant chapter.

WANT A QUICK OVERVIEW? Read the outline of major principles and the shaded key points in the area of interest.

WANT A CLINICAL CHALLENGE? Choose from the list of cases on page xi. Each case is discussed in detail after you have had a chance to form your opinions.

WANT TO BECOME AN EXPERT? Begin with the chapter on the relevant physiology, and then read the appropriate chapter, using the questions to indicate where you need more work. Additional reading is recommended at the end of each section.

Contents

List of Cases

CHAPTER 12
Hyperglycemia

List of Flow Charts

Acid-Base

1

Principles of Acid-Base Physiology

CONCEPTS IN ACID-BASE PHYSIOLOGY

1. Identify H⁺ production by counting new anions
2. Buffers work physiologically to keep added H⁺ from binding to proteins; instead, H⁺ are forced to react with HCO_3^-

3. The [HCO_3^-] is regulated by the kidney, which can excrete HCO_3^- and/or generate new HCO_3^-

OBJECTIVES

☐ To provide an understanding of how H^+ may be a threat to the body and how physiologic responses minimize this threat.

☐ To present a background enabling the recognition of both the production and removal of H^+ by *metabolic processes*.

☐ To develop the vocabulary required to "speak" the acid-base language.

☐ To emphasize the magnitude of H^+ production and removal in normal metabolism, thus elucidating the potential for the development of major acid-base disturbances.

Outline of Major Principles

1. The [H^+] is very tiny; if this concentration rises, H^+ will bind to proteins and change their charge, shape, and possibly function.

2. To quantitate the rate of production or removal of H^+, count the *valences* of substrates and products of metabolic processes.

3. H^+ are produced when certain amino acids in proteins are metabolized. They are also produced if there is insufficient oxygen (L-lactic acid) or insulin (ketoacid).

4. H^+ are produced at a very rapid rate, but only during hypoxia.

5. Buffering of H^+ occurs initially via the bicarbonate buffer system; this system removes H^+ when HCO_3^- are converted to CO_2 + H_2O. A large H^+ load obliges a larger proportion of buffering by intracellular proteins.

6. In people consuming a typical Western diet, the kidney regenerates new HCO_3^-, largely via the excretion of NH_4^+. The kidney must also "reabsorb" all filtered HCO_3^-.

7. The kidney contributes to the elimination of HCO_3^- largely as a result of the excretion of organic anions; there is also some excretion of HCO_3^-.

8. It is important to integrate H^+ with the physiology of sodium, potassium, energy metabolism, and the need to avoid the formation of kidney stones—the latter centers around control of the urine pH.

INTRODUCTORY CASE
Lee Wants to Know the Acid Truth
(Case discussed on pages 35–36)

Lee, a 70-kg insulin-dependent diabetic, did not take insulin for the past 2 days because a gastrointestinal (GI) upset prevented her from

Metabolic processes
A way of examining the overall impact of metabolism by considering only the substrates and products and ignoring all intermediates.

Note
Square brackets denote concentration.

Valence
The net electrical charge on a compound or element.

HCO_3^- (bicarbonate ion)
The conjugate base of carbonic acid (H_2CO_3) and the major H^+ acceptor in the extracellular fluid. New HCO_3^- are made in the kidney when H^+ are excreted or when ammonium ions (NH_4^+) are formed and excreted.

pH
The logarithm of 1/[H^+]. It rises when the [H^+] falls and vice versa.

Note
First-time readers should skip to page 5 and read Parts A and B and then return to this case.

Mole
The weight in grams of a compound when a given number (6.023 × 10^{23}) of molecules is present. One nanomole (nmol) is 10^{-9} mole.

$Paco_2$
The partial pressure of CO_2 in arterial blood.

eating. The relevant values from a sample of plasma were the following:

H^+	60 nmol/L (pH 7.22)	$Paco_2$	25 mm Hg
HCO_3^-	10 mmol/L	Anion gap	27 mEq/L

The relevant values in the urine on admission were:

NH_4^+	200 mmol/day	HCO_3^-	0 mmol/day

Ketoacid anions: strongly positive

What acid-base abnormality is present?
Were acids (H^+) added?
Have H^+ been buffered? If so, how many?
Have the lungs and the kidneys responded appropriately?
Is the acid-base abnormality a major threat to the body? If so, why?
Is it possible to estimate how quickly more H^+ will accumulate?
Do H^+ kill? If so, how do they do it?

Anion gap in plasma
• Calculated as:

$[Na^+] - ([Cl^-] + [HCO_3^-])$

• Used to detect new anions in the body (see pages 54–57). New anions are added with H^+ for the most part.

Normal values in plasma

$[H^+]$ = 40 ± 2 nmol/L
pH = 7.40 ± 0.02
$[HCO_3^-]$ = 25 ± 2 mmol/L
$Paco_2$ = 40 ± 2 mm Hg, or
5.3 ± 0.2 kPa
(1 mm Hg = 0.133 kPa)
Anion gap = 12 ± 2 mEq/L
(excluding K^+)

Characteristics of H⁺

H⁺ and the Potential Threat to Survival

> • The free $[H^+]$ is tiny and must be kept so for survival.
> • A very large accumulation of H^+ may kill by binding to proteins in cells and changing their charge, shape, and possibly their function.

The control of the $[H^+]$ in the body is of central importance; this concentration must not be allowed to rise or fall appreciably because H^+ binds avidly to proteins. When bound, they increase the net positive charge of these proteins, thereby changing their shape and possibly their function. The maintenance of the normal very low $[H^+]$ in the face of enormous turnover depends very heavily on *buffers* and on the mechanisms for excretion of CO_2 and nitrogenous wastes. These points will be discussed in the remainder of this chapter.

Think of H^+ from three perspectives.

1. In relation to the concentrations of other major ions in the extracellular fluid (ECF), the $[H^+]$ is very small. Table 1.1 shows that the normal plasma $[H^+]$ is 40 ± 2 nmol/L and that deviations from this value (halving or doubling) are clinically very significant; larger changes may become life-threatening.

2. $[H^+]$ should be examined relative to the "affinity" of H^+ for chemical groups on organic and inorganic compounds in the body. This comparison will provide insights as to whether H^+ will be bound or remain free.

3. It is important to gain a quantitative perspective by examining

Buffers
Compounds that bind H^+ when the $[H^+]$ rises and release them when the $[H^+]$ falls. Thus, buffers minimize the change in $[H^+]$. They require a high concentration of both the H^+ donor and acceptor in solution.

TABLE 1.1   **Range of [H⁺] in Plasma in Clinical Conditions**

Condition	[H⁺] nmol/L	pH	Importance
Acidemia	>100	<7.00	Can be lethal
Acidemia	50–80	7.1–7.30	Clinically important
Normal	40 ± 2	7.40 ± 0.02	Normal
Alkalemia	20–36	7.44–7.69	Clinically important
Alkalemia	<20	>7.70	Can be lethal

Number of H⁺ in the body
ECF: 15 L × 40 nmol/L = 600 nmol
ICF: 30 L × 80 nmol/L = 2400 nmol

the relative rates of production and removal of H⁺. For example, an enormous number of H⁺ are formed and consumed daily (70,000,000 nmol) in comparison with the amount of free H⁺ in the body at any one time (close to 3000 nmol); discrepancies between the rate of formation vs removal can result in major changes in [H⁺].

The [H⁺] Relative to the Concentration of Other Ions

The concentrations of major ions in the ECF (Na⁺, K⁺, Cl⁻, HCO₃⁻) are close to a million times higher than that of H⁺ (Table 1.2). Nevertheless, this very small [H⁺] is important from a biologic perspective, as discussed later. H⁺ are produced in millimolar amounts in biochemical reactions and during the transport of CO_2, yet their concentration must always remain in the nanomolar range (i.e., must always be a millionfold lower than that of H⁺ produced or the [HCO₃⁻] in the ECF or ICF).

Note
Normal values for the [HCO₃⁻] depend on whether the arterial blood (25 mmol/L) or the venous blood (28 mmol/L) is examined.

The [H⁺] Relative to the Affinity of H⁺ for Their Acceptors

In Certain Locations, H⁺ Remain Free and Do Not Bind

- For digestion, a high [H⁺] (no buffering) is needed in the lumen of the stomach.

Acids and bases
Acids are compounds that are capable of donating a H⁺, bases are compounds that are capable of accepting a H⁺. When an acid (HA) dissociates, it yields a H⁺ and its conjugate base (anion, A⁻).

$$HA \leftrightarrow H^+ + A^-$$

To initiate the digestion of proteins, a very high [H⁺] is needed. Accordingly, the anion secreted by the stomach along with H⁺ is Cl⁻ because Cl⁻ will not bind H⁺. Because HCl dissociates completely in aqueous solutions, and there are no major buffers in

TABLE 1.2   **Normal Concentrations of Cations and Anions in Plasma**

The sum of mEq/L of cations and anions must be equal.

Cations (mEq/L)		Anions (mEq/L)	
Na⁺	140	Cl⁻	103
K⁺	4	HCO₃⁻	25
Ca²⁺	5 (2.5 mmol/L)	Proteins	16
Mg²⁺	2 (1 mmol/L)	Organic	4
H⁺	0.000040 (40 nmol/L)	Other inorganics	3

gastric fluid, H^+ bind avidly when they come in contact with ingested proteins. Binding of H^+ makes the protein much more positively charged and alters its shape so that pepsin can gain access to the sites it will hydrolyze in that protein.

QUESTIONS

(Discussions on page 37)

1.1 *Why doesn't the HCl secreted by gastric cells denature proteins in the cell membrane of the stomach?*

1.2 *What might permit H^+ to bind to the H^+ pump inside cells at a concentration of 0.0001 mmol/L yet dissociate in the lumen of the stomach at a concentration of 100 mmol/L?*

1.3 *What is the rationale for stating that only weak acids kill?*

In Cells, H^+ May Be Bound to Proteins or Phosphates

> • When *acidosis* is severe, binding of H^+ to proteins is a major component of H^+ buffering.

The $[H^+]$ in cells is such that proteins have "just the right net charge" to perform essential functions (e.g., enzyme activities). A rise in the $[H^+]$ means that more H^+ binds to proteins; the converse is also true. There are two points to emphasize: (1) the change in function of proteins with a change in charge; and (2) the enormous number of binding sites for H^+.

Inorganic phosphate can bind an important quantity of H^+ in some circumstances but not others (see margin note). In the ICF, the ECF, and the urine, the difference in degree of binding of H^+ is due to the $[H^+]$ in these three environments relative to the pK for phosphate. In most conditions, binding of H^+ is lowest in the ECF and highest in the urine, where almost every phosphate ion usually has bound H^+ (Table 1.3). The authors return to this phenomenon when discussing buffering in cells and the excretion of bound H^+ in the urine (titratable acid).

Strength of acids
Chemists classify an acid as strong or weak on the basis of its dissociation constant, or pK (the pH at which the acid is 50% dissociated); strong acids have a much lower pK. Hydrochloric acid is a very strong acid. This differentiation is of little importance biologically because at a pH of 7 the dissociation of both weak and strong acids is much greater than 99%.

Note
Question 1.2 is for the more curious.

Acidosis and alkalosis
Acidosis is a process that adds acids to the blood or removes bases from the blood; alkalosis is the converse.

Compartmental $[H^+]$
ECF = 40 nmol/L
ICF = 80–100 nmol/L
Urine = 10,000 nmol/L

Note
The content of inorganic phosphate is quite low in the ECF and the ICF, so little buffering of H^+ occurs by this buffer in these locations.

HPO_4^{2-} = divalent inorganic phosphate ion
$H_2PO_4^-$ = monovalent dihydrogen inorganic phosphate ion

$$\mathbf{pH} = pK + \log \frac{HPO_4^{2-}}{H_2PO_4^-}$$

pH	Compartment	Ratio of $HPO_4^{2-}/H_2PO_4^-$
7.4	ECF	4/1
7.1	ICF	2/1
5.8	Urine	1/10

TABLE 1.3 **Physiology of Phosphate Buffers**

The pK for inorganic phosphate is close to 6.8 at physiologic ionic strength and temperature. Organic phosphates (e.g., ATP) have too low an affinity for H^+ at the $[H^+]$ in cells to act as physiologic buffers.

Compartment	Total Inorganic Phosphate	% as $H_2PO_4^-$	Equation
ECF	1 mmol/L	20%	$H^+ + HPO_4^{2-} \longleftrightarrow H_2PO_4^-$
ICF	4–5 mmol/L	33%	$H^+ + HPO_4^{2-} \longleftrightarrow H_2PO_4^-$
Urine	30 mml/day	90%	$H^+ + HPO_4^{2-} \longleftrightarrow H_2PO_4^-$

The [H⁺] Relative to the Production and Removal of H⁺ During Metabolism

Valence
The number of charges a compound or ion bears in solution, expressed in mEq/L. The term *milliequivalent* (mEq) reflects the number of charges or valences; therefore, multiply mmol by the valence to obtain mEq. Valence is especially important for albumin, which has a large valence on each molecule.

NH_4^+
A cation formed in the kidney during metabolism. When NH_4^+ are excreted, the new HCO_3^- formed along with the NH_4^+ are added to the body.

- Production or removal of H⁺ is best understood by examining the "net charge," or *valence,* of substrates and products of a metabolic process—ignore cofactors.
- Two processes indicate net H⁺ production in metabolism—accumulation of new anions in the body and the excretion of anions without a H⁺ or NH_4^+.
- H⁺ can be classified as "fast" H⁺ or "slow" H⁺ depending on their net rate of production.

An enormous number of H⁺ are produced and removed during the usual metabolic reactions in the body. When are these H⁺ important? The authors offer the following ways to simplify the approach to understanding the clinical significance of H⁺.

Definition of a Metabolic Process

In general, a metabolic process starts with either dietary or stored fuels and ends with *adenosine triphosphate* (ATP) or an energy store (glycogen, triglyceride). A metabolic process can span more than one organ. In the example in Figure 1.1, H⁺ will accumulate if the ketoacid anions are retained in the body or if they are excreted with a cation other than H⁺ or NH_4^+ (e.g., Na⁺ or K⁺). If part of the pathway generates H⁺ and is intimately linked to another part that removes H⁺, both parts can be ignored from an acid-base perspective. For example, H⁺ are formed when ATP is hydrolyzed to perform biologic work (e.g., reabsorb Na⁺). As soon as ATP is regenerated in mitochondria of that cell, H⁺ are removed. Hence, the cycle has no net acid-base impact.

Adenosine triphosphate (ATP)
The useful form of energy in cells that enables biochemical work to be performed. The need for regeneration of ATP limits the flux through ATP-producing reactions because of a limited availability of adenosine diphosphate (ADP).

$$ATP^{4-} \leftrightarrow ADP^{3-} + P_i^{2-} + H^+ \quad \text{(pump Na}^+\text{)}$$
$$ADP^{3-} + P_i^{2-} + H^+ \leftrightarrow ATP^{4-} \quad \text{(mitochondria)}$$

When examining a series of metabolic pathways occurring in a number of organs (Figure 1.1), consider all the substrates and products to determine their acid-base impact. By counting the net charge, or valence, of substrates and products of the overall series of metabolic reactions, the number of H⁺ produced or removed can be deduced.

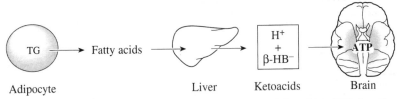

Figure 1.1   Illustration of a metabolic process. The starting point is triglycerides (TG) in adipose tissue and the final product is ATP (and CO_2 + H_2O) in the brain. Ketoacids (H⁺ + β-*hydroxybutyrate anion*) are produced in the liver and removed by the brain. (Reproduced with permission of the authors—Halperin and Rolleston, *Clinical Detective Stories* [London: Portland Press, 1993]).

Adipocyte: Triglyceride $\leftrightarrow$ 3 Palmitate$^-$ + 3 H$^+$ + Glycerol
Liver: 3 Palmitate$^-$ + 3 H$^+$ + 18 O$_2$ $\leftrightarrow$ 12 Ketoacid anions + 12 H$^+$
Brain: 12 Ketoacid anions + 12 H$^+$ $\leftrightarrow$ CO$_2$ + H$_2$O + ATP

Overall: Triglyceride yields ATP, CO$_2$, and H$_2$O in the brain but causes no net production or removal of H$^+$.

β-Hydroxybutyrate anion (β-HB$^-$)
There are two ketoacids formed during the partial oxidation of fatty acids in the liver, acetoacetic acid and β-hydroxybutyric acid (Hβ-HB); the conjugate base of Hβ-HB is β-HB$^-$.

QUESTION

(Discussion on page 37)

1.4 *In the metabolic process in Figure 1.1, under what circumstances will H$^+$ accumulate?*

Examples of the Production and Removal of H$^+$

> - H$^+$ production: Conversion of a neutral compound to anions (usually via oxidation of amino acids) generates most H$^+$.
> - H$^+$ removal: Conversion of dietary anions to neutral products removes most H$^+$. In the kidney, generation and excretion of a new cation (NH$_4^+$) removes H$^+$.

The following generalizations can be made. When a neutral compound is converted to an anion, or when a cation is converted to a neutral compound, H$^+$ are produced; conversely, when an anion is converted to a neutral compound, or when a neutral compound is converted to a cation, H$^+$ are removed. Examples follow:

Concept
1. Identify H$^+$ production by counting new anions.

1. **All of the following yield H$^+$ (more net negative charge):**

   Glucose $\leftrightarrow$ Lactate$^-$ + H$^+$ (new anion)
   Fatty acid $\leftrightarrow$ 4 Ketoacid anions + 4 H$^+$ (new anions)
   Cysteine $\leftrightarrow$ Urea + CO$_2$ + H$_2$O + SO$_4^{2-}$ + 2 H$^+$ (new anion)
   Lysine$^+$ $\leftrightarrow$ Urea + CO$_2$ + H$_2$O + H$^+$ (loss of cation)

2. **All of the following remove H$^+$ (more net positive charge):**

   Lactate$^-$ + H$^+$ $\leftrightarrow$ Glucose (anion removed)
   Citrate^{3-} + 3 H$^+$ $\leftrightarrow$ CO$_2$ + H$_2$O (anion removed)
   Glutamine $\leftrightarrow$ Glucose + NH$_4^+$ + CO$_2$ + H$_2$O + HCO$_3^-$ (generation of a new cation)

Note
Conversion of glutamine to NH$_4^+$ will have a net yield of HCO$_3^-$ only if NH$_4^+$ is made as an end-product of metabolism (i.e., is excreted in the urine).

3. **None of the following yields or removes H$^+$ (no change in net charge):**

   Glucose $\leftrightarrow$ Glycogen + CO$_2$ + H$_2$O (neutrals to neutrals)
   Triglyceride $\leftrightarrow$ CO$_2$ + H$_2$O (neutrals to neutrals)
   Alanine $\leftrightarrow$ Urea + Glucose or CO$_2$ + H$_2$O (neutrals to neutrals)

A quantitative description of H$^+$ balance from metabolism of a typical Western diet is provided in Table 1.4.

Anion for excretion
If a H$^+$ is accompanied by an anion with which it can be excreted in bound form, the acid-base impact of the H$^+$ is eliminated. For example, H$_2$PO$_4^-$ is formed from the metabolism of dietary constituents; it yields H$^+$ and HPO$_4^{2-}$ at a pH of 7.4. Because the kidney secretes H$^+$, H$_2$PO$_4^-$ is excreted when the urine pH is less than 6.8 (see page 16).

Rate of Production of H$^+$

The production of L-lactic acid via anaerobic glycolysis is the only circumstance in which the rate of production of H$^+$ is so rapid that

TABLE 1.4 **Dietary Acid-Base Impact**

The following H^+ load is calculated on the basis of the ingestion of 100 g of protein from beefsteak. The net dietary H^+ load is approximately 70 mmol/day, but 40 mmol of H^+ is produced with an anion such as SO_4^{2-} that does not help in their removal (there is virtually no metabolism or excretion of H_2SO_4) so NH_4^+ must be excreted to maintain acid-base balance.

Nutrient	Product	H^+ (mEq/day)
Reactions Generating H^+		
• Sulfur-containing amino acids		
Cysteine/cystine, methionine	H^+	70
• Cationic amino acids		
Lysine, arginine, histidine ($\frac{1}{2}$)	H^+	140
• Organic phosphates	$HPO_4^{2-} + H^+$	30
Reactions Removing H^+		
• Anionic amino acids		−110
Glutamate, aspartate	HCO_3^-	
• Organic anions (e.g., citrate^{3-})	HCO_3^-	−60
• Organic phosphate excretion with H^+	$H_2PO_4^-$ excreted	−30
Net Total H^+ Load to be Excreted as NH_4^+		40

it might constitute a serious acid-base threat in minutes to hours. The authors consider this rate of production to be "fast." Examples of the rate of H^+ production in clinical conditions are provided in Table 1.5.

TABLE 1.5 **Rates of Production and Removal of H^+**

The total quantity of H^+ that can be buffered per day is close to 1000 mmol in a 70-kg person. With very large acid loads, most of the buffering occurs in the ICF.

Event	Rate (mmol/min)	Comments
Production of H^+		
L-Lactic acid (hypoxia)	72	• Rate reflects complete anoxia
	7.2	• Rate reflects 10% hypoxia
Ketoacids	1	• Production requires lack of insulin
Toxic alcohols	<1	• Poisonous metabolites rather than H^+ are usually the major threat
Removal of H^+		
Kidney (by excretion of NH_4^+)	0–2	• Has a lag period
Metabolism		
L-Lactic acid	4–8	• Half by oxidation and half by glucogenesis
Ketoacids	0.8	• Oxidized primarily in the brain and kidneys

Clinical Classification of Metabolic Reactions Influencing Acid-Base Balance

An overall approach to the net production of H^+ is provided in Figure 1.2; its basis is that only those H^+ that accumulate provide a

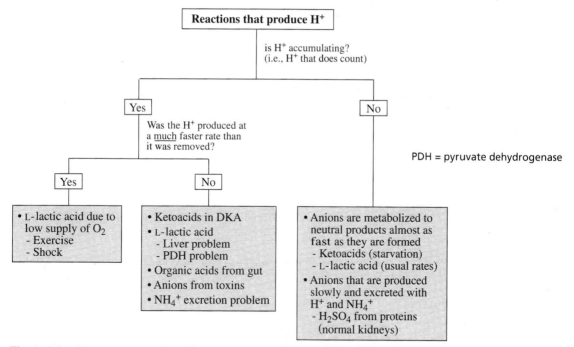

Figure 1.2   Overview of the net production of H⁺. Only anions that accumulate or are excreted without H^+ or NH_4^+ count from an acid-base perspective.

H^+ load to the body. The clinical threat of H^+ accumulation is proportional to the magnitude of the H^+ load and the speed with which H^+ accumulate. If H^+ are being formed very rapidly, production of H^+ must be stopped as soon as possible. Therapy with HCO_3^- will at best buy a little time from an acid-base viewpoint. If H^+ are accumulating slowly, there is time for more thorough investigation.

Note
The rate of H^+ formation is evident from the rate of appearance of anions and the fall in the $[HCO_3^-]$.

H⁺ That Do Not Count

- Because there is a balance between rates of production and removal of H^+ during the normal metabolism of carbohydrates and fats, protons do not accumulate in most of energy metabolism.

Most of the H^+ that do not count are formed along with a partner that aids in their removal. Examples are found in the normal metabolism of carbohydrates and fats and in the metabolism of 13 of the 20 amino acids in proteins. When considering organic phosphates, the anion produced (HPO_4^{2-}) can bind H^+ at most usual $[H^+]$ in the urine so that H^+ do not accumulate in the body.

Carbohydrates

Because all substrates and products of the normal metabolism of carbohydrates have the same net charge, they do not yield a surplus or deficit of H^+. When glucose is converted to pyruvate or L-lactate anions, H^+ are formed but are then removed when these anions are

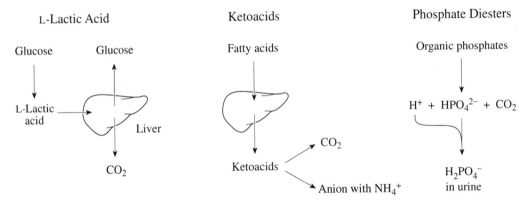

Figure 1.3 **H⁺ that are removed as fast as they are formed.** In each of these examples, an anion is formed but is readily metabolized to a neutral end-product or is excreted with a bound H⁺ at the [H⁺] in urine.

metabolized to the neutral end-products glucose, glycogen, triglycerides, or CO_2 and H_2O (Figure 1.3).

Fats

Despite the fact that fatty acid and ketoacid anions are metabolic intermediates of fat metabolism, neither they nor H^+ accumulate in normal metabolism (see Figure 1.3).

Proteins

The majority (13 of 20) of the amino acids are neutral, and their products (urea, glucose, CO_2, and H_2O) are also neutral. Hence, their metabolism does not contribute to net accumulation of H^+.

Anions That Help H⁺ Excretion

The major anions of the ICF are organic phosphates. These compounds are primarily phosphate diesters (DNA, RNA, phospholipids, and high-energy phosphates). The products of their metabolism are HPO_4^{2-} + H^+ (see Figure 1.3). The divalent phosphate anion (HPO_4^{2-}) is filtered by the kidney. Because the kidney raises the [H⁺] in the urine appreciably above that of the plasma, the filtered HPO_4^{2-} is excreted as $H_2PO_4^-$; this process is called *titratable acid excretion*. Thus, organic phosphates represent production of H^+ with a partner that aids in their excretion.

H⁺ That Do Count

In the following two sections, the net production of H^+ is considered by examining the properties of the accompanying anions.

Anions That Are Formed Faster Than They Are Metabolized

> **Key Point**
> A gain of anions signals a positive balance for H⁺. In this context, the authors are referring to anions other than HCO₃⁻.

- The only time that H^+ are formed very rapidly is during anaerobic metabolism.

Carbohydrates. When oxygen is lacking, carbohydrates cannot be metabolized to the neutral end-products CO_2 and H_2O, so the anion L-lactate and a H^+ accumulate (*L-lactic acidosis*). Two general conditions cause L-lactic acidosis: first, when the demand for oxygen is extremely high (e.g., during a sprint or convulsion); second, when the supply of oxygen is very low (e.g., from a low cardiac output; quantitative considerations appear in Chapter 3, pages 103–104).

At times, one of the enzymes involved in the oxidation of L-lactate may limit its oxidation. In this case, there is usually an inborn error of metabolism or a dietary deficiency of a cofactor such as vitamin B_1 (*thiamine*). See Chapter 3, pages 107–108, for discussion.

Fats. When there is a lack of insulin, ketoacid anions and H^+ accumulate (*ketoacidosis*). A relatively small accumulation occurs during chronic fasting. For a large accumulation to occur, β cells of the pancreas must be destroyed (as in diabetic ketoacidosis) or inhibited (during alcoholic ketoacidosis; see Chapter 3, pages 99–103). In addition, the oxidation of ketoacids must be slower than usual (coma, low GFR; see Chapter 3, pages 91–92).

Unusual Anions. Bacteria in the GI tract produce a variety of organic acids that are absorbed (D-lactic, butyric, acetic, and propionic acids, among others). Each is metabolized to neutral end-products, so there is usually no net H^+ load. Should their production rise dramatically or their metabolism be slower than usual (a liver or kidney problem), H^+ will accumulate.

L-Lactic acidosis
The accumulation of acid produced from the incomplete oxidation of glucose.

Thiamine
A vitamin that is required for the activity of the enzyme pyruvate dehydrogenase.

Ketoacidosis
The accumulation of ketoacids that results from incomplete oxidation of fatty acids and occurs when there is a relative lack of insulin.

QUESTIONS

(Discussions on pages 38–39)

1.5 *Red blood cells produce 200 mmol of L-lactic acid per day. Why doesn't this production cause severe acidemia?*

1.6 *When ATP is used to perform biologic work, H^+ are formed. Should these H^+ be considered as part of the quantity that can cause acidosis?*

1.7 *Acetate is added to the hemodialysis fluid to minimize the net production of H^+. What is the rationale for this maneuver?*

1.8 *During hemodialysis, β-hydroxybutyric acid is formed from acetate anions and is lost in the dialysis fluid. Does this process result in the net production or removal of H^+?*

1.9 *What might permit bacteria in the GI tract to overproduce organic acids?*

1.10 *Does consumption of citrus fruits, which contain a large quantity of citric acid and K^+ citrate, cause an acid or alkali load?*

Anions That Cannot Be Metabolized

Sulfate. Amino acids containing the element sulfur (cysteine/cystine and methionine) can be oxidized to yield the terminal anion SO_4^{2-} plus neutral end-products (glucose, urea, and CO_2 and H_2O). Because the affinity of SO_4^{2-} for H^+ is so low (i.e., SO_4^{2-} has a very low pK), SO_4^{2-} cannot help in removing H^+ by urinary excretion (nor can it help by metabolism). Hence, other ways are needed to

TABLE 1.6 **Production of Anions That Cannot Help in the Removal of H$^+$**

Substrate	Anion Formed
Methanol	Formate
Ethylene glycol	Glycolate, oxalate
Toluene	Hippurate
Protein	Sulfate

remove these H$^+$ (renal excretion of NH$_4^+$; see pages 29–33). For each mEq of SO$_4^{2-}$ that accumulates or is excreted without NH$_4^+$, H$^+$ accumulate. Only 20–40 mmol of H$^+$ is produced as H$_2$SO$_4$ each day in people who consume a typical Western diet (obliging a similar excretion of NH$_4^+$); lower quantities are produced in people who consume a low-protein diet.

Anions From Toxins. Metabolism of methanol, ethylene glycol, and toluene will all yield anions that cannot undergo further metabolism (Table 1.6, Figure 1.4). The affinity of these anions for H$^+$ is also so low that they cannot be excreted with H$^+$ in the urine. Of greater importance, the production of toxic products, such as formaldehyde from methanol, is a much greater threat to the patient than is the production of H$^+$ (see Chapter 3, pages 110–112).

Cations That Are Oxidized to Neutral End-Products

Three cationic amino acids (lysine, arginine, histidine) are metabolized to neutral end-products in normal metabolism (net negative charge); as a result, H$^+$ accumulate. Thus, these H$^+$ also require the excretion of NH$_4^+$ to prevent the accumulation of protons. The net production of H$^+$ from protein oxidation is relatively small (see Table 1.4) but constitutes the majority of the usual daily net H$^+$ production.

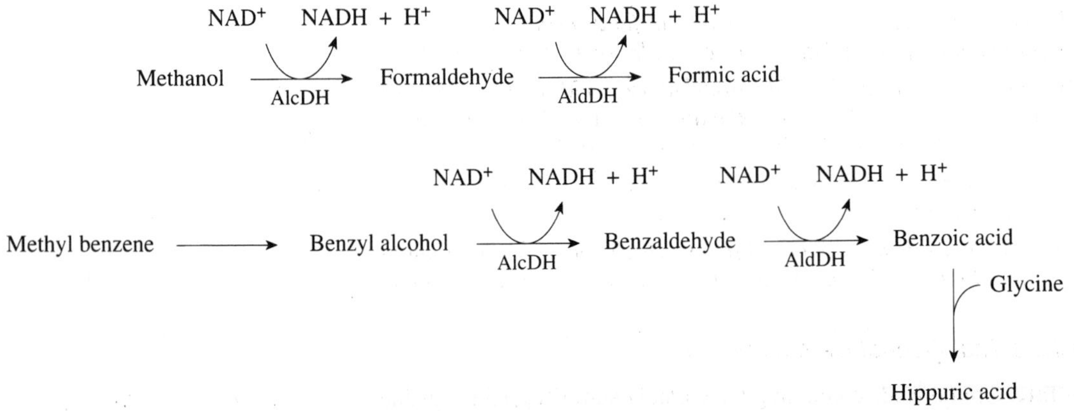

Figure 1.4 Production of acids from alcohols. The initial metabolism of methyl benzene (toluene) takes place in the cytosol of the liver via cytochrome P-450; the resulting alcohol and other alcohols such as methanol are acted on by alcohol dehydrogenase (AlcDH). The aldehydes formed enter mitochondria where aldehyde dehydrogenase (AldDH) converts them to carboxylic acids. In the case of benzoic acid, conjugation with glycine yields hippuric acid.

Physiologic Analysis of Endogenous H⁺ Production

The oxidation of specific components of the diet induces the usual daily net production of H⁺. The authors identify the following two major groups:

Dietary-Acid-Precursor–Driven H⁺ Production

This requires net acid excretion to rise to eliminate these H⁺. Examples include compounds such as divalent phosphate esters, which yield a H⁺ load together with a conjugate base that directly aids the excretion of these H⁺ as HPO_4^{2-} because the latter can bind H⁺ at the pH of urine (more titratable acid). Also in this group is production of H⁺ with the anion SO_4^{2-}, nevertheless, the SO_4^{2-} anion does not aid H⁺ excretion. To eliminate these H⁺, an equivalent amount of NH_4^+ or less HCO_3^- must be excreted.

Dietary-Base–Driven H⁺ Production

This alkali load stimulates the production of organic acids, the H⁺ of which can be used to titrate the alkali. There is one other necessary step: the organic anions that were produced along with these H⁺ must be made into end-products of metabolism by being excreted in the urine as their Na^+ or K^+ salts. By ensuring that some of the organic anions are divalent or trivalent species, this can help minimize the risk of formation of those Ca^{2+} stones that are likely to precipitate in alkaline urine. Moreover, by avoiding the obligatory excretion of HCO_3^-, this will still permit modulation of the excretion of K^+ and thereby retain this as a potential control mechanism for the excretion of K^+ (see Figures 9.10 and 9.11).

Overall. Although the two preceding groups of net acid production represent diet-driven endogenous acid production, they serve different purposes and, as a result, have very different control mechanisms with impacts that are felt in areas broader than just acid-base balance.

PART B

Daily Physiology of H⁺

There are three major components to the daily turnover of H⁺ (Figure 1.5). Each will be considered briefly to demonstrate the overall picture, and then the latter two will be discussed in more detail.

Diet and the Production of H⁺

- The majority of net production of H⁺ occurs because protein is metabolized.
- Close to 60 mmol of H⁺ is removed when fruits and vegetables are metabolized.

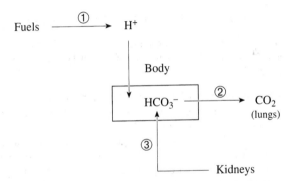

Balance
The difference between input and output. Positive balance is net accumulation and negative balance is net loss.

Figure 1.5   Components of acid-base balance. The body is represented as an HCO_3^- buffer (in the rectangle). There are three components to acid-base balance:

1. A H^+ load is derived from oxidation of fuels.
2. Bicarbonate buffers ultimately buffer this H^+ load. Buffering of H^+ by HCO_3^- leads to production of CO_2, which is removed by the lungs.
3. The kidney regenerates HCO_3^- when glutamine is metabolized to yield HCO_3^- plus NH_4^+. The new HCO_3^- return to the blood when NH_4^+ are excreted in the urine.

An individual eating the usual North American diet is faced with a net daily H^+ load of approximately 1 mmol/kg/day. As listed in Table 1.4, the net production of H^+ is largely from the metabolism of 7 of the 20 amino acids from the proteins of the diet. Metabolism of certain dietary constituents adds H^+, whereas metabolism of other constituents removes H^+; examples of the latter group include the organic anions (usually as their K^+ salts) in fruits and vegetables consumed (citrate^{3-}, malate^{2-}, acetate$^-$, etc.). Quantitatively, some 50–60 mEq of H^+ is removed each day as a result of this metabolism.

Buffering of H^+

Bicarbonate buffer system (BBS)
The major buffer in the ECF and an important buffer in the ICF (providing that the lungs can lower the P_{CO_2}).

The effectiveness of buffering is remarkable. The input of H^+ is more than 1,000,000 nmol per liter of body water, yet the $[H^+]$ is remarkably stable (40 ± 2 nmol/L). Two types of buffers are the proteins in the body and the *bicarbonate buffer system* (*BBS*). In a later section (page 19), the authors discuss how the ability of the lungs to lower the $[CO_2]$ (P_{CO_2}) in the body permits the BBS to be the primary means of alleviating a modest H^+ load.

Generation of New HCO_3^- by the Kidney

- The kidneys must generate 1 mmol of new HCO_3^- per kg body weight each day.
- New bicarbonate is generated when NH_4^+ and $H_2PO_4^-$ are excreted.

Only the kidneys excrete acid or alkali on a continuing basis; therefore, they can regulate the balance of HCO_3^- (called *net acid excretion*). They do so by adjusting the rates of excretion principally of NH_4^+ and HCO_3^-. Each day, 70 mmol of H^+ is derived from the normal oxidative metabolism of dietary constituents and is buffered initially by the BBS. To achieve acid-base *balance*, the kidneys must generate 70 mmol of new HCO_3^- to replace the HCO_3^- consumed by the buffering process (Figure 1.6). Should this process of new HCO_3^- generation fail, the patient will become progressively acidemic, as a result of the continued net negative balance for HCO_3^-.

A More In-Depth Look at Buffering of H^+

> • Buffers minimize the change in $[H^+]$ when an acid or alkali is added.
> • Buffers are a very effective but temporary means of removing H^+ from the body.

The ability of a compound to bind or release H^+ depends on the affinity of that compound for H^+ and the $[H^+]$ in that compartment of the body. The $[H^+]$ when the concentrations of the H^+ donor (acid) and H^+ acceptor (base) are equal is called the *buffer constant* (the pK in negative log terms). At this $[H^+]$, the buffer is best poised to donate or accept H^+ (see Table 1.7 for a quantitative example and Figure 1.7 for a visual representation). The other important factor determining the effectiveness of a given buffer is its concentration in the compartment in which it is to act as a buffer (e.g., inorganic phosphate in the ICF has an appropriate pK, but the concentration is too low to be a physiologically important buffer).

The body contains many substances that can bind or release H^+; some of these are effective buffers at $[H^+]$ that are in the physiologic range. For buffering to be effective, the quantity of H^+ acceptors

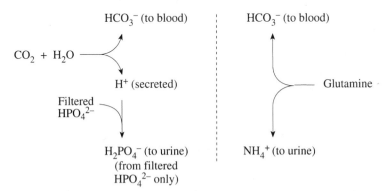

Figure 1.6 Generation of new HCO_3^- in the kidneys. The kidneys generate new HCO_3^- in two ways—by converting CO_2 to H^+ and HCO_3^- and by converting glutamine to NH_4^+ plus HCO_3^-. In the former case (left side of figure), the H^+ must be excreted bound to HPO_4^{2-}, whereas in the latter (right side of figure), NH_4^+ must be excreted in the urine. The net result is that for every mmol of NH_4^+ as well as every mmol of *new* $H_2PO_4^-$ excreted, one mmol of new HCO_3^- will be added to the blood.

Net acid excretion (NAE)
This excretion is the same as HCO_3^- balance across the kidney.
NAE = HCO_3^- gain minus HCO_3^- loss via the kidney.
NAE = NH_4^+ plus $H_2PO_4^-$ minus HCO_3^- excreted in the urine.

Chemistry of buffers
All buffers depend on a simple equilibrium. Each buffer has its unique dissociation constant (K_d or pK), which determines the range of $[H^+]$ at which the buffer is effective. A buffer is most effective at a $[H^+]$ or pH that is equal to its K_d or pK, i.e., when $[HA] = [A^-]$ (A^- is the conjugate base of the weak acid buffer).
   $^*K_{eq}$ is the equilibrium constant for the dissociation of HA to $A^- + H^+$.

$$H^+ + A^- \leftrightarrow HA$$
$$K_{eq} = [H^+] \times [A^-]/[HA]$$
$$[H^+] = K_{eq} \times [HA]/[A^-]$$

New $H_2PO_4^-$
There are two species of inorganic phosphate: divalent (HPO_4^{2-}) and monovalent ($H_2PO_4^-$) ions. To generate new HCO_3^-, HPO_4^{2-} must be converted to $H_2PO_4^-$ via H^+ secretion by the kidney. A $H_2PO_4^-$ that is both filtered and excreted will not contribute to the generation of new HCO_3^-.

TABLE 1.7 **Illustrative Example of Buffering**

When 100 new H^+ are added to two buffer solutions poised at different ratios of proton donor (HA) to proton acceptor (A^-), there is a lesser absolute change in free [H^+] when this ratio is closer to 1 ([H^+] is near the pK of that buffer).

	At the pK	Far from the pK
Starting Point		
Total HA + A^-	1000	1000
Ratio of HA to A^-	500:500	800:200
[H*]	500/500 × K_{eq}	800:200 × K_{eq}
Add 100 new H^+		
Total HA + A^-	1000	1000
Ratio of HA to A^-	600:400	900:100
[H^+]	600:400 × K_{eq}	900:100 × K_{eq}

Idea
Instead of considering the location of buffers, classify the buffers as BBS or non-BBS.

obviously must exceed the quantity of H^+ added. The two most important buffer systems are the protein buffer system and the BBS.

The traditional approach to buffering is based on "geography"—ECF vs ICF. It is said that just over half of the H^+ load is buffered in the ICF; however, this approach ignores the type of buffer, its physical and chemical properties, and whether it is possible to change the buffer capacity. These points will be considered in the following sections.

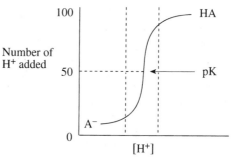

Figure 1.7 Buffer curve describing the buffering of H^+. When H^+ are added, the [H^+] rises quickly until it approaches the pK (between dotted lines) where H^+ can be added with little change in [H^+] (efficient buffering).

Protein Buffer System

- The major non-BBS buffer is protein in the ICF (imidazole group in histidines).
- Recall that when H^+ bind to proteins, the charge, shape, and possibly function of the proteins may change.

Carnosine and anserine
Compounds that act as a major buffer in skeletal muscle. They contain two amino acids, β-alanine and histidine. The β-alanine permits each compound to have a high pK of its terminal amino group; these compounds can therefore remain with no net charge in cells.

The major buffers of the ICF are histidines (in proteins and in the dipeptides *carnosine* and *anserine*). The total content of histidines is close to 2400 mmol in a 70-kg individual. Because the pH of the ICF is close to the mean pK of histidine, only half of these histidines (1200 mmol) are potential H^+ acceptors. With a change in ICF pH of 0.3 units (twofold rise in [H^+]), about 400 mmol of H^+ can be buffered via histidines (the ratio of H^+ donors to H^+ acceptors in histidine changes from 1200:1200 to 1600:800).

Bicarbonate Buffer System (BBS)

- The BBS is the initial buffer for a H^+ load.
- The BBS is virtually the only buffer of the ECF, but it is also important in the ICF.
- A clinical evaluation of acid-base balance is made by examining the $[H^+]$, $[HCO_3^-]$, and the P_{CO_2} in plasma.

$$H^+ + HCO_3^- \leftrightarrow H_2CO_3 \leftrightarrow H_2O + CO_2$$

BBS (Henderson) Equation

$$[H^+] = \frac{23.9}{[HCO_3^-]} \times P_{CO_2}$$

The units are nmol/L for H^+, mmol/L for HCO_3^-, and mm Hg for P_{CO_2}.

Some prefer to express this in log terms (Henderson-Hasselbalch equation).

$$pH = pK + \log \frac{HCO_3^-}{H_2CO_3}$$

There are two ways to consider the BBS—a view related to body geography (ECF vs ICF) and a view related to physiology (BBS is used before proteins for the most part); both will be considered in the following sections.

Quantities

- Close to 1000 mmol of H^+ can be buffered: 350 mmol via the BBS in the ECF, 250 mmol via the BBS in the ICF, and 400 mmol via intracellular histidines.

Given the $[HCO_3^-]$ in plasma (25 mmol/L) and the volume of the ECF (15 L in a 70-kg adult), the ECF can buffer close to 375 mmol of H^+ (see Table 1.8 and the margin note). The ICF contains almost the same amount of HCO_3^- as the ECF (close to half the $[HCO_3^-]$ but twice the volume). The critical question is this: What permits preferential buffering of H^+ by the BBS?

Content of HCO_3^- in the ECF
The total content is the $[HCO_3^-] \times$ the ECF volume (25 mmol/L $\times$ 15 L = 375 mmol). Each mmol of HCO_3^- can remove 1 mmol of H^+.

Physiology: a Reinterpretation

- A function of the BBS is to prevent H^+ from binding to proteins in the ICF.
- The BBS is used first to remove a H^+ load, providing that hyperventilation occurs.
- The key to the operation of the BBS is the control of the P_{CO_2}.

Concept
2. Buffers work physiologically to keep added H^+ from binding to proteins; instead, H^+ are forced to react with HCO_3^-.

TABLE 1.8 **Buffers for an Acid Load**

Values are reported as normal and are approximate for a 70-kg person. The maximum quantity of buffering is close to 1000 mmol. Additional buffering occurs in skeletal muscle during exercise.

Location	Buffers (mmol)			
	HCO_3^-	Protein	Phosphate	Other
ECF	375	<10	<15	0
ICF (muscle)	330	400	<50	CrP*

*Creatine phosphate (CrP) is hydrolyzed to inorganic phosphate, which removes H^+ during anaerobic exercise (see "'Metabolic' Buffering in Skeletal Muscle," page 23).

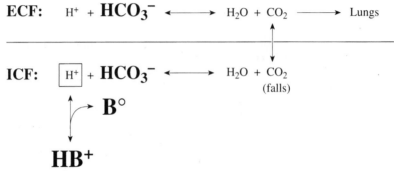

Figure 1.8 Teamwork in buffering. The top of this figure represents events in the ECF, a compartment with only a minor contribution of protein buffers. The main effect of hyperventilation (a lower $[CO_2]$) in the ECF is to lower the $[H^+]$ in this compartment. In contrast, the lower part of the figure represents events in the ICF. When acid is added, H^+ are buffered by proteins (HB^+ rises and $B°$ falls). When the PCO_2 falls, there is an initial small fall in the $[H^+]$ in the ICF, which leads to *back-titration* of the large content of protein buffers (HB^+) and the subsequent consumption of HCO_3^-. The net effects are to raise the concentration of nonprotonated intracellular proteins ($B°$) toward normal and to lower the $[HB^+]$ and $[HCO_3^-]$ in this compartment.

Following an acid load, there is a coordinated operation of the BBS in the ECF and the ICF. It should be appreciated that the fall in PCO_2, which occurs in metabolic acidosis, not only increases the effectiveness of the BBS in the ECF but also prevents a large rise in the net positive charge on intracellular proteins following an acid load; the key to understanding this relationship is summarized in Figure 1.8. When an acid is generated, the $[H^+]$ rises, the respiratory center is stimulated, alveolar ventilation rises, and the PCO_2 falls. The major effect of this fall in PCO_2 differs in the ECF and ICF because the ICF contains a large quantity of non-BBS buffers that is virtually absent in the ECF. Accordingly, with a fall in the PCO_2 there will be a decrease in the $[H^+]$ in the ECF and little change in the $[HCO_3^-]$ because the $[HCO_3^-]$ is 10^6-fold greater than the $[H^+]$, yet they are consumed in a 1:1 stoichiometry with CO_2 formation. In contrast, in the ICF, there will be a decrease in the $[HCO_3^-]$ and an increase in the nonprotonated proteins ($B°$). The reasons for these changes in the ICF are as follows: when the PCO_2 fell, the $[H^+]$ began to fall. As soon as this $[H^+]$ fell, the equilibrium of protein buffers was driven from HB^+ to $B°$ plus H^+. Recall that there is a very large quantity of groups in proteins that are capable of binding H^+ relative to the content of HCO_3^- in the ICF. Accordingly, this cycle will continue and lead to the consumption of HCO_3^- and the generation of $B°$ with only a small fall in the $[H^+]$ in the ICF.

The BBS is the first buffer to remove almost all of the H^+ load when the PCO_2 falls (Table 1.9). The BBS in the ICF removes about one-third of the H^+ load. In the absence of hyperventilation, close to half of the H^+ is buffered by intracellular proteins. With a much larger acid load, the bulk of the BBS buffers will have already been consumed so that most additional buffering will occur in the ICF using the protein buffer capacity. This information forms the basis for the following statements:

1. The volume of distribution of H^+ is larger in more severe metabolic acidosis.
2. Compared with a milder degree of metabolic acidosis, a severe degree of metabolic acidosis requires a greater quantity

Back-titration
The release of H^+ that were previously bound to a buffer.

TABLE 1.9   **Bicarbonate Buffer System: Importance of CO_2 Removal—A Quantitative Example**

If the lungs were not present and a patient had a H^+ load that reduced the $[HCO_3^-]$ in the ECF from 25 to 12.5 mmol/L, the P_{CO_2} would be 455 mm Hg and the resultant $[H^+]$ would be lethal. Because ventilation removes CO_2, and ventilation is stimulated by acidemia, patients with a $[HCO_3^-]$ of 12.5 mmol/L should have a P_{CO_2} of 27 mm Hg, which produces a $[H^+]$ of 52 nmol/L. Had the P_{CO_2} been maintained at 40 mm Hg, the $[H^+]$ would be considerably higher (77 vs 52 nmol/L).

Impact of CO_2 removal on the $[H^+]$ in plasma during metabolic acidosis

Condition	$[H^+]$ (nmol/L)	pH	P_{CO_2} (mm Hg)	HCO_3^- (mmol/L)
Closed system (P_{CO_2} rises)	871	6.06	455	12.5
No change in P_{CO_2}	77	7.11	40	12.5
Lower P_{CO_2}	52	7.29	27	12.5

of HCO_3^- to be given to raise the $[HCO_3^-]$ by a given amount.

Importance of the Venous P_{CO_2}

- A low P_{CO_2} in tissues ensures H^+ buffering by the BBS in the ICF.

The P_{CO_2} in tissues is the net result of two major factors, the rate of production of CO_2 and its rate of disposal—the latter being by diffusion into capillary blood.

Production of CO_2

CO_2 is the carbon end-product of energy metabolism. Therefore, if there is an increased demand to generate ATP (more work), the rate of production of CO_2 will rise. Conversely, when the demand for metabolic work declines, less CO_2 will be produced. Examples that contribute to a low production of CO_2 are a low metabolic rate (hypothermia, hypothyroidism, sedation) and a decreased metabolic rate in individual organs (see Chapter 5 for more discussion).

Another factor to consider is that different fuels yield different amounts of CO_2 per ATP formed. The highest CO_2 yield per ATP comes from fatty acids (8.3 CO_2/ATP) vs glucose (6 CO_2/ATP). Nevertheless, if too much carbohydrate is ingested, the resultant stimulation of lipogenesis will cause much more production of CO_2 (see Chapter 5).

There is one other way to produce CO_2 at a rapid rate: anaerobic metabolism. Now the rate of production of CO_2 is 1 mmol/mmol ATP starting from glucose.

$$\text{Glucose} + 2\,\text{ADP} \rightarrow 2\,\text{lactate} + 2\,H^+ + 2\,\text{ATP}$$
$$2\,H^+ + 2\,HCO_3^- \rightarrow 2\,CO_2 + 2\,H_2O$$

Bottom Line. CO_2 production rate is 10 mmol/min in the absence of hypoxia in normal subjects, and much higher rates are found with anaerobic exercise.

CO₂ Removal

> • CO_2 diffuses from cells to blood. Therefore, the tissue P_{CO_2} exceeds the venous P_{CO_2}.

Note
This may be part of the explanation as to why a sprinter at the end of a race may have an arterial blood pH of 6.9 and be perfectly well, whereas a patient in shock with a similar arterial blood pH may die with a similar degree of L-lactic acidosis.

The venous P_{CO_2} and hence the tissue P_{CO_2} is a function of CO_2 production and blood flow rate. A quantitative example illustrates the overall importance of blood flow rate on the tissue P_{CO_2}. In diabetic ketoacidosis there is a high H^+ load to buffer in the ICF. When Lee was normal and producing 10 mmol of CO_2/min, each of her 5 L of blood carried 2 mmol CO_2 (normal cardiac output is 5 L/min). Assume her CO_2 production rate remains unchanged and her cardiac output is half the normal value (low ECF volume due to a deficit of NaCl). Now, her 10 mmol of CO_2/min must be carried in 2.5 L of blood flow per minute, so each liter carries 4 mmol CO_2/min. As a result, each liter has a higher P_{CO_2}. The higher venous P_{CO} causes a higher tissue P_{CO_2}, a higher ICF $[H^+]$, and more buffering by proteins in the ICF (Figure 1.9). A similar analogy holds for a cardiac arrest (see margin note).

NORMAL CARDIAC OUTPUT   LOW CARDIAC OUTPUT

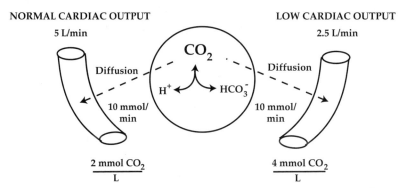

Figure 1.9   Role of blood flow rate on the tissue P_{CO_2}. The circle represents all the cells in the body, and the blood vessels (capillaries) are on either side. On the left side, the cardiac output is normal (5 L/min), and the rate of production of CO_2 is the usual 10 mmol/min. Each liter of blood must transport 2 mmol CO_2. In contrast, the cardiac output is halved on the right. Now each liter of blood must carry 4 mmol of CO_2 (same production rate) and have a higher P_{CO_2}—hence, the P_{CO_2} and thereby the $[H^+]$ in cells is higher in this setting and more H^+ are buffered on ICF proteins.

QUESTIONS

(Discussions on page 39)

1.11 *How much would the $[HCO_3^-]$ in the ECF decrease when a load of 70 mmol of H^+ is retained in a 70-kg person who lacks renal generation of new HCO_3^-?*

1.12 *The following results for a blood sample arrive from the laboratory: $[H^+]$ = 60 nmol/L, pH = 7.22, P_{aCO_2} = 50 mm Hg, $[HCO_3^-]$ = 32 mmol/L. What do you conclude?*

1.13 *What would the P_{aCO_2} be in a normal man if his alveolar ventilation rate decreased by half (assume no change in his* *metabolic rate)? What must you do to keep his pH ([H⁺]) from changing?*

1.14 *Some say that hyperventilation is "maladaptive" because in an experimental situation, there was a fall in the pH of plasma after hyperventilation occurred. How might this phenomenon be interpreted?*

1.15 *Can a patient have a very low arterial P_{CO_2} yet have respiratory acidosis in the cells?*

1.16 *Why is the brain "protected" from a higher mixed venous P_{CO_2} in a patient with diabetic ketoacidosis?*

"Metabolic" Buffering in Skeletal Muscle

- During ischemia in skeletal muscle, metabolic reactions take place that result in the formation of HPO_4^{2-}, a new H^+ acceptor.

Buffering during a sprint or a convulsion (explosive, vigorous exercise) differs from buffering in other circumstances of metabolic acidosis, the main issue being the role of creatine phosphate as a precursor for a H^+ acceptor.

During a sprint or convulsion, the following events occur:

1. When ATP breaks down to provide energy for the contraction-relaxation cycle, it produces a divalent phosphate ion (HPO_4^{2-}) and a H^+.

$$ATP^{4-} \leftrightarrow ADP^{3-} + HPO_4^{2-} + H^+$$

2. The rise in ADP and fall in ATP drives the breakdown of creatine phosphate. This process consumes a H^+ and regenerates ATP without using the divalent phosphate ion.

$$\text{Creatine phosphate}^{2-} + ADP^{3-} + H^+ \leftrightarrow \text{Creatine} + ATP^{4-}$$

3. Combining the first two reactions reveals that creatine phosphate is converted to creatine and divalent inorganic phosphate.

$$\text{Creatine phosphate}^{2-} \leftrightarrow \text{Creatine} + HPO_4^{2-}$$

4. Divalent inorganic phosphate picks up a H^+ avidly at the intracellular [H^+] so that the concentrations of monovalent and divalent phosphates are equal.

$$0.5\ HPO_4^{2-} + 0.5\ H^+ \leftrightarrow 0.5\ H_2PO_4^-$$

5. Overall: These initial events in a cell provide ATP for a sprint and "parking-spots" (divalent phosphate) for the H^+ (in L-lactic acid) made during anaerobic glycolysis. Thus, more ATP can be generated with less net accumulation of free H^+. With a rise in intracellular [H^+], virtually all the inorganic phosphate becomes monovalent dihydrogen phosphate. The reverse occurs on recovery.

$$0.5\ HPO_4^{2-} + 0.5\ H^+ \leftrightarrow 0.5\ H_2PO_4^-$$

QUESTIONS

(Discussions on pages 41–42)

1.17 *Is it more important to control the [H+] in the ECF or in the ICF?*

1.18 *What should the pH of the ICF of muscle be in the first 10 seconds of a sprint in a normal person and in a patient with a defect in the hydrolysis of glycogen?*

A More In-Depth Look at the Kidney and HCO₃⁻ Balance

Concept

3. The $[HCO_3^-]$ is regulated by the kidney, which can excrete HCO_3^- and/or generate new HCO_3^-.

- The first component of renal regulation of plasma $[HCO_3^-]$—preventing the loss of the large quantity of filtered HCO_3^-—is primarily the task of the proximal convoluted tubule (PCT).
- The PCT has a high capacity to secrete H^+ but cannot generate steep $[H^+]$ gradients. Components include a Na^+ and a H^+ story.

Glomerular filtration rate (GFR)
The volume of plasma filtered at the glomerulus per unit time (usually mL/min or L/day); in SI units, mL/sec is now used.

There are two components of renal generation of HCO_3^-:
1. Indirect reabsorption of filtered HCO_3^-, which is achieved primarily by proximal H^+ secretion.
2. Generation of new HCO_3^-, which is achieved principally by NH_4^+ production and excretion.

Indirect Reabsorption of Filtered HCO₃⁻

Quantities

At a normal *glomerular filtration rate* (GFR) (180 L/day), 4500 mmol of HCO_3^- is filtered, and approximately 85% (4000 mmol/day) is reabsorbed in an indirect fashion by the proximal convoluted tubule (PCT) (Table 1.10).

Physiology

The bulk of filtered HCO_3^- is reabsorbed in an indirect fashion in the PCT as a result of H^+ secretion. Molecules of HCO_3^- disappear

TABLE 1.10 **Quantity of HCO₃⁻ Indirectly Reabsorbed in the Nephron**

The numbers are estimates for a 70-kg adult based on micropuncture data in rats.

Event	HCO_3^- (mmol/day)
Filtered	4500
Reabsorbed	
Proximal	4000
Loop	400
Distal	100

from the tubular lumen and reappear in the blood. Because there is neither net HCO_3^- gain nor loss, there is no direct acid-base impact of the indirect *reabsorption of HCO_3^-* (Figure 1.10). The events in the PCT result in conservation of both Na^+ and HCO_3^- and can be viewed as two parallel stories—one dealing with the reabsorption of Na^+ and the other dealing with the secretion of H^+.

The Na^+ Story. This story has three components: one at the luminal membrane, one in the cell, and another at the basolateral membrane. In the luminal membrane, Na^+ are transported on a special transporter, the Na^+/H^+ exchanger-3 (NHE-3). For every Na^+ reabsorbed, one H^+ must be secreted into the lumen. The intracellular component is the very low [Na^+] inside these cells, which permits this NHE-3 to reabsorb Na^+. The basolateral story focuses on the $Na^+K^+ATPase$ in the basolateral membrane. This ion transport system provides the driving force for the overall process—maintaining the low [Na^+] in these cells by transporting 3 Na^+ out of the cell in conjunction with the entry of 2 K^+. In general, this component of the process will be driven by the amount of Na^+ that is reabsorbed.

The H^+ Story. This story also has three components: one at the luminal membrane, one in the cell, and one at the basolateral membrane. On the luminal membrane, there are two unique features: the NHE-3 and the luminal carbonic anhydrase. The latter enzyme hydrolyzes carbonic acid that is formed in the lumen to CO_2 and H_2O; the enzyme-catalyzed rate of hydrolysis is virtually as fast as the rate of generation. If this catalysis did not occur, indirect reabsorption of HCO_3^- would be retarded, and urinary excretion of HCO_3^- would ensue (see the discussion of Question 1.18).

Inside the cell, there are two important components of the story: a different carbonic anhydrase enzyme species that prevents the accumulation of OH^- (or that makes HCO_3^- available inside cells) and a second modifier site on NHE-3 for H^+ that activates this transporter. On the basolateral membrane, there is a unique transport system for the exit of HCO_3^- from these cells—a channel that permits a complex of Na^+ and HCO_3^- to exit as an anionic form: $Na(HCO_3)_3^{2-}$.

"Reabsorption" of HCO_3^-
As shown in Figure 1.10, HCO_3^- are not truly reabsorbed; they disappear from the lumen and reappear in the peritubular blood. The authors call this process *indirect reabsorption*.

Molecular story
See Appendix to Chapter 1.

Abbreviation
NHE: Na^+, H^+ exchanger.

Note
A smaller quantity of Na^+ also exits this cell as $Na(HCO_3^-)_3^{2-}$ down an electrochemical gradient. This is the main exit step for HCO_3^- from cells of the PCT.

Figure 1.10 H^+ secretion in the PCT. There are two components to H^+ secretion in the PCT: reabsorption of Na^+ and secretion of H^+; they are linked via the NHE-3 in the luminal membrane. (CA = carbonic anhydrase.)

Renal threshold for reabsorption of HCO_3^-

The "apparent" renal threshold for reabsorption of HCO_3^- represents that maximum $[HCO_3^-]$ in plasma at which proximal H^+ secretion is sufficient to "reabsorb" all the HCO_3^- that were filtered. In truth, there is no real threshold because factors such as ECF volume expansion (which limits Na^+ reabsorption) and a fall in the $[H^+]$ in the ICF independently diminish proximal H^+ secretion (see Figure 4.5).

Acetazolamide

A drug used for patients with glaucoma. These patients may develop a modest degree of metabolic acidosis from inhibition of luminal carbonic anhydrase.

$[H^+]$ in the ICF

In hypokalemia, K^+ leave the ICF; to maintain electroneutrality, Na^+ or H^+ enter the ICF, and the $[H^+]$ in the ICF rises.

Substrate effect

When an enzyme is not saturated with its substrate, its velocity increases with an increase in substrate concentration.

Regulation of Proximal H^+ Secretion

- The NHE-3 is a pump with high capacity, but the "leaky" luminal membrane in the PCT prevents the generation of steep $[H^+]$ gradients.
- Regulators include the luminal $[H^+]$, the intracellular $[H^+]$, the stimuli for Na^+ reabsorption, and hormonal influences.

The NHE-3 in the luminal membrane of PCT cells has a very large capacity for H^+ secretion, but it cannot generate steep $[H^+]$ gradients. Therefore, the following regulating influences should be evident.

The Filtered Load of HCO_3^-. When the plasma $[HCO_3^-]$ is 25 mmol/L and the glomerular filtration rate is 180 L/day, 4500 mmol of HCO_3^- is filtered and 4000 is indirectly reabsorbed proximally each day (see Table 1.10). With metabolic acidosis, lowering the plasma $[HCO_3^-]$ to 10 mmol/L reduces its filtered load to 1800 mmol/day. In this case, H^+ secretion in the PCT will be reduced by more than 50% (there are no other H^+ acceptors of quantitative importance).

Luminal $[H^+]$. If a patient is given a drug that inhibits luminal carbonic anhydrase (e.g., *acetazolamide*), the luminal $[H^+]$ will rise abruptly and bring H^+ secretion to a halt long before 85% of the filtered HCO_3^- is reclaimed (see discussion of Question 1.18).

$[H^+]$ in PCT Cells. A rise in the *$[H^+]$ in the ICF* stimulates proximal tubular H^+ secretion here for two reasons: first, the addition of H^+ causes a *substrate effect* on the NHE-3, which increases secretion in proportion to the degree of rise in $[H^+]$; second, the binding of H^+ to a separate site on the NHE-3 causes an additional direct activation of this antiporter. This second site permits amplification of the stimulus of a small rise in $[H^+]$. Contrary to intuition, this activation is not very important during metabolic acidosis because of the small filtered load of HCO_3^-. Nevertheless, a modest increase in NHE-3 activity can be seen during hypokalemia and an elevated $Paco_2$—conditions that may be associated with a higher $[H^+]$ in the ICF. In contrast, when a $NaHCO_3$ load is administered, there is a fall in the $[H^+]$ in the ICF that does not permit an augmented flux through the NHE-3 despite an increase in the number of H^+ acceptors in the lumen. Thus, there is a prompt excretion of the excess HCO_3^-.

$[HCO_3^-]$ in the ECF

A very recent finding is that a high Pco_2 in the ECF indirectly stimulates the reabsorption of HCO_3^- in the PCT by alkalinizing the cells. This is surprising because a high Pco_2 should acidify these cells. The authors hypothesize that there is a link between this high Pco_2 and stimulation of NHE-3. Thus, if the Pco_2 rises with metabolic alkalosis, renal reabsorption of HCO_3^- will increase. Hence, the endogenous addition of HCO_3^- during the secretion of HCl by the stomach (Chapter 4, Figure 4.1) creates a setting where there is a loss of Cl^- and a gain of HCO_3^- with no change in the ECF volume. If these HCO_3^- were excreted, there would have to be a loss of Na^+ and/or K^+ plus an enhanced excretion of NH_4^+ later on when the HCl was absorbed from the intestinal tract. To avoid all these difficulties, it is "lucky" that a high P_{CO_2} can stimulate the reabsorption of filtered HCO_3^- by the kidney.

This story should be contrasted with the events following an exogenous load of $NaHCO_3$. In this latter circumstance, the load of Na^+ with its resultant ECF volume expansion overwhelms the direct effect of the $[HCO_3^-]$ to stimulate the indirect reabsorption of HCO_3^- in the PCT. The low level of angiotensin II inhibits the reabsorption of HCO_3^- in the PCT.

Avidity for Na^+ Reabsorption. With an $NaHCO_3$ load, the increased Na^+ load via ECF volume expansion seems to depress net indirect reabsorption of $NaHCO_3$, contributing to the failure to increase H^+ secretion. In contrast, with a contracted ECF volume, proximal Na^+ reabsorption (and thereby H^+ secretion) tends to rise. The mediator of this effect is probably *angiotensin II*, acting through a phosphorylation/dephosphorylation mechanism on NHE-3.

Minor Factors. Hypercalcemia and low parathyroid hormone levels tend to augment proximal H^+ secretion. Perhaps the mechanism involves cyclic AMP and phosphorylation of the NHE-3 by protein kinases; phosphorylation inhibits the antiporter.

Angiotensin II
The active messenger synthesized when renin levels are high. It stimulates the release of aldosterone, is a vasoconstrictor, and increases the indirect reabsorption of $NaHCO_3$ in the PCT (see Figure 9.10).

Proximal Renal Tubular Acidosis (pRTA)

- The failure of proximal H^+ secretion is called *pRTA*.

The failure of proximal renal H^+ secretion results in the following:
   A fall in the plasma $[HCO_3^-]$, caused by renal excretion of HCO_3^-.
   Inability to increase the plasma $[HCO_3^-]$ with administration of HCO_3^- because of low proximal HCO_3^- reabsorption (i.e., HCO_3^- excretion rather than retention).
   Alkaline urine (pH>7.0) in the presence of acidemia when the plasma $[HCO_3^-]$ is below its normal concentration.

Distal H^+ secretion in pRTA
In pRTA, distal H^+ secretion is normal but overwhelmed by the large distal HCO_3^- delivery (distal H^+ secretion is a low-capacity system).

QUESTIONS

(Discussions on pages 42–43)

1.19 *What other role might the NHE-3 have in the PCT?*

1.20 *How do carbonic anhydrase inhibitors compromise the indirect reabsorption of HCO_3^-?*

1.21 *If the patient with pRTA develops diarrhea and the $[HCO_3^-]$ in the ECF drops 2 mmol/L below its usual value, how will the urine pH and $[HCO_3^-]$ change?*

1.22 *How would you establish whether a patient with a low $[HCO_3^-]$ and diarrhea has pRTA?*

Loop of Henle H^+ Secretion

Because 10–15% of filtered HCO_3^- (500 mmol) leaves the PCT, and approximately 100 mmol enters the distal convoluted tubule, close to 400 mmol is removed either in the pars recta of the PCT or in the thick ascending limb of the loop of Henle. H^+ secretion is via an NHE-3.

Generation of New HCO_3^-

There are two processes by which new HCO_3^- are generated, the excretion of titratable acid and the excretion of NH_4^+ (*net acid excretion [NAE]*). Common to both processes is the secretion of H^+. In the following section, secretion of H^+ in the distal nephron is considered, followed by a discussion of the excretion of NH_4^+.

Distal Nephron H^+ Secretion

> - H^+ATPases have a low capacity but can generate steep $[H^+]$ gradients because the luminal membrane has tight junctions.
> - Luminal H^+ acceptors (NH_3) are needed to continue pumping H^+.

Quantities. Distal nephron H^+ secretion is required to reabsorb 100 mmol of HCO_3^- and promote the net secretion of close to 20 mmol of NH_4^+. Most of the HPO_4^{2-} were titrated in earlier nephron segments.

H^+ Pumps. H^+ pumps are located primarily in the mitochondria-rich intercalated cells; those involved in secretion of H^+ are located in the luminal membranes of α-intercalated cells (Figure 1.11). There are two major H^+ pumps in this segment, an *H^+ATPase* (in contrast to the NHE-3 of the proximal nephron) and an *H^+/K^+ATPase*. The H^+ATPase helps to reabsorb any remaining filtered HCO_3^- and also permits an increased renal excretion of NH_4^+. In the absence of an H^+ acceptor in the lumen, however, the free $[H^+]$ in the tubular fluid rises quickly (but is only 0.1 mmol/L), and H^+ secretion by these cells ceases when a gradient limit for H^+ secretion has been reached (the urine pH cannot be lowered below 4.0). With an excess of H^+ acceptors, the $[H^+]$ in the lumen does not rise as markedly because of the limited capacity of the H^+ATPase in the distal nephron.

Net acid excretion (NAE)
- Calculate the urine NAE rate by adding the rates of excretion of NH_4^+ and $H_2PO_4^-$ and subtracting that of HCO_3^-. NAE regenerates the HCO_3^- consumed by the H^+ load from the diet.
- NH_4^+ is quantitatively the most important component of NAE in metabolic acidosis.

H^+ATPase
The major H^+ pump in the distal nephron. It is important for NH_4^+ excretion.

H^+/K^+ATPase
A pump of low capacity that seems to be important primarily for the reabsorption of K^+ in states of K^+ depletion and hypokalemia.

HCO_3^- transport
There is a second type of intercalated cell, the β-intercalated cell. It is a 180° reversed cell in that it secretes H^+ into the peritubular capillaries via an H^+ATPase and secretes HCO_3^- in exchange for luminal Cl^- (the Cl^-/HCO_3^- exchanger). The function of these cells is not really clear; some believe that they are important in excreting a load of HCO_3^-, but they may be important for K^+ secretion (see Chapter 9).

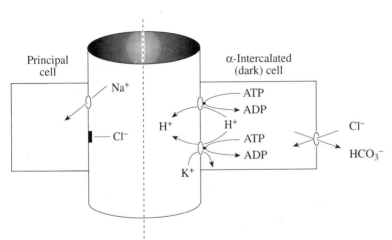

Figure 1.11 H^+ secretion in the distal nephron. The main H^+ pump is an H^+ATPase located in the luminal membrane and in secretory vesicles (precursors or stores of H^+ pumps) inside α-intercalated cells. H^+ secretion generates a steep $[H^+]$ gradient because the luminal membrane is relatively impermeable to H^+. The principal cell is important for K^+ secretion.

Principal cell

α-Intercalated (dark) cell

Na^+

Cl^-

H^+

H^+

K^+

ATP

ADP

ATP

ADP

Cl^-

HCO_3^-

Excretion of NH_4^+

> • Renal NH_4^+ excretion can be equated with HCO_3^- generation on a 1:1 basis.

From a practical point of view, for every NH_4^+ excreted, one new HCO_3^- is added to the body (Figure 1.12); knowing this relationship serves the needs of the clinician.

The NH_4^+ system in the kidney can be considered from two perspectives: first, from those factors leading to a high $[NH_3]$ in the renal medullary interstitium; second, from those factors determining transfer of this NH_3 to the lumen of the collecting duct.

Generating a High $[NH_3]$ in the Renal Medullary Interstitium. There are four components to this story (Figure 1.13):

1. **Production of NH_4^+.** The metabolic process of NH_4^+ excretion begins with proteins from dietary or endogenous sources (Figure 1.14). These proteins release the amino acid glutamine, which, when metabolized in PCT cells, yields NH_4^+ and HCO_3^-. Proteins, when broken down, also yield the amino acids that generate H^+ (see page 9), but, because glutamine is very abundant in most proteins (and it can be made in the liver and muscle), its supply exceeds that of the amino acids that generate H^+.

   The metabolism of glutamine to glucose or CO_2 proceeds via the *TCA cycle,* so ATP must be generated when NH_4^+ are formed. The generation of ATP has several implications for *ammoniagenesis* (Figure 1.15). First, ATP cannot be stored; it is produced in response to demand. In the kidney, the major ATP-utilizing function is Na^+ reabsorption. Second, the rate of ammoniagenesis can also be limited if other fuels are present to regenerate ATP. Third, ammoniagenesis is located in PCT cells because they have the largest rate of turnover of

TCA cycle
The pathway in mitochondria that results in the oxidation of acetyl-CoA and the production of the precursors to regenerate ATP.

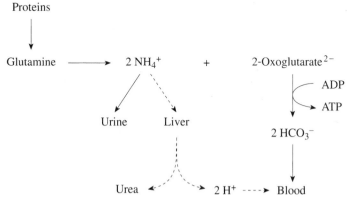

Figure 1.12 Biochemistry of new HCO_3^- synthesis. Glutamine, a neutral compound, is converted to the cation NH_4^+ plus the anion 2-oxoglutarate^{2-} (TCA cycle intermediate) in PCT cells. Further metabolism of 2-oxoglutarate^{2-} results in the formation of HCO_3^- and requires that ATP be formed. If the NH_4^+ are not excreted in the urine, they will be delivered to the liver (dashed line), where subsequent metabolism will yield H^+ plus urea; thus, there is no net HCO_3^- gain if NH_4^+ are not excreted (dashed lines).

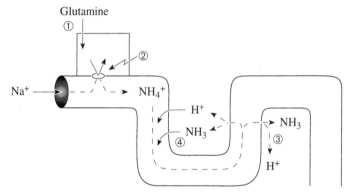

Figure 1.13   Generation of a high [NH₃] in the medullary interstitium. Four steps are required: (1) production of NH₄⁺ in PCT cells; (2) secretion of NH₄⁺ into the lumen of the PCT via NHE-3 (replacing H⁺); (3) reabsorption of NH₄⁺ in the thick ascending limb of the loop of Henle via the Na⁺, K⁺, 2 Cl⁻ cotransporter (NH₄⁺ replace K⁺); and (4) secretion of NH₄⁺ into the descending limb of the loop of Henle together with the operation of a countercurrent system. All of these events lead to the trapping of NH₃ in the medulla.

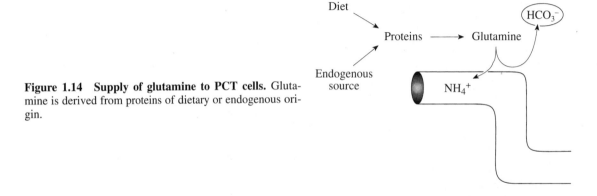

Figure 1.14   Supply of glutamine to PCT cells. Glutamine is derived from proteins of dietary or endogenous origin.

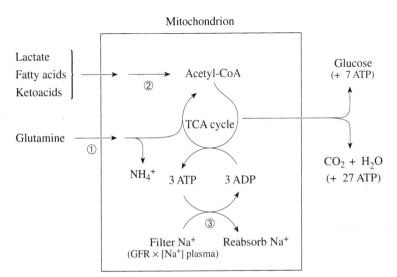

Figure 1.15   Control of ammoniagenesis by ATP turnover and fuel selection. There are three major constraints on the production of NH₄⁺: (1) the amount of glutamine that enters the mitochondrion; (2) the "competition" between glutamine and other fuels to generate the quantity of ATP needed at that moment; (3) the turnover of ATP to perform biologic work (Na⁺ reabsorption, which reflects the GFR).

ATP. Fourth, acidosis may occur in some situations when very high rates of ammoniagenesis do not confer an advantage to the host (i.e., during acute L-lactic acidosis of exercise and in ketoacidosis of fasting). These aspects are explored further in Questions 1.21–1.25.

The specific pathway involved in the production of NH_4^+ requires that glutamine enter mitochondria of PCT cells. This entry process is probably the major barrier that prevents high rates of conversion of glutamine to NH_4^+ by the enzyme phosphate-dependent glutaminase (PDG) in mitochondria. Two stimuli for the entry of glutamine into mitochondria and its subsequent metabolism via PDG are chronic metabolic acidosis and hypokalemia. Although other pathways exist to generate NH_4^+, they do not appear to be quantitatively important.

2. **Secretion of NH_4^+ into the lumen of the proximal nephron.** There are two theoretical ways NH_4^+ can enter the lumen of the PCT, by nonionic diffusion or via a transporter. In the former, the uncharged NH_3 readily crosses the membrane down its difference in concentration. For this movement to occur, NH_3 must be permeable and the concentration difference favorable. It has been demonstrated that these criteria have not always been met, so the general feeling is that NH_4^+ enters the lumen by replacing H^+ on the NHE-3.

3. **Reabsorption of NH_4^+ in the loop of Henle.** To have a very high $[NH_3]$ in the renal medullary interstitium, NH_4^+ are reabsorbed in the thick ascending limb of the loop of Henle (the single effect). Reabsorption occurs via the Na^+, K^+, 2 Cl^- cotransporter, with NH_4^+ taking the place of K^+. This replacement has two implications for regulation of NH_4^+ excretion. First, as more NH_4^+ are reabsorbed, the $[NH_3]$ rises in the medullary interstitium (see point 4 following). A second implication concerns K^+ in the lumen of the thick ascending limb (see margin note). As the $[K^+]$ rises (it is higher in hyperkalemia), fewer NH_4^+ are reabsorbed because of competition between NH_4^+ and K^+. As a result, the $[NH_3]$ in the renal medullary interstitium falls (the NH_4^+ not reabsorbed in the loop are delivered to the distal convoluted tubule and are probably reabsorbed there, not raising the medullary interstitial $[NH_3]$). Accordingly, with hyperkalemia, the rate of NH_4^+ excretion will be lower, but the $[H^+]$ in the urine will be high because H^+ secretion is normal, and there is less H^+ acceptor present.

4. **Recycling of NH_4^+ in the loop of Henle:** The NH_4^+ reabsorbed in the loop of Henle are also secreted into the early descending limb of the loop of Henle. Given the very low medullary blood flow, NH_3 is concentrated in the medullary interstitium. This high $[NH_3]$ is essential for excretion of large quantities of NH_4^+ (see margin note).

Hypokalemia and ammoniagenesis
The most likely reason for the stimulation of ammoniagenesis is the entry of H^+ into PCT cells when K^+ exit; the converse may apply in hyperkalemia.

Other regulators of ammoniagenesis
Alkalemia, a low GFR, and a low supply of glutamine or a high supply of fat-derived fuels may also inhibit production of NH_4^+.

Clinical pearl
A low rate of excretion of NH_4^+ that is secondary to hyperkalemia (from low production of NH_4^+ or low reabsorption in the loop of Henle) is corrected by lowering the $[K^+]$. In contrast, if the low rate of excretion of NH_4^+ is caused by a process that reduces the lumen negative potential difference in the cortical collecting duct (CCD) (see Chapter 9), an action that also leads to hyperkalemia, correction of the hyperkalemia will not reverse the low rate of excretion.

Clinical pearl
Patients who have diseases that damage their renal medulla may have low rates of excretion of NH_4^+.

QUESTIONS

(Discussions on pages 43–44)

1.23 *Why is the production of NH_4^+ low in renal insufficiency?*

1.24 *In the ketoacidosis of chronic fasting, the rate of excretion of NH_4^+ is lower than in chronic metabolic acidosis caused by* *ingestion of HCl. What teleologic advantages might this lower rate of excretion provide and what mechanisms might be involved?*

1.25 *There is a lag period between the net addition of acids and induction of ammoniagenesis. Why might this time be advantageous to a sprinter?*

1.26 *Why might ammoniagenesis be low in a patient with hyperkalemia?*

1.27 *Why is Na^+ acetate added to total parenteral nutrition solutions? Answer from the perspective of NH_4^+ excretion.*

Total parenteral nutrition
A form of therapy in which patients who are unable to obtain adequate nutrients from their GI tract are given intravenous feeding.

Transfer of NH_3 to the Lumen of the Collecting Duct. To excrete NH_4^+, the lumen of the collecting duct must "attract" NH_3. This action is achieved by the presence of a low $[NH_3]$ in the lumen consequent to the secretion of H^+ by collecting duct cells (Figure 1.16). The H^+ATPase produces a high $[H^+]$ in the lumen, which in turn lowers the $[NH_3]$ in the lumen by driving the equation below to the right.

$$H^+ + NH_3 \leftrightarrow NH_4^+$$

HCO_3^- and the NH_4^+ Story

There are two HCO_3^- stories.

New HCO_3^-. All new HCO_3^- are produced in the PCT when glutamine is converted to $NH_4^+ + HCO_3^-$. These HCO_3^- are added to the renal venous blood (see Figure 1.14).

Indirect Reabsorption of HCO_3^- in Later Nephron Segments. Approximately 500 mmol of the filtered HCO_3^- is not reabsorbed in the PCT. Most of them are reabsorbed by H^+ secretion in the loop of Henle (see Table 1.10). There is a second pathway to reabsorb some of these HCO_3^- using NH_4^+ generated and secreted

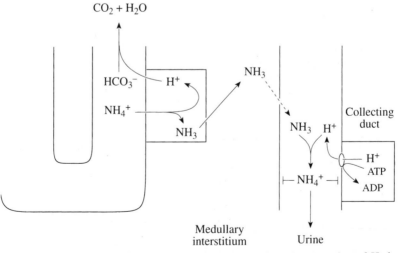

Figure 1.16   Transfer of NH_3 to the final urine. The major feature is active secretion of H^+ by collecting duct cells, which raises the $[H^+]$ and lowers the $[NH_3]$ in the luminal fluid. NH_3 then diffuses (dashed line) from its high concentration (medullary interstitium) to where its concentration is low (lumen of the collecting duct). This process is called *diffusion trapping* or *nonionic diffusion*.

in the PCT (Figure 1.17). In this process, $NaHCO_3$ is filtered. The Na^+ are reabsorbed via NHE-3 in the PCT, but NH_4^+, not H^+, are the countertransporting cations in this case, so that NH_4^+ and HCO_3^- remain in the luminal fluid of the PCT. In the loop of Henle, several events occur. NH_4^+ are reabsorbed and then split into NH_3 and H^+ in the cells of the thick ascending limb. The NH_3 exits via the basolateral membrane, and the H^+ are secreted into the lumen. These secreted H^+ react with luminal HCO_3^- so that filtered HCO_3^- disappear from the lumen, but HCO_3^- do not return to the blood. Carbonic acid (or CO_2 plus H_2O) is delivered to the cortical distal nephron. In α-intercalated cells of the collecting duct, CO_2 is converted to H^+ and HCO_3^-; when the H^+ are secreted, the $[H^+]$ in the luminal fluid increases, and as a result, the $[NH_3]$ in this fluid decreases. Because of the large concentration difference for NH_3, it diffuses from the medullary interstitium to the luminal fluid, where it is trapped as NH_4^+. The HCO_3^- exit via the basolateral membrane and enter the blood, thereby completing the "tricky" indirect reabsorption of filtered HCO_3^- using the NH_4^+ system (see Figure 1.17).

Distal Renal Tubular Acidosis. Renal generation of bicarbonate (excretion of NH_4^+) can fail for two major reasons:

1. Failure to raise the $[NH_3]$ in the renal medullary interstitium (medullary disease or impaired ammoniagenesis).
2. Failure to trap NH_3 in the lumen of the collecting duct because of impaired secretion of H^+ in these nephron segments.

Whatever the basis, a low rate of excretion of NH_4^+ and renal generation of new HCO_3^- is known as *distal renal tubular acidosis* (*dRTA*). As one can appreciate, there are many possible pathogenic mechanisms to explain the presence of dRTA; the specific basis must be established in each case. Nevertheless, the hallmark is a relatively low rate of excretion of NH_4^+ in the urine. The various causes of dRTA are described in Chapter 3.

Acid-Base Balance Viewed from the Perspective of HCO_3^-

An important and often overlooked component of acid-base balance is the disposal of the daily alkali load. When alkaline salts are

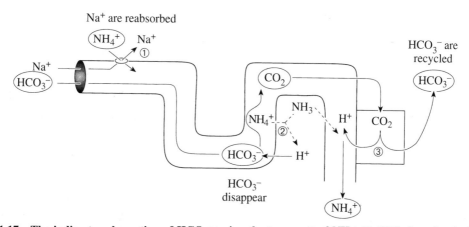

Figure 1.17   The indirect reabsorption of HCO_3^- using the transport of NH_4^+. $NaHCO_3$ is reabsorbed in three separate steps: (1) Na^+ are reabsorbed, and NH_4^+ are secreted in the PCT; (2) HCO_3^- disappear in the loop of Henle as a result of H^+ secretion, but there is no addition of HCO_3^- to the blood; (3) HCO_3^- are finally indirectly reabsorbed once H^+ are secreted in the collecting duct. NH_4^+ made in the PCT end up in the final urine via an indirect route.

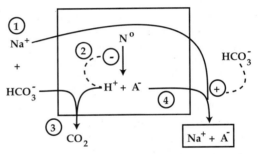

Figure 1.18   Base balance in the body. The production of organic acids and the excretion of organic anions rather than HCO_3^- avoid bicarbonaturia. There are four steps. First, most diets have a significant alkali load (point 1). When presented to cells, this "deinhibits" the production of a variety of organic acids (point 2). The H^+ so produced react with HCO_3^-, and both are eliminated as CO_2 + H_2O (point 3). The organic anions are made end-products of metabolism by having their renal reabsorption inhibited by a higher plasma $[HCO_3^-]$. An example of this type of organic acid is citric acid, which is excreted as Na^+ or K^+ citrate (point 4).

ingested (e.g., K^+ citrate) the citrate is metabolized, yielding HCO_3^-. These HCO_3^- are removed by titration with endogenous organic acid production (Figure 1.18). The story does not end here. HCO_3^-, if present in excess, make these organic anions end-products of metabolism (obligates their excretion without H^+ or NH_4^+ in the urine).

Potential Dangers of Inducing Bicarbonaturia

Bicarbonaturia might be disadvantageous for three major reasons:

1. Obligated loss of Na^+ and a potential for ECF volume contraction if the diet is Na^+-poor.

2. Obligated loss of K^+ (K^+ excretion is promoted by bicarbonaturia; see Chapter 9); K^+ depletion is induced if the diet is K^+-poor.

3. Bicarbonaturia could cause calcium-containing renal calculi as a consequence of an alkaline pH (this may be part of the reason for an increased frequency of renal stones in patients with distal renal tubular acidosis who cannot lower their urine pH appropriately).

Review of Data on Alkali Ingestion and Bicarbonaturia or Organic Aciduria

The traditional concept of acid-base balance, by focusing on a daily H^+ load and its excretion, misses the need to deal with a temporary load of HCO_3^-. This view is supported by the following facts:

1. The diets of humans, rats, and rabbits have an *alkaline ash,* yet overall, net acid is excreted. Hence, dietary anions are either not absorbed or metabolized, or alkali is destroyed.

2. HCO_3^- are added to the body every day when HCl is sequestered in the stomach.

3. Humans on a normal diet excrete 20–30 mEq of organic anions daily. Organic anion excretion is the only part of the daily acid load not matched by the excretion of NH_4^+ (deals with sulphuric acid) or titratable acid (deals with organic monovalent phosphates). These observations could imply that the organic anions in the urine were not added (net) with H^+. Alternatively, the organic anions could have been produced and excreted in re-

sponse to an alkali load and thus did not require an increase in the excretion of net acid to dispose of their protons. Parenthetically, organic anions are also excreted if there was no dietary intake and the alkali was given intravenously in rats.

Physiologic Implications

HCO_3^- should not be delivered in large amounts to the distal segments of the kidney and/or be excreted in the urine even if the diet provides much more HCO_3^- than the net H^+ load in any period during the day. The rationale is that Ca^{2+} salts precipitate much more readily in an alkaline environment. By producing organic acids in response to the alkalemia, bicarbonaturia is prevented throughout most of the 24-hour period.

Quantities

Each day, normal people filter at least 400 mEq of organic anions per day (GFR 180 L/day, $[OA^-]$ 2–4 mEq/L). Of these anions, 90% is reabsorbed and 10% is excreted. If the renal reabsorption of anions could be modulated by an alkali load, this would provide a way to make these potentially metabolizable anions the end-products of metabolism.

PART C

Review

DISCUSSION OF INTRODUCTORY CASE
Lee Wants to Know the Acid Truth

(Case presented on page 4)

What acid-base abnormality is present?

Lee has acidemia ($[H^+]$ = 60 nmol/L) and a plasma $[HCO_3^-]$ that is low (10 mmol/L); therefore, metabolic acidosis is present.

Were acids (H^+) added?

The fact that acids have accumulated is reflected by two observations: the fall in plasma $[HCO_3^-]$ and the increase in the anion gap in plasma (accumulation of the anion that accompanied the H^+—in this case, ketoacid anions undoubtedly).

Have H^+ been buffered? If so, how many?

The fact that H^+ have been buffered is indicated by the fall in $[HCO_3^-]$ of 15 mmol/L and the rise in the anion gap in plasma of 15 mEq/L. Despite the large input of H^+, the $[H^+]$ has only increased by 0.000020 mmol/L. The H^+ have been buffered by HCO_3^- in the ECF, which has lost 15 mmol of HCO_3^- per liter (some H^+ have been buffered by HCO_3^- in the ICF as well). Assuming an ECF volume of 15 L, then the H^+ load in the ECF was 225 mmol (15 L

Note
There is no fixed percentage of buffering of a H⁺ load in the ECF vs the ICF. At smaller H⁺ loads, most buffering is by the BBS. With very large H⁺ loads, all new buffering is via proteins because there are too few HCO_3^- remaining to buffer the H⁺ load. In the introductory case, it was assumed that 40% of the H⁺ was buffered in the ECF at this given [H⁺].

$\times$ 15 mmol/L). Because close to 40% of the H⁺ load was buffered in the ECF at this [H⁺], the total H⁺ load was 563 mmol.

Have the lungs and the kidneys responded appropriately?

The lungs have responded to the acidemia because the $Paco_2$ has fallen to 25 mm Hg (normal $Paco_2$ is 40 mm Hg). The kidneys have also responded, as evidenced by the increased excretion of NH_4^+ from the normal 40 mmol/day to 200 mmol/day.

Is the acid-base abnormality a major threat to the body? If so, why?

This acid-base abnormality is a potential threat to Lee's life. The H⁺ load has already consumed just over half of the total buffer capacity. Whereas the overall H⁺ production in ketoacidosis is close to 1 mmol/min, the rate of accumulation of ketoacids depends heavily on their rate of removal by oxidation. Therefore, ketoacids can accumulate at an appreciable rate if the rate of ketoacid anion metabolism declines. Such a decline would occur if the patient's GFR is low (the need for ATP to reabsorb Na^+ would be reduced) or if the patient develops coma (the need for ATP to maintain cerebral activity would be reduced). Hence, ketoacidosis may become a major threat if Lee becomes comatose and has prerenal failure (a low GFR).

Is it possible to estimate how quickly more H⁺ will accumulate?

Clinical pearl
One can calculate how many H⁺ are accumulating by counting new anions in the body plus anions excreted without H⁺ or NH_4^+.

Lee is currently regenerating 200 mmol of HCO_3^- per day via the excretion of NH_4^+. If the net ketoacid production increases much more, H⁺ will accumulate (production is 1500 mmol/day, and metabolism is 1200 mmol/day via normal brain and kidneys). One can estimate how many H⁺ will accumulate by quantitating the number of new anions that appear in Lee over time. These anions may remain in the body (rise in the plasma anion gap $\times$ total body water) or be excreted in the urine without H⁺ or NH_4^+ (urine ([Na^+] + [K^+] − [Cl^-]) $\times$ urine flow rate).

Do H⁺ kill? If so, how do they do it?

If H⁺ kill, they do so by binding to intracellular proteins and altering their charge and function. The authors are not sure that H⁺ actually kill most patients with metabolic acidosis. Their rationale is that people who sprint vigorously can have very low pH values, but all survive.

Summary of Main Points

- Count the number of charges on substrates and products of the reactions to see if H⁺ are produced or removed in the metabolic process.
- H⁺ accumulates when anions are formed and cannot be metabolized or when they are metabolized more slowly than they are produced.

- H$^+$ accumulates during the metabolism of proteins because the number of sulfur-containing amino acids (methionine, cysteine/cystine $\times$ 2) plus cationic amino acids (lysine, arginine, histidine) exceeds the number of anionic amino acids (glutamate and aspartate).
- Incomplete metabolism of carbohydrates (usually due to hypoxia) or of fats (due to a lack of insulin) causes H$^+$ to accumulate.
- "Fast" H$^+$ are produced only during hypoxia.
- H$^+$ accumulate when alcohols (or neutral compounds that are converted to alcohols) are oxidized to anions in the body. Of greater importance, metabolic intermediates of this metabolism may accumulate, and they are very toxic to humans.

Discussion of Questions

1.1 Why doesn't the HCl secreted by gastric cells denature proteins in the cell membrane of the stomach?

The [H$^+$] is so high in gastric fluid that proteins in cell membranes will be denatured if exposed to this [H$^+$]. The defense mechanisms include a protective mucous barrier along the luminal lining of the stomach and, located below this lining, a relatively alkaline solution that contains HCO$_3^-$. On secretion, H$^+$ are "channeled" quickly through this mucous barrier. Hence, H$^+$ in the lumen are kept away from the gastric mucosa.

1.2 What might permit H$^+$ to bind to the H$^+$ pump inside cells at a concentration of 0.0001 mmol/L, yet dissociate in the lumen of the stomach at a concentration of 100 mmol/L?

The chemical group that binds H$^+$ in the cell must have its pK changed by local influences (structural changes), but this change is probably not enough to alter the pK so drastically. The authors believe that other forces are operating. Perhaps the binding of K$^+$ in the lumen helps "repel" the positively charged proton from the carrier. This theory might provide a rationale for having a special type of H$^+$ pump in the stomach, an H$^+$/K$^+$ antiporter.

1.3 What is the rationale for stating that only weak acids kill?

The major consideration from a clinical perspective is the size of the H$^+$ load. Because strong acids are 99.999% dissociated and weak acids are close to 99% dissociated at the [H$^+$] in the body, the strength of acids is not an important determinant of the number of H$^+$ released. Of greater importance is the quantity of acid produced; weak acids (L-lactic acid, ketoacids) are produced at a much higher rate than strong acids (HCl and H$_2$SO$_4$). Hence, there will be a larger total load of H$^+$ with weak acids.

1.4 In the metabolic process in Figure 1.1, in what circumstances will H$^+$ accumulate?

If the rate of production of ketoacids equals their rate of oxidation, then H^+ does not accumulate. Nevertheless, if the rate of ketogenesis increases or the rate of oxidation of ketoacids declines, H^+ will accumulate (see Chapter 3 for details).

1.5 Red blood cells produce 200 mmol of L-lactic acid per day. Why doesn't this production cause severe acidemia?

Acidemia does not usually result because the hepatic metabolism of the L-lactate anions to neutral end-products consumes all the H^+ that were produced. As long as L-lactate metabolism occurs as quickly as this acid is formed, there is no net production of H^+.

1.6 When ATP is used to perform biologic work, H^+ are formed. Should these H^+ be considered as part of the quantity that can cause acidosis?

This question and answer illustrate the difference between net and absolute rates of production of H^+; the former is very small (but important) and the latter is enormous (and not so important). As soon as ATP is hydrolyzed to perform biologic work, it is regenerated by metabolic reactions. Hence, there is a large turnover of H^+ but no net production of H^+. Because the quantity of ATP in tissues is quite small, there would be only a minor change in the maximum rate of H^+ accumulation even if all the ATP in cells was converted to ADP. Therefore, the answer to the question is no.

$$ATP^{4-} \rightarrow ADP^{3-} + P_i^{2-} + H^+ + work$$
$$ADP^{3-} + P_i^{2-} + H^+ \rightarrow ATP \text{ (regeneration)}$$

1.7 Acetate is added to the hemodialysis fluid to minimize the net production of H^+. What is the rationale for this maneuver?

Acetate anion as its Na^+ salt is added to the dialysis fluid so that H^+ can be removed by metabolic pathways that yield CO_2 as a final product.

$$\text{Acetate anion} + 2\,O_2 + H^+ \rightarrow 2\,CO_2 + 2\,H_2O$$

1.8 During hemodialysis, β-hydroxybutyric acid is formed from acetate anions and is lost in the dialysis fluid. Does this process result in the net production or removal of H^+?

Two molecules of acetate anion (Na^+ salt) are converted to one molecule of β-hydroxybutyrate anion in the liver. In this process, the product has less anionic charge than its substrates, so H^+ are removed despite the fact that a ketoacid (β-hydroxybutyric acid) is the product.

$$2\text{ Acetate anion} + 2\,H^+ \rightarrow \text{β-hydroxybutyrate anion} + H^+$$

Note
In contrast to acetate anions, conversion of neutral triglycerides to β-hydroxybutyrate anions does result in the net production of H^+ (see pages 89–99).

1.9 What might permit bacteria in the GI tract to overproduce organic acids?

The normal digestive process, with largely neutral foodstuff, feces, and absorbed fuels, does not pose a net acid load. However, changes in the normal bacterial content of the intestines (e.g., from new flora produced by the actions of antibiotics or from stasis, which permits more bacterial growth) can potentiate the release of an unusual quantity of organic acids into the body. The production of organic acids might become limited if these bacteria lack a carbohydrate fuel; when the intestines contain more bacteria, eating foods that contain carbohydrates can suddenly increase the rate of production of these acids (see Case 3.5).

$$\text{Carbohydrate} \rightarrow \text{organic anions} + H^+$$

1.10 Does consumption of citrus fruits, which contain a large quantity of citric acid and K$^+$ citrate, cause an acid or alkali load?

Very early on, before citrate anions are metabolized, there is an initial H$^+$ load because citric acid dissociates into H$^+$ and citrate anions

$$(\text{Citric acid} \rightarrow \text{citrate}^{3-} + 3\ H^+).$$

Later, when all citrate anions are removed by metabolism to neutral end-products, there will be a net alkali load because some citrate anions are added to the body with K$^+$ and not H$^+$

$$(\text{Citrate}^{3-} + 3\ H^+ + 4.5\ O_2 \rightarrow 6\ CO_2 + 4\ H_2O).$$

1.11 How much would the [HCO$_3^-$] in the ECF decrease when a load of 70 mmol of H$^+$ is retained in a 70-kg person who lacks renal generation of new HCO$_3^-$?

The kidneys normally regenerate 70 mmol of HCO$_3^-$ per day. If the body gains 70 mmol H$^+$ per day, and just over half is buffered in cells, 30 mmol of H$^+$ would be buffered in the ECF by HCO$_3^-$. Because the ECF volume is close to 15 L, the [HCO$_3^-$] will fall by close to 2 mmol/L each day while the BBS is still a major buffer system operating in the body.

1.12 The following results for a blood sample arrive from the laboratory: [H$^+$] = 60 nmol/L, pH = 7.22, Pa$_{CO_2}$ = 50 mm Hg, [HCO$_3^-$], = 32 mmol/L. What do you conclude?

The values are inconsistent with the Henderson equation. An analytical error may have occurred, measurements may have been made on two different samples of blood, or there may have been a problem with the temperature or ionic strength of the sample. Repeat the analysis and then decide.

Henderson equation

$$[H^+] = \frac{24 \times P_{CO_2}}{HCO_3^-}$$

$$60 \neq \frac{24 \times 50}{32}$$

1.13 What would the Pa$_{CO_2}$ be in a normal man if his alveolar ventilation rate decreased by half (assume no change in his metabolic rate)?

If the rate of formation of CO$_2$ by the body is kept constant, halving the alveolar ventilation will temporarily slow the rate of excretion of CO$_2$. This decreased rate of excretion will cause the P$_{CO_2}$ in each liter of alveolar air to increase so that all the CO$_2$ produced will be excreted and a new steady state will exist (compare with clearance of creatinine—when the GFR is halved, the serum creatinine doubles, so the daily creatinine production is excreted with half the GFR).

The alveolar ventilation during hypoventilation will fall from 5 to 2.5 L/min in this example.

CO_2 removal = [CO_2] in alveolar air × volume of alveolar air exhaled/min

Normal: 10 mmol/min = 2 mmol/L × 5 L/min
Hypoventilation: 10 mmol/min = 4 mmol/L × 2.5 L/min

Therefore, halving the alveolar ventilation will lead to a doubling of the Pa_{CO_2} to 80 mm Hg.

What must you do to keep his pH ([H$^+$]) from changing?

In order to keep the [H$^+$] normal at a Pa_{CO_2} of 80 mm Hg, the [HCO_3^-] must be increased twofold to 48 mmol/L.

1.14 Some say that hyperventilation is "maladaptive" because in an experimental situation, there was a fall in the pH of plasma after hyperventilation occurred. How might this phenomenon be interpreted?

The key question is this: What is the purpose of hyperventilation—to change the [H$^+$] in the ECF or to influence events in the ICF (return the valence of proteins toward normal)?

The authors seem preoccupied with events in the ECF because they measure samples from this compartment. As judged from the ability of subjects to perform vigorous exercise with a very high [H$^+$] in the ECF (the sprint), there is little cause to worry if the [H$^+$] rises in the ECF.

In the authors' opinion, the crucial compartment is the ICF. When the tissue P_{CO_2} falls, the BBS equation is driven to the right, and H$^+$ is removed from proteins and transferred to HCO_3^- (see Figure 1.8). Thus, there can be a major advantage of a lower P_{CO_2} because now proteins will have a valence that is closer to normal and perhaps their charge, shape, and functions will return to normal.

Regarding the question of a maladaptive response with a lower P_{CO_2}: if, as a result of a more normal ICF environment after hyperventilation, there is additional net loss of some HCO_3^-, the [H$^+$] in the ECF might not fall and may even rise a bit. This response is the "price to pay" for a better environment in cells. Therefore "maladaptive or not" depends on where you stand on this issue.

1.15 Can a patient have a very low arterial P_{CO_2} yet have respiratory acidosis in the cells?

Yes. Respiratory acidosis at the cell level is a high tissue P_{CO_2} that elevates the [H_2CO_3] and thereby the [H$^+$]. Even though the arterial P_{CO_2} is low (appropriate ventilation), either a high local CO_2 production rate in cells (anaerobic metabolism or strenuous exercise for muscle cells, for example) or a very low blood flow rate (cardiogenic shock, for example) will cause the tissue P_{CO_2} to be unduly high. These points emphasize that an evaluation of the BBS in cells is not revealed by simply the arterial blood gas result; this information must be integrated with the venous blood P_{CO_2}.

1.16 Why is the brain "protected" from a higher mixed venous P_{CO_2} in a patient with diabetic ketoacidosis (DKA)?

The venous P_{CO_2} is a function of the arterial P_{CO_2}, the rate of production of CO_2, and the rate of blood flow. In a patient with DKA, all three of these parameters lead to a lower P_{CO_2} in the internal jugular vein. The arterial P_{CO_2} is low due to hyperventilation in response to acidemia. The rate of production of CO_2 may be lower in the brain of this patient due to confusion and coma. One might expect the ECF volume contraction to lower blood pressure and blood flow rate to all organs. Notwithstanding, there is autoregulation of cerebral blood flow rate that maintains cerebral blood flow rate despite generalized hypotension. This latter factor protects the brain in DKA. Nevertheless, if the blood pressure falls sufficiently, this latter mechanism can no longer maintain cerebral blood flow rate. At this time, the patient will develop a severe degree of intracellular acidosis and have an abrupt deterioration in clinical status.

1.17 Is it more important to control the [H⁺] in the ECF or in the ICF?

It is more important to control the [H⁺] in the ICF.

[H⁺] in the ECF. There are three major ways in which a high [H⁺] in the ECF can compromise cellular function and limit survival:

1. By virtue of the high [H⁺], hormone receptors on the cell surface can be protonated and thereby compromise signal transduction and cellular function. Examples include the lower affinity for the binding of insulin and of adrenaline to their receptors in severe acidemia; impaired binding of adrenaline to its receptor could compromise myocardial function.
2. It is also possible that protonation of other cell membrane proteins can compromise function.
3. A high [H⁺] in the ECF could bring about a shift of K⁺ from the ICF to the ECF. In this setting, acute hyperkalemia could induce a cardiac arrhythmia.

In spite of the preceding theoretical arguments, during a sprint the [H⁺] rises markedly in the ECF, yet cardiac performance is close to normal.

[H⁺] in the ICF. It is more likely that the detrimental effect of a high [H⁺] may be related to titration of intracellular proteins. When more H⁺ are bound to these proteins, they will have a more positive charge, which could alter their shape and function. Therefore, whereas the traditional clinical view in the assessment of the acid-base status has focused on the assessment of the [H⁺] and [HCO_3^-] in the ECF, a broader view would consider the impact of H⁺ not only on the titration of the BBS but also (and maybe more importantly) on the non-BBS buffers (intracellular proteins for the most part). Therefore, the authors believe that it is more important to defend the [H⁺] in the ICF.

1.18 What should the pH of the ICF of muscle be in the first 10 seconds of a sprint in a normal person and in a patient with a defect in the hydrolysis of glycogen?

Vigorous muscle activity requires a large supply of ATP, which is provided by the metabolism of glucose and glycogen. Because there is insufficient O_2 to regenerate the needed ATP, anaerobic metabolism proceeds (glucose → L-lactic acid). The $[H^+]$ in the ICF rises markedly in a sprint in a normal person because of the huge production of L-lactic acid.

In contrast, if only a small quantity of glycogen in muscle cells can be broken down during a sprint (which is the case in the patient with a defect in hydrolysis of glycogen), little L-lactic acid will be formed during the sprint. Exercise induces the hydrolysis of creatine phosphate, thereby producing HPO_4^{2-}, a H^+ acceptor that causes the muscle cell to become more alkaline. Thus, normally, the impact of the excess local L-lactic acid production in muscle during vigorous exercise is diminished somewhat by the generation of an additional H^+ buffer, HPO_4^{2-}. Parenthetically, the content of creatine phosphate is very high in skeletal muscle cells (20 mmol/kg).

Therefore, in the normal person, the $[H^+]$ in the ICF will be increased during vigorous exercise, but in a patient with a defect in glycogenolysis, the $[H^+]$ in the ICF will be decreased from the increased HPO_4^{2-} coupled with the low H^+ load.

1.19 What other role might NHE-3 have in the PCT?

NHE-3 helps in the excretion of NH_4^+. NH_4^+ replaces H^+ on NHE-3 in PCT cells so that NH_4^+ can be added to the lumen. If too many NH_4^+ are secreted, they can be reabsorbed via the diffusion-trapping mechanism.

1.20 How do carbonic anhydrase inhibitors compromise the indirect reabsorption of HCO_3^-?

Carbonic anhydrase inhibitors inhibit carbonic anhydrase in the lumen of the PCT. In so doing, H_2CO_3 builds up in the lumen. As a result of the carbonic acid dissociation, the $[H^+]$ in luminal fluid increases and prevents further net secretion of H^+ (which would reabsorb more of the filtered HCO_3^-).

1.21 If the patient with pRTA develops diarrhea and the $[HCO_3^-]$ in the ECF drops 2 mmol/L below its usual value, how will the urine pH and $[HCO_3^-]$ change?

In some circumstances (e.g., after a $NaHCO_3$ load), the patient with pRTA has alkaline urine because the filtered load of HCO_3^- exceeds the reduced capacity of the proximal H^+ secretory process to reclaim it. Thus, HCO_3^- are delivered to the distal convoluted tubule. At this point, some (but not all) is reabsorbed because distal H^+ secretion is a low-capacity system. The rest of the HCO_3^- that were not reabsorbed is excreted, and the urine becomes alkaline. If some process (e.g., loss of $NaHCO_3$ via the GI tract) lowers the filtered load of HCO_3^- so that it does not exceed the proximal H^+ secretory capacity, most of the HCO_3^- are then reabsorbed indirectly in the PCT (some HCO_3^- always leaves the PCT because the membrane is leaky, and steep $[H^+]$ gradients cannot be generated by the proximal nephron; i.e., the pH of the luminal fluid at the end of the PCT is in the mid-6 range). In these circumstances, a small enough quantity of HCO_3^- is delivered to the distal tubule so that distal H^+ secretion is sufficient to reabsorb these HCO_3^-; the urine

Note
The urine pH is generally low in patients with pRTA. This low pH permits them to excrete NH_4^+ for daily acid-base balance.

is rendered free of HCO_3^-. The remaining H^+ secretion will lower the urine pH to well below 6; how low the urine pH falls is determined by the quantity of NH_3 available to react with secreted H^+ (see margin note).

1.22 How would you establish whether a patient with a low $[HCO_3^-]$ and diarrhea has pRTA?

Administer a load of $NaHCO_3$. If the patient continues to reabsorb HCO_3^- normally, little if any HCO_3^- will be excreted until the plasma $[HCO_3^-]$ approaches 25 mmol/L. In contrast, with pRTA, bicarbonaturia will be prominent at concentrations of HCO_3^- in plasma that are distinctly subnormal.

1.23 Why is the production of NH_4^+ low in renal insufficiency?

The concentration of ADP, the precursor for ATP, is present in very tiny amounts in cells. Thus, no organ or organelle can generate more ATP than it consumes to perform biologic work (hydrolysis of ATP yields ADP). Because renal work is largely the reabsorption of filtered Na^+, a low GFR means fewer filtered Na^+, less work, and less ATP turnover. Hence, in renal insufficiency, less fuel (glutamine) can be oxidized and fewer NH_4^+ will be produced.

1.24 In the ketoacidosis of chronic fasting, the rate of excretion of NH_4^+ is lower than in chronic metabolic acidosis caused by ingestion of HCl. What teleologic advantages might this lower rate of excretion provide, and what mechanisms might be involved?

Excretion of more NH_4^+ during fasting requires a source of nitrogen. This source is body protein. Hence, excessive catabolism of lean body mass could occur and, from a teleologic viewpoint, might not be advantageous during fasting. With respect to mechanisms, the lower GFR and the oxidation of fat-derived fuels (ketoacids) by PCT cells could limit the rate of production of NH_4^+ because there would be less ATP to regenerate from the metabolism of glutamine (see the discussion of Question 1.23).

1.25 There is a lag period between the net addition of acids and induction of ammoniagenesis. Why might this time be advantageous to a sprinter?

During sprinting, L-lactic acid is formed. During the subsequent period of rest (minutes to hours), all this L-lactic acid will be removed by metabolism. Hence, there is no need for extra HCO_3^- to be made by the kidney.

1.26 Why might ammoniagenesis be low in a patient with hyperkalemia?

Hyperkalemia resulting from a K^+ load can cause K^+ to enter cells. For electroneutrality, some H^+ will exit. This cell alkalinization will lower NH_4^+ production. Hyperkalemia may also lower the rate of excretion of NH_4^+ by mechanisms independent of ammoniagenesis. In addition, K^+ and NH_4^+ compete for reabsorption in the thick

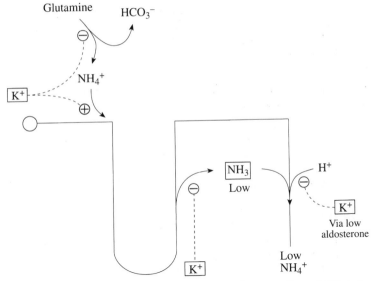

Figure 1.19   Influence of hyperkalemia on the excretion of NH₄⁺. In the PCT, hyperkalemia has two effects: it decreases the production of NH_4^+ but enhances their secretion so that there is little reduction in the quantity of NH_4^+ leaving the luminal fluid in the PCT. In the loop of Henle, hyperkalemia causes a higher $[K^+]$ in the luminal fluid and thereby decreases the reabsorption of NH_4^+. This action leads to a low $[NH_3]$ in the medullary interstitium. Both the low medullary $[NH_3]$ and the low distal H^+ secretion (results of the low aldosterone if that was the cause of the hyperkalemia) lead to a low excretion of NH_4^+.

ascending limb of the loop of Henle. As a result, there is less NH_3 in the medullary interstitium (Figure 1.19).

1.27   Why is Na⁺ acetate added to total parenteral nutrition (TPN) solutions? Answer from the perspective of NH₄⁺ excretion.

Patients on TPN develop metabolic acidosis with a low rate of renal excretion of NH_4^+. A possible explanation for the low rate of NH_4^+ excretion (and hence the acidemia) is that perhaps fuels provided during TPN (other than glutamine) regenerate ATP, but not NH_4^+, in cells of the PCT. When the acetate anion added to the TPN is metabolized to CO_2 and H_2O, the result is consumption of H^+ (or production of HCO_3^-) and correction of the acidemia.

Appendix

Molecular Advances Concerning H⁺ Transport

Na⁺, H⁺ Exchangers (NHE)

Overall, NHE export H^+ from cells in conjunction with importing Na^+ into cells (Figure 1.20). NHE have three bindings sites: two are

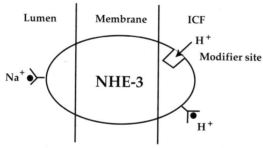

Figure 1.20 NHE-3 in the proximal convoluted tubule. The central area is the luminal membrane of PCT cells; NHE-3 spans this membrane, with part residing in the cytosol and part outside the cell (in the lumen). The net effect is to reabsorb Na^+ and secrete H^+ (shown as solid dots); the activity of NHE-3 is enhanced when the $[H^+]$ rises in PCT cells and H^+ bind to the modifier site.

involved in transport (one for Na^+ and one for H^+), and the third modulates the activity of the NHE (when there is a high $[H^+]$ in cells, H^+ bind to the modifier site and activate the NHE to export H^+).

General Families of NHE. Only two will be mentioned because their physiologic roles are defined. They are distinct entities, being coded for on different chromosomes.

1. **NHE-1.** The main role of NHE-1 is the defense of the ICF $[H^+]$ and thereby the charge on intracellular proteins. NHE-1 may also play an important role in regulating cell growth.
2. **NHE-3.** NHE-3 is present in the luminal membrane of the PCT and in the small intestine; its primary function is to reabsorb $NaHCO_3$ (see Figure 1.10).

Regulation by Phosphorylation. This is a complex issue. NHE-1 and NHE-3 are phosphorylated by three different protein kinases: protein kinase C (PKC) and protein kinase A (PKA), and the Ca-calmodulin system (Ca/CaM). Their effects differ on the two NHEs.

Regulation of NHE by Phosphorylation

	PK_A	PK_C	Ca/CaM
NHE-1	Increased	Decreased	Increased
NHE-3	Decreased	Decreased	Increased

Exit of HCO_3^- from Renal Tubular Cells

There are two different strategies used to export alkali from cells in nephron segments of the kidney involved in H^+ secretion.

1. **Events in the PCT.** Because a large quantity of HCO_3^- must be exported from cells of the PCT, the system used is linked to Na^+ because this process can carry Na^+ out of cells without expending extra energy via the Na^+, K^+, ATPase. Moreover, HCO_3^- must be transported from a site where their concentration is lower (10–15 mmol/L in cells) to a location where the $[HCO_3^-]$ is higher (25 mmol/L in the ECF). To do so without expending extra energy, the net negative voltage in cells is used as the driving force (Figure 1.21). All this can be achieved by having 3 HCO_3^- ions plus 1 Na^+ ion form an ion

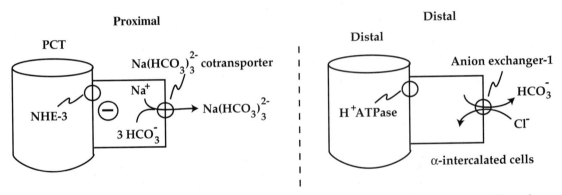

Figure 1.21   Exit of HCO$_3^-$ from cells. The events in the PCT are shown on the left of the dashed line, whereas those in the distal nephron are shown on the right of the dashed line. The major transporters for HCO$_3^-$ into the ECF are on the basolateral membrane of these cells.

complex; indeed, 3 HCO$_3^-$ ions plus 1 Na$^+$ ion form an ion complex spontaneously.

2. **Events in the distal nephron.** The cells responsible for the export of HCO$_3^-$ in the distal nephron are the α-intercalated cells. The mechanism involved is a Cl$^-$/HCO$_3^-$ anion exchange by the ubiquitous anion exchanger (AE-1, which is linked to band-3 protein family in red blood cells; Chapter 2). The driving force is the much higher [Cl$^-$] in the ECF (103 mmol/L) as compared with cells (<20 mmol/L).

Overall. There are a number of transporters, hormone receptors, and enzymes involved in carrying out renal responses to an acid-base perturbation; these are illustrated in Figure 1.22.

Diseases That May Be Associated with Abnormal Transport of HCO$_3^-$ Across the Basolateral Membrane

Proximal

In the PCT, if the Na(HCO$_3$)$_3^{2-}$ exit step proceeds more slowly (lower Vmax) or needs a higher [HCO$_3^-$] in cells (higher Km [the concentration of substrate needed for half-maximal velocity (Vmax)]) to transport all reabsorbed HCO$_3^-$, the cell will be more alkaline (higher [HCO$_3^-$] in the ICF). Thus, one would anticipate less secretion of H$^+$ by NHE-3 (lower reabsorption of NaHCO$_3$), a lower rate of production of NH$_4^+$, and citraturia despite metabolic acidosis—characteristic findings seen in patients with isolated proximal renal tubular acidosis (Chapter 3, page 119).

Distal

In the distal tubule, either a hereditary defect in AE-1 (as in hereditary ovalocytosis) or the presence of abnormal globulins that may inhibit this transporter (perhaps in Sjögren's syndrome) can lead to an alkaline α-intercalated cell and thereby less H$^+$ secretion

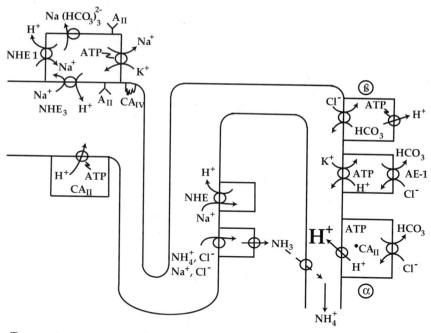

Figure 1.22 Transporters, enzymes and hormone receptors involved in acid-base balance. The structure is a nephron.

PCT: Two cells are represented in the PCT for convenience. There are two receptors for angiotensin II (A_{II}), one in the lumen and one on the basolateral membrane. There are two carbonic anhydrases (CA), one in cells (CA_{II}) and one with its catalytic site in the lumen (CA_{IV}).

Loop of Henle (LOH): In the LOH, NH_4^+ are reabsorbed by replacing K^+ on the *NKCC* cotransporter.

Distal: In the collecting ducts, there are α- and β-intercalated cells (α-cells have their H^+ATPase in the luminal membrane and AE-1 on the basolateral surface; the converse occurs in β-intercalated cells).

by the H^+ATPase in its luminal membrane. The net result will be a low excretion of NH_4^+ and a high urine pH; the disease is called distal RTA (see margin note).

Defense of the Intracellular pH

With hypoxia, for example, a heart cell could have a rise in its $[H^+]$ that compromises its function. In response to the rise in $[H^+]$, H^+ can be exported as a result of two major changes in ion pumps (Figure 1.23).

1. **NHE-1.** H^+ can be exported by activation of NHE-1 in the plasma membrane when the $[H^+]$ rises in these cells. The advantage is that a fall in the ICF $[H^+]$ will cause less H^+ binding to proteins in cardiac myocytes and thereby preserve

Note
There are many causes of distal RTA. One subgroup has low distal H^+ secretion. An alkaline α-intercalated cell pH is one hypothetical basis for this disorder (see Chapter 3, page 122).

Figure 1.23 Defense of the ICF $[H^+]$. When the $[H^+]$ rises in cells (e.g., hypoxia with lactic acid production), the rise in $[H^+]$ may be less than expected due to export of H^+ by NHE-1 or import of HCO_3^- by AE-1.

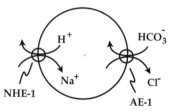

their functions. For this to be "effective," other cells must take up the exported H^+ and buffer them with their BBS.

2. **Anion exchange.** Most cells have a Cl^-:HCO_3^- anion exchanger (AE-1). In response to a lower $[HCO_3^-]$ in cells, HCO_3^- enter and Cl^- ions exit. The net effect is removal of H^+ from the ICF.

C H A P T E R

2

The Clinical Approach to Acid-Base Disorders

OBJECTIVES

☐ To provide the background so that the four primary acid-base disturbances if present can be identified.

☐ To illustrate the expected physiologic responses to a primary acid-base disorder and thereby enable the recognition of mixed acid-base disorders.

□ To provide a group of tools including several "gaps" to assist in the diagnosis of individual acid-base disturbances.

Outline of Major Principles

Henderson equation

$$[H^+] = \frac{24 \times P_{CO_2}}{[HCO_3^-]}$$

Normal values in plasma
pH: 7.40 ± 0.02
[H⁺]: 40 ± 2 nmol/L
Paco₂: 40 ± 2 mm Hg
[HCO₃⁻]: 25 ± 2 mmol/L
Anion gap: 12 ± 2 mEq/L
     (excluding K⁺)
([Na⁺] − ([Cl⁻] + [HCO₃⁻]))

1. The parameters of plasma that describe the patient's acid-base status are summarized in the margin.
2. The *Henderson equation* relates three parameters; one can calculate the third knowing the other two. This equation also helps identify errors in measurement.
3. There are four primary acid-base disorders:

   Metabolic acidosis: increased $[H^+]$ and reduced $[HCO_3^-]$ in plasma;

   Metabolic alkalosis: reduced $[H^+]$ and increased $[HCO_3^-]$ in plasma;

   Respiratory acidosis: increased $[H^+]$ and P_{aCO_2} in plasma;

   Respiratory alkalosis: reduced $[H^+]$ and P_{aCO_2} in plasma.
4. Specific physiologic responses occur as the result of acid-base disorders. In the extracellular fluid (ECF) these responses return the plasma $[H^+]$ toward normal, but not into the normal range. It is more instructive to consider their impact on events in the intracellular fluid (ICF).
5. The clinical and laboratory data must be evaluated together to reach an acid-base diagnosis.
6. Several acid-base disorders may coexist in a patient.

INTRODUCTORY CASE
Lee's Acidosis is Mixed Up
(Case discussed on page 67)

When Lee, an insulin-dependent diabetic, developed abdominal pain and diarrhea, her food intake was curtailed, and the insulin dose was reduced. Because the diarrhea persisted, Lee saw a physician, and the following results were obtained from blood tests.

Na⁺	140 mmol/L	H⁺	60 nmol/L (pH = 7.22)
K⁺	5.0 mmol/L	Paco₂	25 mm Hg
Cl⁻	103 mmol/L	HCO₃⁻	10 mmol/L

What is the acid-base diagnosis?
Is there a primary respiratory acid-base disorder?

PART A

Background

Methods to Interconvert pH and [H⁺]

At times, values may be reported in pH units; at others, the [H⁺] is utilized. Therefore, it is important to know how to interconvert these forms of expression. Methods for this interconversion are provided in the following sections.

Rule of Thumb #1: Drop the 7 and Decimal Point

There is a near-linear relationship between the [H$^+$] and the pH in the range of pH 7.28–7.55. At a pH of 7.40, the [H$^+$] is 40 nmol/L (note that if you drop the 7 and the decimal point you have the [H$^+$] of 40 nmol/L). Next, after dropping the 7 and the decimal point, take the difference of the number from 40. Add that value to 40 if the pH is less than 7.40, and subtract it if the pH is greater than 7.40; the result is the [H$^+$].

pH	Drop 7 and Decimal Point	Difference From 40	[H$^+$] nmol/L
7.40	40	0	40
7.38	38	2	42
7.42	42	2	38

Reference
Kassirer, J. P., and H. L. Bleich. 1965. *N Engl J Med* 272:1067.

The 0.1 pH Change Rule

For every 0.1 unit increase in pH, multiply the [H$^+$] by 0.8. Given that a pH of 7.00 equals a [H$^+$] of 100 nmol/L, a rise in pH of 0.1 (pH 7.10) equals 0.8 × 100, or a [H$^+$] of 80 nmol/L. For values less than 7.00, divide by 0.8 (or multiply by 1.25). Intermediate values are calculated by interpolation.

pH	Conversion Factor	[H$^+$] nmol/L
6.90	100 × 1.25	125
7.00	100	100
7.10	100 × 0.8	80
7.20	100 × 0.8 × 0.8	64

Reference
Fagan, T. J. 1973. *N Engl J Med* 288:915.

Log Table

A log table (Table 2.1) is provided to aid in interconverting the [H$^+$] and pH.

Making an Initial Acid-Base Diagnosis by Examining Parameters in Plasma

- Integrate clinical and laboratory pictures.
- Examine all four parameters in plasma ([H$^+$], [HCO$_3^-$], Paco$_2$, anion gap).

pH vs [H$^+$]
The authors prefer to think in terms of the [H$^+$] rather than the pH, but the principles are the same: a low [H$^+$] is a high pH, and vice versa.

In making an acid-base diagnosis, there are two points to stress. First, one must integrate the clinical picture and the laboratory values to make a proper diagnosis. For example, finding acidemia, a high Paco$_2$, and an elevated [HCO$_3^-$] does not indicate that

TABLE 2.1 **Interconversion of pH and [H$^+$]**

pH	[H$^+$]	pH	[H$^+$]	pH	[H$^+$]	pH	[H$^+$]
.01	9772	.26	5495	.51	3090	.76	1738
.02	9550	.27	5370	.52	3020	.77	1698
.03	9333	.28	5248	.53	2951	.78	1660
.04	9120	.29	5129	.54	2884	.79	1622
.05	8913	.30	5012	.55	2818	.80	1585
.06	8710	.31	4898	.56	2754	.81	1549
.07	8511	.32	4786	.57	2692	.82	1514
.08	8318	.33	4677	.58	2630	.83	1479
.09	8128	.34	4571	.59	2570	.84	1445
.10	7943	.35	4467	.60	2512	.85	1413
.11	7762	.36	4365	.61	2455	.86	1380
.12	7586	.37	4266	.62	2399	.87	1349
.13	7413	.38	4169	.63	2344	.88	1318
.14	7244	.39	4074	.64	2291	.89	1288
.15	7079	.40	3981	.65	2239	.90	1259
.16	6918	.41	3890	.66	2188	.91	1230
.17	6761	.42	3802	.67	2138	.92	1202
.18	6607	.43	3715	.68	2089	.93	1175
.19	6457	.44	3631	.69	2042	.94	1148
.20	6310	.45	3548	.70	1995	.95	1122
.21	6166	.46	3467	.71	1950	.96	1096
.22	6026	.47	3388	.72	1905	.97	1072
.23	5888	.48	3311	.73	1862	.98	1047
.24	5754	.49	3236	.74	1820	.99	1023
.25	5623	.50	3162	.75	1778	1.00	1000

Examples

pH	[H$^+$] nmol/L
7.01	97.7
7.00	100
6.90	125.9

chronic respiratory acidosis is present in a patient who does not have a chronic problem with ventilation; in this case, more than one acid-base disturbance is likely to be present. Second, from the laboratory perspective, the authors recommend that four parameters in plasma be examined, the pH or [H$^+$], the PaCO_2, the [HCO$_3^-$], and the anion gap; the authors usually start with the plasma [H$^+$], as illustrated in Figure 2.1.

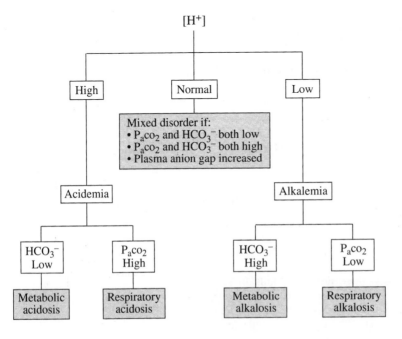

Figure 2.1 Initial diagnosis of acid-base disorders. Start with the plasma [H$^+$]. The information to be interpreted to make a final diagnosis is indicated in open boxes; the final diagnoses are shown in the shaded boxes (see the text for details).

Pao$_2$

The Pao$_2$ has no direct application with respect to the acid-base analysis; however, calculating the alveolar-arterial (A-a) O$_2$ difference provides additional important information (see Chapter 5, pages 203–205 for more discussion).

High [H⁺]

If the [H⁺] is increased, the patient has acidemia, and there are two potential causes—metabolic or respiratory acidosis.

Metabolic acidosis is the result of a process that lowers the [HCO₃⁻] and raises the [H⁺]; the expected adjustment is a low Paco₂.

Respiratory acidosis is characterized by an increased Paco₂ and [H⁺]; the expected adjustment is an increased [HCO₃⁻]. This adjustment is minimal in acute respiratory acidosis and larger in chronic respiratory acidosis.

Low [H⁺]

If the [H⁺] is low, the patient has alkalemia. Again, there are two potential causes—metabolic or respiratory alkalosis.

Metabolic alkalosis is the result of a process that raises the [HCO₃⁻] and lowers the [H⁺]; the expected adjustment is a rise in the Paco₂, which is usually modest because of respiratory stimulation from the resultant hypoxia. Nevertheless, if the patient is receiving O₂, and hypoxia is prevented, hypoventilation can be more profound.

Respiratory alkalosis is characterized by an unexpectedly low Paco₂, which results in a lower [H⁺]. The expected physiologic response is a reduction in plasma [HCO₃⁻]. As in respiratory acidosis, this response is modest in acute disorders and more significant in chronic disorders.

Normal [H⁺]

A normal [H⁺] implies either no acid-base disorder or the presence of two acid-base disorders—one tending to raise the [H⁺] and the other tending to depress the [H⁺].

QUESTION

(Discussion on page 68)

2.1 *A patient has diabetic ketoacidosis and the following laboratory data: pH = 7.10, Paco₂ = 30 mm Hg, [HCO₃⁻] = 13 mmol/L, anion gap = 25 mEq/L. What do you conclude?*

Tests Used in Making Acid-Base Diagnoses

Most hospital-based biochemistry laboratories do not routinely perform all the tests needed to make a definitive acid-base diagnosis. In this section the authors provide the rationale for some tests that can supply additional information at the bedside (Table 2.2).

In almost every case, the tests are performed in patients with metabolic acidosis. The specific questions to be addressed are as follows:

TABLE 2.2 **Tools Used at the Bedside to Make Acid-Base Diagnosis**

The tests described help establish the basis of the metabolic acidosis.

Test	Major Function Assessed	Disadvantages
Anion gap in plasma	Accumulation of acids other than HCl and H_2CO_3	Several laboratory measurements, so errors are possible [Albumin] must be known
Osmolal gap in plasma	Presence of alcohols in plasma	Osmolality method may cause a problem
Urine net charge	$[NH_4^+]$ in urine	Interpretation is confounded by the excretion of anions other than Cl^-
Osmolal gap in urine	$[NH_4^+]$ in urine	May not know [urea] or [glucose] in urine
Urine P_{CO_2}	Distal H^+ secretion	Not quantitative Many quibbles with this test
Urine citrate	Proximal ICF pH	Indirect
Fractional excretion of HCO_3^-	Proximal H^+ secretion	Imprecise
NH_4^+ excretion after furosemide	Proximal NH_4^+ production	Indirect

Anion gap in plasma
$[Na^+] - [Cl^-] - [HCO_3^-]$
- The normal value is 12 ± 2 mEq/L.
- Expect close to a 1:1 reciprocal change in anion gap and $[HCO_3^-]$.
- The anion gap changes with blood pH, but this change is small (0.5 mEq/L for a 0.1 unit change in pH).
- An increased anion gap may be the only clue that metabolic acidosis is present in a mixed acid-base disorder.

Distal RTA
A renal disorder characterized by a low rate of excretion of NH_4^+.

Note
The rate of increase in plasma anion gap and the rate of decrease in plasma $[HCO_3^-]$ provide insights into the rate of H^+ accumulation.

1. Is the net production of acids occurring at an unusually rapid rate?
   Measuring the *anion gap in plasma* and the net charge in urine may indicate the presence of new anions added to the blood or urine (see margin note).

2. Have alcohols accumulated in the body?
   Measuring the osmolal gap in plasma will indicate whether many uncharged particles are present in plasma.

3. In a patient with metabolic acidosis, what quantity of NH_4^+ is being excreted?
   To determine if the disease distal renal tubular acidosis (*distal RTA*) is present, two indirect tests are performed in tandem: the urine net charge is used to estimate NH_4^+ excreted with Cl^-, and the urine osmolal gap is used to detect the excretion of NH_4^+ with all anions.

4. Is H^+ secretion by the distal nephron reduced?
   To determine the basis of the lesion in a patient who has a low rate of excretion of NH_4^+, measure the P_{CO_2} in alkaline urine.

The Anion Gap in Plasma

- The anion gap ($[Na^+] - [Cl^-] - [HCO_3^-]$), a calculation for diagnostic convenience:
  1. normally equals 12 ± 2 mEq/L;
  2. indicates the quantity of added acids (the fall in $[HCO_3^-]$ equals the rise in anion gap);
  3. is useful in following the patient's response to therapy;
  4. helps in detecting laboratory errors, cationic proteins, and mixed acid-base disorders.

In every solution, the number of positive charges on cations must equal the number of negative charges on anions. If measurements indicate an imbalance, either the measurements are wrong, or not all the ionized materials are identified.

Although physiologic fluids may contain many anions and cations, only a few are present in significant amounts, and the concentrations of others usually undergo only minor changes. Hence, by measuring the concentrations of only a few cations and anions, and by making assumptions about the other ions normally found in plasma, it is possible to obtain a rough measure of whether large amounts of unsuspected anions or cations are present. The term *plasma anion gap* is used to signify the difference between the $[Na^+]$ and the sum of $[Cl^-] + [HCO_3^-]$. This shortfall in the number of anions is due to the fact that a significant number of the anions are unmeasured (e.g., albumin; note the quantity of unspecified anions in Table 1.2). The concentrations of the cations K^+, Ca^{2+}, and Mg^{2+} are usually almost constant (minor variations are life-threatening). The concentration of albumin, the only quantitatively important protein that is routinely present, is usually assumed to be constant (although some clinical situations, such as cirrhosis of the liver or nephrotic syndrome, lead to significant changes). The concentrations of other unmeasured anions—primarily SO_4^{2-} and HPO_4^{2-}—do not change appreciably except in renal insufficiency. Hence, subtraction of the measured values for $[Cl^-]$ and $[HCO_3^-]$ from that for $[Na^+]$ will normally yield a value of 12 ± 2 mEq/L, the normal anion gap. Values for the plasma anion gap that are significantly larger than normal indicate the presence of and approximate total concentration of one or more abnormal unmeasured anions (Figure 2.2).

An Example

When lactic acid dissociates into H^+ and lactate anions in the ECF, H^+ are buffered by HCO_3^-, leaving lactate anions as the "footprint" of the lactic acid added to the ECF. These events are depicted below, with values before and after the addition of 10 mmol of lactic acid (HL) to each liter of ECF.

Plasma (mEq/L)	$[Na^+]$	$[Cl^-]$	$[HCO_3^-]$	Anion Gap
Normal	140	103	25	12
+ 10 mmol/L lactic acid	140	103	15 = 25 − 10	22 = 12 + 10

The patient begins with a normal plasma anion gap of 12 mEq/L (140 − [103 + 25]). The protons accompanying 10 mmol of lactate anion per liter of ECF react with HCO_3^-; the result is a decline in plasma $[HCO_3^-]$ to 15 mmol/L and an increase in the plasma anion gap to 22 mmol/L. This value, best thought of as the increment over normal (i.e., 12 + 10), forces one to think of the normal plasma anion gap and to ask whether the patient has any reason not to have a normal anion gap (see the discussions of Questions 2.2 to 2.4). Thus, the increase in the plasma anion gap reflects, in a semiquantitative fashion, the presence of the anion of the organic acid (in this case, 10 mmol of lactate per liter of ECF).

If, in the preceding example, the increase in the anion gap was

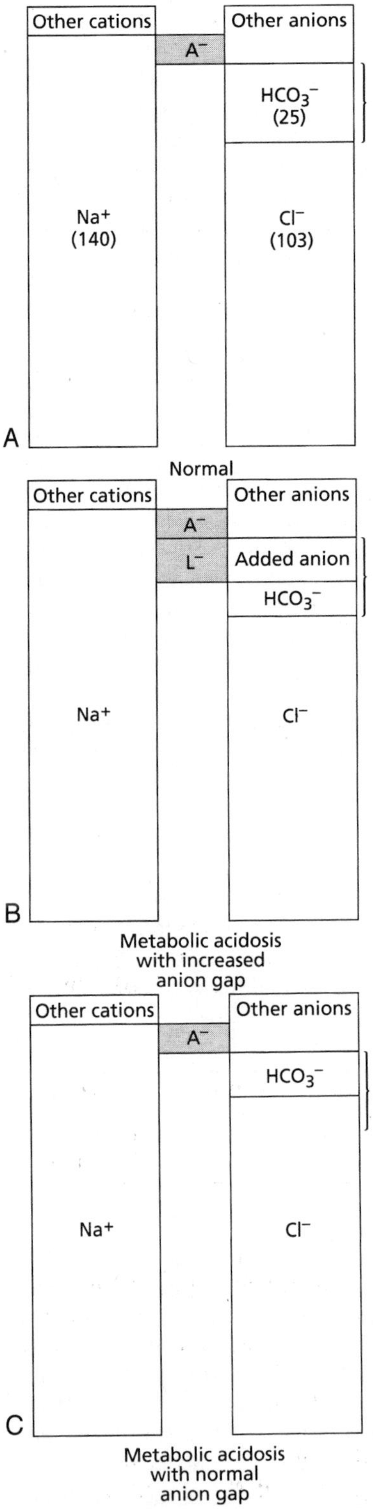

Figure 2.2 The anion gap in plasma. *A*, In this portion of the figure, the concentrations of ions in plasma are shown. The difference between the [Na$^+$] and the sum of [Cl$^-$] and [HCO$_3^-$] is the anion gap, shown as the shaded area between the columns (A$^-$). *B*, When an acid such as lactic acid is added, the [HCO$_3^-$] will fall, and the HCO$_3^-$ will be replaced with an anion such as lactate anion (L$^-$). The bracketed area represents the normal [HCO$_3^-$]. *C*, Note that with a loss of NaHCO$_3$, the [HCO$_3^-$] will fall, but no new anions will be added.

the same 10 mEq/L, but the concentration of lactate in plasma was only 5 mmol/L, lactic acidosis would not be the sole cause of the metabolic acidosis; the patient must have also accumulated other acids and their unmeasured anions (e.g., ketoacid anions).

QUESTIONS

(Discussions on pages 68–69)

2.2 *If the concentration of albumin in plasma is half of normal, what adjustments should be made when interpreting the plasma anion gap?*

2.3 *Patients with multiple myeloma may have a protein in plasma that bears a net positive charge. What is the impact of this protein on the value of the plasma anion gap?*

2.4 *Are there other reasons for having a low value for the plasma anion gap in patients with multiple myeloma?*

The Osmolal Gap in Plasma

- The osmolal gap in plasma is used to reveal alcohols in blood.
- This gap is the measured osmolality minus the calculated osmolality ($2[Na^+]$ + [Glucose] (mmol/L) + [Urea] (mmol/L)).

Rule
Doubling the $[Na^+]$ closely approximates the number of ions in plasma. This includes two errors that cancel out:
- Albumin is 0.5 mmol but has a valence of 16 mEq/L.
- There are cations other than Na^+ (K^+, Ca^{2+}, Mg^{2+}).

Clinical note
If there is a laboratory error with the $[Na^+]$ (i.e., hyperlipidemia), the formula for the osmolal gap will have an error introduced.

The osmolal gap is a useful means of detecting the presence of uncharged molecules in the plasma. The osmotic pressure of a solution is determined by the concentration of dissolved particles in the water; a protein molecule, a molecule of glucose, and a Na^+ make virtually equal contributions to the osmotic pressure. Because the numbers of anions and cations must be equal in any solution, and the concentrations of K^+, Ca^{2+}, and Mg^{2+} in plasma are low and approximately constant, the value of $2 \times [Na^+]$ will account for the osmotic pressure of normal anions plus cations in plasma. Glucose and urea are the two major nonionized molecules in plasma that are likely to change in concentration. Hence, the calculated osmolality is $2 \times [Na^+]$ + [glucose] + [urea] (all measurements in mmol/L; see Table 2.3 for conversion of concentrations in mg/dL to mmol/L). The difference between the measured and the calculated osmolality is the osmolal gap. A high plasma osmolal gap indicates the presence of an unmeasured compound; because the unmeasured compound is not charged, it is probably an alcohol.

TABLE 2.3 **Conversion Between mg/dL and mmol/L**

Constituent	Molecular Weight	Sample Concentrations	
		mg/dL	*mmol/L*
Glucose	180	90	5
Urea	60	30	5
Urea nitrogen (2 × 14)	28	14	5

Notes on Table 2.3
To convert mg/dL to mmol/L, multiply mg/dL by 10, then divide by molecular weight.
In certain circumstances, molality is more useful (e.g., urine osmolality), but in others, knowing the weight is valuable (e.g., what weight of protein was oxidized).

The Urine Net Charge

> - The urine net charge is usually used to detect NH_4^+ excreted with Cl^- in the urine.
> - Sometimes the urine net charge reveals the excretion of unusual anions.

Because most hospital biochemistry laboratories do not routinely measure the $[NH_4^+]$ in urine, it is useful to have an indirect way to estimate this concentration (Figure 2.3). In normal urine, the major cations are Na^+, K^+, and NH_4^+, and the major anions are Cl^- and HCO_3^-. The principle is that NH_4^+ are usually excreted along with Cl^-. Therefore, if NH_4^+ are plentiful in that urine, there will be a much greater quantity of Cl^- than the measured cations Na^+ plus K^+, so that "electrical" room will remain for NH_4^+. On the other hand, if the sum of Na^+ and K^+ is greater than Cl^-, there will be no "electrical" room for NH_4^+ unless there are large amounts of unmeasured anions in that urine.

Urine net charge
Measures NH_4^+ excreted with Cl^-.

$[Cl^-] > [Na^+] + [K^+] =$ High $[NH_4^+]$
$[Cl^-] < [Na^+] + [K^+] =$ Either a low $[NH_4^+]$ or excretion of NH_4^+ with an anion other than Cl^-

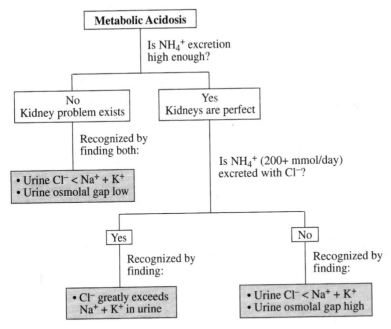

Figure 2.3 Sequence of steps in evaluating the rate of excretion of NH_4^+. These tests are performed in a patient with metabolic acidosis. The expected value for NH_4^+ in the urine is more than 200 mmol/day with normal kidneys and less than 40 mmol/day when the kidneys are the sole cause of the acidosis. These tests provide rough estimates, not precise values.

Assumptions Required to Interpret the Urine Net Charge

1. No cations other than Na^+, K^+, and NH_4^+ are quantitatively important.
   This statement is true unless intake is very unusual.

2. There are no anions in the urine other than Cl^-.

This statement is not true, but the usual anions (phosphate, sulfate, organic anions) do not vary appreciably in most cases.

Alkaline urine contains HCO_3^-, but NH_4^+ is not sought in alkaline urine. A urine pH that is less than 6 eliminates bicarbonaturia.

In some cases of metabolic acidosis (ketoacidosis, glue-sniffing), the urine contains a large quantity of anions other than Cl^-. In these cases, the urine osmolal gap must be examined to estimate NH_4^+ excretion.

Estimate of 24-hour urine
- Creatinine excretion is relatively constant for the 24-hour period.
- Normal individuals excrete 200 μmol (20 mg) of creatinine per kg body weight in 24 hours.
- Divide the $[NH_4^+]$ in urine by the concentration of creatinine in urine and multiply by the 24-hour value for creatinine (see the discussion of Question 2.5 for an example).

Precautions for the Urine Net Charge

1. Only a rough estimate of the $[NH_4^+]$ in the urine is obtained (see margin note).
2. The volume of urine must be known to estimate NH_4^+ excretion. Because most adults excrete 80 mEq of anions other than Cl^- per day, if the urine volume is close to 1 L in a 24-hour period, the following formula applies:

$$NH_4^+ \text{ (mEq/day)} = 80 + (Cl^- - Na^+ - K^+), \text{ all in mEq/day}$$

The Osmolal Gap in Urine

- The osmolal gap in the urine is used to detect NH_4^+.

In a patient with chronic metabolic acidosis and normal renal function, one expects to find more than 200 mmol of NH_4^+ excreted each day. In most circumstances where this excretion is high (e.g., loss of $NaHCO_3$ in diarrhea fluid), the NH_4^+ are excreted with Cl^-, and the urine net charge is very negative. Now consider a second circumstance where there is overproduction of acids, but the anion produced with H^+ is not retained because it is excreted in large quantities in the urine (see the discussion of Case 3.2). For instance, the following values (all in mEq/L) might be measured:

$$[Na^+] = 50, [K^+] = 50, [Cl^-] = 25, [NH_4^+] = 200, A^- = 275$$

Note that the sum of the concentrations of Na^+ plus K^+ exceeds that of Cl^-, yet the $[NH_4^+]$ is high. In this circumstance, the urine net charge does not reflect NH_4^+ excretion; a calculation of the osmolal gap in the urine, however, would provide a more accurate estimate of the $[NH_4^+]$ in the urine. More data are required, though—namely, the concentrations of glucose and urea, the major organic molecules that might be present in the urine.

$$[Glucose] = 0 \text{ mmol/L}, [Urea] = 250 \text{ mmol/L},$$
$$Osmolality = 850 \text{ mosm/kg } H_2O$$

In this example, the measured urine osmolality (850) exceeds the calculated osmolality—urea (250) + glucose (0) + 2 × ($[Na^+]$ + $[K^+]$) (200)—by 400 milliosmoles. Because the osmolal gap contains NH_4^+ and equal number of anions, the quantity of NH_4^+ (if accompanied by a monovalent anion) would be half the difference

Notes
The formula to use to calculate $[NH_4^+]$ in this case is 0.5 (measured minus calculated osmolality) where the calculated osmolality = [Urea] + [Glucose] + 2($[Na^+]$ + $[K^+]$), all in mmol/L (for mg/dL values, see Table 2.3).

One other point is obvious: in this case, the number of NH_4^+ (plus Na^+ and K^+) greatly exceeds the $[Cl^-]$, so there are many unmeasured anions in the urine, and the sum of their concentrations is close to 275 mEq/L. The unmeasured anions one might generally encounter are ketoacid anions, drug metabolites, or hippurate (in toluene "intoxication").

of measured and calculated osmolalities, or 200 mmol/L (see margin note).

The Urine pH

If the $[H^+]$ or the $[NH_3]$ is high, the $[NH_4^+]$ will rise. Therefore, with a separate measure of two of these parameters (NH_4^+, H^+), you can deduce the third (NH_3). This calculation will become important when examining the urine in patients who have a low excretion of NH_4^+ during metabolic acidosis.

$$NH_3 + H^+ \leftrightarrow NH_4^+$$

QUESTIONS

(Discussions on page 69)

2.5 *How can the urine creatinine concentration be used to estimate the rate of excretion of NH_4^+?*

2.6 *A patient has a bladder infection with bacteria that release the enzyme urease. The enzyme urease catalyzes the following reaction:*

$$Urea \longrightarrow 2\ NH_4^+ + 2\ HCO_3^-$$

Which test would you select to determine how many of the NH_4^+ excreted were of renal origin: (a) direct assay of NH_4^+ in urine; (b) urine osmolal gap; (c) urine net charge?

The Urine P_{CO_2}, A Test Reflecting Secretion of H^+ by Collecting Ducts

> • Once you know that NH_4^+ excretion is low, the urine P_{CO_2} in alkaline urine can help you decide if the cause is low distal H^+ secretion.

Another test used to determine the probable cause of a low excretion of NH_4^+ is the urine P_{CO_2}. In a very alkaline urine, the secretion of H^+ by the collecting duct leads to the formation of H_2CO_3. As there is no luminal carbonic anhydrase here, H_2CO_3 is slowly dehydrated to CO_2 in the medulla; the result is an increased P_{CO_2} in the renal medulla and bladder. Patients with a defect in secretion of H^+ have a urine P_{CO_2} close to that of their blood (Figure 2.4).

The test is valid only when the urine pH exceeds 7.40 or the urine $[HCO_3^-]$ is greater than 50 mmol/L. These levels can usually be achieved by giving an oral load of $NaHCO_3$ (0.5 to 2 mmol/kg body weight) on the morning of the test. The patient's K^+ deficit should be corrected before giving HCO_3^-.

The patient with normal secretion of H^+ from collecting ducts should have a urine P_{CO_2} that exceeds 70 mm Hg. This test also enables the identification of patients with a gradient limit to H^+ secretion (back-diffusion of H^+, e.g., resulting from the use of amphotericin B); these patients may have a low urine NH_4^+ excretion but have a normal urine P_{CO_2}.

Notes on the urine P_{CO_2} test
The urine is collected in a bottle with a small surface area relative to volume to minimize CO_2 loss. No oil is necessary if the P_{CO_2} in the urine is measured promptly. The sample is aspirated from the bottom of the bottle into a sealed syringe. The pH and P_{CO_2} are measured anaerobically.

Because this test requires the administration of sufficient $NaHCO_3$ to render the urine frankly alkaline, you can rule out proximal RTA (a disorder in which the urine pH rises long before the $[HCO_3^-]$ in plasma becomes normal).

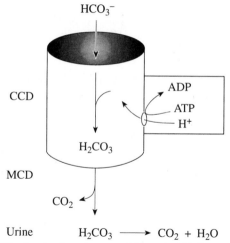

Figure 2.4   The basis of an increased P_{CO_2} in alkaline urine. Because the urine is alkaline, virtually the only H^+ acceptor is HCO_3^-. Any H^+ secretion in the cortical collecting duct (CCD) leads to the formation of H_2CO_3. Because there is no carbonic anhydrase present in the lumen of this nephron segment, the H_2CO_3 dehydrates slowly in the medullary collecting duct (MCD) and the urine; the result is an increase in the urine P_{CO_2}. If H^+ secretion in the CCD and MCD is absent, the urine P_{CO_2} will be close to that of the blood.

QUESTION

(Discussion on pages 69–70)

2.7 *In the following examples of urine excreted by a patient with chronic metabolic acidosis, what is the rate of excretion of NH_4^+, and what might the urine P_{CO_2} be?*

Osmolality mOsm/kg H_2O	Na$^+$ mmol/L	K$^+$ mmol/L	Glucose mmol/L	Urea mmol/L
600	50	50	0	100
600	50	50	0	350

PART B

Identifying Acid-Base Disorders

Expected Responses to Primary Acid-Base Disorders

It has been empirically observed that when a patient has one of the four primary acid-base disturbances, a predictable response occurs to return the [H^+] toward normal (Table 2.4). Only in chronic respiratory alkalosis may the [H^+] actually return to the normal range as a result of the expected response.

TABLE 2.4 **Expected Responses to Primary Acid-Base Disorders**

Disorder	Response
Metabolic acidosis	• For every mmol/L fall in plasma [HCO_3^-] from 25, the $Paco_2$ should fall by 1 mm Hg from 40, or use the Rule of Thumb #2.
Metabolic alkalosis	• For every mmol/L rise in plasma [HCO_3^-] from 25, the $Paco_2$ should rise by 0.7 mm Hg from 40, or use the Rule of Thumb #2.
Respiratory acidosis	
• Acute	• For every mm Hg rise in $Paco_2$ from 40, the plasma [H^+] should rise by 0.8 nmol/L from 40.
	• Alternatively, for every twofold increase in $Paco_2$, the plasma [HCO_3^-] should increase by 2.5 mmol/L.
• Chronic	• For every mm Hg rise in $Paco_2$ from 40, the [H^+] should rise by 0.3 nmol/L, or the plasma [HCO_3^-] should rise by 0.3 mmol/L from 25.
Respiratory alkalosis	
• Acute	• For every mm Hg fall in $Paco_2$ from 40, the plasma [H^+] should fall by 0.8 nmol/L from 40.
• Chronic	• For every mm Hg fall in $Paco$ from 40, the plasma [H^+] should fall by 0.2 nmol/L, or the plasma [HCO_3^-] should fall by 0.5 mmol/L from 25.

How to Recognize Mixed Acid-Base Disorders

1. **Examine the $Paco_2$ in metabolic acidosis and alkalosis to identify the presence of a respiratory acid-base disturbance.**

   If the $Paco_2$ is much higher than expected (see Table 2.4), there is a coexistent respiratory acidosis. If the $Paco_2$ is much lower, respiratory alkalosis is also present.

2. **Compare the increase in anion gap with the fall in [HCO_3^-] in plasma.**

   In metabolic acidosis of the increased anion gap type, the fall in [HCO_3^-] is generally equal to the rise in the plasma anion gap. If the rise in the plasma anion gap substantially exceeds the fall in [HCO_3^-], there must be an additional source of HCO_3^- (e.g., coexistent metabolic alkalosis—see margin note). On the other hand, if the fall in [HCO_3^-] markedly exceeds the increase in the plasma anion gap, there must be two processes contributing to the fall in [HCO_3^-]: a normal anion gap type and an increased anion gap type of metabolic acidosis.

3. **Integrate the clinical picture and laboratory tests with the acid-base disturbances.**

4. **Assess the metabolic adjustment in respiratory acid-base disorders, differentiating between acute and chronic disorders on clinical grounds.**

   (a) With all the respiratory disturbances, if the plasma [HCO_3^-] is unexpectedly high, there is a coexistent metabolic alkalosis; if the plasma [HCO_3^-] is lower than expected, there is also a metabolic acidosis.

Mixed acid-base disorders
When faced with an acid-base disorder, one should ensure that the expected response has occurred; its absence indicates the presence of a second primary acid-base disturbance.

Rule of Thumb #2
This rule helps in identifying if the expected change of ventilation is present.
• Drop the 7 and the decimal point from the pH
• The number remaining is the expected $Paco_2$ in patients with metabolic acidosis or metabolic alkalosis (e.g., if the plasma pH is 7.30, the expected $Paco_2$ is 30 mm Hg).

Note
Be sure to rule out other factors, such as a low concentration of albumin, that lead to a low value for the plasma anion gap (page 54).

Note
See Case 6.1 for a possible exception to this rule.

(b) In acute respiratory acidosis or alkalosis, there should be only a slight change in $[HCO_3^-]$.

(c) In chronic respiratory acidosis or alkalosis, the slope of $[H^+]$ vs $PaCO_2$ is much flatter because of a change in the $[HCO_3^-]$ in plasma (see Table 2.4 for expected changes).

QUESTION

(Discussion on page 70)

2.8 *Consider the following values in a patient who complains of diarrhea and vomiting.*

Na^+	140	mmol/L	H^+	40	nmol/L
K^+	2.3	mmol/L	$PaCO_2$	40	mm Hg
Cl^-	103	mmol/L	Anion gap	12	mEq/L
HCO_3^-	25	mmol/L			

What are the acid-base disorders?

Guidelines for the Diagnosis of Mixed Disorders

1. Clearly, a correct analysis of the laboratory results presumes that the data are accurate. There are two ways to detect laboratory errors. The first way is to calculate the plasma anion gap. If it is very low or negative, there is probably an error in one of the electrolyte values, unless the patient has multiple myeloma or hypoalbuminemia. The second way to evaluate the laboratory results is to insert the $[H^+]$, PCO_2, and $[HCO_3^-]$ (as reflected in the plasma electrolyte values) into the Henderson equation. If there is a substantial error (>10%), one of the three parameters is incorrect; if the discrepancy is great enough to change the diagnosis, the tests should be repeated and the error identified.

2. Calculate the plasma anion gap; if it is increased by more than 5 mEq/L from the expected value, the patient probably has metabolic acidosis.

3. Compare the magnitude of the fall in plasma $[HCO_3^-]$ with the increase in the plasma anion gap. These changes should be similar in magnitude. If the change in $[HCO_3^-]$ differs from the change in the plasma anion gap by more than 5 mEq/L, a mixed disturbance may be present. A rise in the plasma anion gap that is less than the fall in plasma $[HCO_3^-]$ suggests that a component of the metabolic acidosis involves loss of $NaHCO_3$ or renal tubular acidosis. On the other hand, an increase in the plasma anion gap that is much greater than the fall in $[HCO_3^-]$ suggests that there is a coexistent metabolic alkalosis (i.e., an additional source of HCO_3^-).

4. In metabolic acidosis or alkalosis, look for the expected change in $PaCO_2$. If the $PaCO_2$ is significantly lower, the patient has coexistent respiratory alkalosis; if higher, respiratory acidosis.

5. In respiratory acid-base disturbances, one must distinguish between acute and chronic (more than 3–4 days) conditions on

Strong ion difference
Every decade or so, a new way to analyze acid-base disorders is proposed. The impetus for these approaches is that the traditional measures described in this chapter do not permit a total explanation for all the pathophysiology (these newer ways also do not provide a more comprehensive analysis).

An approach in some centers is to use the strong ion difference (SID) proposed by Stewart (difference between measured values for (Na^+ + K^+) minus (Cl^- + negative charges) on albumin for the most part). It is based on the sound chemical principles of electroneutrality, dissociation, and reliance on independent variables, such as the SID and the PCO_2. Chemically, its unfortunate but necessary weakness is that it assigns an arbitrary and fixed valence to all proteins. In the authors' opinion, the SID offers no major advantage, and it has some disadvantages. Radical changes in the clinical approach described in this chapter are therefore not indicated. We have stressed that the laboratory values interpreted by any approach are just one step in an acid-base analysis. To make rational decisions, one must correlate these values with the clinical picture and a knowledge of the underlying biochemistry and physiology.

Delta $[HCO_3^-]$: delta anion gap
Some people rely on the ratio of these changes when defining mixed disorders, but the authors do not believe this practice adds anything of value. Instead, we prefer to consider the difference in the magnitude of these changes and, even then, not to rely too heavily on the 1:1 relationship (see Case 6.1).

clinical grounds, because different degrees of physiologic compensation are present. Table 2.4 summarizes the expected changes in $[HCO_3^-]$ for a given acute or chronic change in $Paco_2$.

Mixed Acid-Base Disturbances

> • The clinical and laboratory data must be integrated.

Objectives

1. To demonstrate that more than one acid-base disturbance can be present in a patient at one time.
2. To demonstrate how to identify the simultaneous presence of even four acid-base disturbances from the history, physical examination, and laboratory results.

Three Simultaneous Acid-Base Disturbances

A 24-year-old woman has an abnormal protein in her circulation that caused a marked reduction in her distal renal H^+ secretion. As a result, she could not reabsorb all the $NaHCO_3$ delivered distally (proximal nephron sites do not reabsorb all filtered $NaHCO_3$). Her clinical picture is shown sequentially in Table 2.5 and Figure 2.5.

As a result of the continuing loss of Na^+ and HCO_3^-, her ECF volume becomes contracted. All the NaCl in her diet is reabsorbed, but there is still a negative balance for Na^+ overall. The net results of these changes are shown in Table 2.5, column 2.

As a result of her low ECF volume, her circulating volume is low—so low, in fact, that she did not deliver enough oxygen to her tissues to meet their demand for aerobic production of adenosine triphosphate (ATP). The net result was a gain of L-lactic acid—10 mmol/L of ECF in this example (Table 2.5, column 3, and Figure 2.5). This accumulation of 10 mmol of L-lactate$^-$ anion per liter of plasma should raise the plasma anion gap by 10 mEq/L. Simultaneously, the 10 mmol of H^+ added per liter will lower the $[HCO_3^-]$ by 10 mmol/L.

$$10 \text{ L-lactate}^- + 10 \text{ H}^+ + 25 \text{ HCO}_3^- \leftrightarrow 10 \text{ CO}_2 \uparrow$$
$$+ 10 \text{ H}_2\text{O} + 10 \text{ L-lactate} + 15 \text{ HCO}_3^-$$

In patients with distal RTA who have the release of aldosterone

TABLE 2.5   **Identification of a Mixed Acid-Base Disorder**

For details, see text. The value for albumin in plasma is 4 g/dL (40 g/L), a normal level that does not change throughout the course of illness in this patient.

$H \cdot L$ = L-lactic acid.

Column		1	2	3	4
Plasma		*Normal*	*Loss NaHCO$_3$* (10 mmol/L)	**Gain H·L** (10 mmol/L)	**Effect of** **K$^+$ Deficit**
pH		7.40	7.30	7.13	6.83
HCO$_3^-$	mmol/L	25	15	5	5
Anion gap	mEq/L	12	12	22	22
Pco$_2$	mm Hg	40	30	15	30

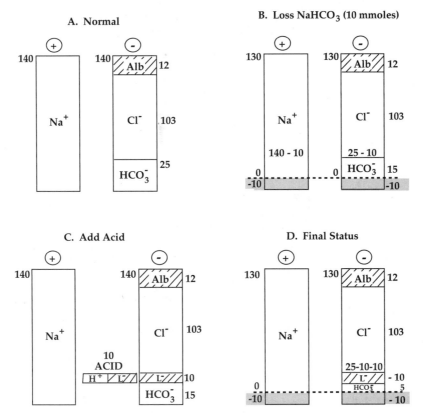

Figure 2.5   Mixed acid-base disturbance: Recognizing two types of metabolic acidosis. The sums of the cations and anions are always equal. In this example, the missing anions (due largely to the anionic charge on albumin shown by the hatched symbol) are constant at 12 mEq/L; this value is 16 mEq/L if K^+ is included in the sum of cations in plasma. When Na^+ and HCO_3^- are lost (shaded area in panels B and D), there is no change in the plasma anion gap. When lactic acid is added, there is a fall in the concentration of HCO_3^- together with an equal rise in the plasma anion gap (panel C). The combination of both types of metabolic acidosis is shown in panel D.

(due to a contracted ECF volume) together with the excretion of HCO_3^- in the urine, there is a very large excretion of K^+. A deficit of K^+ occurs and this could lead to muscular weakness. Eventually, this weakness could involve respiratory muscles and be manifest as an inability to lower the arterial blood PCO_2 to the expected degree (see Table 2.5, column 4).

In summary, if you work backwards beginning at the far right of Table 2.5, you should identify each of the three acid-base disorders.

1. **Respiratory acidosis.** The PCO_2 in blood should be as low as possible (less than 20 mm Hg) with such a low value for the plasma $[HCO_3^-]$ (5 vs 25 mmol/L). Therefore, the arterial PCO_2 is too high for this clinical setting.
2. **Metabolic acidosis due to a gain of acid.** The elevated value for the anion gap of 10 mEq/L in the face of a normal albumin value suggests that 10 of the 20 mmol/L fall in plasma $[HCO_3^-]$ was due to the added L-lactic acid.
3. **Metabolic acidosis due to loss of NaHCO₃.** The fact that the fall in $[HCO_3^-]$ is much greater than the rise in the plasma anion gap suggests a loss of NaHCO₃.

Four Simultaneous Acid-Base Disorders
A patient vomits very frequently and for several days. As shown in Figure 4.1, the loss of HCl during vomiting results in a gain of

TABLE 2.6 **Mixed Acid-Base Disorders:**
Metabolic and Respiratory

For details, see text. Column 5 represents venous rather than arterial blood.

		1	2	3	4	5
		Normal	*Vomiting*	*Lactic Acid Added*	*Hyper-ventilation*	*Low ECFV*
pH		7.40	7.50	7.40	7.50	7.27
HCO_3^-	mmol/L	25	40	25	25	27
Anion gap	mEq/L	12	12	27	27	27
P_{CO_2}	mm Hg	40	50	40	30	60

HCO_3^- together with a commensurate loss of Cl^-. Assume there was a gain of 15 mmol of HCO_3^- and a loss of 15 mmol of Cl^- per liter of plasma (Table 2.6, column 2).

With vomiting, the ECF volume is often very contracted. As a result, there was hypotension and tissue hypoxia with the gain of 15 mmol of L-lactic acid per liter of ECF. The net effect is normal values for pH, P_{CO_2}, and $[HCO_3^-]$ but an elevated value for the plasma anion gap, which is the telltale sign of the two acid-base disorders (see Table 2.6, column 3).

During the vomiting, some fluid was aspirated into the lungs. This caused the patient to breathe faster and somewhat more deeply. As a result, the arterial P_{CO_2} is too low; overventilation is another basis for the alkalemia (see Table 2.6, column 4).

Remember that low blood volume caused a slow circulation and, as a result, not enough delivery of oxygen to the patient's tissues. The CO_2 produced from metabolism plus that formed when H^+ were buffered by HCO_3^- led to a higher venous P_{CO_2} per liter of blood flow (reduced cardiac output). The higher capillary P_{CO_2} leads to a higher tissue P_{CO_2}, a form of tissue respiratory acidosis (see Table 2.6, column 5, and see Figure 1.9).

To summarize, the patient had metabolic alkalosis (vomiting), metabolic acidosis (L-lactic acid), hyperventilation (aspiration), and tissue respiratory acidosis (low cardiac output). The rapid reexpansion of the patient's ECF volume with saline and replacing the deficit of K^+ will deal with most of the mixed acid-base disorders.

QUESTIONS

(Discussions on pages 70–71)

2.9   *A 23-year-old woman with rheumatoid arthritis increased her dose of salicylates because of a flare-up. She then developed epigastric pain and vomited frequently for 2 days. She went to the local hospital, where the following blood results were obtained:*

H^+	20 nmol/L (pH = 7.70)	Pa_{CO_2}	25 mg Hg
Anion gap	17 mEq/L		

What is (are) her acid-base disorder(s)?

2.10 *A 50-year-old woman underwent intestinal bypass for morbid obesity. Because she was having 10–15 watery stools per day, she was treated with tincture of opium and was found somnolent and somewhat hypotensive the next morning. Plasma values were:*

Na$^+$	130 mmol/L	H$^+$	96 nmol/L (pH = 7.02)	
K$^+$	3.2 mmol/L	Paco$_2$	40 mm Hg	
Cl$^-$	102 mmol/L	HCO$_3^-$	10 mmol/L	
Albumin	40 g/L			

What is (are) her acid-base disorder(s)?

What treatment would you consider for her very high [H$^+$] in plasma?

PART C

Review

DISCUSSION OF INTRODUCTORY CASE
Lee's Acidosis Is Mixed Up
(Case presented on page 50)

What is the acid-base diagnosis?

The parameters necessary to make an acid-base diagnosis are the [H$^+$] or pH, [HCO$_3^-$], Paco$_2$, and the anion gap ([Na$^+$] − [Cl$^-$] − [HCO$_3^-$]) in plasma. Given the high [H$^+$] and low [HCO$_3^-$], the major acid-base diagnosis is metabolic acidosis with an increased anion gap. Because the *increase in anion gap* is 15 mEq/L, and the decrease in [HCO$_3^-$] from its expected value of 25 mmol/L is also 15 mEq/L, the basis of the metabolic acidosis is added acids, most likely diabetic ketoacidosis.

Increase in anion gap

[Na$^+$] − [Cl$^-$] − [HCO$_3^-$] − 12
(The expected value for the normal anion gap is 12 because the concentration of albumin is normal.)

Is there a primary respiratory acid-base disorder?

Because the fall in Paco$_2$ (15 mm Hg from 40) equals the fall in [HCO$_3^-$] (15 mmol/L from the normal value of 25), there is no primary respiratory acid-base disorder.

Summary of Main Points

- To identify acid-base disturbances, evaluate the [H$^+$], [HCO$_3^-$], Paco$_2$, and the anion gap and correlate them with the clinical picture. The reliability of the data should be confirmed using the Henderson equation.

- Each primary acid-base disorder is characterized by a specific physiologic response, which should be evaluated. Absence of the expected response signals the coexistence of a second acid-base disorder.
- In metabolic acidosis, additional clues concerning the basis of the acidosis can be obtained from the plasma anion gap, the urine net charge, the plasma and urine osmolal gaps, and the urine P_{CO_2}.
- In all acid-base disturbances, diagnosis of the presence of the acid-base disorder is only the first step; the underlying basis of the specific acid-base disorder must be established and then a plan of management must be developed.

Discussion of Questions

2.1 A patient has diabetic ketoacidosis and the following laboratory data: pH = 7.10, Pa_{CO_2} = 30 mm Hg, [HCO_3^-] = 13 mmol/L, anion gap = 25 mEq/L. What do you conclude?

When the numbers are inserted in the Henderson equation, it appears that at least one of the three parameters is in error (see margin note). When faced with these laboratory results, be cautious; repeat the blood tests to clarify the basis of the discrepancy.

Whatever the scenario, the patient has metabolic acidosis with an increased plasma anion gap and presumably diabetic ketoacidosis. This diagnosis should be confirmed with the appropriate tests (serum ketones, blood glucose), and initial treatment should be instituted.

$$[H^+] = 24 \times P_{CO_2}/[HCO_3^-]$$
$$80 \neq 24 \times 30/13$$
$$80 \neq 56$$

2.2 If the concentration of albumin in plasma is half of normal, what adjustments should be made when interpreting the plasma anion gap?

When correcting for a change in the concentration of albumin, use a value of 16 for the normal plasma anion gap to include all the major positive charges in solution (K^+ of 4 mmol/L). Therefore, if the concentration of albumin is 20 g/L, or 2 g/dL (half the normal concentration), the expected value for the plasma anion gap should be reduced to 8 mEq/L.

2.3 Patients with multiple myeloma may have a protein in plasma that bears a net positive charge. What is the impact of this protein on the value of the plasma anion gap?

With a lysine-rich or arginine-rich protein in plasma (IgG myeloma), this paraprotein carries a net positive charge, and, if high enough, it can actually render the value for the plasma anion gap negative because these "unmeasured" positive charges are associated with "measured" Cl^-.

2.4 Are there other reasons for having a low value for the plasma anion gap in patients with multiple myeloma?

Although hypercalcemia may be seen with multiple myeloma, hypercalcemia generally is not severe enough to have a significant impact on the plasma anion gap. Patients may have an unexpectedly low plasma anion gap because of hypoalbuminemia, quirks of the laboratory methods, or actual laboratory errors. The plasma [Cl^-] will be overestimated in patients with halide intoxication (bromide or iodide may elevate the reported value for Cl^- depending on the method used to measure Cl^-) and hyperlipidemia (techniques for measurement depend on turbidity). Similarly, a simple error in the measurement of [Na^+], [Cl^-], or [HCO_3^-] will make the calculation of the plasma anion gap invalid.

2.5 How can the urine creatinine concentration be used to estimate the rate of excretion of NH_4^+?

Creatinine is excreted at a relatively constant rate throughout the day; its rate of excretion in an adult male is close to 0.2 mmol/day/kg of body weight (20 mg/day/kg of body weight). Thus, estimating the proportion of the 24-hour urine contained in a sample is possible if the concentration of creatinine and the urine volume are known. In fact, the rate of excretion of NH_4^+ can be calculated without knowing the urine volume.

> [NH_4^+] = 40 mmol/L, [Creatinine] = 10 mmol/L
> [NH_4^+]/[Creatinine] = 4 mmol/mmol
> A 70-kg person excretes 14 mmol of creatinine per day.

Therefore, NH_4^+ excretion is 56 mmol/day if there is no diurnal variation in NH_4^+ excretion (see margin note).

Calculation
Multiplying 4 mmol of NH_4^+ per millimole of creatinine by 14 mmol of creatinine per day equals 56 mmol of NH_4^+ per day.

2.6 A patient has a bladder infection with bacteria that release the enzyme urease. The enzyme urease catalyzes the following reaction:

$$\text{Urea} \rightarrow 2\ NH_4^+ + 2\ HCO_3^-$$

Which test would you select to determine how many of the NH_4^+ excreted were of renal origin: (a) direct assay of NH_4^+ in urine; (b) urine osmolal gap; (c) urine net charge?

The urine contains NH_4^+ from two sources, the kidney and urea via urease.

(a) Total NH_4^+ assay cannot determine how much was from each source, so it is not the best test to use.
(b) Urine osmolal gap just estimates total NH_4^+, so it is not the best test to use.
(c) Urine net charge does not reveal NH_4^+ if its salt is HCO_3^-. Therefore, if renal NH_4^+ was excreted with Cl^-, the urine net charge would provide the only real estimate of the renal component of NH_4^+ excretion (see margin note).

Note
Humans do not excrete NH_4^+ with HCO_3^-, but alligators do. This excretion provides a way for alligators to excrete more water at the same urine osmolality (alligators do not have a loop of Henle, and although urea has one particle, four particles are excreted when these ions are excreted as 2 NH_4^+ and 2 HCO_3^-).

2.7 In the following examples of urine excreted by a patient with chronic metabolic acidosis, what is the rate of excretion of NH_4^+, and what might the urine Pco_2 be?

Osmolality mOsm/kg H_2O	Na^+ mmol/L	K^+ mmol/L	Glucose mmol/L	Urea mmol/L
600	50	50	0	100
600	50	50	0	350

To obtain the calculated urine osmolality, double ($[Na^+] + [K^+]$) and add the concentration of urea. The $[NH_4^+]$ is half the difference of the measured and calculated urine osmolality. In the first example, the urine osmolal gap suggests that the $[NH_4^+]$ is high (150 mmol/L). Because a high distal H^+ secretion is needed to have a high rate of excretion of NH_4^+, the urine PCO_2 should be high in alkaline urine (following a $NaHCO_3$ load).

Conversely, in the second example, the estimated concentration of NH_4^+ is low (25 mmol/L). In this case, a low PCO_2 in alkaline urine suggests a defect in H^+ secretion, and a high PCO_2 in alkaline urine suggests a very low $[NH_3]$ in the medulla (either impaired ammoniagenesis or impaired function of the loop of Henle).

2.8 Consider the following values in a patient who complains of diarrhea and vomiting.

Na^+	140	mmol/L	H^+		40 nmol/L
K^+	2.3	mmol/L	$Paco_2$		40 mm Hg
Cl^-	103	mmol/L	Anion gap		12 mEq/L
HCO_3^-	25	mmol/L			

What are the acid-base disorders?

Note
In the presence of a contracted ECF volume, a normal plasma $[HCO_3^-]$ implies a reduced HCO_3^- content—evidence of metabolic acidosis.

On the surface, most of the laboratory data do not suggest an acid-base disturbance, but the hypokalemia must be explained (see margin note). It is most likely that the patient has a mixed metabolic acidosis (HCO_3^- loss due to diarrhea) and metabolic alkalosis (HCO_3^- gain due to vomiting) with the hypokalemia associated with excessive renal loss of K^+. The acid-base status, which results from the combination of these two disorders, is normal when judged solely by the four parameters in plasma (pH, $Paco_2$, $[HCO_3^-]$, and anion gap). The physical examination test results were not normal; the ECF volume was contracted. In therapy, the ECF should be reexpanded with an isotonic solution containing K^+ (40–60 mmol/L). Half-normal saline plus KCl is a good initial solution.

2.9 A 23-year-old woman with rheumatoid arthritis increased her dose of salicylates because of a flare-up. She then developed epigastric pain and vomited frequently for 2 days. She went to the local hospital, where the following blood results were obtained:

H^+	20 nmol/L (pH = 7.70)	$Paco_2$	25 mm Hg
Anion gap	17 mEq/L		

What is (are) her acid-base disorder(s)?

The pH of her blood is very alkalemic ($[H^+]$ = 20 nmol/L, pH = 7.70). Her $[HCO_3^-]$ can be calculated from the Henderson equation:

$$[HCO_3^-] = 24 \times Paco_2/[H^+] = 30 \text{ mmol/L}$$

Thus, she has metabolic alkalosis (low $[H^+]$ and elevated plasma $[HCO_3^-]$). However, her $Paco_2$ is low (the expected response during metabolic alkalosis is hypoventilation to return the $[H^+]$ in cells toward normal), and she is hyperventilating; therefore, she has a second primary acid-base disorder—respiratory alkalosis—which is why she is so alkalemic. Her metabolic alkalosis was secondary to vomiting and HCl loss (see Figure 4.1), and her respiratory alkalosis was secondary to salicylate intoxication. In addition, the small rise in her plasma anion gap raises the possibility of a third acid-base disorder, metabolic acidosis resulting from added acids (salicylic acid and the more negative valence of albumin, most likely).

2.10 A 50-year-old woman underwent intestinal bypass for morbid obesity. Because she was having 10–15 watery stools per day, she was treated with tincture of opium and was found somnolent and somewhat hypotensive the next morning. Plasma values were:

Na^+	130 mmol/L		H^+	96 nmol/L (pH = 7.02)
K^+	3.2 mmol/L		Pa_{CO_2}	40 mm Hg
Cl^-	102 mmol/L		HCO_3^-	10 mmol/L
Albumin	40 g/L			

What is (are) her acid-base disorder(s)?

The patient is very acidemic ($[H^+]$ = 96 nmol/L, pH = 7.02). The $[HCO_3^-]$ is low (10 mmol/L); therefore, she has metabolic acidosis. The plasma anion gap (18 mEq/L) is increased by about 6 mEq/L because her albumin level is normal; however, the $[HCO_3^-]$ has fallen by 15 mmol/L (from 25 mmol/L). Thus, the fall in $[HCO_3^-]$ exceeds the increase in the plasma anion gap and indicates two components to the metabolic acidosis: part is due to the accumulation of an organic acid, as reflected by the increase in the plasma anion gap (presumably D-lactic acidosis, L-lactic acidosis, or ketoacidosis), and part is due to $NaHCO_3$ loss in the diarrhea.

The patient's Pa_{CO_2} is 40 mm Hg, which is higher than expected during metabolic acidosis with a plasma $[HCO_3^-]$ of 10 mmol/L (the Pa_{CO_2} should be 40 − 15 = 25 mm Hg). Thus, this patient also has a respiratory acidosis.

Therefore, this patient has three acid-base disturbances:
1. metabolic acidosis resulting from $NaHCO_3$ loss (diarrhea);
2. D-lactic acidosis (abnormal bowel flora and GI motility suppression), L-lactic acidosis (hypotension), or ketoacidosis (starvation);
3. respiratory acidosis (suppression of ventilation).

What treatment would you consider for her very high $[H^+]$ in plasma?

The treatment is determined by the underlying causes for the acid-base disturbances. Presumably the respiratory acidosis is due to the central nervous system suppression by the narcotic. Therefore, treatment with naloxone (a morphine antagonist) would be an appropriate first step. One could also stimulate the patient (verbally and physically) to breathe. If the patient does not respond to the naloxone, or if her condition deteriorates, mechanical ventilation will give the quickest control of the acidemia. Reducing her Pa_{CO_2} to 25 mm Hg will lower her plasma $[H^+]$ to 24 × 25/10, or 60 nmol/L (pH = 7.22).

The patient is very acidemic and has lost some $NaHCO_3$; therefore, one could also give $NaHCO_3$ to alleviate the severe acidemia, but the danger of more severe hypokalemia makes this option unattractive.

Time is required to slow the rate of production of D-lactic acid. Do not give food (carbohydrate) by mouth because the bacteria may make more D-lactic acid and other toxic metabolites. Restoring the ECF volume and giving thiamine, if indicated, could alleviate L-lactic acidosis. Giving glucose will correct ketoacidosis if the patient is hypoglycemic; otherwise, reexpansion of the ECF volume with an isotonic solution containing KCl and $NaHCO_3$ will be effective.

Metabolic Acidosis

OBJECTIVES

Metabolic acidosis
A process that tends to lower the $[HCO_3^-]$ and to increase the $[H^+]$ in plasma. Metabolic acidosis is defined in terms of the bicarbonate buffer system (BBS) in plasma.

☐ To provide a diagnostic classification of *metabolic acidosis* based on:
1. acid accumulation;
2. HCO_3^- loss;
3. failure of the kidneys to generate new HCO_3^-.

☐ To explain the roles of hyperventilation in metabolic acidosis. Hyperventilation not only defends the plasma $[H^+]$ but also reduces the binding of H^+ on intracellular fluid (ICF) proteins.

☐ To emphasize the critical importance of disturbances in the plasma $[K^+]$ in the genesis of metabolic acidosis and in the response to therapy.

☐ To elucidate the pathogenesis of the various forms of lactic acidosis, ketoacidosis, and the acidosis associated with certain intoxications.

☐ To provide a therapeutic approach to metabolic acidosis based on physiologic priorities and to consider the controversy concerning therapy with $NaHCO_3$.

Outline of Major Principles

1. Metabolic acidosis occurs with acid gain (other than H_2CO_3) or loss of HCO_3^- plus Na^+ and/or K^+. Both result in a rise in the $[H^+]$ and a fall in the $[HCO_3^-]$ in plasma.

2. Metabolic acidosis often occurs as a complication of catastrophic illness (shock, sepsis) and adds to the seriousness of the clinical setting.

3. Because metabolic acidosis is not a primary diagnosis, the underlying cause must be sought; specific therapy may be life-saving (e.g., insulin for diabetic ketoacidosis, ethanol for methanol intoxication).

Threats to life
• Severe acidosis
• Poisonous products
• Changes in $[K^+]$

4. The rate of H^+ input may be very high (hypoxia) or normal (renal failure). In the latter case, the plasma $[HCO_3^-]$ declines

slowly but progressively; thus, on admission to the hospital, both types of acidemia might be equally severe.

5. The accumulation of new anions in the plasma or the urine indicates an overproduction of acids. The plasma anion gap provides a useful clue to determine the basis of the metabolic acidosis. It is elevated in most patients whose metabolic acidosis results from overproduction of acids.

6. The impact of metabolic acidosis may depend on the quantity of H^+ bound to intracellular proteins. This quantity is minimized by a reduction in the tissue P_{CO_2}. Normally, there is a predictable decline in Pa_{CO_2} for a given degree of metabolic acidosis.

7. Profound derangements in plasma $[K^+]$ may accompany either metabolic acidosis or its therapy. At times, the abnormal level of K^+ may pose a greater threat than the acidemia.

8. The therapeutic role of $NaHCO_3$ in metabolic acidosis varies; for example, its use is important when the degree of acidemia is very severe, but it may endanger patients who have a severe degree of hypokalemia along with metabolic acidosis. The decision whether to give $NaHCO_3$ must be individualized.

INTRODUCTORY CASE
To Make a Diagnosis, Step on the Gas
(Case discussed on pages 128–130)

The following results in plasma were obtained in Lee, a diabetic patient who presented with weakness.

Na$^+$	mmol/L	140	H$^+$	nmol/L	144	(pH 6.84)
K$^+$	mmol/L	1.8	Pa$_{CO_2}$	mm Hg	30	
Cl$^-$	mmol/L	125	HCO$_3^-$	mmol/L	5	

What is (are) your acid-base diagnosis(es)?

What would the plasma $[H^+]$ be if the respiratory response were appropriate?

What are the likely causes for the metabolic acidosis in Lee?

What is the significance of the hypokalemia?

Must all patients with metabolic acidosis have a high plasma $[H^+]$?

Can a patient have a low plasma $[HCO_3^-]$ and not have metabolic acidosis?

Is it possible to have a persistently alkaline urine (i.e., no renal HCO_3^- generation) and maintain acid-base balance?

PART A

Background

Development of Metabolic Acidosis

The BBS equation shown in Figure 3.1 reveals two major ways that one can have a high $[H^+]$ and a low $[HCO_3^-]$ (metabolic acidosis).

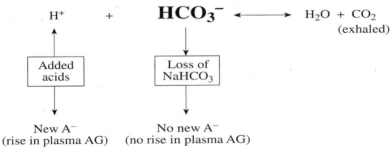

Figure 3.1 Basis of metabolic acidosis. Metabolic acidosis (a rise in the [H⁺] and a fall in the [HCO₃⁻]) is recognized by examining the bicarbonate buffer system in plasma. When acids are added and H⁺ are retained, "new anions" appear in the plasma or in the urine. Failure to find new anions suggests that there is a loss of NaHCO₃ (AG = anion gap).

Indirect loss of HCO₃⁻
When an acid is produced and dissociates, if its H⁺ are titrated by HCO₃⁻ and its anion is excreted with an Na⁺ or a K⁺, an indirect loss of HCO₃⁻ has occurred (see Figure 3.3).

Acid accumulation
Addition of acids to the body faster than they can be removed. H⁺ are produced when anions without a cation such as Na⁺ or K⁺ are made from a neutral substance.

$$N° \longrightarrow A^- + H^+$$

First, the addition of H⁺ (acid) will consume HCO₃⁻ and drive this equilibrium to the right. Conversely, if there is a loss of HCO₃⁻ (i.e., when NaHCO₃ is excreted in the urine or is *lost indirectly*), the [H⁺] will be increased along with the decline in the [HCO₃⁻]. In this case, the BBS equilibrium is shifted to the left. Making this distinction between *acid accumulation* and loss of NaHCO₃ is the first step to take in the differential diagnosis of metabolic acidosis (Table 3.1).

Use of the Anion Gap in Plasma to Detect the Net Addition of Acids

- In patients with a metabolic acidosis associated with an increase in the plasma anion gap, there are two possible reasons for the metabolic acidosis:
  1. overproduction of an organic acid;
  2. renal failure (low glomerular filtration rate [GFR]).

Overproduction of Organic Acids

Patients may produce organic acids as a result of the excess activity of a normal metabolic pathway. For example, there is an exceedingly rapid rate of L-lactic acid production during hypoxia and a modest rate of production of ketoacids during states with a relative deficiency of insulin (Table 3.2). In addition, the metabolism of an ingested substance (methyl alcohol, ethylene glycol) may lead to a moderate rate of acid production (see Table 3.2). In *salicylate* intoxication, the usual problem is respiratory alkalosis, but overproduction of acids may be a problem, especially in children.

Salicylate
Acetylsalicylic acid (ASA), the active moiety of aspirin, causes harm to the body via direct toxicity to cells rather than injury from acidosis. ASA stimulates the respiratory center and disturbs a variety of metabolic processes.

Note
In renal failure, there is no obvious relationship between the plasma anion gap and the [HCO₃⁻]. In some patients, the degree of rise in the plasma anion gap is much less than the fall in the plasma [HCO₃⁻]; the converse is also true.

Renal Failure

During renal failure, metabolic acidosis is usually accompanied by an increase in the plasma anion gap. This condition is an exception to the rule that an increase in the plasma anion gap signals a large overproduction of acids. As illustrated in Figure 3.2, the cause of the rise in the plasma anion gap is a decrease in the GFR, but the cause of the acidosis is a tubular problem—a low rate of excretion of NH₄⁺.

TABLE 3.1 **Overview of the Etiology of Metabolic Acidosis**

Each disorder is discussed in more detail in later sections of this chapter.

Overproduction of Acids

- **Retention of anions in the plasma (increased plasma anion gap)**
  L-Lactic acidosis (L-lactic acid)
  Ketoacidosis (largely *β-hydroxbutyric acid*)
  Overproduction of organic acids in the GI tract (D-lactic acidosis)
  Conversion of alcohols (methanol, ethylene glycol) to acids and poisonous aldehydes

- **Excretion of anions in the urine (no increase in the plasma anion gap)**
  Ketoacidosis and impaired renal reabsorption of β-HB$^-$
  Inhalation of toluene (hippurate)

Actual Bicarbonate Loss (Normal Plasma Anion Gap)

- **Direct loss of NaHCO$_3$**
  Gastrointestinal tract (e.g., diarrhea, ileus, fistula or T-tube drainage, villous adenoma, ileal conduit combined with delivery of Cl$^-$ from urine)
  Urinary tract (e.g., proximal renal tubular acidosis, use of carbonic anhydrase inhibitors)

- **Indirect loss of NaHCO$_3$**
  Failure of renal generation of new bicarbonate (low NH$_4^+$ excretion)
  Low production of NH$_4^+$ (e.g., renal failure [low GFR], hyperkalemia)
  Low transfer of NH$_4^+$ to the urine (e.g., medullary interstitial disease, low distal net H$^+$ secetion)

Metabolic Acidosis and a Normal Plasma Anion Gap

When metabolic acidosis is not associated with an increase in the plasma anion gap, it is due to a direct or indirect loss of NaHCO$_3$.

TABLE 3.2 **Rates of Production and Removal of H$^+$**

The total quantity of H$^+$ that can be buffered is close to 1000 mmol in a 70-kg person. With very large acid loads, most of the buffering occurs in the ICF.

	Rate (mmol/min)	Comments
Production of H$^+$		
L-Lactic acid (hypoxia)	72	• Rate reflects complete anoxia.
	7.2	• Rate reflects 10% hypoxia.
Ketoacids	1	• Production requires lack of insulin.
Toxic alcohols	<1	• Poisonous metabolites rather than H$^+$ are the threat.
GI organic acids		• Antibiotics, stasis, and feeding increase their production rate.
Removal of H$^+$		
Kidney (by excretion of NH$_4^+$)	0–0.2	• Has a lag period. • Metabolic acidosis is needed for rapid rates of excretion.
Metabolism		
L-Lactic acid	4–8	• Half by oxidation and half by glucogenesis.
Ketoacids	0.8	• Oxidized primarily in the brain ($\frac{2}{3}$) and kidneys ($\frac{1}{3}$).

β-Hydroxybutyric acid
One of the so-called ketoacids produced in the liver when levels of insulin are low. (β-HB$^-$ = β-hydroxybutyrate anion.)

Generation of new bicarbonate
The usual diet generates approximately 1 mmol of H$^+$ per kilogram of body weight. The normal kidney regenerates 1 mmol of "new" HCO$_3^-$ per kilogram of body weight; failure to regenerate this new HCO$_3^-$ results in metabolic acidosis.

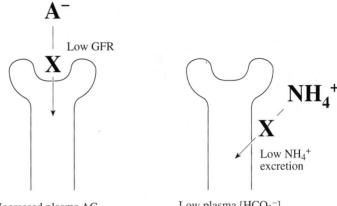

A^-

Low GFR

X

NH_4^+

X

Low NH_4^+
excretion

Increased plasma AG   Low plasma $[\text{HCO}_3^-]$

Figure 3.2   Basis of high plasma anion gap and acidosis in renal failure. The basis of the increased plasma anion gap (AG) is the low GFR with the need for higher levels in plasma to excrete anions such as phosphate or sulfate (left side). The acidosis is due to a low rate of excretion of NH_4^+ (right side).

Direct HCO_3^- loss occurs either via the gastrointestinal (GI) tract or in the urine. Indirect loss of HCO_3^- occurs as follows: an organic acid is produced and dissociates into an organic anion plus a H^+; when more organic anions than H^+ or NH_4^+ are excreted in the urine, there is a net gain of H^+ (or loss of HCO_3^-) in the body. Two major subgroups can be identified:

1. A large number of organic anions are filtered and not reabsorbed so that their excretion exceeds the quantity of NH_4^+ that can be excreted.

2. Only a modest number of anions are filtered and escape reabsorption, but this quantity exceeds the amount of NH_4^+ excreted because there is a major reduction in the rate of excretion of NH_4^+; consequently, the kidneys are unable to generate enough "new" HCO_3^- (Figure 3.3).

Because the generation of "new" HCO_3^- is largely the result of the urinary excretion of NH_4^+, tests to measure the rate of excretion of this cation are important (see Chapter 2, pages 58–60).

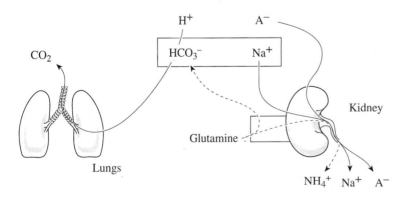

CO_2

H^+ A^-

HCO_3^- Na^+

Kidney

Glutamine

Lungs

NH_4^+ Na^+ A^-

Figure 3.3   Indirect loss of NaHCO₃. The body is represented by a rectangle and contains Na^+ and HCO_3^- for simplicity. An acid ($\text{H}^+ + \text{A}^-$) is produced. The H^+ is titrated by a HCO_3^-, and the A^- is excreted with a Na^+. The net result is loss of Na^+ and HCO_3^- involving the lungs and the kidneys. As shown in the dashed line, there is no net loss of HCO_3^- if the anion is excreted with NH_4^+ rather than Na^+.

Respiratory Response During Metabolic Acidosis

- Acidemia stimulates ventilation and lowers the Pa_{CO_2}.
- In metabolic acidosis, there is an empiric, predictable relationship between the fall in the Pa_{CO_2} and the degree of acidemia.

Acidemia is a potent stimulus to the respiratory center. In metabolic acidosis, hyperventilation (lowering the Pa_{CO_2}) displaces the equilibrium of the BBS equation downward and lowers the $[H^+]$ (see margin note). As discussed in Chapter 1, the net effect of this fall in Pa_{CO_2} is to minimize binding of H^+ to intracellular proteins (page 19). The relationship between the Pa_{CO_2} and the fall in $[HCO_3^-]$ is predictable from empiric data. Two ways to remember this relationship are as follows:

1. **Rule of thumb:** The Pa_{CO_2} should equal the value after the 7 in the pH (page 62).
2. **Relationship between Pa_{CO_2} and $[HCO_3^-]$:** As the $[HCO_3^-]$ in the extracellular fluid (ECF) falls, the Pa_{CO_2} also falls; the slope of the line is approximately 1, which means that the Pa_{CO_2} falls 1 mm Hg from 40 mm Hg for every 1 mmol/L fall in plasma $[HCO_3^-]$ from 25 mmol/L.

Detrimental Effect of an Inadequate Degree of Hyperventilation

- When the $[HCO_3^-]$ is very low, small changes in the Pa_{CO_2} or the $[HCO_3^-]$ will result in large changes in the $[H^+]$.

In patients who are incapable of appropriately lowering the arterial Pa_{CO_2} during metabolic acidosis, the degree of rise in $[H^+]$ is greater (see the discussion of Question 3.1 and Tables 3.3 and 3.4). Although the $[H^+]$ and $[HCO_3^-]$ in the ECF are the variables that are clinically evident, the impact of hyperventilation on the defense of the net charge on intracellular proteins must also be kept in mind

$$H^+ + HCO_3^-$$
$$\updownarrow$$
$$H_2CO_3$$
$$\updownarrow$$
$$H_2O + CO_2$$

Expected Pa_{CO_2}

If the Pa_{CO_2} is significantly lower than predicted by the relationship between Pa_{CO_2} and $[HCO_3^-]$, the patient has another primary stimulus to the respiratory center in addition to the acidemia (respiratory alkalosis). Similarly, if the Pa_{CO_2} is significantly higher than predicted, there is a compromised ability to ventilate in response to normal stimuli (respiratory acidosis).

TABLE 3.3 **Plasma $[H^+]$ in Patients Who Have Progressive Metabolic Acidosis with and Without an Appropriate Degree of Hyperventilation**

Patients without hyperventilation in this table are assumed to have a Pa_{CO_2} of 40 mm Hg.

$[HCO_3^-]$ (mmol/L)	Status with Appropriate Hyperventilation			Status Without Hyperventilation		
	Pa_{CO_2} (mm Hg)	$[H^+]$ (nmol/L)	pH	Pa_{CO_2} (mm Hg)	$[H^+]$ (nmol/L)	pH
20	35	42	7.38	40	48	7.32
15	30	50	7.30	40	64	7.19
10	25	60	7.22	40	96	7.02
5	20	96	7.02	40	191	6.72

TABLE 3.4 **Impact of Small Changes in the [HCO$_3^-$] or Paco$_2$ on the Acid-Base Status of the Patient with a Plasma [HCO$_3^-$] of 7 mmol/L**

A small increase in Paco$_2$ in patient B or a small fall in [HCO$_3^-$] in patient C converts a modest degree of acidemia into a severe one.

Patient	Condition	[H$^+$] nmol/L	pH	Paco$_2$ (mm Hg)	[HCO$_3^-$] (mmol/L)
A	Stable metabolic acidosis	72	7.13	20	7
B	Small reduction in hyperventilation	102	6.99	30	7
C	Further fall in plasma [HCO$_3^-$]	96	7.02	20	5

whenever a patient with metabolic acidosis is subjected to any procedure that may interfere with ventilation (see the discussions of Questions 3.2 and 3.3).

QUESTIONS

(Discussions on pages 145–146)

3.1 *Which patient has a primary respiratory acid-base disorder? How should each patient be managed from an acid-base point of view?*

Patient	[H$^+$] nmol/L	pH	Paco$_2$ (mm Hg)	[HCO$_3^-$] (mmol/L)
A	64	7.20	20	8
B	120	6.90	40	8
C	30	7.50	10	8

3.2 *Does the arterial or venous Pco$_2$ best reflect the degree of protonation of intracellular proteins during metabolic acidosis?*

3.3 *How can reexpansion of the ECF volume affect the Pco$_2$ in vital organs?*

Diagnostic Approach to Metabolic Acidosis

The overall diagnostic approach to the patient with metabolic acidosis is outlined in Figure 3.4. There are four steps to take:

1. **Confirm that metabolic acidosis is present:** The presence of metabolic acidosis is confirmed by finding a higher [H$^+$] and a lower [HCO$_3^-$] in plasma than expected. Alternatively, metabolic acidosis is present in virtually all cases when the plasma anion gap is unexpectedly high.

2. **Has the ventilatory system responded appropriately?** In patients with an elevated [H$^+$], a fall in the tissue Pco$_2$ is necessary to minimize binding of H$^+$ to intracellular proteins. If the Paco$_2$ does not fall by the appropriate amount (see margin), a coexistent respiratory acid-base disorder is also present.

3. **Does the patient have metabolic acidosis and no increase**

Note

In metabolic acidosis, for every mmol/L decrease in plasma [HCO$_3^-$] expect a 1 mm Hg decrease in Paco$_2$.

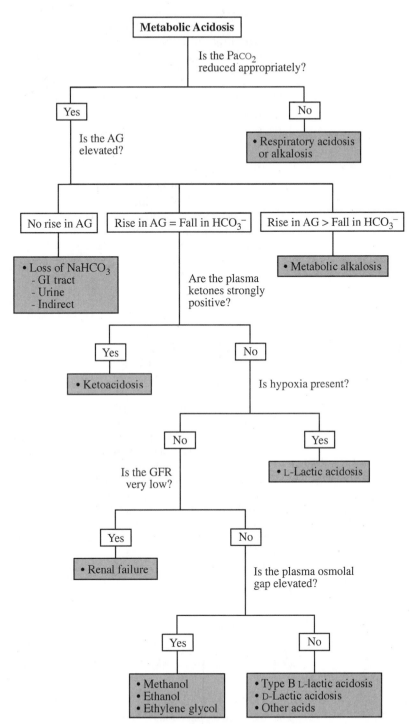

Figure 3.4 Diagnostic approach to metabolic acidosis. Metabolic acidosis is present when the [H⁺] in plasma is higher than expected and the [HCO₃⁻] in plasma is lower than expected. The first step is to assess the respiratory response to acidosis and then to define the basis of the acidosis—a gain of acid vs a loss of HCO₃⁻. The final diagnoses are shown in the shaded boxes (AG = plasma anion gap). One may have more than one acid-base disturbance in a patient—even if there is a coexistent respiratory acid-base disorder or metabolic alkalosis, proceed to discover the basis for the metabolic acidosis.

in the plasma anion gap? In patients with metabolic acidosis and no increase in the plasma anion gap, begin by ruling out an occult accumulation of organic acids because another condition (e.g., hypoalbuminemia) obscured the expected rise in the plasma anion gap.

The two major diagnostic possibilities are the loss of $NaHCO_3$ and the overproduction of acids with anions that do not appear in plasma; either these anions were excreted without H^+ or NH_4^+ or the plasma anion gap was underestimated. If the kidneys are not the cause of the metabolic acidosis, the rate of excretion of NH_4^+ should be high (>200 mmol/day in a 70-kg adult). The *urine net charge* can be used to estimate the $[NH_4^+]$ in urine (Chapter 2, pages 58–59). A nonrenal basis of metabolic acidosis (e.g., diarrhea) is suggested when the urine NH_4^+ excretion is greater than 200 mmol/day. In this case, the urine $[Cl^-]$ will exceed the urine $[Na^+] + [K^+]$. In contrast, with a low urine $[NH_4^+]$, suspect distal renal tubular acidosis (RTA) (urine $[Na^+] + [K^+]$ exceeds $[Cl^-]$). Rarely, NH_4^+ may be in the urine in conjunction with an anion other than Cl^- (β-HB^-, hippurate anion). If a patient excretes β-HB^- with NH_4^+, the marked ketonuria will remove an important clue for the diagnosis of ketoacidosis as there may be no increase in the plasma anion gap. In this case, a high rate of excretion of NH_4^+ may be revealed by calculating the *urine osmolal gap* (Chapter 2, pages 59–60).

4. **Has the plasma anion gap risen appropriately?** If the rise in the plasma anion gap is approximately equal to the fall in $[HCO_3^-]$ in plasma, the patient has a gain of acids or renal failure. Now the basis of the added acids must be detected: the presence of ketoacids, hypoxia, or a very low GFR. In the absence of these findings, suspect the presence of toxic products from unusual alcohols (an increased plasma osmolal gap). If the plasma osmolal gap is normal, the most likely diagnoses are a low rate of removal of L-lactic acid (usually a liver problem) and the accumulation of D-lactic acid (a GI problem).

The detailed approach to each category will be provided later.

Urine net charge
Detects $NH_4^+ + Cl^-$.

Urine osmolal gap
Detects NH_4^+ + any anion.

Clinical pearls
- Always suspect methanol or ethylene glycol poisoning in an intoxicated patient with metabolic acidosis.
- In a patient with metabolic acidosis, an increased plasma anion gap, and a normal ECF volume, be extremely suspicious of methanol or ethylene glycol poisoning especially if the GFR, GI tract, and the liver are normal.

PART B

Treatment of Metabolic Acidosis

The therapeutic decisions about patients with metabolic acidosis revolve around the following issues:

1. What emergency measures are required?
2. How can the threats to life be avoided?
3. What are the options for treating the acidosis per se?
4. How should one deal with an abnormal $[K^+]$ in plasma?

Emergency Measures

Before the biochemical results are available, measures to ensure a proper airway, adequate circulation, and O_2 delivery must be pursued vigorously. These measures are not discussed further.

Avoiding Threats to Life

There are three critical reasons for making a specific diagnosis:

1. It is important to determine the rate of H^+ production, which may be so high that the most effective means of arresting it is to increase the delivery of O_2 (e.g., L-lactic acidosis caused by a low cardiac output; see Table 3.2).

2. The cause of the metabolic acidosis may pose a serious but independent threat to the patient (e.g., methanol overdose). Its specific therapy (ethanol administration) is the most important therapeutic measure.

3. In certain types of metabolic acidosis that are associated with hypokalemia (low distal tubular H^+ secretion, diarrhea), K^+ replacement may be necessary before or along with administration of $NaHCO_3$ in order to avoid serious cardiac arrhythmias or respiratory failure (the HCO_3^- administered might promote entry of K^+ into cells). In patients with kidney failure, the danger is hyperkalemia.

Stop H^+ Production

Arresting H^+ production is critical in conditions with a very rapid rate of H^+ production (Figure 3.5). This rate can be 72 mmol/min in L-lactic acidosis from anoxia. Because the rate of production of H^+ is much lower in diabetic ketoacidosis and methanol overdose (1 mmol/min), it is less urgent to stop the production of H^+ in these situations (see Table 3.2). Instead, other measures can be lifesaving: delivery of oxygen in L-lactic acidosis (so that adenosine triphosphate (ATP) can be regenerated), stopping the production of toxins by ethanol administration in methyl alcohol intoxication, and possibly gastric lavage in certain intoxications.

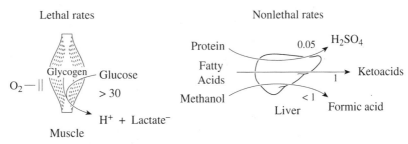

Figure 3.5   The production of acids. The numbers next to the arrows represent the rate of production of H^+ in mmol/min.

Lower the Quantity of H^+ Bound to Proteins by Lowering the Venous P_{CO_2}

There are two therapeutic options for rapidly lowering the quantity of H^+ bound to intracellular proteins. First, ensure an adequate degree of hyperventilation. Second, increase the rate of blood flow to vital organs (see discussion of Questions 3.2 and 3.3). These options are most useful in coexistent respiratory and metabolic acidosis and are the initial treatments of choice.

Increase Endogenous HCO_3^- Formation

Increasing the formation of endogenous HCO_3^- is a therapeutic option only in patients with metabolic acidosis and an increased plasma anion gap (Figure 3.6). The only emergency measure of value is to increase the metabolism of the circulating organic anions (renal new HCO_3^- formation can occur only at a rate of 0.3 mmol/min with perfectly adapted kidneys). Net removal of L- or D-lactate anions and β-HB$^-$ by metabolism requires that the rate of their removal exceed their ongoing production.

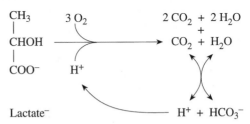

Figure 3.6 Oxidation of organic anions and the generation of HCO_3^-. Oxidation of an organic anion to a neutral end-product consumes a H$^+$ and yields a HCO_3^-. One CO_2 plus one H_2O is converted to a H$^+$ and a HCO_3^- and leads to the net yield of a HCO_3^-.

Treatment of the H$^+$ Load

To assess the need for $NaHCO_3$ therapy, use the plasma $[HCO_3^-]$ instead of the pH to avoid being misled by an unusually low Pa_{CO_2} (see margin note). The major dangers of this therapy are summarized in Figure 3.7.

The Use of $NaHCO_3$ in L-Lactic Acidosis

Treatment with $NaHCO_3$ is a controversial area. Some strongly advocate the use of $NaHCO_3$, but others consider it harmful. The following comments reflect the authors' view.

The Database Is Weak

Humans. L-Lactic acidosis is an acid-base "cough." It is a common finding that results from a heterogeneous group of disorders (see Table 3.12). Even the subgroup of type A L-lactic acidosis is not homogeneous; there are many different causes for inadequate delivery of O_2 to tissues, as well as varying degrees of tissue hypoxia. Further, delivery and demand do not remain constant from minute to minute. Hence, evaluating modes of therapy is fraught with hazard, and the conclusions drawn are not really justified.

Animals. The basis of L-lactic acidosis in animals differs markedly from that seen in clinical situations. For example, in rats breathing

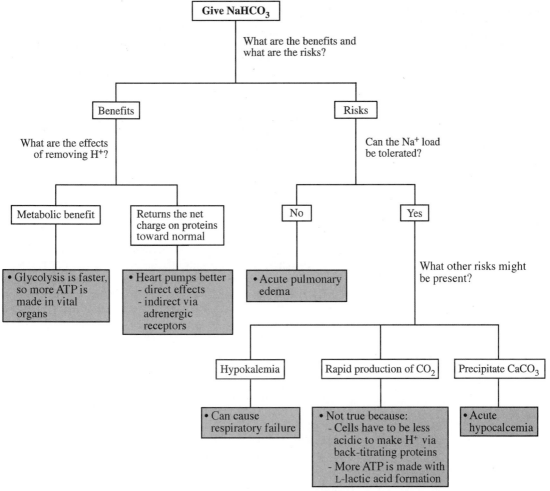

Figure 3.7 Dangers of therapy with NaHCO₃. The dangers of therapy with NaHCO₃ are ECF volume expansion, hypokalemia, hypocalcemia, excessive production of CO_2, and possibly hypoglycemia. Benefits may be the back-titration of proteins primarily in the ICF and the generation of more ATP because of a fall in the [H⁺] in the ICF.

air with a low P_{O_2}, the cardiac output was markedly reduced (see margin note). Nevertheless, what NaHCO₃ might or might not do in this setting cannot be translated reliably to the bedside, where most cases with L-lactic acidosis are caused by a failing, diseased heart.

Note
1996. *Am J Physiol* 271: R381–387. The point raised in this reference is that survival for extra minutes rather than clinical or laboratory measurements is what should be most important for decision-making.

Stoichiometry

One mmol of HCO_3^- is needed to titrate each millimole of H⁺ produced, or each millimole of H⁺ will be bound to intracellular proteins. The following statements illustrate some of the problems.

1. The quantity of H⁺ produced in each subtype of metabolic acidosis is not constant and may vary considerably (see Table 3.2).

2. The quantity of H⁺ bound to intracellular proteins rises with increased severity of the acidosis. For example, when acidosis is very severe, several hundred millimoles of NaHCO₃ is needed to raise the [HCO_3^-] in the ECF even by 1–2 mmol/L (see the example in the margin note on the next page).

Quantitative example
If you want to raise the [HCO$_3^-$] so that the [H$^+$] is halved, the [HCO$_3^-$] must be doubled if the Pco$_2$ does not change. In a patient with a [HCO$_3^-$] of 2 mmol/L, a [H$^+$] of 125 nmol/L, and a pH of 6.9, the [HCO$_3^-$] needs to be raised only to 4 mmol/L to halve the [H$^+$] (62.5 nmol/L, pH 7.20; assume the Pco$_2$ remained close to 10 mm Hg). To raise the [HCO$_3^-$] 2 mmol/L in this setting, more than 200 mmol of NaHCO$_3$ may have to be given (the content of HCO$_3^-$ in the ECF expands by only close to 30 mmol). Therefore, there is a large H$^+$ content in the ICF that is being titrated.

Paco$_2$ and effectiveness of BBS
The BBS requires CO$_2$ removal by ventilation in order to provide effective buffering.

H$^+$ + HCO$_3$ ↔ H$_2$CO$_3$ ↔ H$_2$O + CO$_2$ ↑

Clinical note
At times, the Na$^+$ load will limit how much NaHCO$_3$ can be given. In these settings, diuretics are rarely helpful, and alternate measures are needed.

Use of NaHCO$_3$ in a patient with metabolic and respiratory acidosis
Liberalize the goal of a plasma [HCO$_3^-$] of 5 mmol/L in a patient with chronic lung disease because this patient's ability to hyperventilate during metabolic acidosis might be severely compromised.

Basics of NaHCO$_3$ Therapy

1. **Treatment of patients with a normal plasma anion gap and a defect in NH$_4^+$ excretion (moderate degree of acidosis):** Because these patients have no renal or metabolic source of HCO$_3^-$, they must receive exogenous HCO$_3^-$ if their acidemia is to be corrected. When calculating the amount of NaHCO$_3$ to administer to a patient with a moderate degree of metabolic acidosis, assume a volume of distribution of 50% of total body weight. This figure is derived from experimental data and reflects the fact that 60% of buffering occurs in the ICF with a modest degree of metabolic acidosis. This assumption is not valid for a more severe or a less severe degree of metabolic acidosis (illustrated in the calculation in the margin note) because much more than 70 mmol of NaHCO$_3$ would be needed to raise the plasma [HCO$_3^-$] by 2 mmol/L from 2 to 4 mmol/L (0.5 × 70 kg × 2 mmol/L).

2. **Treatment of patients with a severe degree of metabolic acidosis:** In these patients, the initial therapy with NaHCO$_3$ should remove the patient from immediate danger. It should raise the plasma [HCO$_3^-$] to close to 5 mmol/L if the Paco$_2$ is less than 20 mm Hg (see margin note). With a higher Paco$_2$, the alveolar ventilation should be increased by means of intubation and ventilation. The rapidity with which the NaHCO$_3$ should be given is determined by the severity of the acidemia, the rate of H$^+$ production, and the [K$^+$] and cardiac status of the patient. The tonicity of the NaHCO$_3$ administered should be determined primarily by the patient's tonicity and the quantity to be administered. The administration of NaHCO$_3$ in an acidemic patient is a CO$_2$-producing process. If the patient is being artificially ventilated, the Paco$_2$ will rise if the alveolar ventilation is not increased appropriately.

Therapeutic Options in Patients with Metabolic Acidosis, Renal Failure, and ECF Volume Expansion

Gastric HCO$_3^-$ Generation. Each day the stomach usually generates 150 mmol of HCO$_3^-$, which can be mobilized as a therapeutic tool in certain challenging patients. One can insert a nasogastric tube, stimulate gastric acid secretion with pentagastrin (provided that the patient has not received H$_2$-receptor blockers and is not achlorhydric), and remove significant amounts of HCl (see Figure 4.1). One must ensure that the nasogastric tube is well situated to remove most of the acid. The periodic instillation of antacids down the tube helps in preventing complications secondary to excess HCl secretion. Should sufficient Na$^+$ be removed via this route, some NaHCO$_3$ could be administered intravenously.

Phlebotomy and Dialysis. If a patient with a severe degree of metabolic acidosis also has pulmonary edema, an additional therapeutic maneuver is a phlebotomy to permit the administration of NaHCO$_3$ (acidemia may also impair cardiac function). The phlebotomized blood should be packed and the cells returned to the patient after dialysis is instituted. Early dialysis with a HCO$_3^-$ bath should be planned.

Ventilation. One should ventilate patients to lower their Paco$_2$ if it is unduly high. This treatment can influence the acid-base state much faster than can administration of $NaHCO_3$. In patients with pulmonary edema, ventilation is also beneficial for the pulmonary edema (provided the patient can tolerate positive end-expiratory pressure, which might decrease the cardiac output).

Guidelines for $NaHCO_3$ Therapy

The authors propose the following guidelines for the use of $NaHCO_3$. The issues concerning the use of $NaHCO_3$ in specific diagnostic categories will be considered in Part C of this chapter.

Ketoacidosis. In ketoacidosis, the rate of H^+ production is slow, and $NaHCO_3$ therapy may carry the risk of provoking severe hypokalemia; therefore, $NaHCO_3$ should be avoided in most cases. Cases in which $NaHCO_3$ (along with K^+ if significant hypokalemia exists) should be considered are as follows:

1. when hyperkalemia is severe despite insulin therapy;

2. in very severe acidemia ($[HCO_3^-]$ <5 mmol/L) to raise the plasma $[HCO_3^-]$ close to twofold;

3. when acidemia worsens despite insulin therapy (perhaps insulin resistance is a result of acidemia).

Type A L-Lactic Acidosis. In type A L-lactic acidosis, the primary efforts should be directed at improving delivery of O_2. $NaHCO_3$ should be used when the $[HCO_3^-]$ is less than 5 mmol/L.

In states of low cardiac output, raising the cardiac output will have a larger impact on the pH of the ICF via a reduction in tissue P_{CO_2} than will therapy with $NaHCO_3$ (see the discussions of Questions 3.2 and 3.3 and Figure 1.9).

In cases with low alveolar ventilation, increase ventilation to lower the tissue P_{CO_2}.

QUESTION

(Discussion on page 146)

3.4 *Some recommend that a 50:50 mixture of $NaHCO_3$ and Na_2CO_3 (Carbicarb) be used as a source of alkali to minimize CO_2 production. If a patient has L-lactic acidosis and is producing 12 mmol of L-lactic acid per minute, how much less CO_2 (expressed in percentage form) will be produced by titrating the H^+ produced with Carbicarb instead of $NaHCO_3$? (Assume 12 mmol of O_2 is consumed each minute by the body.)*

Stoichiometry

$H^+ + HCO_3^- \rightarrow CO_2 + H_2O$

$2 H^+ + CO_3^{2-} \rightarrow CO_2 + H_2O$

K^+ and Metabolic Acidosis

- One must avoid a severe degree of hypokalemia when $NaHCO_3$ is given to a patient with a severe degree of metabolic acidosis.

The principal cation in the ICF is K^+. There is normally a very large electrochemical gradient for K^+ across cell membranes by

TABLE 3.5 **Potassium Depletion and Metabolic Acidosis**

In all three settings, there is a deficit of K^+. In diabetic ketoacidosis (DKA), hyperkalemia is usually present despite K^+ depletion (due to insulin deficiency); be wary if the diabetic patient has normokalemia or hypokalemia.

Disorder	Basis of K^+ Depletion
Distal RTA (low H^+ secretion type)	Renal K^+ loss
Loss of $NaHCO_3$ from the GI tract	Mainly renal K^+ loss, but some GI loss too
DKA	Renal K^+ loss (osmotic diuresis)

Resting membrane potential

$$-61 \times \log\frac{[K^+]_{in}}{[K^+]_{out}}$$

virtue of the $Na^+K^+ATPase$ in cells, the selective permeability of cell membranes to Na^+ (very low) and K^+ (high), and the fact that most intracellular anions are macromolecular and do not cross cell membranes. This K^+_{in}/K^+_{out} ratio is largely reflected by the *resting membrane potential*, with hyperkalemia diminishing the magnitude of this negative voltage and hypokalemia increasing it. Cells are more excitable during hyperkalemia and less excitable during hypokalemia. Notwithstanding, there is a tendency for cardiac arrhythmias in both cases. The challenge in therapy for metabolic acidosis is that correction of the acidemia will be associated with movement of K^+ into the ICF as H^+ move in the opposite direction.

Hypokalemia

There are two general features leading to a K^+ deficit and/or hypokalemia in a patient with metabolic acidosis: altered release of K^+ from cells, and increased renal excretion of K^+ (Table 3.5). A severe degree of hypokalemia has two major negative consequences: cardiac arrhythmias and respiratory failure from muscle weakness. In either case, the aim of therapy is to infuse K^+ quickly (Table 3.6). The authors recommend the following treatment:

1. Give K^+ rapidly in the case of an arrhythmia or respiratory arrest. Also, when a patient with a very severe degree of metabolic acidosis has hypokalemia and/or a deficit of K^+, promptly administer K^+ with HCO_3^- (see margin note).

2. Give K^+ more slowly (0.5–1 mmol/min) in the absence of

Aggressive intravenous K^+ therapy

1. Calculate the increment between the current plasma $[K^+]$ and 3.0 mmol/L; multiply this value by the plasma volume (plasma volume is close to 20% of the ECF volume) and give this amount over 1 minute via a central line.
2. Reduce the infusion rate to 1 mmol/min, and recheck the ECG and plasma $[K^+]$ in 5 minutes.
3. Repeat steps 1 and 2 if the $[K^+]$ remains well below 2.5 mmol/L.

TABLE 3.6 **Principles of Therapy in Patients with Acidemia and K^+ Depletion**

Principle	Comments
Use oral route for K^+ whenever possible (bowel sounds present).	• Giving large amounts of K^+ orally may prevent the IV problems.
Use several IV sites.	• Using different sites allows the dissociation of K^+ vs HCO_3^- infusion rates and permits more aggressive administration of K^+ by peripheral vein.
Use a cardiac monitor.	• A monitor will enable early detection of arrhythmias.
Ensure adequate K^+ output via the urine for continued infusion of K^+.	• If the patient has renal failure, give K^+ more cautiously.

important electrocardiogram (ECG) changes or respiratory failure.

Hyperkalemia

In the patient with hyperkalemia in the presence of important ECG abnormalities (Table 3.7), administer Ca^{2+} to minimize the electrical disturbance, and give HCO_3^- and insulin to shift K^+ into cells (see Chapter 11 for details).

TABLE 3.7　**Hyperkalemia and Metabolic Acidosis**

Although some patients with metabolic acidosis have hyperkalemia and a total body surfeit of K^+, others have a deficit of K^+. Obviously, treatment differs in the long run, but not necessarily in the acute situation if the ECG is very abnormal.

Cause	Total Body K^+	Comment
Renal failure	Increased	Excretion of K^+ is low.
Low aldosterone	Increased	Administer aldosterone and assess bioactivity by the degree of kaliuresis.
DKA	Decreased	The shift to ECF reflects the low level of insulin, not the acidosis.

PART C

Specific Disorders

Ketoacidosis

- The basis of ketoacidosis is relative insulin deficiency.

In order to understand why ketoacidosis develops and why it might be so severe, one must evaluate in a quantitative fashion the rates of production and removal of *ketoacids*. Production of ketoacids occurs in the liver if there is a lack of insulin and/or a resistance to its actions (Table 3.8).

TABLE 3.8　**Causes of Ketoacidosis**

Ketoacidosis with normal β-cell function (i.e., physiologically low release of insulin):
- Hypoglycemia
- Inhibition of β cells (α-adrenergics)
- Excessive lipolysis

Ketoacidosis with abnormal β-cell function:
- Insulin-dependent diabetes mellitus
- Pancreatic destruction

Ketoacids
- The most abundant ketoacid, β-HB^-, is really a hydroxy acid.

$$CH_3-\overset{OH}{\underset{H}{C}}-CH_2-COO^- + H^+$$

- Acetoacetate (AcAc) is the only real ketoacid.

$$CH_3-\overset{O}{C}-CH_2-COO^- + H^+$$

- Acetone is made from AcAc; it is not an acid.

$$CH_3-\overset{O}{C}-CH_3$$

Production of Ketoacids

Insulin acts at two major sites to influence the rate of ketogenesis: an extrahepatic site (adipocyte) and an intrahepatic site.

Extrahepatic Effects

Low levels of insulin combined with high levels of hormones whose actions oppose insulin (e.g., adrenaline, ACTH) lead to *activation of hormone sensitive lipase* (HSL) in adipocytes and the release of larger quantities of fatty acids (Figure 3.8).

Intrahepatic Effects

Low levels of insulin and, more importantly, elevated levels of glucagon lead to a fall in the level of malonyl-CoA, the key intermediate in the hepatocyte. This fall permits fatty acids to enter mitochondria, where they are oxidized to acetyl-CoA. Acetyl-CoA has three possible fates:

1. oxidation via the tricarboxylic acid (TCA) cycle to yield the important product, ATP (inhibited by the low adenosine diphosphate (ADP) levels that result from fatty acid oxidation);

2. reconversion to fatty acids (inhibited by a lack of insulin);

3. conversion to ketoacids (Figure 3.9).

When more acetyl-CoA is produced than can be oxidized to regenerate ATP and when fatty acid synthesis is blocked, the only major fate left for acetyl-CoA is to be converted to ketoacids, a pathway driven by a high level of acetyl-CoA (see Figure 3.9).

Control of the Production of Ketoacids

There are two major features in the control of ketogenesis:

1. Low levels of insulin give permission for a high rate of production of ketoacids by activating HSL, which provides more fatty

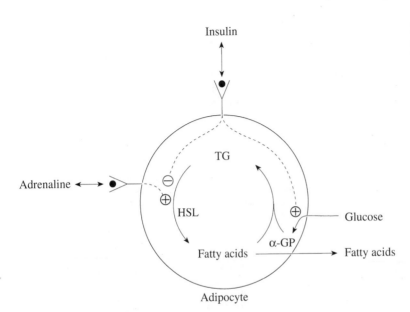

Adipocyte

Figure 3.8 Release of fatty acids from adipocytes. When levels of hormones such as adrenaline are high, HSL is activated and fatty acids are released. If insulin levels are low, HSL is more active and reesterification of fatty acids is low because less α-glycerol phosphate (α-GP) is available. (TG = triglyceride; + = stimulated; − = inhibited.)

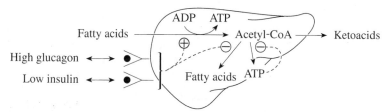

Figure 3.9   Control of ketoacid production in the liver. The hormonal setting of low levels of insulin and high levels of glucagon, via intrahepatic signals (low level of malonyl-CoA), promotes the entry of fatty acids into mitochondria and the formation of intramitochondrial acetyl-CoA. The rate of regeneration of ATP limits the ultimate fate of acetyl-CoA (i.e., it is converted to ketoacids at a controlled rate).

acids for the liver, promotes fatty acyl entry into hepatic mitochondria, and inhibits fatty acid synthesis from acetyl-CoA.

2. Once fat-derived fuels are "selected," the rate of turnover of ATP in hepatocytes sets the upper limit on ketogenesis, a pathway that must regenerate ATP. The key features in understanding the constraints on ketogenesis by the turnover of ATP are as follows: (1) The pathway must generate ATP and consumes ADP in the process (see Figure 3.9). (2) Cells contain a very tiny amount of ADP, the precursor of ATP. Hence, for ketogenesis to proceed, ADP must be reformed—via hydrolysis of ATP when hepatic work is performed (i.e., biosynthesis or ion pumping).

The rate of turnover of ATP in hepatocytes permits the generation of only 1.3 mmol of ketoacids per minute at the usual rates of O_2 consumption in the liver (see margin note).

Ketogenesis and hepatic O_2 consumption
- Hepatic blood flow is 1 L/min.
- Each liter of portal blood contains 6 mmol of O_2 and 0.6 mmol of fatty acid.
- The liver extracts 2 mmol of O_2/min (33% of delivery).
- Stoichiometry: 6 O_2 needed per C_{16} fatty acid → 4 ketoacids. Therefore, with 2 mmol of O_2 consumed per minute, only 1.3 mmol of ketoacids can be formed per minute; this formation requires that 0.3 mmol fatty acids be extracted per minute, a difficult task because fatty acids are sparingly soluble in water.

Removal of Ketoacids

Oxidation of Ketoacids

Two organs—the brain and the kidneys—are primarily involved in the oxidation of ketoacids (Figure 3.10).

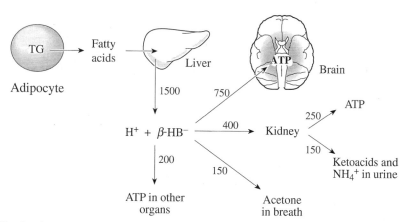

Figure 3.10   Production and removal of ketoacids: an overview. Ketoacids are produced in the liver at a maximum rate of 1 500 mmol/day in the absence of insulin; half are oxidized in the brain, and one-fourth are removed by the kidney. The numbers beside the arrows refer to mmol/day and are approximate values. The pathways leading to ATP generation will be limited by the rate of ATP utilization in the organ concerned. Reproduced with permission from *Clinical Detective Stories*, Portland Press Inc., London, 1993.

Brain. The brain can oxidize 750 mmol of ketoacids per day, half the quantity of ketoacids produced when ketogenesis is most rapid. The following influence the oxidation of ketoacids:

> The brain will oxidize ketoacids preferentially if their levels are high because the products of their metabolism (NADH, acetyl-CoA) inhibit the key step in the oxidation of glucose (pyruvate dehydrogenase; see Figure 12.1).

> If the utilization of ATP declines in the brain (less ion pumping in the central nervous system), fewer ketoacids can be oxidized. In the presence of coma, anesthetics, or sedation, the brain consumes less O_2 (and utilizes less ATP). Sedation might be important during the generation of alcoholic ketoacidosis because alcohol may act as a depressant of metabolism in the brain.

Kidney. The kidneys remove about 350–400 mmol of ketoacids per day. If renal work (largely the reabsorption of Na^+) is normal, the kidneys will oxidize 250 mmol ketoacids per day. Because more ketoacids are filtered than reabsorbed, close to 150 mmol of ketoacid anions will be excreted per day during the ketoacidosis of prolonged fasting. Because virtually all of these anions are excreted along with NH_4^+ (major) and H^+ (minor), acid-base balance results (Figure 3.11). Much lower renal removal of β-HB$^-$ and H^+ occurs if the filtered load of Na^+ declines (from prerenal failure secondary to loss of Na^+ in the glucose-induced osmotic diuresis) because the rates of both NH_4^+ production and β-HB$^-$ oxidation are both reduced.

Other Organs. The intestinal tract will oxidize ketoacids. If digestion and absorption are proceeding, this utilization can be appreciable (200–300 mmol/day). Notwithstanding, absorption is low in fasting and during diabetic ketoacidosis (DKA).

Skeletal muscle does not seem to oxidize ketoacids if fatty acid levels are high.

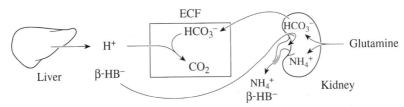

Figure 3.11   Excretion of β-HB$^-$ + NH$_4^+$ has no net acid-base effect. The liver produces H^+ with β-HB$^-$. H^+ are removed after reacting with HCO_3^- to form CO_2 + H_2O; the result is a deficit of HCO_3^-. When glutamine is metabolized in the kidney, NH_4^+ and HCO_3^- are produced. If NH_4^+ are excreted, HCO_3^- are added to the body, and balance for H^+ and HCO_3^- is restored. To the degree that β-HB$^-$ are excreted with Na^+ or K^+, a deficit of HCO_3^-, Na^+, and K^+ may occur.

Conversion of Ketoacids to Acetone

When the level of AcAc is high, this ketoacid is converted spontaneously to acetone and CO_2. High levels of AcAc require both a high total ketoacid level and a low level of NADH, as shown in the following equations:

$$\text{Acetoacetate}^- + H^+ + NADH \leftrightarrow \beta\text{-HB}^- + NAD^+$$
$$\text{Acetoacetate}^- + H^+ \rightarrow \text{Acetone} + CO_2$$

Bottom line
Because hepatic O_2 consumption rarely rises appreciably, ketogenesis is a rather slow way to generate H^+. This rate will be even slower if other fuels are used to regenerate ATP in the liver (e.g., the conversion of amino acids to glucose).

Hepatocytes use O_2 primarily during biosynthesis and to pump Na^+ via the Na^+K^+ATPase.

Note
High levels of NADH occur most commonly when the supply of O_2 is low or during the oxidation of ethanol.

Causes of a Relative Deficiency of Insulin

The causes of relative deficiency of insulin are listed in Tables 3.8 and 3.9. Two groups are evident, those with normal β cells of the pancreas that either lack a stimulus or are inhibited and those with damage to these β cells (diabetes mellitus). Diabetic and alcoholic ketoacidosis are discussed in detail in the next section because of their clinical importance.

Clinical pearl

In ketoacidosis, production of acetone not only leads to an important diagnostic clue (acetone in the breath) but also is a H^+-removing process. Therefore, a high $NADH/NAD^+$ provides the following four negative effects:

1. less acetone on the breath;
2. fewer H^+ removed with acetone formation;
3. false-negative test for ketoacids (see page 97);
4. overproduction of lactic acid.

TABLE 3.9 **Etiologic Classification of Ketoacidosis**

For details, see the text.

Cause	Special Features	Treatment
Insulin Deficiency with Normal β Cells		
Hypoglycemia	• With fasting, $[HCO_3^-]$ is >18 mmol/L; anion gap <19 mEq/L; plasma concentration of glucose is 3 mmol/L.	• The intake of glucose cures hypoglycemia and ketoacidosis.
Liver problem, e.g., glycogen storage disease or a defect in gluconeogenesis (GNG)	• Hypoglycemia can be marked. • Plasma $[HCO_3^-]$ can be <18 mmol/L. • If there is a defect in GNG, the patient may also have L-lactic acidosis.	• Glucose eliminates ketoacidosis. • Provide special therapy for the underlying disease.
Inhibited insulin release by α-adrenergics; an example is vomiting with marked ECF volume contraction in the alcoholic	• The ECF volume is very low. • Ketoacidosis may be severe. • Mixed acid-base disorders, K^+ depletion, and phosphate depletion will be present.	• Give NaCl to restore ECF volume. • Give KCl to replace K^+, but do not give insulin. • Give vitamin B. • Give glucose only if the patient is hypoglycemic.
β Cell Destruction (Diabetes Mellitus)		
Insulin-dependent diabetes mellitus	• Patient has severe hyperglycemia and ketoacidosis, a low ECF volume, K^+ depletion, and hyperkalemia.	• Give NaCl and insulin. KCl later • Hypokalemia will become a threat in 2 hours. • Glucose will be needed in 6 hours. • Treat precipitating factors.
Other Causes		
Excessive lipolysis: After exercise	• Although fatty acid mobilization is high, oxidation rate slows.	• Because no real danger exists, no special treatment is needed.
Salicylate overdose	• Excess salicylates activate hepatic lipase and cause hyperventilation, CNS toxicity, and K^+ depletion.	• Remove salicylates by promoting excretion plus GI lavage; dialysis may be necessary. • Replace K^+ deficit.

QUESTIONS

(Discussions on pages 146–147)

3.5 *Why is the rate of production of ketoacids so much lower than that of L-lactic acid if both are regulated by the rate of turnover of ATP?*

3.6 *The rates of ketoacid production and removal are usually equal in a person who lacks insulin. Why is this equality beneficial?*

3.7 *What makes DKA severe in degree compared with the ketoacidosis of chronic fasting?*

Diabetic Ketoacidosis

Clinical Features

Although diabetic ketoacidosis (DKA) often occurs in the previously diagnosed insulin-dependent diabetic (often with a precipitating event), it may be the initial mode of presentation in young patients with *insulin-dependent diabetes mellitus* (IDDM).

Hormonal Events

Look for the cause of the lack of insulin and the high levels of counterinsulin hormones. Failure of a patient with IDDM to take insulin is the most common reason for lack of insulin; an associated illness (e.g., infection, stress, or even pancreatitis) can lead to elevated concentrations of hormones such as adrenaline and glucocorticoids.

Consequences of Hyperglycemia

The major complaints are polyuria, which is secondary to the osmotic diuresis, and thirst, which accompanies contraction of the ECF volume. Because lean body mass is catabolized during *gluconeogenesis,* there is excessive weight loss and a loss of the sense of well-being.

The severity of hyperglycemia is influenced mainly by the degree of contraction of the ECF volume (a low GFR impairs the excretion of glucose) and to a lesser degree by the quantity of glucose ingested (see Chapter 12, page 487).

Signs of the Ketoacidosis

The major signs of the ketoacidosis are ECF volume contraction, the smell of acetone on the breath, and an extreme degree of hyperventilation (*Kussmaul's respirations*).

Insulin-dependent diabetes mellitus (IDDM)
A form of diabetes mellitus that occurs most commonly in young, thin patients. Those with IDDM are prone to ketoacidosis.

Noninsulin-dependent diabetes mellitus (NIDDM)
A form of diabetes mellitus that is most common in older, obese patients; ketoacidosis is rare. Complications focus on long-term disorders.

Gluconeogenesis
The synthesis of glucose in the liver (or kidney) from compounds not derived directly from glucose—predominantly, the conversion of proteins to glucose. Urea is the other product.

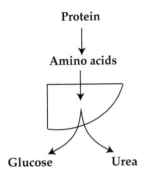

Kussmaul's respirations
Deep and rapid breathing, stimulated by acidemia.

Symptoms Related to Specific Organs

The most important signs and symptoms occur in the central nervous system (CNS). As DKA becomes more severe, confusion and even coma may develop. Other symptoms and signs that can be attributed to hyperglycemia include problems with vision from swelling of the lens of the eye, nausea and vomiting from poor gastric emptying, and symptoms such as abdominal pain secondary to hyperlipidemia. There may also be complications related to long-standing diabetes mellitus (autonomic or peripheral neuropathy, visual problems, nephropathy, and atherosclerosis).

Natural History

The signs and symptoms of DKA develop very slowly in the initial 12–24 hours after stopping the administration of insulin. This time course can be accelerated if there are high levels of counterinsulin hormones and/or ethanol present. When hyperglycemia and acidosis become more prominent, a vicious cycle develops. As the patient starts to become confused, cerebral metabolism of ketoacids declines, and the degree of ketoacidosis suddenly becomes even more severe. The GFR and renal work also decline as a result of a lesser filtered load of Na^+, so fewer ketoacids are oxidized and excreted by the kidney. Taken together, these factors largely account for the later accelerated phase of DKA.

Ethanol and DKA
Metabolism of ethanol, by producing acetyl-CoA, obviates the usual lag period in ketoacid production (see page 97 for more detail).

Changes in Body Composition

The features of hyperglycemia and ketoacidosis have been discussed. As a consequence of the osmotic diuresis, there are major changes in Na^+, water, and K^+.

Sodium

As a result of the osmotic diuresis, there is a major loss of Na^+ in the urine, a loss that exceeds any reasonable intake of Na^+. Accordingly, a major feature of DKA is a significant degree of ECF volume contraction. This aspect may dominate the clinical picture. Deficits of Na^+ are close to 5–10 mmol/kg body weight unless renal failure is present (Table 3.10).

Hyponatremia

Hyponatremia reflects the $Na^+:H_2O$ ratio in the ECF; it means that Na^+ were lost and/or water was gained in the ECF (see Chapter 6). Hyponatremia may be present for four major reasons:

1. Hyperglycemia induces the movement of water to the ECF from the ICF of cells that require insulin for glucose transport (osmoles restricted to the ECF attract water from the ICF; see Chapter 12, page 494).

2. Na^+ are lost in the urine in the osmotic diuresis and may be excreted with β-HB$^-$.

3. Water is ingested (because of thirst) while ADH is present.

Summary
1. Osmotic shift
2. Loss of Na^+ in the urine
3. Thirst plus ADH
4. Laboratory error

TABLE 3.10 **Deficits in Diabetic Ketoacidosis**

The deficits represent typical values in an adult with DKA. As a result of a
continuing osmotic diuresis, anticipate a further renal excretion of at least 100
mmol of Na^+.

Substance	Typical Deficit	Therapy
Na^+	5–10 mmol/kg	Give 1–2 L isotonic saline plus >2 L ½ isotonic saline.
K^+	5–10 mmol/kg	Add 20–40 mmol/L KCl to the IV once plasma $[K^+]$ <5.0 mmol/L.
Water	3 L from ECF and 3 from ICF	Give EFW, especially if the patient is hypernatremic.
HCO_3^-	2–3 mmol/kg	Give $NaHCO_3$ initially only if there is life-threatening acidemia ($[H^+]$ >100 nmol/L) and later only if the excretion of NH_4^+ is low or hyperkalemia persists.
Phosphate	0.5 mmol/kg	A deficit is not life-threatening, but therapy is advisable (6 mmol/h).

4. There may be a laboratory error secondary to hyperlipidemia if
   certain techniques are used to measure the $[Na^+]$ (see Chapter 8,
   page 331). Although patients are hyponatremic, they are still
   hyperosmolar because of the hyperglycemia.

Potassium

The plasma $[K^+]$ is usually somewhat elevated (5.3–5.7 mmol/L),
but there is a large overall total body deficit of K^+ from prior renal
loss early during the osmotic diuresis (see Table 3.10). Hyperkalemia is due to insulin deficiency, which causes K^+ to shift out of
cells; hyperkalemia may be aggravated by tissue catabolism. Some
patients may be hypokalemic if they had large prior loss of K^+
(vomiting or a prolonged osmotic diuresis with high aldosterone
bioactivity; see margin note).

Diagnosis of DKA

The diagnosis of DKA is usually not a difficult one to establish. It
should be ruled out in all patients with metabolic acidosis and an
increase in the plasma anion gap. Hyperglycemia and ketonemia
(positive qualitative test for acetoacetate in a serum dilution of 1:8)
are sufficient criteria in a patient likely to have IDDM. The fall in
plasma $[HCO_3^-]$ should initially approximate the increase in the
plasma anion gap, but this equality is fortuitous and misleading
(Table 3.11).

Pitfalls in the Laboratory Diagnosis of DKA

β-Hydroxybutyric Acidosis but Little Acetoacetic Acidosis. The
β-HB$^-$ and acetoacetate (AcAc$^-$) are in equilibrium because of
high activity of the enzyme β-hydroxybutyrate dehydrogenase in
mitochondria. The quick screening test for ketoacids (nitroprusside
reaction) detects only AcAc$^-$ and acetone. Therefore, if the patient

Note
On admission, a patient with
diabetes in poor control has a
compromised ability to excrete K^+,
even though aldosterone is present
and Na^+ are being excreted; this
patient has an unexpectedly low
TTKG (see Chapter 9, pages
390–393).

Note
"Early treatment" refers to the
expected response in the first 4–6
hours after insulin action, whereas
"later treatment" is 12–15 hours
after the initial therapy.

TABLE 3.11   **Changes in [HCO₃⁻] and Anion Gap During Treatment of DKA**

The content of ketone body anions (KB^-) in the ECF is their concentration multiplied by the ECF volume. The sum of the contents of HCO_3^- plus KB^- is lower than normal in DKA (content is only 300 mmol vs 375 mmol), even though the rise in $[KB^-]$ equals the fall in $[HCO_3^-]$. Despite the conversion of KB^- to HCO_3^-, there is not an equivalent rise in the $[HCO_3^-]$ in the ECF. This inequality reflects three processes: (1) the infusion of HCO_3^--free solution to reexpand the ECF volume; (2) the entry of H^+ in excess of KB^- into the ECF from the ICF, where they were buffered on ICF proteins; and (3) continued excretion of KB^- with Na^+ and K^+. With increased renal new HCO_3^- generation (excretion of NH_4^+), the HCO_3^- deficit will be repaired.

| Condition | ECF Volume (L) | Concentration in ECF | | Content in ECF | | |
| | | HCO₃⁻ | KB⁻ | HCO₃⁻ | KB⁻ | Sum |
		(mmol/L)		(mmoles)		
Normal	15	25	0	375	0	375
Admission	12	10	15	120	180	300
Early treatment	15	12	5	180	75	255
Later treatment	15	18	1	270	15	285
Recovery	15	25	0	375	0	375

has NADH accumulation in mitochondria (e.g., in hypoxia or during alcohol metabolism; Figure 3.12), the equilibrium of this equation is displaced to the right and $[AcAc^-]$ falls (see margin). Because this test may yield only a weakly positive serum ketone result, it is possible to underestimate the degree of ketoacidosis. If hyperglycemia and glycosuria are present without ketonemia or with only moderate ketonemia, suspect coexistent ketoacidosis and L-lactic acidosis. This suspicion is supported by a strongly positive test for ketones in the urine. Enzymatic determinations for β-HB⁻ and L-lactate anions in blood confirm that diagnosis.

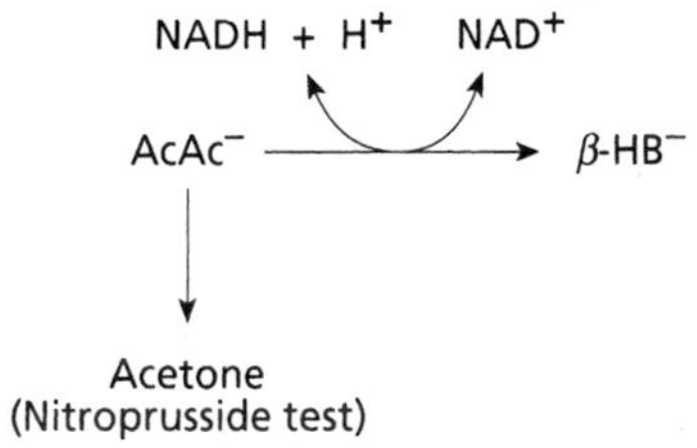

A Plasma Anion Gap that is Not Sufficiently Increased. An unexpectedly low plasma anion gap may result from hypoalbuminemia, an unusual degree of ketonuria, or therapy with NaCl.

1. Hypoalbuminemia resulting from diabetic glomerulosclerosis is common in long-standing diabetes mellitus and can obscure the expected increase in the plasma anion gap. Thus, if a patient has hyperglycemia, ketonemia, metabolic acidosis, ketonuria, glycosuria, and proteinuria, do not be deterred from

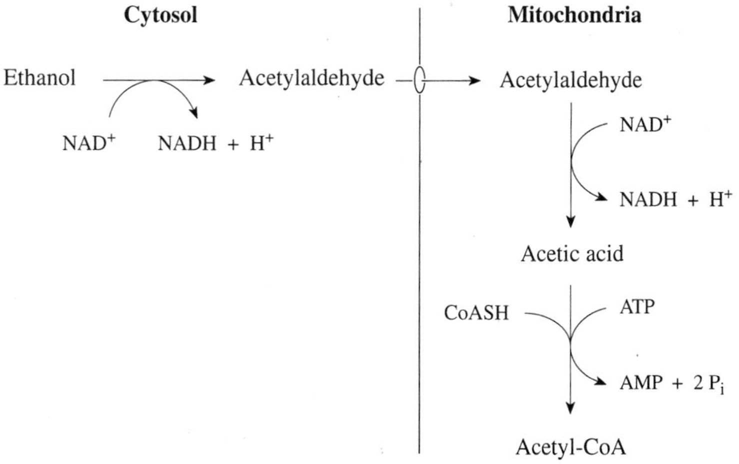

$$NADH + H^+ \quad NAD^+$$
$$AcAc^- \longrightarrow \beta\text{-HB}^-$$
$$\downarrow$$
Acetone
(Nitroprusside test)

Figure 3.12   Synthesis of acetyl-CoA from ethanol. The conversion of ethanol to acetyl-CoA generates 2 ($NADH + H^+$) (equivalent to 6 ATP) and uses the equivalent of two ATP bonds when acetyl-CoA is formed.

Cytosol | Mitochondria

Ethanol → Acetylaldehyde → Acetylaldehyde

NAD^+ $NADH + H^+$

NAD^+

$NADH + H^+$

Acetic acid

CoASH   ATP

AMP + 2 P_i

Acetyl-CoA

Urine net charge and osmolar gap in DKA

Urine net charge and osmolar gap in DKA

If ketoacid anions are excreted with Na^+ and K^+, the urine net charge will be positive; if they are excreted with NH_4^+, the urine osmolal gap will be high.

the diagnosis of DKA by the normal or only slightly elevated level of the plasma anion gap.

2. If the patient has impaired proximal tubular reabsorption of ketoacid anions, the plasma anion gap may not be very high in the presence of ketoacidosis. The clue to the diagnosis is metabolic acidosis and ketonuria. Suspect DKA if an analysis of the urine electrolytes reveals an unusually high urine osmolal gap and a positive urine net charge ($Na^+ + K^+ > Cl^-$; see Chapter 2, pages 58–60). To confirm the diagnosis, quantitate β-HB^- excretion.

3. As shown in Table 3.11, even though the fall in $[HCO_3^-]$ equals the rise in the plasma anion gap in a patient with DKA, there is still a large indirect loss of $NaHCO_3$ (see Figure 3.3). This latter loss is somewhat occult because of the marked difference in the ECF volume (15 L in the normal adult and close to 12 L in the patient presenting with a severe degree of DKA). This difference becomes obvious when one considers the content instead of the concentration of HCO_3^- in the ECF, and it is unmasked when saline is infused and the ECF volume is restored; this therapy lowers both the concentration of HCO_3^- and the anion gap in plasma.

Treatment of the Patient with DKA

Before dealing with the details of treatment, the clinician should recognize the deficits present (see Table 3.10). The therapeutic approach to DKA involves attention to four major issues. First, the ECF volume must be reexpanded; second, the rate of H^+ production must be diminished; third, the deficit of K^+ must be replaced, but timing is critical; fourth, an underlying event that precipitated DKA or was a complication of it must be sought.

Reexpand ECF Volume

If the patient is in impending shock (systolic blood pressure <90 mm Hg with tachycardia), use isotonic saline at 1000 mL/30 minutes until systolic blood pressure is greater than 100 mm Hg or for the first 2–3 L. If the patient is severely acidemic ($[HCO_3^-]$ <5 mmol/L), give some of the Na^+ as isotonic $NaHCO_3$ instead of NaCl until the plasma $[HCO_3^-]$ is in the 5–6 mmol/L range. Once the patient is hemodynamically stable (systolic blood pressure >100 mm Hg), use 1/2 isotonic NaCl at 0.5–1 L/h, depending on the remaining degree of ECF volume depletion.

In the first several hours of treatment, the fall in blood glucose will be largely due to dilution (reexpansion of the ECF volume) and renal excretion (from the rise in GFR)—actions that are not caused by insulin (see Table 12.3); the rate of fall is close to 100 mg/dL/h (5.5 mmol/L/h). Glucose should be added to the infusion once the blood sugar reaches 250 mg/dL (12–15 mmol/L).

Clinical pearls
- The fall in glucose early in therapy reflects the actions of IV saline rather than insulin.
- Do not permit too great a fall in glycemia. Give glucose once the blood sugar approaches 250 mg/dL (12–15 mmol/L).

Stop Ketoacid Production

Regular (crystalline) insulin is needed to stop the formation of ketoacids. An initial bolus of 5–10 units should be given intravenously, and a continuous infusion of 0.1 U/kg body weight/h (in normal saline) should be started. Even though the lipolytic rate declines promptly, there is a lag period of several hours before there is a net decline in the degree of ketoacidosis. Hence, expect little rise in the [HCO_3^-] in plasma in the first several hours, despite the actions of insulin. The plasma anion gap should return to normal in 8–10 hours (the time required for ketoacid anions to disappear).

K^+ Status

The major parameter to guide K^+ replacement therapy is the plasma [K^+]. Patients with DKA usually are quite severely K^+-depleted but have hyperkalemia due to insulin deficiency. Therefore, if the plasma [K^+] is less than 5 mmol/L, add 20 mmol KCl to each liter of infusion once insulin is given. If the plasma [K^+] is less than 4 mmol/L, use $NaHCO_3$ with caution (HCO_3^- cause K^+ to enter into the ICF).

If the plasma [K^+] is greater than 5 mmol/L, wait at least 1 hour before initiating K^+ replacement. If the plasma [K^+] is less than 3.5 mmol/L, the patient is profoundly K^+-depleted, and special precautions should be taken (aggressive replacement of K^+, cardiac monitoring, and attention to alveolar ventilation), as the plasma [K^+] will fall with insulin administration.

Underlying Illness

Always look for the factors (such as infection or myocardial infarction) responsible for initiating this metabolic emergency, and consider the events secondary to DKA, such as thrombotic complications or possibly aspiration.

Alcoholic Ketoacidosis

Some subjects who consume ethanol in large amounts develop ketoacidosis (see Figure 3.12; Figure 3.13). The following features are required to develop this metabolic picture:
1. **Lack of insulin:** A lack of insulin may be due to IDDM, but this disease need not be present. Although destruction of β cells by pancreatitis is also possible, the most important cause of lack of insulin is inhibition of its release from β cells by an intense adrenergic response (see Table 3.8). Hence, an extreme degree of ECF volume contraction from excessive vomiting is almost always part of the clinical picture of alcoholic ketoacidosis (AKA).
2. **Synthesis of acetyl-CoA in hepatic mitochondria:** The usual precursor of large quantities of acetyl-CoA in hepatic mitochondria is fatty acyl-CoA (acetyl-CoA prevents rapid synthesis via pyruvate dehydrogenase, so glucose cannot be a precursor of appreciable quantities of ketoacids). A considerable lag period is required to activate this step (via low malonyl-CoA levels). Notwithstanding, if ethanol is oxidized, acetyl-CoA is generated in hepatic mitochondria, and a lag period is not required (see Figure 3.12).
3. **Conversion of ethanol to Hβ-HB:** The oxidation of ethanol occurs in the liver, for the most part, and is catalyzed by the enzyme alcohol dehydrogenase. The affinity of ethanol for its dehydrogenase is high so that it functions at its *Vmax* with a concentration of ethanol of just several millimoles per liter.

K^+ excretion
Early in therapy, the excretion of K^+ is trivial. Consider the following example: the [K^+] in urine is 30 mmol/L, and the urine flow rate is 2 mL/min. In 2 hours (0.24 L excreted), K^+ excretion is only 7.2 mmol—a tiny amount vs the quantity of K^+ infused.

Phosphate and K^+
In the first 6 hours of therapy, it is also reasonable to use some K^+ with phosphate (up to 6 mmol/h) because these patients are also phosphate-depleted. Nevertheless, it takes a considerable time before anabolism (synthesis of RNA, etc.) will occur in a patient during a catabolic state, even after insulin is administered. Hence, it is too optimistic to think that cells will incorporate much of the administered phosphate (the deficit is close to 100 mmol, yet only 50 mmol is needed in the first 12 hours).

Clinical pearls
- When diagnosing alcoholic ketoacidosis, look for the cause of the inhibited release of insulin from β cells; IDDM or NIDDM are not necessarily present.
- The concentration of glucose in plasma is usually lower in AKA than in DKA.

Hβ-HB
β-Hydroxybutyric acid

Vmax:
The maximum rate catalyzed by an enzyme.

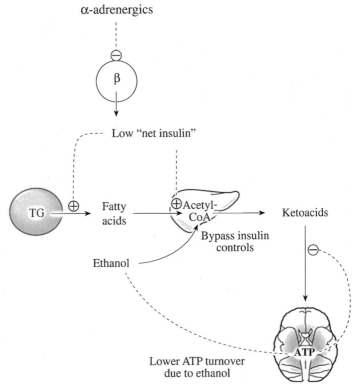

Figure 3.13 Pathophysiology of AKA. The important features are a low level of insulin (α-adrenergic response to a low ECF volume), a high rate of formation of acetyl-CoA in the liver, and a lower rate of oxidation of ketoacids in the brain (effect of ethanol) and kidneys (low GFR, not shown).

Net yield of ATP when ethanol is converted to β-HB⁻:

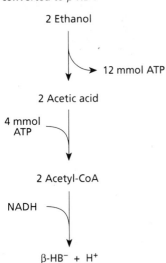

The limit on ethanol metabolism is via the rate of removal of the other product, NADH (see Figure 3.12). The following quantitative example could illustrate why β-HB⁻ is the predominant product of ethanol metabolism when insulin levels are low.

- Hepatic oxygen consumption is 2 mmol/min, or 3000 mmol/day (18,000 mmol of ATP produced daily).
- When ethanol is oxidized in the TCA cycle, 16 mmol of ATP is produced per millimole of ethanol oxidized. Therefore, only 113 mmol (5 g) of ethanol could be metabolized by this route in a day.
- When acetic acid is the product, 2 NADH (6 mmol of ATP) is produced per millimole of ethanol consumed. Thus, this pathway could remove 3000 mmol (138 g) of ethanol per day.
- When β-HB⁻ is the product of ethanol metabolism, 0.5 mmol of NADH is consumed for each millimole of ethanol converted to β-HB⁻. Thus, the net yield is 2.5 mmol of ATP formed per millimole of ethanol consumed in this pathway (see margin). Now 7200 mmol (close to 350 g) of ethanol can be consumed per day, and this value is close to the rate of ethanol metabolism in vivo. Thus, AKA is commonly seen in states where ethanol is present in abundant amounts and insulin levels are low.

4. **Low oxidation of ketoacids:** Both suppression of CNS me-

tabolism (intoxication) and a low GFR (prerenal failure) decrease the rate of oxidation and excretion of ketoacids.

5. **Low conversion of ketoacids to acetone:** The high NADH:NAD⁺ ratio in the liver causes a lower concentration of AcAc⁻ relative to β-HB⁻. This low level of AcAc⁻ leads to decreased synthesis of acetone. Hence, the quick test for ketoacids, which measures AcAc⁻ and acetone, might be unduly low given the degree of ketoacidosis (β-hydroxybutyric acidosis; see margin note).

6. **Other features:** The impact of the metabolism of ethanol on the concentration of glucose is considered in Chapter 12 (see also Figure 3.15).

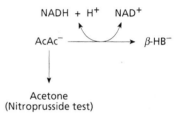

Acetone
(Nitroprusside test)

QUESTIONS

(Discussions on page 147)

3.8 *In hepatic mitochondria, acetyl-CoA is formed from ethanol and from fatty acids at about the same rate. Why are these rates so similar?*

3.9 *Must ethanol levels be elevated on admission for metabolism of ethanol to be an important cause of ketoacidosis?*

Diagnosis of AKA

The major clinical features include the recent ingestion of ethanol together with a relative lack of insulin from a marked contraction of the ECF volume; this contraction, similar to shock, is often due to excessive vomiting related to alcoholic gastritis or possibly pancreatitis.

Biochemically, ketoacidosis is present by definition, but the patient might not be acidemic because of the metabolic alkalosis consequent to vomiting. The key to the diagnosis of this *mixed acid-base disturbance* is the discovery of an unusually large increase in the plasma anion gap. A note of caution must be inserted here because *hypoalbuminemia* may make the rise in the plasma anion gap less apparent (for every 10 g/L decline in the concentration of albumin in plasma, the anion gap will fall by 4 mEq/L). Given the high propensity to aspiration pneumonitis and the fact that alcohol withdrawal may stimulate ventilation, it is not uncommon to see a respiratory acid-base disorder as well.

Several other biochemical features merit emphasis. From an acid-base perspective, there may be L-*lactic acidosis* if the metabolism of ethanol raises the NADH:NAD⁺ in the cytosol of hepatocytes; the lower [AcAc⁻] that results may give a false-negative or weakly positive test result for ketoacids in plasma. L-Lactic acidosis may be present for a number of other reasons besides ethanol metabolism; two of the most common causes are hypoxia in tissues because of the very low ECF volume, and muscular contraction (delirium, tremors, or convulsions). The most important cause, however, is thiamine deficiency, which may cause permanent cerebral damage if it is not recognized and treated (Figure 3.14).

As regards K⁺, the insulin deficiency tends to raise the [K⁺] in plasma, but the excessive vomiting leads to a large kaliuresis. Therefore, the K⁺ deficit is usually much larger in AKA than in DKA, and it is not uncommon to see a plasma [K⁺] in the 3–4

Mixed acid-base disturbance
- When ketoacids are added, H⁺ are added to the body. The "footprint" of the added acid is the β-HB⁻ or a rise in the plasma anion gap.
- With vomiting, Cl⁻ are lost and HCO₃⁻ are added to the body (see Figure 4.1).
- Overall, HCO₃⁻ are lost and added, so the [HCO₃⁻] may not change, but the plasma anion gap will be higher.

Hypoalbuminemia
A low level of albumin in plasma that may be due to liver damage or poor nutrition.

Causes of L-lactic acidosis related to ethanol intake
1. Raised NADH/NAD⁺
2. Thiamine deficiency
3. Low ECF volume and hypoxia
4. Muscular contraction

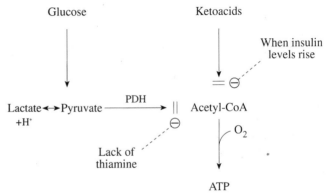

Figure 3.14   Treatment of AKA with thiamine. Thiamine is a cofactor for PDH. Without this vitamin B, oxidation of ketoacids, but not glucose, can provide the ATP needed by brain cells. Infusion of glucose and the subsequent release of insulin could lead to local overproduction of L-lactic acid and a local deficit of ATP with subsequent harm to brain cells due to the lack of fuel for oxidation.

Insulin release in AKA
In the setting of AKA, excessive vomiting leads to ECF volume contraction, an α-adrenergic response, and an inhibited release of insulin from β cells of the pancreas. Reexpansion of the ECF volume will remove this inhibition.

mmol/L range (an alarming K^+ deficit is present). In parallel, there is a large deficit of phosphate, as in DKA. Finally, the blood glucose level can be low, normal, or high, depending primarily on the quantity of glucose ingested. Ethanol levels in plasma can be measured directly or inferred from the plasma osmolal gap. An important point to keep in mind is that other alcohols (methanol, ethylene glycol) might also be present (see pages 110–112).

Treatment of the Patient with AKA

There are several life-threatening components to the clinical picture of AKA, and each requires urgent attention.

ECF Volume Reexpansion

Rapid infusion of saline that is isotonic to the patient will take care of this potential danger. The first liter should be given as quickly as possible (30 minutes) and, depending on the blood pressure, the next liter can be given over 30 or 60 minutes. Anticipate that perhaps one more liter of isotonic fluid will be needed; renal losses should be small.

K^+ Deficit

Once the ECF volume is reexpanded, insulin will be released, and K^+ will move rapidly from the ECF to the ICF. Accordingly, replacement of part of the K^+ deficit should begin early in treatment, but the actual amount given will depend on the plasma $[K^+]$.

Nutritional Therapy

Thiamine. It is critical that B vitamins be added to the first IV solution to replace a potential thiamine deficit. This addition will permit aerobic oxidation of glucose in the brain once ketoacids disappear (see Figure 3.14).

Phosphate. Although phosphate depletion is quite marked, it will take time before anabolic reactions occur subsequent to the actions of insulin. Hence, as in DKA, replacing the majority of the phosphate deficit must be delayed.

Glucose. Glucose is needed only if hypoglycemia is present. In this situation, just give enough glucose to achieve normal values because metabolism of glucose will be slow in this setting (see margin note). Further, the advantage of avoiding very high levels of insulin once normovolemia is achieved is the prevention of a sudden fall in glycemia and plasma [K$^+$].

Insulin. Insulin need not be given initially unless there is a severe degree of hyperkalemia or acidemia. Otherwise, delay giving insulin, especially in the patient with hypokalemia.

Dose of glucose
Assume that the concentration of glucose must rise by 3 mmol/L (54 mg/dL) in a 70-kg patient with a volume of distribution of glucose that is close to 20 L.
- 3 mmol/L $\times$ 20 L = 60 mmol.
- 60 mmol of glucose = 10.8 g of glucose.
- Give 200 mL D$_5$W or 20 mL D$_{50}$W.

L-Lactic Acidosis

Background

Although both overproduction and underutilization of L-lactic acid result in L-lactic acidosis, their quantitative dimensions may differ by an order of magnitude.

Overproduction of L-Lactic Acid

Net production of L-lactic acid occurs when the body must regenerate ATP without oxygen. The bottom line is that 1 H$^+$ is produced per ATP regenerated from glucose. Quantitatively, because a patient at rest needs to regenerate 72 mmol of ATP per minute, as much as 72 mmol of H$^+$ can be produced per minute during anoxia (see margin note).

Accumulation of L-lactic acid
- There are two reasons for L-lactic acid to accumulate: overproduction and underutilization.
- Production of L-lactic acid can occur very quickly, but utilization of L-lactic acid occurs slowly.

$$2\ ATP \rightarrow 2\ (ADP + P_i) + \text{biologic work}$$
$$Glucose + 2\ (ADP + P_i) \rightarrow 2\ H^+ + \text{L-lactate}^- + 2\ ATP$$

Underutilization of L-Lactic Acid

There are two major ways to remove L-lactic acid: oxidation and conversion to glucose. To oxidize 1 mmol of L-lactate anion, 3 mmol of oxygen must be consumed (18 mmol of ATP must be formed). Hence, if all organs could be "persuaded" to oxidize L-lactate anion to yield 100% of their requirement to regenerate ATP, only 4 mmol of L-lactate anion could be oxidized per minute at rest (because 72 mmol of ATP is used per minute).

Stoichiometry of ATP and O$_2$
- The ratio of phosphorus to oxygen is 3:1.
- Because there are two atoms of O in O$_2$, 6 ATP can be produced per O$_2$ (3 ATP/0.5 O$_2$).
- Consumption of O$_2$ at rest is close to 12 mmol/min. Therefore, the amount of ATP needed per minute is 12 $\times$ 6, or 72 mmol/min.

$$\text{L-Lactate}^- + H^+ + 3\ O_2 + 3\ (ADP + P_i) \rightarrow$$
$$18\ ATP + 3\ CO_2 + 3\ H_2O$$

The other major metabolic way to remove the L-lactate anion is glucogenesis, a pathway that occurs in the liver and in the kidney cortex. Applying stoichiometry and a quantitative analysis, the maximum rate of glucogenesis is close to 4 mmol/min in either the liver or kidney cortex. This calculation is determined by the rate at which the liver and the kidneys consume oxygen (2 mmol/min in each organ) and their requirements for ATP in this process.

Note
See the margin note on page 151 for extra definitions of glucogenesis, gluconeogenesis, and glucopaleogenesis.

$$\text{L-Lactate}^- + H^+ + 3\ ATP \rightarrow 0.5\ \text{glucose}$$

QUESTION

(Discussion on pages 147–148)

3.10 *An anoxic limb needs to regenerate 18 mmol of ATP per minute (25% of the ATP needed in the body) via anaerobic glycolysis. If the rest of the body were "persuaded" to oxidize L-lactate anions (+ H⁺) to regenerate all needed ATP (54 mmol/min, equivalent to the utilization of 9 mmol of O_2), would L-lactic acid accumulate?*

Clinical Picture

Pathogenesis

L-Lactic acidosis, a common cause of metabolic acidosis, often occurs in a life-threatening situation (Table 3.12). The most common cause of L-lactic acidosis is relative hypoxia (when the O_2 demand exceeds the O_2 supply—type A L-lactic acidosis). Hypoxia may be due to hypoxemia, hypotension, or impaired blood supply to an organ. There are a number of causes of L-lactic acidosis in which hypoxia does not play a major role (type B L-lactic acidosis); almost all patients with type B L-lactic acidosis have liver problems.

TABLE 3.12 **Causes of L-Lactic Acidosis**

Type A: Deficit of oxygen
- Lung problem (low PaO_2)
- Circulatory problem (poor delivery of O_2)
- Hemoglobin problem (low capacity of blood to carry O_2)

Type B: Compromised metabolism of L-lactate without hypoxia
- Excessive formation of L-lactic acid (increased glycolysis as a result of low ATP, e.g., from inhibitors of mitochondrial generation of ATP, such as cyanide, or from the presence of agents that uncouple oxidative phosphorylation)
- Insufficient utilization of L-lactic acid:
  PDH problem (from a deficiency of thiamine or an inborn error)
  Increased availability of other fuels (fatty acids)
  Low flux through the ATP generation system (less biologic work)
- Decreased conversion of L-lactate to glucose, a liver problem:
  Destruction or replacement of cells in the liver (see margin note)
  Defect in glucogenesis (from an inborn error or from inhibitors of glucogenesis, such as drugs, ethanol, tryptophan)

Causes of L-lactic acidosis
- The cause of type A is usually hypoxia (acute problem).
- The cause of type B is usually a liver problem (can be chronic).
- The treatment depends on the cause; in type A, H⁺ production must be stopped (increase O_2 delivery to tissues).

Quantitative Aspects

In type A L-lactic acidosis, the rate of H⁺ production is close to 72 mmol/min with total body anoxia. Hypoxia rather than anoxia is usually the case; thus, survival for more than a few minutes depends entirely on delivering more O_2 to hypoxic tissues. To develop L-lactic acidosis, a supply of glucose is needed. The major endogenous source of glucose is hepatic glycogen, but the glycogen in skeletal muscle can be converted to L-lactic acid if there is a specific stimulus for glycogenolysis in muscle (e.g., a sprint).

L-Lactic acidosis and malignancy
- Malignant cells produce more L-lactic acid than do normal cells under aerobic conditions (mechanism unknown). More L-lactic acid will be produced if the tumor outgrows its blood supply or if there is a nutritional deficit (thiamine).
- Low removal of L-lactate is usually a liver problem resulting from replacement of mass or inhibition of gluconeogenesis by tumor products.
- Drugs used for therapy can aggravate L-lactic acidosis. Even adding $NaHCO_3$ can increase the production of L-lactic acid.

QUESTION

(Discussion on page 148)

3.11 *If a patient has hypoxia but little glycogen in the liver, will L-*

lactic acidosis develop? If not, what changes would you expect to find in the concentration of metabolites in blood?

Diagnosis

The diagnosis of type A L-lactic acidosis must be made quickly because of the high rate of H^+ production or, more likely, the failure to generate ATP quickly enough. This form of L-lactic acidosis is easily established on the basis of the clinical setting of low O_2 content (severe anemia or cyanosis) or, much more commonly, on very poor delivery of O_2 to tissues (shock). There may also be symptoms of ischemia in one region of the body. However, for a severe degree of L-lactic acidosis, the patient must also be hypotensive because of the following:

1. With local arterial inflow obstruction, the reduction in O_2 delivery is accompanied by a reduction in the delivery of glucose, the precursor of L-lactic acid;
2. A normally perfused liver yields glucose at a reasonable rate via metabolism of L-lactic acid.

In type B L-lactic acidosis, the diagnosis may be less obvious. There is usually evidence of a liver problem or of the intake of drugs that interfere with hepatic metabolism. Alternatively, there may be signs of a very large tumor load. In addition, the other causes of metabolic acidosis associated with an increase in the plasma anion gap should be ruled out (see Table 3.1).

The diagnosis of types A and B L-lactic acidosis can be confirmed with an enzymatic determination of the plasma L-lactate concentration.

Treatment of L-Lactic Acidosis

> • In type A L-lactic acidosis, the rate of production of H^+ must be decreased.

Type A L-Lactic Acidosis

The only effective treatment of type A L-lactic acidosis is to stop the production of H^+ by increasing the delivery of O_2. Elevation of blood pressure is usually required if hypotension is present. Blood, plasma, and solutions containing Na^+ and/or albumin are required in many patients with an inadequate circulating volume, depending on the cause. In those patients with cardiogenic shock, myocardial function and thereby tissue perfusion should be improved. Less commonly, hypoxemia may require correction with O_2. Other considerations could include the resection of an ischemic area if it is necrotic; if not, restore its blood supply. Sepsis can cause several circulatory disturbances that lead to tissue hypoxia (it decreases O_2 delivery and interferes with O_2 extraction). Treatment of the vasodilation caused by sepsis may involve vigorous expansion of the circulating volume.

$NaHCO_3$ Therapy in Type A L-Lactic Acidosis. The use of $NaHCO_3$ in total anoxia is of little value because of the magnitude of the H^+ load (H^+ are produced at a rate of 72 mmol/min). Nevertheless, in cases in which hypoxia is marginal and potentially reversible, NaHCO$_3$ may "buy time" to improve myocardial function, although this issue remains controversial. The Na$^+$ load accompanying the HCO$_3^-$ poses a major limit to this type of therapy, and the use of loop diuretics is rarely very beneficial in this regard. If time permits, dialysis against a HCO$_3^-$ bath might be helpful. Hence, more imaginative adjuncts to therapy are required, and some of these are explored in the following questions.

QUESTIONS

(Discussions on pages 148–150)

3.12 *If NaHCO$_3$ was given as treatment for L-lactic acidosis and there was no rise in the plasma [HCO$_3^-$], was the alkali of no help to that patient?*

3.13 *Why might the rate of L-lactic acid production rise with alkali therapy?*

3.14 *What metabolic adaptations prolong survival in hypoxic environments?*

3.15 *Why is the L-lactic acidosis of exercise better tolerated than the L-lactic acidosis of shock, even if the former is more severe in degree?*

3.16 *Is a rise in L-lactic acid production beneficial or harmful to a patient with L-lactic acidosis?*

Type B L-Lactic Acidosis

> • Type B L-lactic acidosis does not have the same urgency as type A L-lactic acidosis because it is not associated with a problem in generating ATP; in addition, the rate of H$^+$ accumulation is much lower.

Ethanol-Induced L-Lactic Acidosis. One cause of L-lactic acidosis in an alcoholic is hepatic ethanol metabolism, which generates NADH and leads to the diversion of pyruvate to L-lactate (Figure 3.15). Ethanol metabolism must be ongoing for this form of L-lactic

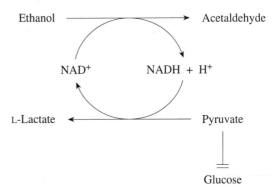

Figure 3.15   Ethanol-induced L-lactic acidosis. The metabolism of ethanol raises the NADH/NAD$^+$, which favors the conversion of pyruvate to L-lactate, not to glucose.

acidosis to occur; furthermore, because all other tissues can oxidize the L-lactate produced, the degree of L-lactic acidosis should be mild if ethanol metabolism is the sole cause. No specific treatment is required.

There are other ways that an alcoholic may develop L-lactic acidosis. For example, L-lactic acid can be produced at the time of a convulsion or extreme agitation, which occurs in delirium tremens. L-Lactic acid is removed at an extremely slow rate because of the ongoing oxidation of fat-derived fuels. Hence, this cause for overproduction of L-lactic acid might be remote from the clinical presentation.

A third cause of L-lactic acidosis in an alcoholic is thiamine deficiency.

L-Lactic Acidosis from Thiamine Deficiency. This form of L-lactic acidosis is entirely preventable by giving *thiamine*. The clinical setting in which this form of L-lactic acidosis is most prevalent is in the alcoholic patient or in the patient with an inadequate nutritional intake. The major danger is not the acidosis but rather the CNS lesion that is caused when glycolysis is accelerated to supply ATP that is no longer supplied by the oxidation of ketoacids. The rate of glycolysis accelerates when ketoacids disappear following a rise in insulin levels (after glucose and NaCl are given; see Figure 3.14).

Drug-Induced L-Lactic Acidosis. The drugs in question (see Table 3.12) accumulate if intake is high or excretion is low (especially when prerenal failure is caused by the use of metformin or phenformin). Although the degree of L-lactic acidosis may be severe, chances of survival are good. The measures required are neutralization of the excess H^+ with $NaHCO_3$, slowing of the H^+ production with insulin in the case of phenformin-induced L-lactic acidosis, acceleration of L-lactate metabolism (via *dichloroacetate*), and elimination of the offending drug by renal excretion or dialysis.

Thiamine (vitamin B₁)

A cofactor for pyruvate dehydrogenase (PDH). A deficiency of thiamine prevents glucose from being oxidized aerobically (Figure 3.14). Thiamine is also a component of 2-oxoglutarate dehydrogenase, a TCA-cycle enzyme; this enzyme is less affected by minor deficits of thiamine.

Dichloroacetate

A drug that activates PDH.

L-Lactic Acidosis Associated with Zidovudine Therapy

An interesting example of drug-induced L-lactic acidosis was described in patients with AIDS who were treated with zidovudine (AZT). Several hypotheses have been offered to explain the pathophysiology of this L-lactic acidosis. Many of these patients have a mitochondrial lesion: a mitochondrial myopathy with ragged red fibers and coarse granular deposits on histologic examination. Biochemical studies have shown that prolonged or high doses of AZT may induce a decrease in enzymes in the electron transport system of mitochondria. This pathophysiology is explored further in the discussions of Questions 3.17 and 3.18.

There is also a large number of conditions, many of them inborn errors of metabolism, that have in common a degree of L-lactic acidosis and the same characteristic findings on muscle biopsy sample: a mitochondrial myopathy. The general belief is that there is a defect in mitochondrial ATP generation; hence, more L-lactic acid accumulates when the glycolytic rate is high because of an increased demand for turnover of ATP (Table 3.13).

TABLE 3.13 **Possible Lesions in Lactic Acidosis with Mitochondrial Myopathy**

Associated with more severe L-lactic acidosis during exercise
- Inadequate generation of NADH aerobically in mitochondria
  Low activity of enzymes in the TCA cycle
  Failure to supply enough acetyl-CoA in mitochondria (low oxidation of fatty acids and/or pyruvate)
- Problem with utilizing NAD to make ATP
  Low activity of the electron transport system
  Problems with oxidative phosphorylation
  Problems with the adenine nucleotide transporter
  Uncouplers of oxidative phosphorylation

Not necessarily associated with more severe L-lactic acidosis during exercise
- Defect in redox transport such that the NADH/NAD$^+$ ratio in cytoplasm reflects that of mitochondria (Figure 3.16)

QUESTIONS

(Discussions on pages 150–151)

3.17 *A 34-year-old male patient with AIDS has extreme muscular weakness and chronic L-lactic acidosis related to AZT. A biopsy revealed a mitochondrial myopathy. When he exercises, his L-lactic acidosis does not become more severe. Did the lesion in his muscle mitochondria cause his L-lactic acidosis?*

3.18 *The L-lactic acidosis of the patient in Question 3.17 was greatly aggravated by ethanol intake. What might this effect of ethanol imply?*

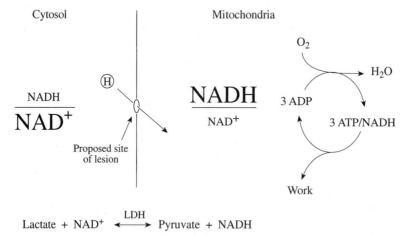

Figure 3.16 Possible defect in redox transport and L-lactic acidosis. This figure depicts the proposed site of the lesion induced by AZT. Normally, the NADH/NAD$^+$ ratio is much lower in the cytosol than in the mitochondria. This difference in ratio is maintained by an energy-dependent transport step in the inner mitochondrial membrane (glutamine/aspartate antiporter). Once the reducing power enters the mitochondria, it is transported down the electron transport system and leads to the conversion of ADP to ATP. Should the above barrier for reducing power be compromised, the high NADH/NAD$^+$ ratio in mitochondria might be "transmitted" to the cytosol and result in much higher L-lactate levels for a given concentration of pyruvate (the LDH reaction is close to thermodynamic equilibrium; LDH = lactate dehydrogenase). Reproduced with permission (*J. Am. Soc. Nephrol.* 3:1212–1219, 1992).

Organic Acid Load from the GI Tract (D-Lactic Acidosis)

Certain bacteria in the GI tract may convert carbohydrate (cellulose) into organic acids. Three factors lead to the overgrowth of bacteria and give them ample time to generate organic acids. First, slow GI transit (from blind loops, obstruction, drugs decreasing GI motility) leads to bacterial growth; second, a change of the normal flora, which occurs with antibiotic therapy, can lead to a large population of bacteria that can form D-lactic acid and other organic acids. Because humans metabolize the D-lactic acid isomer more slowly than L-lactate and production rates can be very rapid, a severe degree of acidosis can result. Third, if these bacteria have an adequate supply of nutrients, they may produce D-lactic acid at rates that exceed its removal. Hence, feeding of carbohydrate-rich food can aggravate D-lactic acidosis in a patient with GI bacterial overgrowth.

There are three additional points with respect to D-lactic acidosis:

1. The usual laboratory test for "lactate" is specific for the L-lactate isomer. Hence, with D-lactic acidosis, the laboratory report for "lactate" will not be elevated. To confirm this diagnosis, measure the plasma D-lactate concentration with a specific enzymatic assay.

2. GI bacteria produce amines and other compounds that may cause clinical symptoms related to central nervous system (CNS) dysfunction (personality changes, gait changes, confusion, etc.). Be wary of the diagnosis in the absence of CNS abnormalities.

3. Some of the D-lactate will be lost in the urine if the GFR is not too low. Hence, the degree of rise in the plasma anion gap may not be as high as expected for the fall in the plasma $[HCO_3^-]$.

Focus treatment on the GI problem, and ensure that the patients do not die of severe metabolic acidosis (give $NaHCO_3$ and possibly insulin or dichloroacetate, if necessary; see margin note).

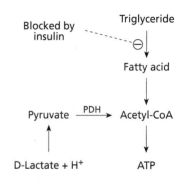

* PDH can be activated by dichloroacetate

QUESTIONS

(Discussions on pages 151–152)

3.19 *If the same number of bacteria are growing in the small bowel rather than the colon, why might more D-lactic acid be formed?*

3.20 *How many of these organic acids are produced each day in the colon?*

3.21 *What useful functions can be attributed to the production of organic acids in the colon?*

3.22 *What measures can be taken to "coax" the body to oxidize organic acids absorbed from the GI tract?*

Metabolic Acidosis Caused by Toxins

Those with an Increased Plasma Osmolal Gap

- Suspect the presence of toxins when an intoxicated patient has metabolic acidosis with an increased plasma anion gap.
- If the *plasma osmolal gap* is increased, treat the patient with ethanol.
- Confirm the diagnosis with a specific assay for the offending alcohols.

Methyl Alcohol (Methanol) Intoxication

Methanol is an inexpensive and widely available alcohol. Overall, methanol should always be suspected in the differential diagnosis of the cause of metabolic acidosis with an increased anion gap in plasma, especially if the ECF volume of the patient is not contracted and renal failure is not present. Methanol is nontoxic, but it is metabolized to a toxic product (formaldehyde) by alcohol dehydrogenase (Table 3.14). One ounce of methanol can yield 1000 mmol of formic acid; when methanol levels in blood exceed 50 mmol/L, 1 mmol of H^+ can theoretically be produced per minute (see the margin). The products of metabolism are particularly toxic to the CNS, especially the optic nerve because of its own alcohol dehydrogenase.

Therapy. The affinity of ethanol for alcohol dehydrogenase is 100-fold greater than either methanol or ethylene glycol. Therefore, the principle of therapy is to diminish the metabolism of methanol with ethanol and thus prevent formation of the toxic products

Plasma osmolal gap (measured osmolality − calculated osmolality)
Calculated osmolality = 2 × [Na⁺] + [glucose] + [urea], in mmol/L. If values are in mg/dL, convert [glucose] to mmol/L by dividing [glucose] by 18 and [urea] by 2.8 (see Table 2.3).

Methanol (wood alcohol)
An alcohol that is used as thinner for shellac and varnish, as windscreen and gasoline antifreeze, and as fuel for alcohol-burning devices.

Methanol → Formic Acid
One oz (32 mL) of methanol is close to 32 g. Because the molecular weight of methanol is 32, 1 oz of methanol can yield 1 000 mmol of formic acid. Hepatic alcohol dehydrogenase has a maximal activity of close to 7 000 mmol/day, but constraints on the removal of NADH will cause a much lower rate of H^+ production (<1 mmol/min).

TABLE 3.14 **Products of Metabolism of Ethanol, Methanol, and Ethylene Glycol**

Because ethanol is the preferred substrate, competition prevents the metabolism of methanol and ethylene glycol. Although ethylene glycol is not really an alcohol, it can be considered as a "dialcohol" because it has two adjacent carbons, each with an hydroxyl group. (AlcDH refers to hepatic alcohol dehydrogenase; AldDH refers to aldehyde dehydrogenase.)

Alcohol	AlcDH ⟶	Aldehyde	AldDH ⟶	Carboxylic Acid
Ethanol	⟶	Acetaldehyde	⟶	Acetic acid
Methanol	⟶	Formaldehyde	⟶	Formic acid
Ethylene glycol	⟶	Glycoaldehyde	⟶	Glycolic acid
				↓
				Glyoxylic acid
				↓
				Oxalic acid

formaldehyde and formic acid. In addition, the removal of methanol by dialysis must be promoted.

1. **Arrest methanol metabolism with ethanol:** Establish therapeutic ethanol levels (100 mg/dL or 22 mmol/L) by giving 0.6 g ethanol/kg intravenously or orally or give 4 oz whiskey orally. Maintain a therapeutic level of ethanol in the blood for the duration of the intoxication. Give chronic drinkers ethanol at a rate of 0.15 g/kg/h intravenously or 2 oz whiskey per hour orally. Give nondrinkers 0.07 g/kg/h intravenously or 1 oz whiskey per hour orally. Monitor the ethanol levels during therapy.

2. **Correct the acidemia:** At high blood methanol levels, acidemia may be severe, although the rate of production of formic acid is not usually that rapid in most cases. Nevertheless, if acidemia is severe, therapy with $NaHCO_3$ might be indicated.

3. **Remove methanol:** If levels of methanol exceed 50 mg/dL (15 mmol/L), dialysis should be instituted. Hemodialysis is most efficient, but, if not available, peritoneal dialysis removes some methanol. Ethanol, which is also removed by dialysis, must be replaced. Adding ethanol to the dialysate is the easiest way to ensure that adequate blood levels are maintained.

Ethylene Glycol (Antifreeze) Intoxication

> • Suspect ethylene glycol intoxication if the patient is intoxicated, has metabolic acidosis with an increased plasma anion gap and osmolal gap, oxalate crystals in the urine, and acute tubular necrosis.

Ethylene glycol, which is readily available, relatively inexpensive, and pleasant-tasting, might be ingested as an intoxicant. It causes fulminant metabolic acidosis, severe CNS toxicity, and acute tubular necrosis. As with methanol, toxicity results from the products of ethylene glycol metabolism (see Table 3.14). Following the initial toxicity associated with profound metabolic acidosis and CNS manifestations (confusion, coma, seizures), patients may develop congestive heart failure during therapy because of the large load of $NaHCO_3$ given coupled with acute renal failure. Those who survive usually have acute tubular necrosis that is generally of the oliguric form. Ethylene glycol intoxication should always be suspected in patients with metabolic acidosis and an increased plasma anion gap, especially if the patient appears intoxicated and denies intake of ethanol or if the odor of ethanol is not evident. The index of suspicion should be increased greatly by the finding of oxalate crystals in the urine. As with methanol, finding an increased plasma osmolal gap is helpful in the absence of ethanol (see the discussion of Question 3.23). The diagnosis is confirmed by detecting ethylene glycol in the blood.

Therapy. The principles of initial therapy using ethanol administration for ethylene glycol intoxication are identical to those for methanol (see margin note). The additional complication of acute tubular

Dose of ethanol
The ethanol in one bottle of beer (15 g) is 1/3 mole (mol wt 46) or close to 330 mmol. If all the ethanol were in the body, its concentration would be 10 mmol/L. Hence, the bolus for treatment is two bottles of beer.

Clinical pearls
• Suspect methanol intoxication if there is:
  1. a history of ingestion in an intoxicated patient;
  2. the sweet odor of methanol;
  3. an increased plasma osmolal gap in a patient with metabolic acidosis, or an increased plasma anion gap in a patient with a normal ECF volume and GFR.
  The diagnosis is confirmed by finding elevated levels of methanol in blood.
• Because chronic drinkers have higher levels of alcohol dehydrogenase, they may metabolize methanol more rapidly. They are therefore exposed to increased toxicity. On the other hand, if they have ingested ethanol as part of the intoxication, they will be protected as long as they have high ethanol levels in their blood.

Toxins from ethylene glycol
One product of the metabolism of ethylene glycol is oxalic acid. This acid precipitates as its Ca^{2+} salt and might be a basis of the development of acute tubular necrosis.

Kinetics of alcohol metabolism

If the concentration of alcohol is several times higher than the K_m, the enzyme proceeds at close to maximum velocity. As the concentration falls below the K_m, the rate of removal falls appreciably. Because the K_m for ethanol is 100-fold lower than for methanol or ethylene glycol, lower levels of ethanol prevent the metabolism of higher levels of methanol or ethylene glycol.

Methanol and ethylene glycol intoxications are characterized by higher rates of H^+ production at high blood levels; at blood levels below 40 mmol/L, rates decline appreciably. Therefore, at a low degree of intoxication, the agent can be removed by renal excretion without undergoing metabolism.

Note

If hippurate is excreted with K^+ that were derived from the ICF in conjunction with entry of Na^+ into cells, the ECF volume will be contracted further.

Note

Some patients with toluene intoxication have been reported to have a low rate of NH_4^+ excretion. In these cases, there is some other process that reduces either NH_3 availability in the renal medullary interstitium or distal nephron H^+ secretion. In these cases, hippurate will be excreted with Na^+ and K^+, and the urine net charge will be very positive (the sum of Na^+ and K^+ greatly exceeds Cl^-).

necrosis may limit the quantity of $NaHCO_3$ that can be given because the patient with this form of intoxication is generally oliguric. The use of nasogastric suction and pentagastrin stimulation of gastric acid secretion may lessen both the acidemia and the pulmonary edema while dialysis is being arranged (see pages 86–87). Early dialysis is critical because of the acute renal failure. All patients who have ingested this toxin should probably be dialyzed because of the toxicity. As with methanol, hemodialysis is the preferred means of removing ethylene glycol; however, if it is not available, peritoneal dialysis should be implemented. Again, ethanol levels should be maintained during hemodialysis by infusion or addition to the bath.

Those with a Normal Plasma Osmolal Gap

Toluene Inhalation (Glue-Sniffing)

- The patient who has sniffed glue has metabolic acidosis, but the plasma anion gap is usually not elevated appreciably.
- Hypokalemia is often present.
- There is an increased osmolal gap in the urine (NH_4^+ + hippurate).

Toluene intoxication has a variable presentation, depending on the clinical setting. Whereas these patients do not have an increased plasma osmolal gap, they share certain clinical and metabolic features with the alcohol intoxications. They might even "enter the back door" of this classification by having an increased plasma osmolal gap from ingestion of ethanol as part of their intoxication.

It has been recognized that the metabolic acidosis of toluene intoxication is indeed due to an acid load (hippuric acid); it had previously been incorrectly classified as distal renal tubular acidosis because of its frequent presentation as a normal plasma anion gap type of metabolic acidosis associated with hypokalemia and a urine pH close to 6.0.

Toluene is methylbenzene, a volatile compound that is inhaled during the sniffing of glue and that accumulates in fat. Its primary routes of removal are metabolism in the liver and exhalation via the lungs. For every mmol of toluene metabolized, 1 mmol of H^+ is added. Metabolism of toluene (Figure 3.17) leads to the formation of benzoic acid and the eventual excretion of hippurate in the urine. When hippurate is excreted in the urine, a cation—NH_4^+, K^+, or Na^+—must also be excreted. To the extent that hippurate is excreted with NH_4^+, the acid load is neutralized by renal production of HCO_3^-; excretion with K^+ will result in metabolic acidosis and hypokalemia. The excretion of hippurate with Na^+ will deplete the ECF volume and decrease the GFR. As a result, the rates of excretion of both NH_4^+ and hippurate will decrease; these low rates of excretion will prolong the acidemia and possibly increase the plasma anion gap (see margin note).

If Na^+ intake is maintained and ECF volume contraction is avoided, toluene intoxication should present as metabolic acidosis with a normal plasma anion gap. On the other hand, if ECF volume contraction is severe, hypokalemia might be significant, the plasma anion gap might increase, and the acidemia might be more severe (from reduced HCO_3^- generation that is due to decreased NH_4^+ excretion).

Despite the lack of an increased plasma anion gap, toluene intoxication causes acidemia from an organic acid load. The specific clue to the diagnosis—excretion of NH_4^+ at an increased rate—may be identified in different ways, depending on the cation(s) accompanying the hippurate (see the discussion of Question 3.25 and the associated margin note).

Therapy. Several therapies should be implemented simultaneously.

1. Correct the K^+ deficits, which may be profound.

2. Correct the ECF volume depletion by using a combination of NaCl and $NaHCO_3$. If hypokalemia is significant, delay aggressive $NaHCO_3$ therapy until the administration of K^+ because $NaHCO_3$ will aggravate the degree of hypokalemia.

3. In most cases, renal NH_4^+ excretion is enhanced, and the acidemia will therefore correct itself in several days without $NaHCO_3$ therapy. If the acidemia is severe at presentation, use some $NaHCO_3$ with the above caveat concerning the plasma $[K^+]$. If the acidemia persists for several days, reassess the rate of excretion of NH_4^+.

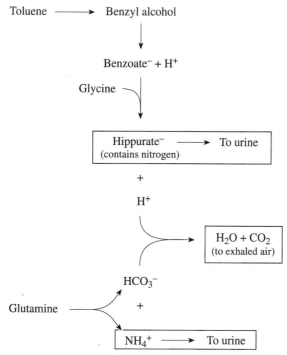

Figure 3.17   Metabolism of toluene. Metabolism of toluene occurs in the liver using a series of cytoplasmic enzymes, cytochrome P-450, alcohol, and aldehyde dehydrogenases. Hippuric acid is formed in hepatic mitochondria. When hippurate is excreted with NH_4^+, there is no acid-base impact. Reproduced with permission from *Clinical Detective Stories,* Portland Press Inc., London, 1993.

Hippurate excretion
Hippurate is excreted at a rapid rate (it is both filtered and secreted), but peak excretion is often 24 hours after exposure to toluene; this delay suggests the need for enzyme induction in the liver (cytochrome P-450). Those who sniff glue frequently have had enzyme induction and therefore may have more severe acidemia as a result of rapid metabolism.

QUESTIONS

(Discussions on pages 153–154)

3.23 *A 26-year-old intoxicated man is brought to the emergency room. His friends state that he ingested several ounces of methanol. Other than intoxication, his physical examination results were normal. His laboratory results were as follows:*

Na$^+$	mmol/L	142	[H$^+$]	nmol/L	40
K$^+$	mmol/L	3.7	Paco$_2$	mm Hg	40
Cl$^-$	mmol/L	105	Osmolality	mOsm/kg	360
HCO$_3^-$	mmol/L	25	Glucose	mmol/L (mg/dL)	7 (126)
Urea	mmol/L (mg/dL)	5 (14)	Albumin	g/L	40

Should one take the allegation of methanol seriously? Explain your reasoning. What should the course of action be?

3.24 *If oxalic acid were formed during the metabolism of ethylene glycol, why might the degree of metabolic acidosis be less severe?*

3.25 *What is the specific clue suggesting glue-sniffing as the diagnosis in a patient presenting with a normal plasma anion gap type of metabolic acidosis and hypokalemia?*

3.26 *What factors contribute to the hypokalemia and K$^+$ depletion in glue-sniffers?*

Salicylate Intoxication

> - Respiratory alkalosis usually accompanies ASA intoxication, but metabolic acidosis may be prominent in children.
> - The problem is ASA$^-$ levels in tissue.
> - The treatment is to promote excretion of ASA$^-$ and avoid both acidemia and severe alkalemia.

Note

ASA = acetylsalicylic acid

ASA$^-$ = salicylate anions

HASA = nonionized salicylic acid

Clinical note

Because the toxic level of ASA$^-$ is only 3–5 mmol/L, the plasma anion gap associated with a severe degree of metabolic acidosis is to a minor extent the result of ASA$^-$; ketoacid anions, L-lactate anions, and possibly other unidentified organic anions are the major causes for an elevated anion gap. Other findings could include adult respiratory distress syndrome, a bleeding disorder (low vitamin K), and hypokalemia.

Although ASA intoxication is very common, it rarely causes an appreciable degree of metabolic acidosis. When metabolic acidosis does occur, children are the most likely to be affected; the younger the child, the more likely the metabolic acidosis. The most common acid-base disturbance associated with ASA intoxication is respiratory alkalosis from central stimulation of respiration. Acid-base disturbances tend to accompany acute ASA intoxication but are less prominent in chronic ASA intoxication (see margin note).

Diagnosis. The diagnosis of ASA intoxication might be suspected from a history of ingestion or symptoms of tinnitus and lightheadedness and the presence of a respiratory alkalosis complicating the metabolic acidosis. The suspicion is increased by finding unexplained ketosis (ASA$^-$ activates hepatic lipase), hypouricemia (high-dose ASA$^-$ is uricosuric), and an increased urine net charge from ASA⁻ excretion (Na⁺ and K⁺ in urine greatly exceed Cl⁻). The diagnosis is confirmed by detecting ASA⁻ in the blood.

Treatment. Generally, metabolic acidosis is not a serious feature of ASA intoxication. Dialysis should be instituted for ASA⁻ levels above 90 mg/dL (6 mmol/L) and should be considered for levels greater than 60 mg/dL (4 mmol/L). In the absence of severe metabolic acidosis, the therapeutic efforts in ASA intoxication are to promote ASA⁻ excretion via the following maneuvers:

1. **Alkali therapy:** If the patient with ASA intoxication has metabolic acidosis, acidemia should be corrected because it increases the concentration of HASA in the blood. Because this uncharged form crosses cell membranes, its diffusion into brain cells is facilitated, and toxicity is promoted (Figure 3.18).

   In an analogous manner, an alkaline urine pH promotes ASA⁻ excretion by converting HASA to ASA⁻ and thereby retards HASA reabsorption by nonionic diffusion. The problem with aggressive HCO_3^- therapy is that the patient with respiratory alkalosis may become very alkalemic. In severe intoxications, hemodialysis or, in its absence, peritoneal dialysis should be used. Infusion of 1/2 isotonic saline containing 50 mmol of $NaHCO_3$ per liter at a rate of 300–500 mL/h may produce an alkaline diuresis. If the patient cannot tolerate that Na⁺ load, a loop diuretic may be used to promote Na⁺ excretion. The blood pH should be monitored hourly, and if it exceeds 7.55, 250 mg acetazolamide should be given to promote HCO_3^- excretion.

2. **Use of acetazolamide:** Acetazolamide, a carbonic anhydrase inhibitor, has been advocated in the therapy for ASA⁻ intoxication, supposedly because of its ability to alkalinize the urine (alkalinization of the urine should enhance ASA⁻ excretion; see Figure 3.18); however, its use has also been condemned. What are the issues? One detrimental effect relates to protein binding. Acetazolamide competes with ASA⁻ for binding to albumin and thus may enhance toxicity by increasing the free ASA⁻ concentration. Second, there is a possibility of inducing acidemia with acetazolamide by means of excess excretion of

Methyl salicylate (oil of wintergreen)
Ingestion of oil of wintergreen provides a large load of readily absorbed ASA⁻ and leads to toxic ASA⁻ levels. Treatment must be aggressive because patients can worsen "before your eyes."

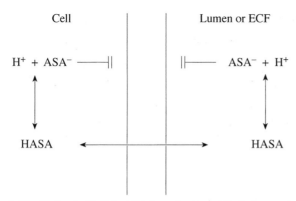

Figure 3.18   Role of alkali in ASA intoxication. Alkali therapy increases the concentration of ionized ASA⁻ in the lumen of the proximal convoluted tubule and in the ECF. This higher concentration should reduce diffusion of ASA⁻ + HASA into cells and thereby reduce the toxicity of ASA⁻ (the bulk of ASA⁻ is in the anionic rather than the HASA form).

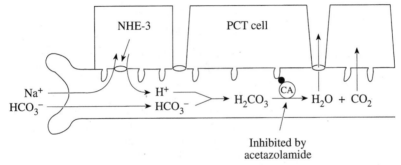

Figure 3.19   Acetazolamide and the decreased reabsorption of ASA⁻ in the proximal tubule. Acetazolamide inhibits the carbonic anhydrase (CA) on the luminal membrane of the PCT and thereby raises the $[H^+]$ in the lumen. Inhibition of ASA⁻ reabsorption is not due to tubular fluid alkalinization and is therefore more likely via another basis—perhaps inhibition of reabsorption on the organic acid transporter.

Increased ASA⁻ excretion with acetazolamide

In the proximal tubule, the impact of acetazolamide is to increase, not lower, the $[H^+]$ of tubular fluid via inhibition of luminal carbonic anhydrase; both the $[H^+]$ and $[HCO_3^-]$ rise (Figure 3.19).

HCO_3^- in the urine. Acidemia will increase the amount of nonionized HASA in the blood, so that more of this acid enters cells, and toxicity increases. On the other hand, the benefit is that acetazolamide enhances ASA⁻ excretion, but the mechanism may not be by nonionic diffusion as a result of alkalinization of the urine (see margin note).

Another important consideration is how much acetazolamide to use. The patient might develop acidemia from the HCO_3^- loss; acidemia will promote higher levels of ASA⁻ in brain cells and thereby increase toxicity. Measuring the levels of NH_4^+ in the urine indicates that 250 mg of acetazolamide has a tubular effect for 15–20 hours. Therefore, very little drug is necessary to achieve beneficial effects.

3. **Dialysis:** If levels of ASA⁻ exceed 60 mg/dL (4 mmol/L), dialysis should be considered, particularly if further absorption is anticipated. In patients with decreased levels of consciousness, dialysis should also be considered because of the poor prognosis. Hemodialysis is more efficient in removal of ASA⁻, but peritoneal dialysis can achieve substantial removal of this toxin.

QUESTION

(Discussion on page 154)

3.27 *Patients A, B, and C each have metabolic acidosis and an increased plasma anion gap. Which one has renal failure, which has methanol intoxication, and which has D-lactic acidosis?*

Patient		A	B	C
Calculated osmolality		290	290	320
2 × plasma [Na⁺]	mmol/L	280	280	280
Urea	mmol/L	5	5	35
Glucose	mmol/L	5	5	5
Measured osmolality		290	320	320

Metabolic Acidosis with a Normal Plasma Anion Gap

> - Classify metabolic acidosis with a normal plasma anion gap by renal response:
>   1. associated with increased loss of HCO_3^-;
>   2. associated with low excretion of NH_4^+.

The normal renal response to acidemia is to reabsorb all of the filtered HCO_3^- and to increase new HCO_3^- generation by increasing the excretion of NH_4^+ in the urine. When the metabolic acidosis is due to the inability of the kidney to respond normally to acidemia, the clues are easily found by assessing renal HCO_3^- reabsorption and NH_4^+ excretion. When either of these functions is compromised, there is a renal cause of metabolic acidosis that is termed *renal tubular acidosis* (RTA) (Table 3.15 and Figure 3.20).

TABLE 3.15 **Metabolic Acidosis with a Normal Plasma Anion Gap**

Excessive excretion of HCO_3^-
- Proximal RTA
- Acetazolamide ingestion

Increased excretion of NH_4^+
- Loss of HCO_3^- via the GI tract
- Ingestion of HCl or NH_4Cl
- Overproduction of acids with the rapid excretion of their conjugate base
  Glue-sniffing
  Ketoacidosis with marked ketonuria
- After hypocapnia

Low excretion of NH_4^+ (distal RTA)
- Reduced NH_3 available in the medullary interstitium
  Decreased ammoniagenesis (from a low GFR or hyperkalemia)
  Medullary interstitial disease
- Reduced collecting duct H^+ secretion
  H^+ pump "failure"
  H^+ back-leak (lumen to cell)
  Failure of voltage augmentation of distal H^+ secretion

Increased Renal NH_4^+ Excretion

An increased excretion of NH_4^+ is identified by either a negative urine net charge (urine $[Cl^-]>[Na^+] + [K^+]$) or a high urine osmolal gap (Chapter 2, pages 59–60). These patients have a "non-renal" basis of their metabolic acidosis because the enhanced renal NH_4^+ excretion should be sufficient to prevent metabolic acidosis from developing from the normal daily H^+ load derived from the diet.

Gastrointestinal HCO_3^- Loss

Diarrhea, unless more than 4 L per day, is not sufficient to cause a significant degree of metabolic acidosis because the normal kidney can generate 200 mmol of HCO_3^- per day as a result of enhanced excretion of NH_4^+ (stimulated by hypokalemia and/or a mild degree of chronic metabolic acidosis). Accordingly, the three factors associ-

Difficulty with proximal RTA
In proximal RTA, the excretion of NH_4^+ is much lower than expected for the degree of chronic acidemia. The acidosis is caused by:
- low reabsorption of HCO_3^-;
- relatively low excretion of NH_4^+.

Laxative abuse
Patients who abuse laxatives may not admit to their habit and thus present a diagnostic challenge, a disorder that resembles distal RTA. The problem is resolved by the presence or absence of a low rate of excretion of NH_4^+. With metabolic acidosis due to laxatives, the urine NH_4^+ excretion rate should be high.

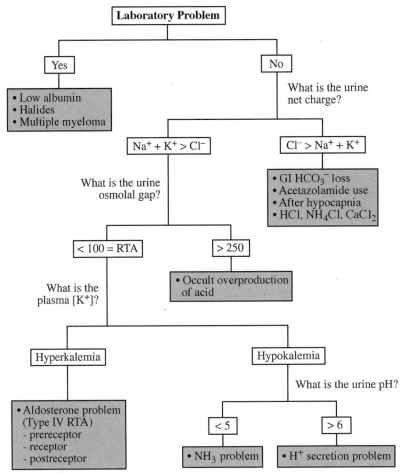

Figure 3.20   Approach to the patient with metabolic acidosis and a normal plasma anion gap. See Figures 3.21, 3.25, 3.26, and 3.27 for further details.

Distal RTA vs diarrhea

Patients with diarrhea often have hypokalemia, ECF volume depletion, a mild degree of metabolic acidosis, and a urine pH that is close to 6.0; therefore, their condition could be confused with distal RTA. Again, the difference is the low rate of excretion of NH_4^+ in distal RTA.

ated with a severe degree of metabolic acidosis in the patient with diarrhea are copious diarrhea, reduced rates of NH_4^+ excretion, and excessive production of organic acids by bacteria in the GI tract. Diarrhea is easily diagnosed; pooling of HCO_3^--rich fluid in the bowel lumen (ileus), however, may not be so evident.

QUESTION

(Discussion on pages 154–155)

3.28 *An 80-year-old man with a history of "pyelonephritis" developed diarrhea after a course of antibiotics. On the basis of the following results, a diagnosis of distal RTA was made. Is it correct?*

Plasma			Urine		
Na^+	mmol/L	134	Na^+	mmol/L	10
K^+	mmol/L	2.8	K^+	mmol/L	40
Cl^-	mmol/L	115	Cl^-	mmol/L	100
HCO_3^-	mmol/L	10	Osmolality	mmol/L	800
H^+	mmol/L	62	Urea	mmol/L	300
pH		7.20	pH		5.9

Acid Ingestion

If the anion of an acid is Cl^-, its intake can cause metabolic acidosis with no increase in the plasma anion gap. HCl, NH_4Cl, lysine$^-$, and arginine-HCl may cause this disorder.

Other Causes

There are several situations in which a patient can have metabolic acidosis with a normal plasma anion gap, no overproduction of acids, and a high rate of excretion of NH_4^+. One example is a subject who ingests acetazolamide, which causes bicarbonaturia. A second example is recovery from chronic hypocapnia. With chronic hypocapnia, there is suppression of renal NH_4^+ excretion, and the plasma $[HCO_3^-]$ will fall. The patient is not acidemic initially because of the low $Paco_2$. When the stimulus for hyperventilation is removed, the $Paco_2$ will rise. The $[HCO_3^-]$ will then be low, and metabolic acidosis with a normal anion gap will be present; NH_4^+ excretion should rise from the stimulus of acidemia. Within a few days, the enhanced renal new HCO_3^- generation will return the plasma $[HCO_3^-]$ to normal. A third example is the so-called expansion acidosis. When the ECF volume is expanded with solutions lacking HCO_3^- (isotonic saline), the plasma $[HCO_3^-]$ will fall. To understand this occurrence, one must distinguish between HCO_3^- content and HCO_3^- concentration in the ECF. In the following table, the patient described had a normal plasma $[HCO_3^-]$ despite severe ECF volume contraction; thus, the HCO_3^- content in the ECF was reduced, but this reduction might not have been appreciated (line 2). Reexpansion of the ECF volume with normal saline (a HCO_3^--free solution) made the reduced HCO_3^- content evident because the $[HCO_3^-]$ was now lower (line 3). For the $[HCO_3^-]$ to return to normal in this patient, the patient must either make new HCO_3^- (excrete NH_4^+) or receive $NaHCO_3$.

Condition	ECF Volume (L)	$[HCO_3^-]$ (mmol/L)	HCO_3^- Content (mmol)
Normal	15	24	360
Contracted ECF volume	10	24	240
Restored ECF volume	15	16	240

Inadequate Indirect Reabsorption of Filtered HCO_3^- (Proximal RTA)

The diagnosis of proximal RTA hinges on the demonstration of impaired indirect reabsorption of filtered HCO_3^- (Tables 3.16 and 3.17). Indirect reabsorption of filtered HCO_3^- is achieved by proximal tubular H^+ secretion. A defect in this H^+ secretion results in a metabolic acidosis with no increase in the plasma anion gap and is due initially to the excretion of $NaHCO_3$ in the urine (called proximal RTA or type II RTA). Later on, the acidosis is maintained because the rate of excretion of NH_4^+ is low considering the fact

NH_4^+ excretion in proximal RTA
The excretion of NH_4^+ is on the low side in most patients with proximal RTA unless there is a second cause for metabolic acidosis (e.g., chronic diarrhea), in which case the rate of excretion of NH_4^+ may rise towards the expected rate.

TABLE 3.16 **Diagnostic Features in Proximal RTA**

The filtered load of HCO_3^- is 4500 mmol/day (see the margin). In all of the examples below, the GFR is presumed to remain normal at 180 liters/day. The major lesion in proximal RTA is reduced proximal H^+ secretion (lines 2–4). Since distal H^+ secretion is of low capacity, all the extra HCO_3^- delivered are not reabsorbed, and the urine pH is >7.0. If an extra acid load is present, NH_4^+ excretion can rise and augment new HCO_3^- formation (line 4).

State	Filtered HCO_3^-	Proximal HCO_3^- Reabsorbed	Distal HCO_3^- Delivery*	HCO_3^- Excretion	NH_4^+ Excretion
			(mmol/day)		
Normal	4500	4000	500	0	30
Proximal RTA					
Onset	4500	3000	1500	>100	0
Established	3600	3000	600	0	20
+ Acid load	3000	2700*	300	0	60

*We assume that distal HCO_3^- delivery must be at least 300 mmol/day, so only half 2700 mmol of HCO_3^- can be absorbed proximally when an extra acid load is given.

Fanconi's syndrome
A defect in proximal tubular reabsorption that leads to glycosuria, aminoaciduria, increased excretion of uric acid and phosphate, and proximal RTA.

Calculation
Normal filtered load of HCO_3^-
= GFR × plasma $[HCO_3^-]$
= 180 L/day × 25 mmol/L
= 4500 mmol/day.

Excretion of citrate
Citrate disappears from the urine in patients with metabolic acidosis. The sole exception to this rule is patients with proximal RTA.

that chronic metabolic acidosis is present and the urine pH is low (see margin note). The H^+ secretory defect may be isolated, but if it occurs in concert with other transport defects, the *Fanconi syndrome* may be the appropriate diagnosis.

Distal H^+ secretion does not have the capacity to reabsorb all the HCO_3^- delivered as a result of the proximal deficit in H^+ secretion, and HCO_3^- excretion ensues if $NaHCO_3$ is given. Notwithstanding, patients with this disorder in steady state have a chronic metabolic acidosis, no bicarbonaturia, and a low excretion of NH_4^+ with a very low urine pH.

Possible Basis of the Findings in Proximal RTA

Possibly, the proximal cells of patients with proximal RTA have a defect that makes these cells uniquely more alkaline. This hypothesis could explain the cardinal features of low reabsorption of HCO_3^-: low synthesis of NH_4^+ despite chronic metabolic acidosis, and a high *excretion of citrate* (unique in metabolic acidosis with

TABLE 3.17 **Conditions Leading to Decreased Indirect Bicarbonate Reabsorption in the Proximal Convoluted Tubule**

Proximal RTA
- Fanconi's syndrome
  Genetic disorders, including cystinosis, galactosemia, hereditary fructose intolerance, Wilson's disease, Lowe's syndrome, tyrosinemia
  Toxin-induced disorders from exogenous toxins (including heavy metals, outdated tetracycline, streptozocin) and endogenous toxins (dysproteinemias, including multiple myeloma, etc.)
  Other disorders, including sporadic, transient proximal RTA of infants
  Disorders secondary to other renal diseases, including amyloidosis, renal transplantation, autoimmune diseases such as chronic active hepatitis, Sjögren's syndrome, etc.
- Isolated proximal RTA
- Combined proximal and distal RTA in carbonic anhydrase II deficiency.

Carbonic anhydrase inhibitors

Other conditions
- Hyperparathyroidism, hypocalcemia, vitamin D deficiency

acidemia). Finally, it could help explain the absence of medullary nephrocalcinosis in untreated patients with isolated proximal RTA.

Technique to Diagnose Proximal RTA

When the patient is acidemic, correct any deficit for K^+ and then administer $NaHCO_3$ and monitor the plasma $[HCO_3^-]$ and urine pH. If the urine pH becomes alkaline (>7.0) while the plasma $[HCO_3^-]$ remains low, impaired proximal H^+ secretion may be present. With continued HCO_3^- administration, the urine pH rises further, and distal H^+ secretion can be assessed by measuring the urine P_{CO_2} (see Chapter 2, pages 60–61, and Figure 3.21). Finally, in patients with proximal RTA, the $[HCO_3^-]$ in plasma falls promptly to subnormal levels once the infusion stops. The *fractional excretion of* HCO_3^- should be measured at this point; it will be greater than 15% in proximal RTA.

Urine pH, $[HCO_3^-]$, and $[NH_4^+]$ in proximal RTA
Because patients are in steady state, 24-hour net acid excretion in proximal RTA is the same as in normal individuals (i.e., HCO_3^- gain equals HCO_3^- loss but at a lower plasma $[HCO_3^-]$). Given these patients' lower urine NH_4^+ excretion, they need either a lower urine pH to have more titratable acid excretion and/or they must have a lower rate of excretion of organic anions to achieve acid-base balance.

Fractional excretion of HCO_3^-

$$\frac{[HCO_3^-]_{urine}/[HCO_3^-]_{plasma}}{[creatinine]_{urine}/[creatinine]_{plasma}}$$

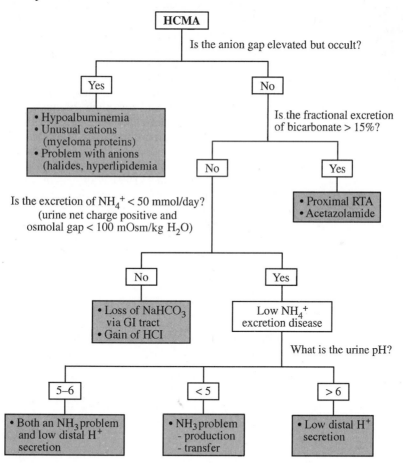

Figure 3.21   Approach to the diagnosis of RTA. The final diagnoses are shown in the shaded boxes. Reproduced with permission from *The ACID truth and BASIC facts with a Sweet Touch, an enLYTEnment*, 4th ed. RossMark Medical Publishers, 1998, Stirling, Ont., Canada. (HCMA = hyperchloremic metabolic acidosis.)

QUESTIONS

(Discussions on page 155)

3.29 *What are the diagnostic features of disorders with reduced indirect reabsorption of filtered* HCO_3^- *?*

3.30 *If a patient with metabolic acidosis is taking acetazolamide, how will the urine test results change once this diuretic is no longer acting (but metabolic acidosis persists)?*

Reduced Renal NH_4^+ Excretion (Distal RTA)

> • In distal RTA, there is metabolic acidosis and an NH_4^+ excretion defect from:
> 1. low NH_3 availability in the renal medullary interstitium;
> 2. low H^+ secretion in the collecting duct.

Distal RTA represents a heterogeneous group of disorders characterized by reduced excretion of NH_4^+ and failure to regenerate the needed HCO_3^- (consumed by the daily H^+ load). Although a number of titles have been applied to these defects (type I RTA, type IV RTA), the authors do not use them because they provide no etiologic insight and in fact may mislead the reader into grouping lesions with different pathophysiologies (Table 3.18).

A high urine pH has been proposed by some as the gold standard in the diagnosis of distal RTA; the authors discourage this approach because the urine pH may sometimes be misleading (Figure 3.22). The urine pH is certainly useful in identifying bicarbonaturia (pH >7.0), which helps in the diagnosis of proximal RTA. Also, a very low urine pH (<5.0) in a patient with metabolic acidosis and a low rate of excretion of NH_4^+ strongly suggests low availability of NH_3 as the basis of the defect. The authors' approach to the differential diagnosis of distal RTA is shown in Figure 3.21. The biologic importance of the urine pH relates to the risk of formation of kidney stones (see page 127).

TABLE 3.18 **Nomenclature Used in the Classification of RTA**

The authors prefer a classification based on the pathophysiology rather than numerical labels.

Lesion: Reduced indirect reabsorption of filtered HCO_3^-	
Current	**Preferred**
• Type II RTA or proximal RTA	• Proximal H^+ secretory defect
Lesion: Low excretion of NH_4^+	
Current	**Preferred**
• Type I RTA, distal RTA, or classic RTA	• Decreased NH_4^+ excretion from: Low medullary NH_3 concentration Low net distal H^+ secretion
• Type IV RTA	• Decreased NH_4^+ excretion related to hyperkalemia

Decreased [NH_3] in the Medullary Interstitium

There are two ways to examine why the rate of excretion of NH_4^+ is low (Table 3.19; see margin note). Hyperkalemia and a very low GFR are the most common causes of a reduced ammoniagenesis; medullary diseases such as pyelonephritis and analgesic nephrotoxicity are common causes of medullary dysfunction. The distinctive features are metabolic acidosis and a normal plasma anion gap, low rates of NH_4^+ excretion, and a low urine pH (arbitrarily set at

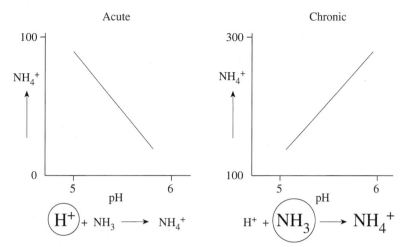

Figure 3.22   **Urine pH and the excretion of NH_4^+.** In acute acidosis, the rate of NH_4^+ excretion is higher when the urine pH is lower; the increased $[H^+]$ traps more NH_3 in the lumen as NH_4^+. Thus, the rate of H^+ secretion exceeds that of NH_3. In chronic metabolic acidosis, both the H^+ secretory rate and the NH_3 availability are greatly increased. The increase in NH_3 is due to augmented ammoniagenesis and is relatively larger than the increment in H^+ secretion. Thus, the urine NH_4^+ excretion rate is increased in conjunction with a higher urine pH because of the increased trapping of H^+ by NH_3. Note the difference in scale for NH_4^+, as shown on the y-axis of each panel.

<5.3). These patients can have a very low urine pH (often <5.0) because the H^+ secretory mechanism of their collecting ducts may be normal. Nevertheless, because they have little NH_3 available to bind the free H^+, they have a reduced overall capacity to excrete NH_4^+. Therefore, despite the low urine pH, there is very little renal H^+ excretion. This normal H^+ secretory mechanism may be revealed by finding a high urine P_{CO_2} with alkali loading (Chapter 2, pages 60–61).

TABLE 3.19   **Causes for a Low Rate of Excretion of NH_4^+ in a Patient with Metabolic Acidosis**

Patients in group 1 will be prone to have a low urine pH, and the urine pH will tend to be greater than 6.0 in patients in group 2.

1. Low $[NH_3^-]$ in the renal medullary interstitium
Low production of NH_4^+ in the proximal convoluted tubule
• Low turnover of ATP (low GFR, i.e., renal failure)
• Hyperkalemia
• Low availability of glutamine (e.g., malnutrition)
• High availability of fat-derived fuels (e.g., total parenteral nutrition)
• Alkaline cell (possibly isolated proximal RTA)

Problems with functions in the loop of Henle
• Interstitial diseases, *hyperkalemia* (see Figure 1.19)

2. Low transfer of NH_3 into the lumen of the collecting duct

H^+ATPase units with low activity
• Medullary destruction
• Inhibition by immune complexes (e.g., Sjögren's disease)

H^+ATPase units without a stimulator
• Less lumen negative voltage (e.g., Cl^- shunt, possibly lithium, amiloride)
• Low aldosterone bioactivity
• Alkaline intercalated cell (e.g., defect anion exchanger for Cl^-/HCO_3^-)

Back-leak of H^+
• Amphotericin B

Notes
• There are two factors that lead to a low rate of excretion of NH_4^+: a low $[NH_3]$ in the renal medulla and a low transfer of NH_3 into the lumen of the collecting duct (i.e., low H^+ secretion in the collecting duct).
• There are two reasons for a low $[NH_3]$ in the medullary interstitium: a low production of NH_4^+ and/or a defect in medullary function.

Decreased Transfer of NH₃ to the Lumen of the Collecting Duct

Less NH_3 is transferred to the lumen of the collecting duct as a result of defects in the H^+ secretory mechanism of the collecting duct. These defects can be considered in four subgroups; examples of each subgroup are shown in Table 3.20.

1. Problems with the H^+ATPase pump.

2. Problems with voltage augmentation of this pump.

3. Low NH_3 availability to neutralize luminal H^+ (a high luminal $[H^+]$ lessens H^+ pumping).

4. An abnormal back-leak of H^+ from the lumen into the cell.

These four subgroups have in common a low rate of NH_4^+ excretion. All but the third group tend to have a high urine pH (>6.0). Groups 1 and 2 can also be distinguished because patients with these problems should have a low urine PCO_2 (<50 mm Hg) in alkaline urine, yet the urine PCO_2 in the other groups should exceed 70 mm Hg. The low-voltage stimulation group tends to have reduced Na^+ reabsorption in the collecting duct, a problem that also interferes with K^+ excretion (a low transtubular $[K^+]$ gradient; see Figure 9.11); these patients therefore have hyperkalemia, which lowers NH_4^+ production and excretion (see margin note).

Diseases involving the renal medulla can destroy collecting duct cells and thereby cause a low H^+ pump activity. Such a lesion also lowers NH_3 availability in the medullary interstitium. Hence, the excretion of NH_4^+ is low, but the urine pH can be less than 5.3 if the NH_3 defect predominates, greater than 6.0 if the H^+ secretory defect predominates, or between 5.0 and 6.0 if neither predominates. In fact, a urine pH of 5.5 would suggest a combined NH_3 and H^+ defect (see Figure 3.21).

Voltage augmentation of the H⁺ pump

H^+ secretion is "electrogenic" in that it renders the lumen voltage positive. It is enhanced by Na^+ reabsorption, which renders the transepithelial voltage negative. On the other hand, if Na^+ reabsorption is "electroneutral," i.e., accompanied by Cl^- reabsorption (Cl^- shunt), H^+ secretion will not be enhanced. This same principle applies to K^+ secretion, which takes advantage of the lumen negative potential difference to enhance its net secretion.

Note

See Case 3.6 for the authors' clinical approach to a patient with RTA.

TABLE 3.20 **Pathophysiologic Approach to Distal RTA**

Defect	Causes of Lesions	Diagnostic Features
H^+ATPase	• Mineralocorticoid deficiency • Medullary damage or infiltration • Immunological basis (e.g., Sjögren's syndrome) • Congenital disorders • Alkaline intercalated cell	Low urine PCO_2, High urine pH
Voltage augmentation of H^+ secretion	• Low distal Na^+ delivery (ECF volume contraction, congestive heart failure, cirrhosis) • Inhibitors of Na^+ reabsorption (e.g., amiloride, lithium, trimethoprim) • Lack of stimulation (e.g., aldosterone deficiency or blockade) • Excess Cl^- permeability	Hyperkalemia with a low transtubular $[K^+]$ gradient
Raising luminal $[H^+]$ by low NH_3 availability	• Low NH_4^+ production (e.g., hyperkalemia, low GFR) • Low medullary $[NH_3]$ (tubulointerstitial diseases)	Low urine pH
Back-leak of H^+	• Increased H^+ permeability (e.g., amphotericin B)	High urine pH, High urine PCO_2

Importance of the Plasma [K⁺] in the Diagnosis of Distal RTA

Hypokalemia. When the cause of distal RTA is low H⁺ secretion in the collecting duct rather than low NH_3 availability, hypokalemia is often present. This hypokalemia is due to an unexpectedly high rate of K⁺ excretion and is associated with a urine pH that is greater than 5.8 (see margin note).

Hyperkalemia. Hyperkalemia may be associated with metabolic acidosis and a low rate of NH_4^+ excretion (Table 3.21); this condition has also been referred to as *type IV distal RTA*. The basis of the reduced NH_4^+ excretion is inhibition of NH_4^+ production by hyperkalemia and low reabsorption of NH_4^+ in the thick ascending limb of the loop of Henle (see the discussion of Question 1.26).

Hyperkalemia and reduced H⁺ secretion coexist for several reasons (see Table 3.21, Table 3.22). Each circumstance can be identified by specific diagnostic features. First, there may be insufficient distal Na⁺ resorption because of low Na⁺ delivery to the "cortical distal nephron." As a result, aldosterone has a smaller quantity of Na⁺ on which to act, so that less secretion of K⁺ and H⁺ occurs here. The low rate of excretion of NH_4^+ should disappear when more Na⁺ are delivered distally (following an infusion of NaCl or the administration of a loop diuretic). A second subgroup has low aldosterone bioactivity and subsequent hyperkalemia. The low rate of NH_4^+ excretion may disappear when hyperkalemia is treated (see margin note). In yet other examples, there is a failure to generate a lumen-negative transtubular voltage. The most common of these

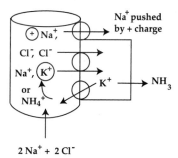

TABLE 3.21 **Hyperkalemia, Metabolic Acidosis, and Low Urine NH_4^+**

Cause	Features	Basis
Decreased Na⁺ reabsorption		
• Low distal delivery	• Urine [Na⁺] <10 mmol/L	• ECF volume depletion • Severe hypoalbuminemia • Congestive heart failure
• Decreased mineralocorticoid bioactivity	• Urine pH <5.3 as a result of hyperkalemia, which causes low NH_3 synthesis	• Hyporeninemia • Converting enzyme inhibitor • Aldosterone antagonists • Adrenal gland problem
Renal failure	• Low GFR	• Low NH_4^+ production
Decreased distal H⁺ secretion	• Urine pH >6.0	• Interstitial disease • Drugs (e.g., amiloride, lithium, trimethoprim) • Immune basis • Alkaline intercalated cell
Chloride shunt	• ECF volume expansion, • Low urine [K⁺], • Urine pH <5.3 as a result of hyperkalemia	• Dissipation of lumen negative transepithelial potential difference (possibly caused by cyclosporine)

TABLE 3.22 **Impaired Voltage Augmentation of H$^+$ and K$^+$ Secretion in the Collecting Duct**

Low distal Na$^+$ delivery
- ECF volume contraction
- Hypoalbuminemia, cirrhosis, nephrotic syndrome

Low aldosterone bioactivity
- Prereceptor defects (e.g., ACE inhibitor, problems with the adrenal gland or low renin)
- Receptor blockage (e.g., spironolactone)
- Postreceptor defects (e.g., amiloride, Cl$^-$ shunt)

Decreased end-organ function
- Interstitial nephritis
- Obstructive nephropathy

Mineralocorticoid deficiency and H$^+$ excretion

Mineralocorticoid deficiencies may bring about decreased NH$_4^+$ excretion by two different means, hyperkalemia and impaired Na$^+$ reabsorption, either of which may predominate.

1. Hyperkalemia may decrease the amount of NH$_3$ in the renal medullary interstitium; as a result, the urine pH will be low. NH$_4^+$ excretion will increase with reduction of the hyperkalemia.
2. Impaired Na$^+$ reabsorption results in a failure of voltage augmentation of H$^+$ secretion. Consequently, the urine pH will be greater than 6.0, the urine Pco$_2$ will not be appropriately elevated, and NH$_4^+$ excretion will not increase with a fall in the plasma [K$^+$] (NH$_4^+$ excretion will increase with hormone replacement, however, as will the transtubular [K$^+$] gradient).

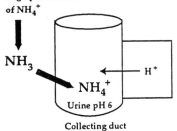

High production of NH$_4^+$

NH$_3$

NH$_4^+$ ← H$^+$

Urine pH 6

Collecting duct

Note

NH$_3$ is the major H$^+$ acceptor in the lumen of the collecting duct, preventing a fall in urine pH.

defects is the failure to reabsorb filtered Na$^+$ at the collecting duct because of a failure to respond to aldosterone or to the presence of drugs that block aldosterone action (e.g., amiloride). Less commonly, a Cl$^-$ shunt type of lesion might be present. The third subgroup is characterized by a renal medullary lesion that impairs medullary function.

Hyperkalemia and metabolic acidosis can also be present in renal failure (discussed in the following section).

Importance of the Urine pH

While it is commonplace to think of the urine pH in the context of acid-base physiology, this is too narrow a viewpoint. The issues are:

1. **Is a low urine pH commonly seen with chronic acidosis and the highest rate of excretion of NH$_4^+$?** In fact, the urine pH in subjects fed NH$_4$Cl on a chronic basis is close to 6, the same value as seen in patients with the chronic ketoacidosis of fasting or those with chronic diarrheal states. The urine pH is not low because the increase in the [NH$_3$] in the medullary interstitial fluid as a result of enhanced ammoniagenesis makes more NH$_3$ available to the collecting ducts than the number of H$^+$ that can be secreted by collecting duct cells (see margin note).

2. **Is a low urine pH required to have a high rate of excretion of NH$_4^+$?** A low urine pH simply lowers the [NH$_3$] in the lumen of the collecting duct so that a larger concentration difference for NH$_3$ can exist to favor the diffusion of NH$_3$ from the interstitial fluid to its lumen. The authors deliberately used a concentration difference, not a concentration gradient (ratio of concentration) term. The relative lack of importance of lowering the urine pH below 6.4 is shown in Figure 3.23. In fact, most of the benefit of this concentration difference is achieved by the time the urine pH reaches 6.4.

Bottom Line. Distal H$^+$ secretion lowers the urine pH and this, by lowering the [NH$_3$] in the lumen of the collecting duct, initiates the excretion of NH$_4^+$. Notwithstanding, the low urine pH is not a critical determinant of the rate of excretion of NH$_4^+$. From the point of view of diagnosis of why excretion of NH$_4^+$ is low, knowing the urine pH is useful to see the relative importance of the availability

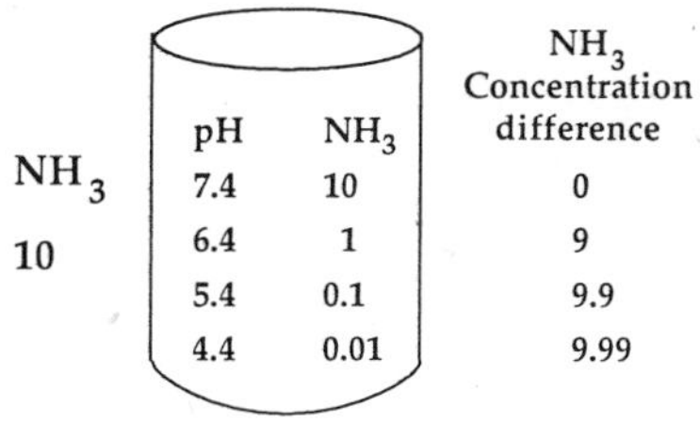

Figure 3.23 Importance of the urine pH for diffusion of NH$_3$. For simplicity, the authors set an arbitrary concentration of NH$_3$ as 10 and a pH of 7.4 in the interstitial fluid.

pH	NH$_3$	NH$_3$ Concentration difference
7.4	10	0
6.4	1	9
5.4	0.1	9.9
4.4	0.01	9.99

of NH$_3$ and distal H$^+$ secretion in a patient with a defect in the rate of excretion of NH$_4^+$.

Urine pH and the Likelihood of Renal Stone Formation

1. **Uric acid:** Uric acid is relatively insoluble as can be determined from bird droppings. The solubility of uric acid in the urine is close to 90 mg/L. Because a typical total urate excretion rate is 450 mg/day, one would need 5 L of urine a day to excrete uric acid if this were its only chemical form.

   The pK of uric acid is 5.3. This means that at a urine pH of 5.3, half of the uric acid will be in its salt form (urate). Hence, to favor the urate form, the urine pH must rise ([H$^+$] fall). For every 0.3 pH unit rise, the ratio of urate/uric acid doubles. Hence, at a urine pH of 5.9, one-fifth of the total urate + uric acid is in the insoluble uric acid form (90 of the 450 mg). Hence, only 1 L of urine at pH 5.9 is needed to dissolve the 450 mg of total urate (see margin note).

2. **Precipitation of Ca with phosphate:** This precipitate requires divalent phosphate. Given its pK of 6.8, as the urine pH approaches 6.8, the greater the likelihood of formation of these Ca stones (Ca oxalate stones, the most common ones, are independent of the urine pH).

Bottom Line. It is best to have a urine pH close to 6 to minimize the risk of renal stone formation. By adjusting the interstitial [NH$_3$], NH$_4^+$ excretion can be high at this urine pH.

Metabolic Acidosis in Renal Failure

- Metabolic acidosis in renal failure progresses slowly, is associated with an increased plasma anion gap, and is usually associated with hyperkalemia.

The acidemia associated with renal failure is due to the usual H$^+$ load from the diet (1 mmol/kg) coupled with a failure of the kidney to generate new HCO$_3^-$ from a reduced rate of synthesis and excretion of NH$_4^+$ (Figure 3.24). Because the body accumulates approximately 70 mmol of H$^+$ per day, the [HCO$_3^-$] can fall by approximately 2.3 mmol/L/day (see margin note). Nevertheless, this

Uric acid stones
- Most commonly seen when the urine pH is low.
  - Low NH$_4^+$ production (e.g., hyperkalemia)
  - Low medullary NH$_3$ (interstitial diseases).
- The best treatment is to give NaHCO$_3$ to raise the urine pH to 6.0.

Calculation
A 70-kg person generates 70 mmol of H$^+$ daily. Approximately one-half is buffered in the ECF by the BBS. Therefore, 35 mmol is buffered in 15 L. The expected decline in plasma [HCO$_3^-$] is therefore 2.3 mmol/L/day when the plasma [HCO$_3^-$] is close to its normal range.

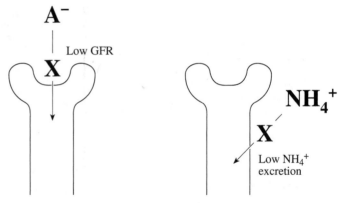

Figure 3.24 Basis of high plasma anion gap and acidosis in renal failure. The basis of the increased plasma anion gap (AG) is the low GFR with reduced excretion of anions such as phosphate or sulfate (left side). The acidosis is due to a low rate of excretion of NH_4^+ (right side).

amount is a gross overestimate of the rate of H^+ accumulation in patients with chronic renal insufficiency because they still have residual net acid excretion.

The increase in the plasma anion gap is a result of the reduced GFR, with accumulation of anions (e.g., HPO_4^-) (see Figure 3.24). Usually the anion gap does not rise appreciably until the GFR has fallen to 20% of normal. If one compares the magnitude of the dietary H^+ load with the degree of reduction in NH_4^+ excretion and in the GFR, one can see discrepancies between the degree of increase in the plasma anion gap and the magnitude and rate of fall of the plasma $[HCO_3^-]$.

The acidemia of renal failure may be complicated by hyperkalemia. Whereas both the acidemia and the hyperkalemia will improve after treatment with $NaHCO_3$, patients with renal failure often have an expanded ECF volume; therapy with $NaHCO_3$ may therefore be hazardous without an option for Na^+ removal.

PART D

Review

DISCUSSION OF INTRODUCTORY CASE
To Make a Diagnosis, Step on the Gas
(Case presented on page 75)

What is (are) your acid-base diagnosis(es)?

Lee has a mixed acid-base disorder: metabolic acidosis ($[HCO_3^-]$ = 5 mmol/L with acidemia) and respiratory acidosis (during acidemia, a $[HCO_3^-]$ of 5 mmol/L should be accompanied by a PCO_2 of 20 mm Hg, not 30 mm Hg).

What would the plasma [H⁺] be if the respiratory response were appropriate?

If the P_{aCO_2} were the expected 20 mm Hg, the [H⁺] would be 96 nmol/L instead of 144 nmol/L (a blood pH of 7.02 instead of 6.84).

What are the likely causes for the metabolic acidosis in Lee?

Lee has a normal plasma anion gap and therefore has lost $NaHCO_3$. Suspect either reduced renal new HCO_3^- generation (low excretion of NH_4^+) or $NaHCO_3$ loss via the GI tract or the urinary tract.

What is the significance of the hypokalemia?

Hypokalemia, unusual among the other causes of metabolic acidosis, is an important diagnostic clue. It suggests that the basis of the metabolic acidosis is most likely a reduced rate of renal NH_4^+ excretion or severe diarrhea. There are two other important aspects of hypokalemia: first, hypokalemia can lead to a cardiac arrhythmia and/or muscle weakness; second, as discussed in the following question, it must be dealt with during treatment because it is likely to become more severe once the acidemia lessens in severity. With hypokalemia, $NaHCO_3$ therapy may be dangerous if it is not accompanied by aggressive K⁺ replacement. In this case, the hypokalemia impairs respiratory muscle function and therefore contributes to the severe acidemia. If the hypokalemia is not treated as aggressively as the acidemia, respiratory arrest may occur.

As HCO_3^- appear in the ECF, H⁺ exit from cells, and, to the extent that K⁺ enter the ICF, the degree of hypokalemia could become much more severe. In patients with metabolic acidosis and a normal plasma anion gap, therapy with $NaHCO_3$ may ultimately be more essential than in patients with an increased plasma anion gap because metabolism of the unmeasured organic anions in the latter case leads to generation of HCO_3^-.

Must all patients with metabolic acidosis have a high plasma [H⁺]?

No. Acidemia is not always present during metabolic acidosis; a coexistent metabolic or respiratory alkalosis may reduce the plasma [H⁺] to a normal or abnormally low value in a patient with metabolic acidosis. Metabolic acidosis and metabolic alkalosis are independent events, not mirror images. Consider the following example: a patient vomits and develops metabolic alkalosis with ECF volume contraction. As vomiting continues, the patient goes into shock and produces L-lactic acid. Although the blood pH is closer to normal, this patient is closer to death.

Can a patient have a low plasma [HCO_3^-] and not have metabolic acidosis?

Yes. If the P_{aCO_2} is lowered by hyperventilation, the bicarbonate buffer equation is shifted to the right; the result is a lower [H⁺] and [HCO_3^-] (i.e., respiratory alkalosis).

Is it possible to have a persistently alkaline urine (i.e., no renal HCO_3^- generation) and maintain acid-base balance?

Henderson equation

$$H^+ = \frac{24}{[HCO_3^-]} \times P_{CO_2}$$
$$= \frac{24}{5} \times 20 = 96$$

Indirect loss of $NaHCO_3$

Patients with reduced renal NH_4^+ excretion will have a low urine negative net charge, whereas patients with GI $NaHCO_3$ loss will have a large excretion of NH_4^+ and usually a large urine negative net charge.

Note

Suppression of the expected hyperventilation due to muscular weakness was life-threatening, demanding acute attempts to lower the P_{aCO_2} and aggressive therapy for the hypokalemia.

Yes. Renal HCO_3^- generation is essential in maintaining acid-base balance only if there is ongoing net HCO_3^- consumption (i.e., a dietary H^+ load). If one consumes a diet that does not present an acid load (e.g., certain vegetarian diets), acid-base balance is maintained without renal HCO_3^- generation; in fact, maintaining this balance now requires organic anion excretion in the urine.

Cases for Review

CASE 3.1
Ken Has a Drinking "Problem"
(Case discussed on pages 136–137)

A 26-year-old man consumed an excessive quantity of alcohol during the past week; in the last 2 days, he has eaten little and has vomited on many occasions. He has no history of diabetes mellitus. Physical examination reveals marked ECF volume contraction. Alcohol is detected on his breath. The laboratory data are as follows:

Blood			Plasma		
Glucose	mmol/L (mg/dL)	5 (90)	Na^+	mmol/L	140
BUN	mmol/L (mg/dL)	10 (28)	K^+	mmol/L	3.0
pH		7.30	Cl^-	mmol/L	93
H^+	mmol/L	50	HCO_3^+	mmol/L	15
Pa_{CO_2}	mm Hg	30			
			Ketones		Strongly positive

What is the total body Na^+ content?
Is there relative insulin deficiency?
Why is the patient hypokalemic, and to what degree is he K^+-depleted?
What are the acid-base diagnoses?
What are the primary considerations for therapy?
The plasma osmolality is 350 mOsm/kg H_2O. Is the ICF volume high, low, or normal?
When ethanol is no longer present, what changes will be observed in the metabolic picture?

CASE 3.2
An Unusual Type of Ketoacidosis
(Case discussed on pages 137–138)

A 21-year-old woman has had diabetes mellitus for 2 years and requires insulin. Six months ago, she presented with lethargy, malaise, headaches, and metabolic acidosis with a normal plasma anion gap. Her complaints and the acid-base disturbance have persisted for 6 months, so she was referred for further evaluation. She denies a past history of diarrhea, abdominal complaints, or ingestion of drugs (acetazolamide, halides, or HCl equivalents). She has no past history of renal disease.

While taking her usual 34 units of insulin per day, she frequently had glycosuria and ketonuria but no major increase in the plasma anion gap. Her physical examination results were unremarkable, and her urinalysis showed no protein and a normal sediment. The results of her laboratory investigations are in the following table.

Plasma

Urea	mmol/L (mg/dL)	7 (20)	Na$^+$	mmol/L	136
Creatinine	μmol/L (mg/dL)	100 (0.9)	K$^+$	mmol/L	2.9
Glucose	mmol/L (mg/dL)	10.6 (190)	Cl$^-$	mmol/L	103
pH		7.35	HCO$_3^-$	mmol/L	19
[H$^+$]	nmol/L	45	Anion gap	mEq/L	14
Paco$_2$	mm Hg	35	β-HB	mmol/L	2.2

Urine

Glucose	mmol/L	5	Na$^+$	mmol/L	47
Urea	mmol/L	50	K$^+$	mmol/L	60
pH		5.3	Cl$^-$	mmol/L	13
Osmolality	mOsm/kg H$_2$O	680			

What is the differential diagnosis of her acid-base disorders?

What investigative plan would be appropriate?

Following the ingestion of NaHCO$_3$ and KCl, the plasma [HCO$_3^-$] rose to 26 mmol/L and did not fall promptly after the intake of HCO$_3^-$ was stopped; the urine Pco$_2$ was 90 mm Hg.

What is the diagnosis now?

Why was this patient hypokalemic?

CASE 3.3
Ketoacidosis: a Stroke of Bad Luck
(Case discussed on pages 138–139)

A 42-year-old man has two medical problems, hypertension and rare alcohol binges; he is not a chronic alcohol abuser. Last night he consumed half a bottle of whiskey. This morning he was found unconscious. Physical examination revealed coma and hemiparesis from an acute intracerebral hemorrhage. There was no ECF volume contraction. Laboratory results in plasma are summarized in the following table; these values were essentially unchanged 2 hours later (before therapy was initiated). He produced only a small amount of urine in this 2-hour period.

Plasma

pH		6.96	Glucose	mmol/L (mg/dL)	9.0 (162)
Paco$_2$	mm Hg	11	Urea	mmol/L (mg/dL)	5.0 (14)
HCO$_3^-$	mmol/L	3	Creatinine	μmol/L (mg/dL)	100 (0.8)
Anion gap	mEq/L	42	Osmolality	mOsm/kg H$_2$O	305
Na$^+$	mmol/L	139	Ethanol	mmol/L	20
K$^+$	mmol/L	6.8	Ketone	(screen)	moderate

What is (are) the most likely cause(s) for his metabolic acidosis?

Are acids being produced rapidly?

What hormonal changes were involved?

Why did ketoacidosis develop so quickly?

CASE 3.4
A Superstar of Severe Acidosis
(Case discussed on pages 139–140)

A patient who had walked into the emergency room was found to have astounding results of blood tests. Physical examination revealed a near-normal ECF volume and hyperventilation. Clinical and laboratory test results for alcohol were negative. His $[HCO_3^-]$ was 1 mmol/L, his pH was 6.69, and he had a markedly increased anion gap of 46 mEq/L. His GFR was not appreciably abnormal.

What are the most likely diagnoses?

What acid-base treatment would be most appropriate?

CASE 3.5
Acute Popsicle Overdose
(Case discussed on page 140)

A 56-year-old man developed diarrhea while traveling abroad for several months. He took antibiotics and a GI motility depressant. His clinical condition deteriorated, and metabolic acidosis developed when he ate popsicles to quench his thirst. The only physical finding of note was confusion and poor coordination. Laboratory results revealed a mixed type of metabolic acidosis (pH was 7.20, $[HCO_3^-]$ was 10 mmol/L, anion gap was increased by 7 mEq/L).

		Plasma	Urine
pH		7.20	5.2
Pa_{CO_2}	mm Hg	25	No data
HCO_3^-	mmol/L	10	0
Anion gap	mEq/L	19	101
Osmolal gap	mOsm/kg H_2O	0	430
Albumin	g/L	38	No data
Ketoacids		Negative	Negative

Could chronic diarrhea have caused the acidosis?

If not, what other diagnosis is likely?

What role did the popsicles play?

CASE 3.6
RTA: No Bones About It
(Case discussed on pages 141–142)

A 3-year-old child was investigated for "failure to thrive" at 1 year of age. Two medical problems were recognized: hypermineralization of his bones (osteopetrosis) and chronic metabolic acidosis (table follows).

Plasma		**Values in Plasma**		
		Usual State	**Acid Load**	**Alkali Load**
pH		7.26	7.22	7.39
HCO_3^-	mmol/L	20	15	25
Anion gap	mEq/L	8	11	8
K^+	mmol/L	3.4	3.7	—
Urine				
FE_{HCO_3}	%	—	—	15 (high)
U-B P_{CO_2}	mm Hg	—	—	7 (low)
NH_4^+	μmol/min/1.73 M^2	12 (low)	43	0
Citrate	mmol/mmol creat	0.35*	0	0.38
Urine pH		7.0	5.8	7.6

*Typical values for someone eating a typical diet and one who has normal plasma values for acid-base parameters.

Is there evidence for proximal RTA? What additional tests are needed to deduce its likely basis?

Is there evidence for distal RTA?

How can a defect in H^+ secretion in both the proximal convoluted tubule and the distal convoluted tubule be incorporated into a single pathophysiologic lesion?

To help with these cases, the authors have provided additional flow charts as Figures 3.25, 3.26, and 3.27 on pages 134–135.

CASE 3.7
The Kidneys Are Seeing Red
(Case discussed on pages 142–143)

A 27-year-old patient noticed progressive weakness when climbing stairs during the past several months. There was no diarrhea or evidence of a problem in the GI tract. There were no special findings in the physical examination.

Values in plasma and urine are shown in the following table.

		Plasma	**Urine**
pH		7.32	7.3
HCO_3^-	mmol/L	17	—
P_{CO_2}	mm Hg	32	—
Na^+	mmol/L	140	57
K^+	mmol/L	2.7	32
Cl^-	mmol/L	115	82
Creatinine	μmol/L (mg/dL)	70 (0.8)	7 mmol/L
Osmolality	mOsm/kg H_2O	290	350

The rate of excretion of NH_4^+ was very low considering the presence of hyperchloremic metabolic acidosis (see Figure 3.25). K^+ excretion was 45 mmol/day, a high value considering the hypokalemia. All other renal function studies were normal.

What is the most likely basis for the metabolic acidosis?

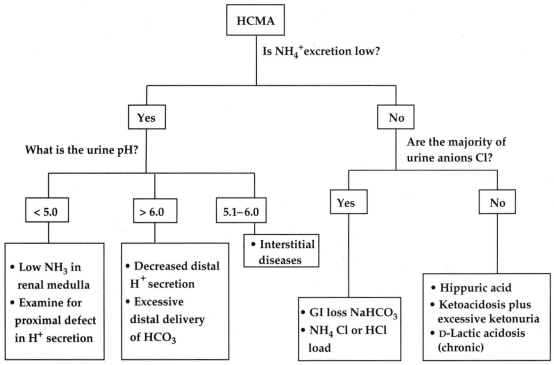

Figure 3.25 Approach to the patient with HCMA considering the rate of excretion of NH_4^+. When the rate of excretion of NH_4^+ is low, the urine pH is helpful to determine whether a low distal and/or proximal H^+ secretion or a low NH_3 availability was the cause for the low rate of NH_4^+ excretion.

The urine P_{CO_2} was 80 mm Hg. What might this imply for the pathophysiology of the lesion?

How might the hypokalemia be explained?

CASE 3.8
Does This Patient Have a Defect in "Urine Acidification"?
(Discussion on page 143)

The only significant past medical history was a single kidney stone in a 12-year-old boy. The only laboratory test result that was unusual was a urine pH that was always in the low 6.0 range. His diet was said to be "normal," and there is no family history of a renal or any other disorder. No abnormalities were detected in the physical examination.

1. **Acid-base data in plasma:** pH 7.42, $Paco_2$ 44 mm Hg, HCO_3^- 28 mmol/L, anion gap 12 mEq/L.
2. **Urine:** pH 6.3, Pco_2 39 mm Hg, flow rate 1 L/day, NH_4^+ excretion rate was 30 mmol/day.

All other tests of renal function were normal.

If there is an acid-base disorder, what is it?

What additional tests are needed to confirm the nephron site involved and the molecular basis of a possible lesion?

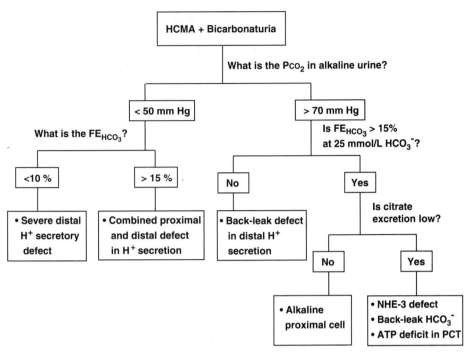

Figure 3.26   Approach to the patient with HCMA and an alkaline urine pH. Any excretion of HCO_3^- during metabolic acidosis is excessive (urine pH > 6.5). To detect the basis for renal loss of HCO_3^-, the Pco_2 in alkaline urine and the FE_{HCO_3} at a plasma $[HCO_3^-]$ near 25 mmol/L are examined. Based on the results, defects are suggested.
    NHE-3 = Na^+/H^+ Exchanger in the PCT.

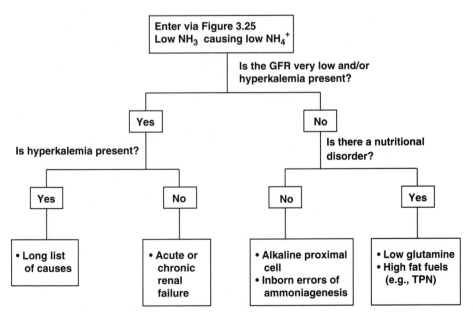

Figure 3.27   Approach to the patient with a low urine pH and a low rate of excretion of NH_4^+. The first step to determine the basis for a low urine pH and NH_4^+ excretion rate is to rule out a low GFR and hyperkalemia (the common causes). In their absence, one could rule out a nutritional problem by measuring the plasma glutamine level and fatty acid metabolites. An alkaline proximal cell is suspected if there is citraturia in the patient with HCMA.

Discussion of Cases

DISCUSSION OF CASE 3.1
Ken Has a Drinking "Problem"
(Case presented on page 130)

What is the total body Na⁺ content?

Because the ECF volume is markedly contracted, there is a large Na⁺ deficit, which was probably partially due to renal Na⁺ excretion ("dragged out by HCO_3^-") from vomiting.

Is there relative insulin deficiency?

Yes. Ketoacidosis signals relative insulin deficiency. If he does not have IDDM, the lack of insulin is probably due to the α-adrenergic response secondary to ECF volume contraction. Hyperglycemia is not present because ethanol has inhibited gluconeogenesis in the liver (high NADH/NAD drives pyruvate to lactate rather than to glucose).

Why is the patient hypokalemic, and to what degree is he K⁺-depleted?

The patient is severely K⁺-depleted because hypokalemia is present during relative insulin deficiency (insulin deficiency is usually associated with hyperkalemia). Vomiting leads to large renal K⁺ loss (see page 423).

What are the acid-base diagnoses?

The acidemia, low $[HCO_3^-]$, and increased plasma anion gap all indicate that metabolic acidosis is present. The most likely cause is alcoholic ketoacidosis plus some L-lactic acidosis from either ethanol or the low circulating volume. In addition, he has metabolic alkalosis from vomiting; the rise in plasma anion gap (32 − 12, or 20 mEq/L) is greater than the fall in the plasma $[HCO_3^-]$ from normal (25 − 15 = 10 mmol/L).

What are the primary considerations for therapy?

Administer the following:

1. isotonic saline to reexpand the ECF volume,
2. KCl (40 mmol/L) to replace the K⁺ deficit,
3. B vitamins (especially thiamine) to replace nutritional deficits.

Phosphate should be given if the patient is severely hypophosphatemic. Do not give insulin now, because the patient may suffer from acute hypokalemia (insulin will probably be released from β cells of the pancreas once the ECF volume is reexpanded).

There is controversy concerning glucose administration; in the authors' opinion, it should be given only to prevent hypoglycemia.

The plasma osmolality is 350 mOsm/kg H₂O. Is the ICF volume high, low, or normal?

Although the plasma osmolality is 350 mOsm/kg H₂O, the calculated value (2 [Na⁺] + mmol/L urea + mmol/L glucose) is 310 mOsm/kg H₂O. The difference is mostly due to the presence of 40 mmol/L ethanol. Because the ethanol concentration (like that of urea) is equal in the ICF and ECF, it does not produce a water shift. The normal [Na⁺] and concentration of glucose suggest that the ICF volume is normal.

When ethanol is no longer present, what changes will be observed in the metabolic picture?

When alcohol is not present, the patient will still have ketoacidosis because of fatty acid mobilization. L-Lactate levels will not be elevated, and the concentration of glucose in plasma will be higher because of reduced impairment of glucogenesis.

DISCUSSION OF CASE 3.2
An Unusual Type of Ketoacidosis
(Case presented on pages 130–131)

What is the differential diagnosis of her acid-base disorders?

The patient's hypokalemia and metabolic acidosis suggest proximal RTA or reduced distal H⁺ secretion. The urine net charge, which suggests little NH₄⁺ excretion, supports a diagnosis of proximal or distal RTA. The differential diagnosis, at this point, would be the causes of low proximal or distal H⁺ secretion associated with hypokalemia.

What investigative plan would be appropriate?

The plan would be to confirm the absence of proximal RTA with HCO₃⁻ administration and then confirm low distal H⁺ secretion by measuring the rate of excretion of NH₄⁺ and possibly the urine P_{CO_2}.

Following the ingestion of NaHCO₃ and KCl, the plasma [HCO₃⁻] rose to 26 mmol/L and did not fall promptly after the intake of HCO₃⁻ was stopped; the urine P_{CO_2} was 90 mm Hg. What is the diagnosis now?

The HCO₃⁻ administration ruled out proximal RTA. Nevertheless, the normal urine P_{CO_2} indicates that either back-diffusion of H⁺ from lumen to cell occurred when the urine pH was low (H⁺ back-leak type of distal RTA) or that there was a normal distal H⁺ secretory process and a more complex disease. Because the patient had not used amphotericin B, back-leak of H⁺ in the collecting duct is an unlikely diagnosis. The other possibility is that the urine net charge is misleading. There may have been high NH₄⁺ excretion that was in conjunction with an anion other than Cl⁻. This possibility can be confirmed by measuring the urine osmolality and comparing it with the calculated urine osmolality.

The measured urine osmolality is 680 mOsm/kg H₂O, but the calculated urine osmolality (2([Na⁺] + [K⁺]) + glucose + urea) is only 269 mOsm/kg H₂O. Therefore, there is an "osmolal gap" in urine of 411 mOsm/kg H₂O that indicates the presence of a large number of unmeasured osmoles (possibly NH₄⁺ + β-HB⁻). Urine is tested for NH₄⁺ and β-HB⁻; later, these values are confirmed to be 120 mmol/L and 234 mmol/L, respectively. Because the urine volume was greater than 1 L/day, the patient had a normal renal response to acidemia and excreted close to 200 mmol of NH_4^+ per day. Ketoacidosis, which caused an ongoing acid load that resulted in acidemia, was not evident because of marked ketonuria (see Figure 3.3). With better diabetic control, the acidemia disappeared. Therefore, she had a renal tubular lesion in β-HB^- reabsorption in the presence of diabetic ketoacidosis.

Why was this patient hypokalemic?

In the face of hypokalemia, the patient had a urine $[K^+]$ of 60 mmol/L. Back-correcting for medullary water abstraction, her $[K^+]$ in the cortical collecting duct was close to 30 mmol/L, about 10-fold greater than her plasma $[K^+]$. Thus, aldosterone was released in response to ECF volume contraction, which was caused by renal Na^+ loss secondary to the ketonuria. Her hypokalemia was therefore secondary to renal K^+ loss. Furthermore, despite insulin deficiency, the plasma $[K^+]$ was 2.9 mmol/L; this value suggests a very large K^+ deficit.

Note
See pages 391–393 for a discussion of "back-correction" for medullary water abstraction to establish the $[K^+]$ in the cortical collecting duct. This calculation allows the detection of mineralocorticoid actions, as reflected by the transtubular K^+ gradient.

DISCUSSION OF CASE 3.3
Ketoacidosis: a Stroke of Bad Luck
(Case presented on pages 131–132)

What is (are) the most likely cause(s) for his metabolic acidosis?

The first question to consider is whether acids are being overproduced. Because the patient's plasma anion gap is markedly elevated at 42 mEq/L (30 higher than expected), and renal failure is not present, he therefore has overproduction of acids. Given this story, alcoholic ketoacidosis seems to be the most likely diagnosis, but his screening test result for ketoacids in plasma is only moderately positive. This result suggests a mixture of L-lactic acidosis (most likely from ethanol) and ketoacidosis, although the very unlikely diagnosis of D-lactic acidosis cannot be ruled out.

Follow-up data reveal very elevated levels of β-HB^- (12 mmol/L) and L-lactate (6 mmol/L), which confirm the clinical impression.

Are acids being produced rapidly?

There are two types of information needed to answer this question, the nature of the acid added and how many new anions are appearing.
1. **Nature of the acid:** L-Lactic acid, which is produced very quickly, requires poor delivery of O_2 to tissues. Given the clinical picture, the delivery of O_2 to all organs except part of the CNS is adequate, so this setting is probably not appropriate for rapid accumulation of acids.
2. **Net appearance of new anions:** For new anions to be present, there must be a rise in the plasma anion gap in the past hour or two (the anion gap did not rise) or the excretion of more $Na^+ + K^+$ than Cl^-. Because the urine output is trivial, there is no major appearance of new anions in the urine.

In conclusion, it appears that the net rate of accumulation of acids is small at this point.

What hormonal changes were involved?

For ketoacidosis to have developed, there must have been a relative lack of insulin. Although the patient could have IDDM, the most likely basis of the lack of insulin is inhibited release of insulin from β cells by the α-adrenergic response to adrenaline. Adrenaline is released in large quantities secondary to the major CNS lesion (intracerebral hemorrhage), the so-called "cerebral diabetes."

Long-term follow-up reveals that he does not have diabetes mellitus.

Why did ketoacidosis develop so quickly?

1. **Increased production:** Usually there is a lag period before the rate of formation of ketoacids begins to rise. This patient may have "by-passed" the rate-limiting step (the supply of intramitochondrial fatty acyl-CoA in hepatocyte mitochondria) by making acetyl-CoA in hepatocytes from ethanol.
2. **Decreased utilization:** The major organ that utilizes ketoacids is the brain. Because the patient is comatose and has a major intracerebral lesion, the oxidation of ketoacids might be diminished appreciably.

DISCUSSION OF CASE 3.4
A Superstar of Severe Acidosis
(Case presented on page 132)

What are the most likely diagnoses?

The patient has a very severe degree of metabolic acidosis. The production of acids should have the following characteristics:

1. **A relatively low rate of production:** A rapid rate of production of acids would have killed the patient. This fact rules out (temporarily) production of L-lactic acid via anaerobic glycolysis.
2. **A near-normal ECF volume:** Ketoacidosis (DKA, alcoholic ketoacidosis) would be an attractive diagnosis, but at this degree, it should be accompanied by an extremely contracted ECF volume. Given the absence of alcohols, both ketoacidosis and ingestion of alcohols are very unlikely diagnoses.
3. **Expected history for D-lactic acidosis:** There is no GI history to support the diagnosis of D-lactic acidosis, and the degree of acidosis is much more severe than one would expect with this diagnosis; hence, although D-lactic acidosis is a remote possibility, it is unlikely.

By exclusion, the most likely diagnosis is type B L-lactic acidosis. The authors suspect a small reduction in gluconeogenesis or a small deficit in vitamin B_1 (thiamine) because a diagnosis with a slow but steady net accumulation of acid is needed. This suspicion was confirmed by finding that the L-lactate level in plasma exceeded 30 mmol/L and that the patient was taking metformin for treatment of his NIDDM (information provided later).

What acid-base treatment would be most appropriate?

The most important point to note is that although the numbers are alarming, the patient walked into the emergency room. Further, the rate of addition of new anions is small. Nevertheless, he would probably benefit from receiving some $NaHCO_3$. Doubling his current plasma $[HCO_3^-]$ (from 1 to 2 mmol/L) will raise his pH to 7.0 if his Pa_{CO_2} stays constant. Tripling the $[HCO_3^-]$ will require 30 mmol of $NaHCO_3$ for his ECF (the ECF volume is 15 L). In addition, he will need a large quantity of HCO_3^- for his ICF, but the authors cannot tell how much. Our guess is to give 100 mmol of $NaHCO_3$ and observe but to be prepared to give 200 mmol of $NaHCO_3$.

To increase the oxidation of L-lactate, administering dichloroacetate, an activator of PDH (Figure 12.1), would be a good choice in this setting.

DISCUSSION OF CASE 3.5
Acute Popsicle Overdose
(Case presented on page 132)

Could chronic diarrhea have caused the acidosis?

[HCO₃⁻] in diarrhea fluid
This concentration is usually <50 mmol/L. Therefore, to lose more than 200 mmol of HCO_3^- per day, the volume of diarrhea must exceed 4 L/day.

For diarrhea to be the sole cause of acidosis, the patient would have to lose 200 mmol of $NaHCO_3$ per day in the stool (see margin note). During chronic metabolic acidosis, the kidneys, if normal, will generate 200 mmol of HCO_3^- each day by excreting this quantity of NH_4^+. Hence, diarrhea per se is an unlikely cause. In addition, diarrhea-induced metabolic acidosis is not associated with an increase in the anion gap.

If not, what other diagnosis is likely?

Note
Low excretion of NH_4^+ is not associated directly with a rise in the anion gap in plasma.

Two major causes are possible in this setting: low excretion of NH_4^+ and overproduction of D-lactic acid by the intestinal bacteria.
1. **Low excretion of NH_4^+:** It is possible that the patient has a renal lesion that compromised the excretion of NH_4^+. Measuring the urine $[NH_4^+]$ did not reveal a low quantity (200 mmol excreted per day), so this less likely possibility was ruled out (see margin note).
2. **Overproduction of D-lactic acid:** Several factors make this diagnosis very likely: the history of a GI problem; the ingestion of antibiotics to alter the GI flora; the ingestion of a motility suppressant to permit a longer time of incubation; the CNS disturbance (bacteria produce other toxins, too); and the unexpectedly small rise in the plasma anion gap (some D-lactate was excreted in the urine). Confirm this diagnosis by measuring the D-lactate level in plasma; this metabolite was markedly elevated (10 mmol/L).

What role did the popsicles play?

The bacteria in his upper GI tract were starved. When fed sugar from the popsicles, they responded by producing D-lactic acid plus CNS toxins.

DISCUSSION OF CASE 3.6
RTA: No Bones About It
(Case presented on pages 132–133)

Is there evidence for proximal RTA? What additional tests are needed to deduce its likely basis?

An approach is summarized in Figure 3.26. There is evidence of proximal RTA because there is a very large excretion of HCO_3^- when the plasma $[HCO_3^-]$ was normal (alkali load). The basis for the low secretion of H^+ in the PCT was not hyperkalemia. The fractional excretion of HCO_3^- was 15% (in normal subjects, this would be close to 0 at this level of plasma HCO_3^-).

Basis for Proximal RTA. Because there was no glucosuria, aminoaciduria, or excessive phosphaturia or uricosuria, there is no generalized PCT dysfunction.

The basis for his proximal lesion could be an alkaline PCT cell because there is citraturia despite acidemia, and citraturia disappears with an acid load; there is also a low NH_4^+ excretion rate, but this could reflect the high urine pH.

Given his bone disease, a defect in carbonic anhydrase II (CA_{II}) was suspected, and this was confirmed by direct assay (both bone and kidney cells have CA_{II}). The basis for the alkaline cell pH with this lesion is illustrated in the figure below. Blocking intracellular CA_{II} leads to an alkaline cell because OH^- is a stronger base than HCO_3^-.

CA_{IV} is a different enzyme in the lumen that lowers the $[H_2CO_3]$ and thereby the luminal $[H^+]$. CA_{IV} was normal in this patient.

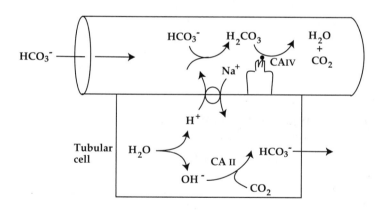

Note
CA_{II} is located inside cells of the PCT and DCT.

Is there evidence for distal RTA?

There is evidence for distal RTA because the urine P_{CO_2} in alkaline urine was so low; the urine P_{CO_2} is high in other patients with proximal RTA. Moreover, the urine pH was high when the patient had metabolic acidosis, consistent with distal RTA.

How can a defect in H^+ secretion in both the PCT and the DCT be incorporated into a single pathophysiologic lesion?

Because the main H^+ pump in the PCT is the NHE-3, whereas the main H^+ pump in the DCT is an $H^+ATPase$, it is unlikely that there is a common lesion with these pumps per se (Figure 1.21). Because the HCO_3^- exit steps also differ in the PCT ($Na(HCO_3)_3^{2-}$) and the DCT (AE-1), there is not a common lesion here. The authors suspect that the common lesion is an alkaline PCT and DCT cell due to a defect in CA_{II} as shown in the figure.

The fact that NH_4^+ excretion could rise and the urine pH fall with an additional acid load supports the premise that the α-intercalated cells, like the PCT cells, are more alkaline (the following reaction is catalyzed by CA_{II} in both these cell types).

$$CO_2 + OH^- \rightarrow HCO_3^-$$

DISCUSSION OF CASE 3.7
The Kidneys Are Seeing Red
(Case presented on pages 133–134)

What is the most likely basis for the metabolic acidosis?

The patient has metabolic acidosis without an elevated value for the anion gap in plasma. Because the rate of excretion of NH_4^+ was low for a patient with chronic metabolic acidosis, the most likely diagnosis is renal tubular acidosis (see Figure 3.27). The very low $[H^+]$ (high pH) in the urine in the context of a low rate of excretion of NH_4^+ implies a low rate of H^+ secretion in the distal nephron or a low rate of indirect reabsorption of HCO_3^- in the PCT (see margin illustration).

When $NaHCO_3$ was given and the plasma $[K^+]$ was normal, there was little excretion of HCO_3^-, so a proximal defect in H^+ secretion is an unlikely diagnosis.

The low value for the urine net charge and the fact that the urine creatinine concentration is high suggests the absence of polyuria and a low rate of excretion of NH_4^+. It is unlikely that overproduction of acids with the excessive production of an organic acid and excretion of the anions with Na^+ or K^+ (like hippurate) played a role in this process.

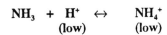

$$NH_3 + H^+ \leftrightarrow NH_4^+$$
$$\text{(low)} \qquad \text{(low)}$$

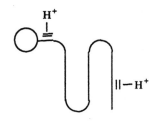

The urine P_{CO_2} was 80 mm Hg. What might this imply for the pathophysiology of the lesion?

The expected value for the urine P_{CO_2} is a low value (~ 40 mm Hg) as the proposed defect was a low rate of H^+ secretion in the distal nephron (high urine pH). To explain a high urine P_{CO_2}, distal HCO_3^- secretion must be postulated. These HCO_3^- react with H^+ in the luminal fluid, and ultimately one H^+ from $H_2PO_4^-$; this generates CO_2 and as shown in the equation below.

$$HCO_3^- + H^+ \leftrightarrow H_2CO_3 \rightarrow CO_2 + H_2O$$

The basis for enhanced HCO_3^- secretion could be:

1. A lack of α-intercalated cells.

2. α-Intercalated cells with absent or inhibited $H^+ATPase$ (due to inhibition of the AE-1 on their basolateral surface by a circulating globulin as may occur in Sjögren's syndrome, or possibly a defective AE-1 protein as in hereditary ovalocytosis); they also need AE-1 in their lumuinal membrane.

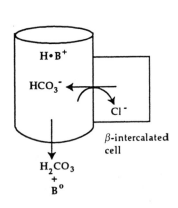

β-intercalated cell

3. A down-regulation of α-intercalated and up-regulation of β-intercalated cells.

How might the hypokalemia be explained?

The basis for the excessive excretion of K^+ is a higher $[K^+]$ in the urine and the cortical collecting duct (see Chapter 9, page 390, for details). This usually requires aldosterone actions and the presence of HCO_3^- in the cortical collecting duct; the latter is due to the defect causing distal RTA.

DISCUSSION OF CASE 3.8
Does This Patient Have a Defect in "Urine Acidification"?
(Case presented on page 134)

If there is an acid-base disorder, what is it?

The patient does not have an acid-base defect when only his plasma values are considered. There does not seem to be a major defect when his urine is examined as well. Nevertheless, there is a problem—he has the same rate of excretion of NH_4^+ as a normal individual, but his urine $[H^+]$ is lower (pH higher) than in normal subjects. Applying these data to the following equation, his $[NH_3]$ is unduly high in the urine if these values are representative of the 24-hour period.

$$H^+ \; + \; NH_3 \; \leftrightarrow \; NH_4^+$$
$$\text{(low)} \quad \text{(high)} \quad \text{(normal)}$$

What additional tests are needed to confirm the nephron site involved and the molecular basis of a possible lesion?

First, ensure that the picture from his 24-hour urine is representative of all urine specimens in the 24-hour period by collecting multiple urine samples (every 2 hours) and assaying each one for NH_4^+, pH, and citrate.

Next, ensure that there is no organism present that has urease in his urine or collecting system.

$$\text{Urea} \xrightarrow{\text{urease}} 2 \; NH_4^+ \; + \; 2 \; HCO_3^-$$

If there is a tubular defect, it will be in the nephron site that produces NH_4^+, the PCT. Enhanced production of NH_4^+ can occur with excessive glutamine, a very high energy (ATP) turnover, a defect in oxidation of the usual substrates (lactate, fatty acids), and/or a stimulus for ammoniagenesis (intracellular acidosis). Evidence for this stimulus would include a higher reabsorption of HCO_3^- and a lower rate of excretion of citrate (an acidified cell). One way to explain why the cell has a lower pH is an abnormally active HCO_3^- exit step (higher Vmax or lower affinity for the $Na(HCO_3)_3^{2-}$ ion complex). These are the findings in the so-called "incomplete" distal RTA (which may originate as a proximal lesion). Studies are planned to test this hypothesis in the near future.

Summary of Main Points

Acid-Base Balance

- Metabolism of proteins and vegetables yields a net of 1 mmol H^+/day/kg body weight. Excessive H^+ are produced during ischemia, if there is a lack of insulin, or during certain intoxications.
- Almost all H^+ are buffered by HCO_3^-, but, if the H^+ load is very large, an appreciable number of H^+ are buffered by intracellular proteins. A low $Paco_2$ signals the appropriate response to an acid load. Drop the 7 and the decimal point of the pH to see the expected value for the $Paco_2$; compare this value with the measured one.
- The expected response to a chronic acid load is excretion of more than 200 mmol of NH_4^+ per day and reabsorption of all filtered HCO_3^- by the kidney. Find NH_4^+ in urine by calculating the urine net charge and/or the urine osmolal gap.

Diagnostic Procedures

- Use the anion gap in plasma to find anions produced with H^+.
- Quantitate new anions added to the body (multiply the rise in anion gap by the total body water) and to the urine (count the anions excreted without H^+ or NH_4^+ by multiplying (Na^+ + K^+ − Cl^-) in urine by urine volume).
- Use the osmolal gap in plasma to detect toxic precursors of acids (alcohols).
- Use the urine net charge and/or osmolal gap to detect NH_4^+ in the urine.
- The urine pH is good for detecting HCO_3^- in the urine but not good for detecting NH_4^+ in the urine. It is useful in determining why the $[NH_4^+]$ is low in the urine.

Overall Summary

Although metabolic acidosis may be the result of a large number of diverse disorders, these disorders can be sorted out easily with an organized approach, as outlined in Figure 3.4. Metabolic acidosis associated with increased H^+ production and with renal failure is identified by an increase in the plasma anion gap. The subgroup associated with methanol or ethylene glycol intoxication also has an increased osmolal gap.

The critical feature in discovering the basis of metabolic acidosis with a normal plasma anion gap is determining whether the excretion of NH_4^+ in the urine is appropriate. The urine $[NH_4^+]$ is reflected by the apparent urine net charge ($[Na^+]$ + $[K^+]$ − $[Cl^-]$) when the urine pH is less than 6.1. A negative apparent urine net charge (i.e., $[Cl^-]$ greatly exceeds the sum of $[Na^+]$ and $[K^+]$), indicates an appropriate urine $[NH_4^+]$, and the diagnosis is $NaHCO_3$ loss, either via the GI tract or some other site (proximal RTA, acetazolamide, NH_4Cl administration). If the apparent net charge is positive (i.e., the sum of [Na$^+$] and [K$^+$] greatly exceeds [Cl$^-$]), the urine [NH$_4$$^+$] may be low. In this setting, the diagnosis is one of three possibilities: the presence of RTA, diabetic ketoacidosis with marked β-hydroxy-butyrate and NH$_4$$^+$ excretion, or toluene toxicity with hippurate and NH$_4$$^+$ excretion (revealed by the urine osmolal gap).

Discussion of Questions

3.1 Which patient has a primary respiratory acid-base disorder? How should each patient be managed from an acid-base point of view?

Patient	[H$^+$] nmol/L	pH	Paco_2 (mm Hg)	[HCO$_3$$^-$] (mmol/L)
A	64	7.20	20	8
B	120	6.90	40	8
C	30	7.50	10	8

Case A represents the appropriate respiratory response to metabolic acidosis. Management involves determining the basis of the metabolic acidosis.

Case B has metabolic acidosis and respiratory acidosis. The coexistent respiratory acidosis has made the acidemia life-threatening, and intervention is indicated. If immediate correction of the basis of the respiratory acidosis is not possible, mechanical ventilation is advisable.

Case C has a significant degree of respiratory alkalosis; management depends on the basis of the hyperventilation.

3.2 Does the arterial or venous Pco_2 best reflect the degree of protonation of intracellular proteins during metabolic acidosis?

The venous Pco_2 best reflects the protonation of intracellular proteins. Because CO_2 must diffuse from tissues to plasma in capillaries, the Pco_2 in tissues must be higher than that in venous blood. Therefore, the venous Pco_2 best reflects tissue Pco_2 and the degree of effectiveness of the bicarbonate buffer system in the ICF. Because the venous Pco_2 is not measured in vital organs, this value must be estimated. Remember that the mixed venous Pco_2 reflects the Pco_2 of the venous blood draining from organs with the largest blood supply. For example, the Pco_2 of venous blood draining from exercising muscles may be close to 100 mm Hg; at the same time, the Pco_2 of venous blood draining from the brain might be close to 46 mm Hg.

Arterial Pco_2 primarily reflects the effect of alveolar ventilation—removal of the CO_2 that is produced. It does not reflect the Pco_2 in the various organs.

3.3 How can reexpansion of the ECF volume affect the Pco_2 in vital organs?

The Pco_2 in venous blood is the result of the rate of production of CO_2 and its rate of removal via the blood. Consider the following example in which the rate of production of CO_2 is 10 mmol/min and the cardiac output is 5 L/min (normal) and 2.5 L/min (reduced by 50% because of ECF volume contraction).

Cardiac Output	CO_2 Production	CO_2 Carried	Venous P_{CO_2}
5 L/min	10 mmol/min	2 mmol/L	46 mm Hg
2.5 L/min	10 mmol/min	4 mmol/L	60 mm Hg

Therefore, in this example, reexpansion of the ECF leads to a rise in cardiac output from 2.5 to 5 L/min and thereby to a fall in venous P_{CO_2} from 60 to 46 mm Hg.

3.4 Some recommend that a 50:50 mixture of $NaHCO_3$ and Na_2CO_3 (Carbicarb) be used as a source of alkali to minimize CO_2 production. If a patient has L-lactic acidosis and is producing 12 mmol of L-lactic acid per minute, how much less CO_2 (expressed in percentage form) will be produced by titrating the H^+ produced with Carbicarb instead of $NaHCO_3$? (Assume 12 mmol of O_2 is consumed each minute by the body.)

Respiratory quotient = CO_2 produced/O_2 consumed.

$$0.8 = \frac{10 \text{ mmol of } CO_2}{12 \text{ mmol of } O_2}$$

First, examine the rate of production of CO_2 before and after buffering. If the *respiratory quotient* is 0.8, approximately 10 mmol of CO_2 is produced each minute via aerobic metabolism. Titrating 12 mmol of H^+ with $NaHCO_3$ will yield 12 mmol of CO_2 and a total rate of CO_2 production of 22 mmol/min. Using Carbicarb, for every 4 mmol of H^+ titrated, 3 mmol of CO_2 will be produced. Thus, to titrate 12 mmol of H^+, 9 mmol of CO_2 will be produced, and 19 mmol of CO_2 will be produced per minute if all the alkali is titrated. Hence, the difference in CO_2 production is small (22 vs 19), close to 15%, and will have a minor effect on the arterial P_{CO_2} unless alveolar ventilation is low and fixed.

3.5 Why is the rate of production of ketoacids so much lower than that of L-lactic acid if both are regulated by the rate of turnover of ATP?

The answer involves the restrictions set by the rate of consumption of oxygen and by stoichiometry. Ketogenesis is restricted to the liver, an organ with little variation in oxygen consumption. Stoichiometry is close to 6 ATP molecules generated per ketoacid formed. In contrast, L-lactic acid is produced by many organs. Consider skeletal muscle, which can increase its demand for O_2 20-fold and thus can have a much greater rate of consumption of O_2 than the liver. The rate of production of ATP and L-lactic acid, although still under ATP feedback control, can be enormous (H^+ production is perhaps 50-fold greater than in ketogenesis). In type A L-lactic acidosis, some of the needs for ATP are not met by aerobic metabolism, hence the need for anaerobic metabolism. Therefore, one might conceptualize that L-lactic acidosis is being pushed by the need for ATP rather than being limited by it.

3.6 The rates of ketoacid production and removal are usually equal in a person who lacks insulin. Why is this equality beneficial?

Ketoacid production is designed to permit one to exist for long periods without the intake of carbohydrates. Ketoacids are formed in the liver so that the brain can oxidize a fat-derived fuel (it cannot oxidize fatty acids from the circulation at appreciable rates). This oxidation of ketoacids prevents major catabolism of lean body mass (the brain alone would oxidize the equivalent of 1–2 lb of muscle per day without ketoacids to oxidize, because gluconeogenesis would have to provide the daily supply of glucose; see margin note). The danger of ketoacids is accumulation of H^+, but the ATP constraints on ketogenesis in the liver permit the rate of ketogenesis to be relatively small and to equal the rates of ketoacid removal in other organs (see Figure 3.10). Hence, the degree of this ketoacidosis is constant and mild when fasting is the cause of low levels of insulin.

Facts
- The brain consumes 120 g of glucose per day in the absence of ketoacids.
- 200 g of protein can yield 120 g of glucose.
- Lean body mass is 80% water (1 kg yields 200 g of protein).

3.7 What makes DKA severe in degree compared with the ketoacidosis of chronic fasting?

The answer is probably the lower rate of ketoacid removal by metabolism in DKA. Although the rate of ketogenesis is similar in DKA and fasting, coma and severe confusion appear with a severe degree of hyperglycemia. These disturbances, along with the low GFR (osmotic diuresis caused loss of Na^+), diminish O_2 consumption in DKA and thereby fuel oxidation in the two major organs that consume ketoacids.

3.8 In hepatic mitochondria, acetyl-CoA is formed from ethanol and from fatty acids at about the same rate. Why are these rates so similar?

The answer lies in the stoichiometry of ATP per acetyl-CoA formed.

C_{16} fatty acid $\rightarrow$ 33 ATP + 8 acetyl-CoA
Ethanol $\rightarrow$ 4 ATP + acetyl-CoA

Therefore, the yield is close to 4 mmol of ATP per acetyl-CoA in both cases (the numbers include the quantity of ATP needed to form CoA derivatives of fatty acids and acetic acid).

3.9 Must ethanol levels be elevated on admission for metabolism of ethanol to be an important cause of ketoacidosis?

No. Although ethanol levels were elevated when ketoacids were formed initially, the source of acetyl-CoA can now be fatty acids. Contraction of the ECF volume causes the release of adrenaline, which results in the stimulation of hormone-sensitive lipase and the subsequent release of more fatty acids.

3.10 An anoxic limb needs to regenerate 18 mmol of ATP per minute (25% of the ATP needed in the body) via anaerobic glycolysis. If the rest of the body were "persuaded" to oxidize L-lactate anions ($+H^+$) to regenerate all needed ATP (54 mmol/min, equivalent to the utilization of 9 mmol of O_2), would L-lactic acid accumulate?

The normal rate of consumption of oxygen is 12 mmol/min, and it is reduced by 25% to 9 mmol/min. Given the stoichiometry of 3 mmol of O_2 per mmol of lactic acid oxidized, only 3 mmol of lactic

Note
Athletes "cool down" by jogging. In
doing so, they can oxidize more
L-lactate anions because of the
higher rate of turnover of ATP.

acid could be oxidized by the rest of the body each minute. The generation of 18 mmol of ATP from glucose in the anoxic limb will result in the formation of 18 mmol of L-lactic acid. Because the maximum rate of glucogenesis is less than 15 mmol/min, L-lactic acidosis must get worse unless oxygen can be delivered to the anoxic limb.

Even if oxygen were delivered to the hypoxic leg and no more L-lactic acid were formed, the rate of decline in the concentration of L-lactate anions in plasma would be very slow. In quantitative terms, a 70-kg patient with lactic acidosis (15 mmol/L) has a pool size of L-lactate of close to 450 mmol (assume a volume of distribution of lactate of 30 L, for simplicity). If all the ATP regenerated were derived from the oxidation of L-lactate anions, only 4 mmol of L-lactate anions could be oxidized per minute at rest. If a maximum rate of glucogenesis of 8 mmol/min is added, the overall clearance of L-lactate anions by metabolic routes would be 12 mmol/min. Hence, the degree of decline in L-lactic acid would be almost 4 mmol/L in 10 minutes, but this rate of metabolism of L-lactate anions is probably a gross overestimate, because the brain consumes about 25% of O_2 at rest and it will burn glucose. Further, it is unlikely that 100% of the rest of the ATP generated will be from the oxidation of L-lactate anions.

3.11 If a patient has hypoxia but little glycogen in the liver, will L-lactic acidosis develop? If not, what changes would you expect to find in the concentration of metabolites in blood?

Development of L-lactic acidosis is not likely. To develop L-lactic acidosis, a supply of glucose is needed. Because glucose distributes in close to half the volume of L-lactate anion but yields two L-lactate anions on a molar basis, only a small rise in L-lactate anion is possible from this source in the absence of hyperglycemia. The usual source of L-lactic acid is muscle or liver glycogen. The former requires a specific stimulus (e.g., exercise) to be hydrolyzed, and there is little glycogen in the liver; this patient will therefore suffer from hypoglycemia and organ malfunction (from less regeneration of ATP) rather than from L-lactic acidosis (Figure 3.28).

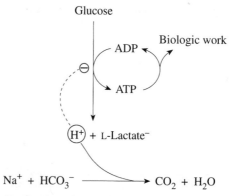

Figure 3.28 Production of L-lactic acid by anaerobic glycolysis. When L-lactic acid is produced, ATP is regenerated so that biologic work can be performed. This pathway is inhibited by a rise in the [H+].

3.12 If NaHCO₃ was given as treatment for L-lactic acidosis and there was no rise in the plasma [HCO₃⁻], was the alkali of no help to that patient?

To be a successful buffer, HCO_3^- must remove H^+ bound to proteins in the ICF or accelerate the rate of production of ATP. In terms of acid-base balance, if HCO_3^- were given and are no longer present, they were titrated or excreted (unlikely). To be titrated, a source of H^+ is needed. Two possible sources are the H^+ bound to proteins (buffered H^+) or new L-lactic acid formed. In both cases, this disappearance of H^+ and HCO_3^- was beneficial because ATP is formed whenever L-lactic acid is formed (see Figure 3.28).

The authors focus on the plasma H^+ and $[HCO_3^-]$ because they are easy to measure. It really does not matter how much the plasma $[HCO_3^-]$ per se rises because it represents untitrated base; in most cases, the $[H^+]$ in the ECF is unlikely to play an important direct role in toxicity.

3.13 Why might the rate of L-lactic acid production rise with alkali therapy?

As background, two molecules of ATP are generated per molecule of glucose metabolized during anaerobic glycolysis. In contrast, 36 molecules of ATP are generated per molecule of glucose oxidized during aerobic metabolism. Hence, glycolytic flux must be 18-fold higher during anaerobic conditions to yield the same quantity of ATP. During anaerobic glycolysis, H^+ accumulate. Because H^+ inhibit the rate-limiting step in glycolysis (*phosphofructokinase-1*), ATP regeneration will be compromised earlier in anaerobic conditions (faster flux is needed). Therefore, removal of H^+ with alkali can "de-inhibit" glycolysis and increase the rate of regeneration of ATP (see Figure 3.28) at a cost of $H^+ + $ L-lactate⁻ generation.

3.14 What metabolic adaptations prolong survival in hypoxic environments?

To prolong survival in hypoxic environments, less anaerobic metabolism must occur, yet enough ATP must be available. Therefore, the demand for ATP (biologic work) must decline. Strategies in individual organs are summarized in Table 3.23. A general strategy is to lower the metabolic rate (hypothermia, hypothyroidism).

Goldfish can make the end-products of anaerobic metabolism uncharged (ethanol) rather than an anion such as L-lactate anion.

3.15 Why is the L-lactic acidosis of exercise better tolerated than the L-lactic acidosis of shock, even if the former is more severe in degree?

TABLE 3.23 **Decreasing the Rate of Metabolism in Specific Organs**

Organ	Strategy
Brain	Anesthetics/sedative to reduce work Drug to decrease Na^+ permeability (adenosine in certain animals)
Kidney	Anything that lowers the GFR will lower Na^+ pumping
Muscle	Paralytic agent

Higher tissue Pco$_2$ in cardiogenic shock
If the rate of production of CO$_2$ in the brain were similar in both settings, the lower cerebral blood flow rate in cardiogenic shock would require that each liter of blood flowing out of the brain carry more CO$_2$ and thus have a higher Pco$_2$ (see the discussion of Question 3.3 and Figure 1.9).

In the L-lactic acidosis of both exercise and cardiogenic shock, L-lactic acid accumulates because the delivery of O$_2$ does not match the demand for it. A major difference is that in exercise, muscle undergoes hypoxia, but the brain does not. In addition, there is no reduction in the rate of cerebral blood flow.

Because tissue Pco$_2$ must be higher than that in the vein for diffusion of CO$_2$ to occur, the Pco$_2$ in the brain (and thereby the [H$^+$] in the ICF) is much higher in cardiogenic shock than in exercise (see margin note). A higher [H$^+$] can limit anaerobic glycolysis (see Figure 3.28). Therefore, the supply of ATP is reduced, and brain cells are more likely to die. This point is valid for all cells that are performing work.

3.16 Is a rise in L-lactic acid production beneficial or harmful to a patient with L-lactic acidosis?

During anaerobic glycolysis, glucose is consumed and both ATP and L-lactic acid are formed. Hence, dangers of glycolysis are H$^+$ accumulation and hypoglycemia; the advantage is ATP generation. If generation of more ATP occurs in the heart, contractility can increase and more O$_2$ can be pumped to other organs. Thus, more production of L-lactic acid can be beneficial at some times and detrimental at others (see Figure 3.28).

3.17 A 34-year-old male patient with AIDS has extreme muscular weakness and chronic L-lactic acidosis related to AZT. A biopsy revealed a mitochondrial myopathy. When he exercises, his L-lactic acidosis does not become more severe. Did the lesion in his muscle mitochondria cause his L-lactic acidosis?

Note
This question is for the more curious.

It has been stated that AZT causes a deletion of part of the mitochondrial system that regenerates ATP (the electron transport system). This disturbance is analogous to having hypoxia as the cause of L-lactic acidosis. In this setting, one would expect L-lactic acidosis to get worse if more regeneration of ATP is required. Because the severity does not increase, there must be another explanation for these results.

The problem is to devise a way in which more ATP can be generated in affected muscle fibers without the accumulation of more L-lactic acid. The authors offer the following speculations:

1. **More L-lactic acid was generated in affected fibers but was oxidized in adjacent normal fibers:** Although this theory is possible, the authors find it unattractive because of the stoichiometry described in the discussion of Question 3.10 (i.e., in terms of ATP turnover, so much more L-lactic acid is formed anaerobically than is oxidized aerobically). Furthermore, one would not expect the L-lactic acidosis to be near steady-state, as exhibited in the patient. Finally, the number of affected muscle fibers would have to be relatively small and perhaps not permit such predominant symptoms of weakness.

2. **Other organs removed the extra L-lactate anions:** While this theory is also possible, the authors believe that it is unlikely because they do not know what would drive the higher flux rates. Surely at such high levels of L-lactate in plasma, metabolic processes for L-lactate anion removal are close to being saturated with their substrate, L-lactate.

3. **A lesion is present in mitochondria of affected myocytes**

that permits the rate of regeneration of ATP to increase but does not allow the accumulation of more L-lactic acid: A rate-limiting lesion in the TCA cycle or the electron transport system would not have this effect. Instead, a lesion would have to permit a high enough level of pyruvate for oxidation and allow a very high level of L-lactate. A high NADH/NAD⁺ ratio would therefore have to exist in the cytosol of myocytes. A possible example is shown in Figure 3.16.

3.18 The L-lactic acidosis of the patient in Question 3.17 was greatly aggravated by ethanol intake. What might this effect of ethanol imply?

When ethanol is metabolized, the NADH/NAD⁺ in the cytosol of hepatocytes rises. This increase diverts pyruvate to L-lactate and may aggravate the degree of L-lactic acidosis if flux rates are particularly rapid (see Figure 3.15). This patient might have had a very high rate of release of L-lactate anions from affected myocytes and now has a compromised removal of L-lactate anions via glucopaleogenesis in the liver.

3.19 If the same number of bacteria are growing in the small bowel rather than the colon, why might more D-lactic acid be formed?

The factors that determine the quantity of D-lactic acid formed are the number of bacteria, their nature, the amount of substrate (glucose, sucrose, etc.) available, and the incubation conditions (e.g., pH and duration of incubation). In the small bowel, the supply of substrate and a higher pH (secretion of NaHCO₃) might favor the production of more organic acids. The authors cannot comment on the number and nature of the bacteria or the length of time that they dwell in the lumen of the bowel because these factors depend on specific details of the case.

3.20 How many of these organic acids are produced each day in the colon?

The GI tract produces close to 300 mmol of organic acids each day; most of this production occurs in the colon, and the limit is primarily the supply of metabolizable carbohydrates (fiber hydrolyzed by other bacteria). Of the acids produced, most are acetic acid (60%); the remainder are equally divided between propionic acid (20%) and butyric acid (20%).

3.21 What useful functions can be attributed to the production of organic acids in the colon?

1. **Butyric acid:** The main function of butyric acid is to provide half the usual fuel for the colon to regenerate its ATP (Figure 3.29). Without butyric acid, the colon may not function properly (starvation colitis) due to a deficiency of ATP.
2. **Propionic acid and D-lactic acid:** Although these are minor constituents of the daily organic acids produced, they enter metabolism at the pyruvate step (see Figure 3.29) so they can be converted to glucose as well as be oxidized.
3. **Acetic acid and butyric acid:** These organic acids are con-

Extra definitions

The authors use three terms to describe the production of glucose in the liver.
1. Glucogenesis: synthesis of glucose from all sources.
2. Gluconeogenesis: synthesis of new glucose (e.g., from amino acids).
3. Glucopaleogenesis: resynthesis of glucose using fuels derived from glucose molecules (e.g., L-lactate anions derived from circulating glucose).

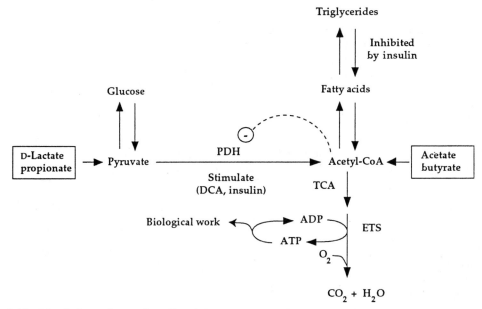

Figure 3.29   Metabolism of organic acids of GI origin. There are two families of organic acids depending on whether they yield pyruvate as a metabolic product. Organic anions that cannot be converted to pyruvate can only be oxidized, converted to storage fat, or be converted to ketoacids; they cannot be substrates for the net synthesis of glucose. Fatty acid synthesis occurs only at appreciable rates when insulin levels are high (with meals).

Abbreviations: PDH = pyruvate dehydrogenase, TCA = tricarboxylic acid cycle, ETS = electron transport system.

verted to acetyl-CoA, the product of pyruvate dehydrogenase. As such, they can be converted only to fatty acids (requiring insulin and a fed state) or oxidized to CO_2 + ATP (see Figure 3.29). For the latter, organs must have a high rate of turnover of ATP (perform biologic work), but the rate will depend on the supply of fatty acids as well.

4. **Other organic acids:** When fiber is hydrolyzed, extra calories can be obtained. Quantitatively, one-third of a mole is close to 25 g or 100 kcal. The products of this fermentation are a wide variety of organic acids.

3.22   What measures can be taken to "coax" the body to oxidize organic acids absorbed from the GI tract?

One could devise two therapeutic strategies to augment the rate of oxidation of these organic acids.

1. **Stop the oxidation of alternate fuels:** This means give an antilipolytic agent (e.g., insulin) to make fatty acid levels fall (see Figure 3.29).
2. **Promote the oxidation of D-lactic acid:** This can be achieved by activating pyruvate dehydrogenase with dichloroacetate or insulin (see Figure 3.29). This will not help the oxidation of acetic acid or byturic acid. To promote their oxidation, more work must be done (e.g., exercise, increase the GFR that is low due to a low blood volume, avoid sedatives).

   Insulin may lead to an increase in the rate of oxidation of D-lactate by decreasing the supply of fatty acids, the alternate fuel.

3.23 A 26-year-old intoxicated man is brought to the emergency room. His friends state that he ingested several ounces of methanol. Other than intoxication, his physical examination results were normal. His laboratory results were as follows:

Na^+	mmol/L	142	$[H^+]$	nmol/L	40
K^+	mmol/L	3.7	Pa_{CO_2}	mm Hg	40
Cl^-	mmol/L	105	Osmolality	mOsm/kg	360
HCO_3^-	mmol/L	25	Glucose	mmol/L (mg/dL)	7 (126)
Urea	mmol/L (mg/dL)	5 (14)	Albumin	g/L	40

Should one take the allegation of methanol seriously? Explain your reasoning. What should the course of action be?

The absence of an increased plasma anion gap and no evidence of metabolic acidosis should diminish the suspicion of methanol intoxication; therefore, one should seek more evidence before embarking on dialysis, which has some risk (insertion of lines is associated with some morbidity). The osmolal gap is readily available. Because it is elevated, some credence is added to the allegation of methanol poisoning; however, this elevation could result from the ingestion of any alcohol, including ethanol. With an increased plasma osmolal gap and the allegation of methanol ingestion, one must proceed with therapy until further data can be obtained. At the very least, one should give ethanol after sending blood and urine tests for toxin screen; then one should await confirmation by the laboratory. In the absence of either an increase in the anion gap or acidosis, it is perfectly safe to treat initially with just ethanol.

Laboratory results revealed that he indeed had toxic levels of methanol, and he also had elevated levels of isopropyl alcohol, but no ethanol was detected. Therefore, the authors assume that it was the ingestion of isopropyl alcohol that had delayed the metabolism of methanol by alcohol dehydrogenase and had protected him from both acidemia and the toxicity of formaldehyde and formic acid. He should undergo hemodialysis to remove methanol while maintaining high levels of ethanol in his plasma.

3.24 If oxalic acid were formed during the metabolism of ethylene glycol, why might the degree of metabolic acidosis be less severe?

The unique property of oxalic acid is that it is insoluble in the presence of Ca^{2+}. Hence, when ionized Ca^{2+} is precipitated in the body as its oxalate salt, the $[Ca^{2+}]$ falls and bone salts will be hydrolyzed. These bone salts are alkaline, and the anions released (PO_4^{3-} and CO_3^{2-}) will remove H^+. The net result is "curing" the acidemia.

3.25 What is the specific clue suggesting glue-sniffing as the diagnosis in a patient presenting with a normal plasma anion gap type of metabolic acidosis and hypokalemia?

The differential diagnosis in this problem includes three main possibilities: distal RTA, diarrhea, and toluene intoxication. A distant fourth is DKA with excessive ketoacid anion excretion.

The important evidence needed to resolve the differential diagnosis is a critical assessment of the urine electrolytes and osmolality to establish the NH_4^+ excretion rate. One should also test for ketoacid anions in the urine.

With distal RTA, the $[Cl^-]$ does not exceed $[Na^+] + [K^+]$, and there is no osmolal gap in the urine (i.e., urine NH_4^+ excretion is not increased).

With diarrhea, the urine $[Cl^-]$ greatly exceeds $[Na^+] + [K^+]$ and indicates an increased NH_4^+ excretion.

With toluene toxicity, there may be significant Na^+ excretion despite ECF volume contraction because of the excretion of the anion hippurate (see pages 112–113 for more details). The $[Cl^-]$ is usually less than $[Na^+] + [K^+]$, but there will be a high urine osmolal gap because of the excretion of hippurate anions with NH_4^+ (see margin note).

With DKA, the qualitative test result for ketoacid anions is positive, and there is also an osmolal gap in the urine (due to NH_4^+ + β-HB^-).

3.26 What factors contribute to the hypokalemia and K^+ depletion in glue-sniffers?

The formation and excretion of hippurate ultimately obliges the excretion of some Na^+. Because glue-sniffers often consume a limited quantity of Na^+, they are frequently ECF-volume–depleted. Once ECF volume depletion is present, aldosterone is released. In response to aldosterone, Na^+ are reabsorbed in an electrogenic fashion because the luminal fluid contains primarily Na^+ and hippurate anions but only a small quantity of Cl^-. The excretion of K^+ ensues, resulting in K^+ depletion. As acidemia persists, NH_4^+ excretion increases. The bulk of hippurate is then excreted with NH_4^+; less is excreted with K^+ and Na^+.

3.27 Patients A, B, and C each have metabolic acidosis and an increased plasma anion gap. Which one has renal failure, which has methanol intoxication, and which has D-lactic acidosis?

Patient	A	B	C
Calculated osmolality	290	290	320
2 × plasma $[Na^+]$ (mmol/L)	280	280	280
Urea (mmol/L)	5	5	35
Glucose (mmol/L)	5	5	5
Measured osmolality	290	320	320

The hallmark of renal failure is an elevated concentration of urea in plasma; only patient C can have renal failure because A and B have normal values for urea.

The hallmark of methanol intoxication is a large difference between measured and calculated osmolalities in plasma; only patient B has a large osmolal gap in plasma, so B has methanol intoxication.

In D-lactic acidosis, there is neither an elevated osmolal gap nor a high level of urea; hence, patient A has D-lactic acidosis.

3.28 An 80-year-old man with a history of "pyelonephritis" developed diarrhea after a course of antibiotics. On the basis of

Clinical pearl
The blood urea nitrogen could be much lower than expected in a glue-sniffer because much of the nitrogen is excreted as NH_4^+ + hippurate, and less is available for the synthesis of urea.

the following results, a diagnosis of distal RTA was made. Is it correct?

Plasma			Urine		
Na^+	mmol/L	134	Na^+	mmol/L	10
K^+	mmol/L	2.8	K^+	mmol/L	40
Cl^-	mmol/L	115	Cl^-	mmol/L	100
HCO_3^-	mmol/L	10	Osmolality	mOsmkg/ H_2O	800
H^+	nmol/L	62	Urea	mmol/L	300
pH		7.20	pH		5.9

Not likely. Both the urine net charge and the estimated osmolal gap in the urine imply that a high concentration of NH_4^+ is present in the urine. If he had distal RTA, the $[Na^+] + [K^+]$ would exceed the $[Cl^-]$ in the urine. His GI disease is the most likely basis of the metabolic acidosis with a normal renal NH_4^+ excretion.

3.29 What are the diagnostic features of disorders with reduced indirect reabsorption of filtered HCO_3^-?

The major finding is metabolic acidosis with a normal plasma anion gap. The degree of acidosis is modest and is not really influenced by administration of $NaHCO_3$. The rate of excretion of NH_4^+ is much lower than expected for the chronic metabolic acidosis. Usually, in an isolated lesion, the urine pH is low, citrate excretion is not reduced, and there are no other renal findings. The patients studied have otherwise normal renal functions, normal bones on x-ray examination, and do not have nephrocalcinosis or hypokalemia if they have not received therapy.

Note
The diagnostic features listed are those of isolated proximal RTA.

3.30 If a patient with metabolic acidosis is taking acetazolamide, how will the urine test results change once this diuretic is no longer acting (but metabolic acidosis persists)?

The expected response in chronic metabolic acidosis is an increase in the rate of excretion of NH_4^+. Therefore, expect to see 200 mmol of NH_4^+ excreted per day, a negative urine net charge ($Cl^- > (Na^+ + K^+)$), a high urine osmolal gap, and possibly a lower urine pH.

4

Metabolic Alkalosis

OBJECTIVES

☐ To provide the background so that the three components of the pathophysiology of metabolic alkalosis can be understood:
  1. Events in the extracellular fluid (ECF): Cl^- loss and HCO_3^- gain;
  2. Events in the intracellular fluid (ICF): K^+ deficit along with a gain of H^+ and Na^+;
  3. Renal "permission" to maintain a high $[HCO_3^-]$ in plasma.

☐ To identify the different clinical scenarios with metabolic alkalosis: those in which a loss of Cl^- and gain of HCO_3^- play a prominent role (low urine Cl^-) and those in which $NaHCO_3$ is retained in conjunction with the excretion of K^+ in the urine (urine Cl^- is not low).

☐ To emphasize that the treatment of metabolic alkalosis depends on the specific deficit involved; KCl is needed to replace a deficit of KCl, and NaCl is needed if there is a deficit of NaCl.

Outline of Major Principles

1. The pathophysiology of metabolic alkalosis involves events in three major areas—the ECF, the ICF, and the urine. Each must be considered for a comprehensive understanding.

2. Metabolic alkalosis is not primarily an acid-base disorder; it is the net result of deficits in the ECF volume (NaCl) and in K^+ for the most part, with secondary acid-base changes.

3. Appropriate treatment of metabolic alkalosis requires a knowledge of the expected deficits of ions.

INTRODUCTORY CASE
Basically, Toby Is Not "OK"
(Case discussed on pages 179–180)

Toby, a 26-year-old dancer, complains of weakness. She denies vomiting and the intake of medications other than vitamins. Physical examination reveals a thin woman who has a contracted ECF volume. Laboratory results are in the following table.

		Plasma	Random Urine
Na^+	mmol/L	133	52
K^+	mmol/L	3.1	50
Cl^-	mmol/L	90	0
HCO_3^-	mmol/L	32	Not determined
pH		7.48	8.0

What acid-base disturbance is present?

Why is the [Na$^+$] in urine not lower, given the presence of ECF volume contraction?

Why is Toby hypokalemic?

What is the basis for the acid-base disturbance?

Pathophysiology of Metabolic Alkalosis

- Metabolic alkalosis is present if the [HCO$_3^-$] rises and the [H$^+$] declines in the ECF.
- The [HCO$_3^-$] = the ratio of the HCO$_3^-$ content in the ECF to the volume of the ECF.
- The three components to assess are the ECF, the ICF, and the renal response.

Metabolic alkalosis, an acid-base disorder, has two hallmarks: an elevated [HCO$_3^-$] and a lower [H$^+$] in the ECF. Although this definition appears to be simple enough, it addresses only one part of the disorder, the ECF. Two other aspects of this disorder also merit emphasis. First, implicit in this definition is the fact that renal mechanisms have been called into play to permit the ECF to have an elevated [HCO$_3^-$]. Second, although not so obvious, is the occurrence of important events in the ICF that may not be directly reflected by variables that are measured in the ECF or in the renal response. Accordingly, the events in the three areas of interest will be addressed in Part A.

Keys to the analysis of metabolic alkalosis
- Electroneutrality,
- Stoichiometry,
- Quantitative analysis.

Events in the ECF

- The plasma [HCO$_3^-$] may be raised in two ways:
  1. by the addition of HCO$_3^-$ to the ECF.
  2. by the loss of ECF volume.

Addition of HCO$_3^-$ to the ECF

With the constraints of electroneutrality, there are only two ways to add a specific anion (HCO$_3^-$) to a compartment: either loss of an anion such as Cl$^-$ or retention of a cation such as Na$^+$.

Loss of Cl$^-$

Another anion must be lost from a compartment for HCO$_3^-$ to "take its place," electrically speaking. In terms of the ECF, the only anion that is present in sufficient quantity to be lost is Cl$^-$. Hence, on mass balance, if a Cl$^-$ is lost without a major cation

(Na^+ or K^+), it will be lost with a H^+ or NH_4^+. Because a loss of H^+ or NH_4^+ is equivalent to a gain of HCO_3^- (Figure 4.1), the net effect is a loss of Cl^- along with a gain of HCO_3^-. Consider the swap of anions that takes place during vomiting or nasogastric suction. Imagine that you are viewing events at point X on the ECF side of the basolateral membrane of stomach cells (see Figure 4.1). You will see Cl^- leaving the ECF and entering stomach cells; HCO_3^- will be moving in the opposite direction.

Two more steps are needed to complete the picture of the development of metabolic alkalosis associated with depletion of Cl^-.

1. **Bicarbonaturia:** As the $[HCO_3^-]$ in plasma rises, more HCO_3^- are filtered by the kidney. Because most but not all this "extra" filtered HCO_3^- can be reabsorbed (reabsorption occurs mainly in the proximal convoluted tubule [PCT]), a few HCO_3^- are excreted. To the extent that the HCO_3^- are lost with Na^+, a degree of contraction of the ECF volume occurs.

2. **Depletion of K^+:** When HCO_3^- are excreted in the urine, they may "drag out" K^+ (see Chapter 9). The resulting depletion of K^+ in the body indirectly contributes to an elevated $[HCO_3^-]$ in the ECF.

Retention of NaHCO₃

The second way to add HCO_3^- to the ECF and maintain electroneutrality is to retain HCO_3^- along with Na^+. When Na^+ are retained in the ECF, its volume is expanded. Hence, "permission of the kidneys" to retain extra Na^+ and HCO_3^- will be required (see the discussion of Question 4.1). It is also possible that some of the Na^+ retained will be located in the ICF (Na^+ enter the ICF while K^+ exit to the ECF with subsequent excretion of KCl). In this case, an underlying feature is a deficit of K^+ (Figure 4.2).

It is possible that instead of ingesting $NaHCO_3$, a subject may consume the Na^+ (or K^+) salt of organic anions (e.g., potassium citrate, potassium malate, potassium acetate). Metabolism of these organic anions to neutral end-products yields HCO_3^- (or removes H^+), as shown in Figure 4.3.

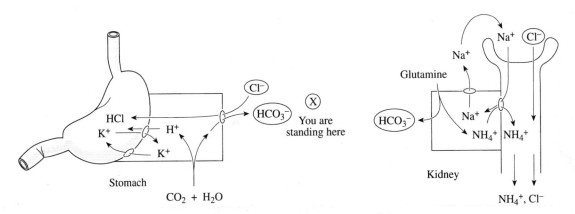

Figure 4.1   Loss of HCl or NH₄Cl is equivalent to a swap of Cl⁻ for HCO₃⁻
The two organs capable of inducing a loss of Cl^- together with a gain of HCO_3^- are the stomach and the kidney; the stoichiometry is 1:1 for Cl^- loss and HCO_3^- gain.

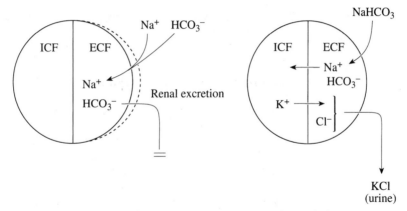

Figure 4.2   Retention of NaHCO₃ in the pathophysiology of metabolic alkalosis
For $NaHCO_3$ to be retained, either expansion of the ECF volume (left-hand figure) or K^+ depletion (right-hand figure) must develop.

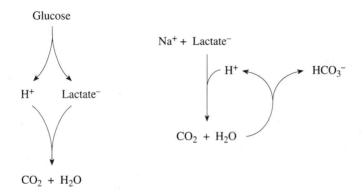

Figure 4.3 Metabolism of organic anions and H⁺ balance
Because organic anions of endogenous origin are synthesized from neutral compounds, metabolism of these anions just restores HCO_3^- balance (figure on left). In contrast, ingestion of the Na^+ or K^+ salts of organic anions yields new HCO_3^- (figure on right) and can produce a net gain of HCO_3^- for the body.

QUESTIONS

(Discussions on pages 186–188)

4.1 *Why will the ingestion of NaHCO₃ not lead to the development of chronic metabolic alkalosis?*

4.2 *For net loss of HCl or NH₄Cl to be the sole cause of metabolic alkalosis, what must the mass balance for Na⁺, K⁺, and Cl⁻ be?*

4.3 *How many liters of emesis must be lost in order to raise the [HCO₃⁻] in plasma by 10 mmol/L in a 70-kg adult?*

4.4 *If a patient has gastric drainage, how can the quantity of new HCO₃⁻ formation be minimized?*

4.5 *How can the progressive rise in the [HCO₃⁻] in plasma and K⁺ depletion be explained in a patient with metabolic alkalosis due to vomiting?*

4.6 *Why might the [HCO₃⁻] in plasma rise in a patient with* *normovolemia who is undergoing plasmapheresis for rapidly progressive glomerulonephritis and renal failure?*

Contraction of the ECF Volume

If the ECF volume is contracted (from removal of NaCl and water), the $[HCO_3^-]$ in the ECF may rise without the addition of new HCO_3^-. In this situation, the $[HCO_3^-]$ rises because the HCO_3^- are distributed in a smaller volume—i.e., the content is unchanged, but the concentration is increased (see the discussion of Question 4.7).

Diuretic ingestion is commonly associated with metabolic alkalosis; diuretics cause NaCl loss in the urine and ECF volume contraction. They may also cause new HCO_3^- formation by increasing production and excretion of NH_4^+ consequent to hypokalemia. The ECF volume contraction results in enhanced proximal tubule H^+ secretion (angiotensin II), which enables the retention of the increased HCO_3^- (see margin note).

Metabolic alkalosis with diuretic use

1. Loss of NaCl leads to ECF volume contraction.
2. ECF volume contraction leads to the release of renin and thereby aldosterone.
3. The delivery of NaCl to the cortical collecting duct (CCD) and the actions of aldosterone lead to excretion of K^+ and thereby to K^+ depletion.
4. K^+ depletion leads to intracellular acidosis.
5. Intracellular acidosis leads to new HCO_3^- generation (NH_4^+ excretion) and increased HCO_3^- reabsorption.
6. Increased renin production leads to increased angiotensin II, which results in enhanced PCT HCO_3^- reabsorption.
7. Metabolic alkalosis is thus due to:
   - ECF volume contraction;
   - K^+ depletion;
   - shift of H^+ into cells;
   - generation of new HCO_3^-;
   - enhanced renal reabsorption of HCO_3^- and a decreased glomerular filtration rate (GFR).

QUESTIONS

(Discussions on page 188)

4.7 *How high might the $[HCO_3^-]$ in plasma rise if a patient has a modest degree of contraction of the ECF volume and no increase in the content of HCO_3^- in the body?*

4.8 *What impact does the loss of 200 mmol of Na^+ and Cl^- from diuretic action have on the content and concentration of HCO_3^- in the ECF? (For simplicity, assume no change in the plasma $[Na^+]$, which is 140 mmol/L.)*

Mechanisms for Renal Retention of HCO_3^-

- The renal mechanisms for maintaining a high $[HCO_3^-]$ are mediated by a lower GFR and/or enhanced reabsorption of filtered HCO_3^-; both usually occur in a given patient.

If a normal person were to ingest substantial amounts of $NaHCO_3$, the $[HCO_3^-]$ in the ECF would increase temporarily before all this extra HCO_3^- would be excreted at a rapid rate (see discussion of Question 4.1). Because patients with metabolic alkalosis often have a plasma $[HCO_3^-]$ in excess of 35 mmol/L, they must have stimulated renal mechanisms to enable them to maintain this very elevated $[HCO_3^-]$ in the ECF. There are two mechanisms that might permit such a high plasma $[HCO_3^-]$ in the presence of normal kidney function—a decreased GFR and enhanced reabsorption of HCO_3^-.

Decreased GFR

One component of the renal mechanism for maintaining an elevated $[HCO_3^-]$ is a reduced filtered load of HCO_3^-. At times, there is a nearly proportionate reduction in the GFR; this reduction keeps the filtered load of HCO_3^- near normal (i.e., when the plasma $[HCO_3^-]$ doubles, the GFR almost halves). This mechanism is an important component of the renal contribution to the maintenance of an elevated plasma $[HCO_3^-]$ in patients with marked ECF volume contraction, especially if there is a large K^+ deficit. The basis of the decreased GFR in many cases is ECF volume contraction. In other cases, such as the metabolic alkalosis consequent to mineralocorticoid excess, however, there is no ECF volume contraction. Nevertheless, a decreased GFR has been demonstrated in animal models of this disorder and has been attributed to the associated hypokalemia.

Enhanced Reabsorption of HCO_3^-

A very important renal mechanism for maintaining an elevated $[HCO_3^-]$ is increased reabsorption of filtered HCO_3^-. The major stimuli are low "effective" circulating volume and intracellular acidosis of cells of the PCT. With respect to a low "effective" circulating volume, the major mediator identified is angiotensin II; this hormone leads to an activation of the Na^+,H^+ exchanger (NHE-3) in the luminal membrane of proximal convoluted cells (Figure 4.4). Distal H^+ secretion may also be stimulated by mineralocorticoid secretion during ECF volume contraction, but the capacity for H^+ secretion in the distal tubule is small relative to proximal H^+ secretion. Regarding the fall in intracellular pH, both hypokalemia and a rise in P_{CO_2} raise the $[H^+]$ in the ICF and could act in concert with the high angiotensin II levels to promote the enhanced reabsorption of filtered HCO_3^-. It is not clear whether Cl^- deficiency per se plays any role in this regard. Some investigators who

GFR, decreased ECF volume, and K^+ deficit

If the patient with ECF volume contraction, metabolic alkalosis, and a K^+ deficit did not have a decreased GFR, there would be increased $NaHCO_3$ delivery to the distal nephron and increased $KHCO_3$ excretion, which would result in a more marked K^+ deficit. Further K^+ depletion causes more ECF volume depletion because Na^+ enter the ICF when K^+ exit the ICF.

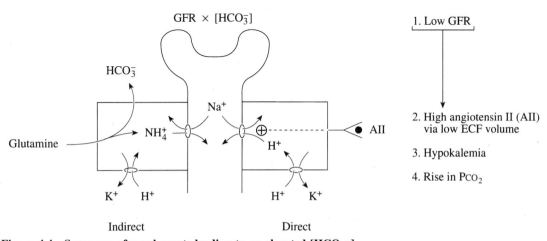

Increase HCO_3^- generation

Decrease HCO_3^- excretion

1. Low GFR

2. High angiotensin II (AII) via low ECF volume

3. Hypokalemia

4. Rise in P_{CO_2}

Figure 4.4　Summary of renal events leading to an elevated $[HCO_3^-]$

The renal events in metabolic alkalosis are a lower filtered load of HCO_3^- (low GFR), more reabsorption of HCO_3^- in the proximal convoluted tubule (angiotensin II, hypokalemia, and an elevated P_{CO_2}), and more excretion of NH_4^+ to generate metabolic alkalosis (hypokalemia).

favor a more direct role of Cl^- deficiency propose that low luminal $[Cl^-]$ in the collecting duct could promote Cl^- secretion via the Cl^-/HCO_3^- exchanger and thereby enhance the distal reabsorption of HCO_3^-. For this hypothesis to be valid, the $[Cl^-]$ would have to be very low in the lumen given the low K_m of this transporter for Cl^-, a requirement not strongly supported by experimental data.

Renal Handling of HCO_3^-: A More Detailed Examination

> • Is there a renal threshold or tubular maximum for the renal reabsorption of HCO_3^-?

Experiment of Pitts

The classic experiment performed by Pitts was to study the renal response to an intravenous infusion of $NaHCO_3$. Both the Na^+ load (via low angiotensin AII) and the HCO_3^- load (via intracellular alkaline pH shift) caused the kidneys to excrete the surplus $NaHCO_3$ (Figure 4.5). This led to the general impression that there is a tubular maximum for the reabsorption of HCO_3^- at close to the normal value for HCO_3^- in plasma (25 mmol/L GFR) and thereby a renal threshold for the reabsorption of HCO_3^-.

Physiologic Load of HCO_3^-

A load of $NaHCO_3$ is rarely encountered in clinical medicine, but if so, it will simply be excreted—as it was for Pitts—until the plasma $[HCO_3^-]$ level returns to its normal value of 25 mmol/L.

Let us now examine a physiologic load of HCO_3, the temporary trapping of, e.g., 1 L of HCl in the stomach (a loss of 150 mmol Cl^- and a gain of 150 mmol HCO_3 in the body [see Figure 4.1]). We first take a teleologic look at the alternatives.

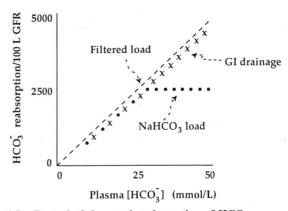

Figure 4.5 Control of the renal reabsorption of HCO_3^-
The horizontal axis is the plasma $[HCO_3^-]$ and the amount of HCO_3^- reabsorbed (with a GFR of 100 L/day for convenience) is shown on the vertical axis. The dashed line represents the filtered load of HCO_3^-. The data from a load of $NaHCO_3$ is shown in solid circles, and the data from selective removal of HCl is shown by the X symbols.

Because the kidney cannot make new Cl^-, the electrolyte abnormality cannot be fully corrected.

Excretion of HCO_3^-. If this were to occur, the net effect would be the loss of 150 mmol of a cation, Na^+, K^+ or NH_4^+, in addition to the HCO_3^-.

Excretion of NH_4^+ and HCO_3^-. Because NH_4^+ cannot be excreted in alkaline urine, and the excretion of NH_4^+ leads to new generation of HCO_3^-, this is not a viable option.

Bottom Line. Do not excrete NH_4^+ plus HCO_3^-.

Excretion of Na^+ and HCO_3^-. If this were to occur, the loss of 150 mmol of Na^+ would cause a loss of 1 L of ECF. Although the plasma $[HCO_3^-]$ will be normal, the ECF volume becomes "volumetrically challenged."

There is yet another danger. The HCl may eventually exit the stomach and be reabsorbed in the small intestine. The host will have a degree of metabolic acidosis along with the ECF volume contraction. Now more NH_4^+ will have to be excreted (150 mmol) to achieve acid-base balance. Having such a high NH_4^+, excretion does not occur. If there was a high rate of excretion of NH_4^+, it could result in a loss of lean body mass and possible damage to the renal medulla by NH_3 itself.

Bottom Line. Do not excrete much $NaHCO_3$.

Excretion of K^+ and HCO_3^-. This again is a poor alternative because a deficit of K^+ could occur. Moreover, when K^+ leave the cell, H^+ (made with HCO_3^- for the most part) or Na^+ must enter cells (contracting the ECF volume).

If a degree of contraction of the ECF volume occurs, the combination of aldosterone actions and distal delivery of HCO_3^- could lead to excessive loss of K^+.

Bottom Line. Do not excrete a large amount of K^+ and HCO_3^-.

Actual Data

As shown in Figure 4.5, the majority of filtered HCO_3^- is reabsorbed. Nevertheless, this reabsorption is not 100%, and there is a small alkaline tide in the late morning urine. In quantitative terms, the amount of HCO_3^- excreted is less than 10 mmol per day.

There is a second physiologic consequence of trapping of HCl at some times and $NaHCO_3$ at other times—a wide range of "normal" values for the plasma $[HCO_3^-]$ (22–31 mmol/L).

HCO_3^- stimulates the reabsorption of HCO_3^- in the PCT. On the surface, having HCO_3^- stimulate its own reabsorption when the subject is already alkalemic seems to be "an acid-base error." Nevertheless, there are reliable data supporting this observation. The authors interpret this observation as follows. When HCl is secreted into the stomach, the $[HCO_3^-]$ in plasma rises and that of Cl^- falls (see Figure 4.1). There is no change in ECF volume, and the alkalemia should depress the reabsorption of HCO_3^- in the PCT. Notwithstanding, HCO_3^- reabsorption rises in this setting (see Figure 4.5). Thus, the stimulation of PCT H^+ secretion by peritubular HCO_3^- could accomplish this aim. In body balance terms, this will avoid a loss of Na^+ and K^+ in the urine as well as prevent a subsequent need for the excretion of NH_4^+ to correct the acidosis that would result from the excretion of HCO_3^- when the HCl from the stomach is reabsorbed in the small intestine.

QUESTIONS

(Discussions on pages 188–189)

4.9 *Why do some patients who vomit have a large deficit of Na^+ in the ECF?*
Hint: In the selective HCl depletion model of metabolic alkalosis, there is no significant deficit of Na^+.

4.10 *Under what circumstances might vomiting cause metabolic acidosis? How might this be recognized as the pathophysiology?*

Events in the ICF

The simplest model of metabolic alkalosis in humans is that produced when HCl is removed from the stomach. In a study, normal human volunteers underwent this procedure for 4–5 days. All ion and water losses other than HCl were replaced. Examination of the mass balance data reveals that the ICF is an important site of involvement in metabolic alkalosis resulting from loss of HCl. The significance of the ICF is best shown by examining events in three phases (see margin illustration).

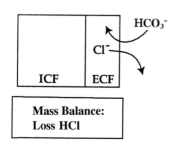

Loss of HCl

As shown in Figure 4.1, loss of HCl results in a net gain of HCO_3^- in the body and metabolic alkalosis. Mass balance in humans and in experimental animals reveals an initial deficit of Cl^- but not Na^+ or K^+, and the ECF volume changes to only a modest degree.

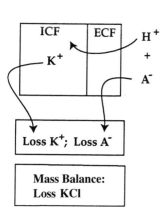

Change of Mass Balance

After losing HCl, subjects were permitted to stabilize in a postdrainage period of 5–7 days. Their deficit of Cl^- was not replaced. During this period, all subjects developed a rather prominent degree of K^+ depletion. It is not clear from the study what anion was excreted with K^+. Nevertheless, the source of the K^+ was the ICF (the ECF did not contain enough K^+ to account for the negative balance). The likely events for the excretion of K^+ with an endogenous anion are shown in the margin and in Figure 4.5. The bottom line is that for every K^+ lost on mass balance without a Cl^-, a net gain of a H^+ (or loss of an HCO_3^-) occurred. The striking feature in the mass balance is the near-equimolar loss of K^+ and Cl^- (Table 4.1); there was little change in mass balance for Na^+. To provide mass balance and electroneutrality in the ICF and ECF, H^+ and Na^+ entered the ICF when K^+ exited (see margin illustration).

H^+ Balance During KCl Depletion

There is an equimolar loss of K^+ and Cl^-. Nevertheless, these two losses are not simultaneous. First, the loss of Cl^- without Na^+ or

TABLE 4.1 **Deficits in the Selective Depletion of HCl Model of Metabolic Alkalosis**

Data were chosen from studies involving selective loss of HCl (or a swap of HCO_3^- for Cl^-) in humans, dogs, and rats, followed by a post-drainage period. Note the near-equimolar losses of Cl^- and K^+ in each example. In each case, chronic metabolic alkalosis was present ([HCO_3^-] was close to 35 mmol/L).

	Species		
	---	---	---
Variable	*Human (mmol)*	*Dog (mmol)*	*Rat (μmol)*
Na^+	− 22	9	− 535
K^+	− 213	− 118	− 2931
Cl^-	− 199	− 110	− 2533
ECF volume	− 0.5 L	—	− 10 mL
% change	− 3	—	− 12

K^+ equates to a gain of HCO_3^- (see Figure 4.1); second, the loss of K^+ without Cl^- equates to a gain of H^+ (Figure 4.6). Although there is acid-base balance, there is a high [HCO_3^-] in the ECF that is largely due to an increase in content of HCO_3^- in this compartment (the ECF volume was not markedly contracted; see Table 4.1). The explanation is that instead of being retained in the ECF (and lowering the [HCO_3^-]), H^+ enter cells concomitant with the exit of K^+ from the ICF. Ultimately, metabolic alkalosis associated with selective loss of HCl (the so-called Cl^--depletion type of metabolic alkalosis) has the following features:

1. a higher content and concentration of HCO_3^- in the ECF;
2. K^+ depletion and intracellular acidosis;
3. enhanced reabsorption of HCO_3^- by the kidney.

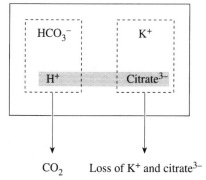

CO_2 Loss of K^+ and citrate^{3-}

Figure 4.6 Loss of K^+ plus an endogenous anion is equivalent to a gain of H^+

As indicated in the horizontal stippled bar, citrate^{3-} are formed in the body along with protons. H^+ may titrate HCO_3^-, yielding CO_2, which is exhaled (dashed rectangle on the left). Citrate^{3-} may be excreted with K^+ (dashed rectangle on the right side of the figure). Taken together, the excretion of K^+ and citrate^{3-} represents the indirect loss of HCO_3^- from the body.

QUESTIONS

(Discussions on pages 189–190)

4.11 *What pathophysiologic mechanisms must be involved to have Cl^--depletion metabolic alkalosis? What is the expected mass balance in each case?*

4.12 *Three factors contributed to the degree of intracellular acidosis in a patient who has vomited on a chronic basis and who has a significant degree of ECF volume contraction. What are they? The pertinent values in plasma are pH 7.48, HCO_3^- 36 mmol/L, and K^+ 2.7 mmol/L.*

PART B

Clinical Clues

> • Metabolic alkalosis occurs most commonly with the loss of gastric contents or diuretic use; mineralocorticoid excess is less commonly the sole cause of metabolic alkalosis.

If the basis for metabolic alkalosis can be established, the expected deficits can be approximated and appropriate therapy can be instituted. The most helpful aspects of the presentation are the history, an assessment of the ECF volume, and certain laboratory data—random urine electrolytes along with the plasma creatinine concentration and $[K^+]$; each will be discussed in turn.

History

Clinical pearls for Cl^- depletion and metabolic alkalosis
• ECF volume is often contracted.
• Urine $[Cl^-]$ < 20 mmol/L, unless diuretics are acting.

The most common causes of metabolic alkalosis are vomiting and diuretics; other causes are listed in Table 4.2. Among the items to explore in the history are issues such as previous investigations, eating habits, drug or unusual ingestions, body image, psychosocial aspects, a knowledge of previous kidney function, family history, gastrointestinal (GI) complaints, hypertension, and the clinical setting (e.g., ventilation for chronic lung disease).

One might think that the diagnosis of metabolic alkalosis would be straightforward, and often it is. Nevertheless, a number of patients, because of personality disorders, are not willing to admit to the self-induction of vomiting or the abuse of diuretics. Therefore, the history cannot be relied upon entirely, and clinicians must often resort to a series of laboratory tests and a degree of subterfuge to establish the diagnosis (Table 4.3).

ECF Volume

ECF Volume Contraction

The major causes of metabolic alkalosis—diuretic abuse or vomiting—usually present with a significant degree of ECF volume

TABLE 4.2   **Causes of Metabolic Alkalosis**

See Table 4.3 for more information concerning urine electrolytes in metabolic alkalosis.

Causes usually associated with a contracted ECF or "effective" circulating volume:

1. Low urine $[Cl^-]$ (unless a diuretic is acting)
   - Loss of gastric secretions (e.g., from vomiting, nasogastric suction)
   - Remote use of diuretics
   - Delivery of nonreabsorbable anions plus a reason for Na^+ avidity
   - Posthypercapnia (see also secondary hyperaldosteronism below)
   - Loss of NaCl via the Gl tract (as in certain diarrheas, e.g., congenital Cl^- loss, some villous adenomas)
2. Persistent high urine $[Cl^-]$
   - Bartter's-like syndromes
   - Current diuretic use

Causes usually associated with a normal or expanded ECF or "effective" circulating volume:

1. Large reduction in GFR plus a source of HCO_3^-
   - Examples include alkali ingestion, ingestion of ion-exchange resin plus nonreabsorbable alkali
2. Enhanced mineralocorticoid activity
   - Primary aldosteronism
   - Secondary hyperaldosteronism (examples include renal artery stenosis, malignant hypertension, renin-producing tumor, low effective arterial blood volume plus an alkali load)
   - Endogenous or exogenous mineralocorticoids, licorice ingestion, ACTH-driven mineralocorticoid secretion (see Chapter 10, pages 423–424)

Causes that are difficult to classify with respect to ECF volume:

1. Hypomagnesemia
2. Excessive alkaline tide with Zollinger-Ellison syndrome

contraction (Table 4.4 lists cautions regarding clinical findings). ECF volume contraction contributes to both the generation and maintenance of an elevated plasma $[HCO_3^-]$ either via a decreased denominator or increased numerator of the HCO_3^-/ECF volume ratio. As pointed out in the discussion of Question 4.7, a decrease in the denominator of this ratio accounts for only a small portion of the elevation in the $[HCO_3^-]$. The primary influence is an increase in the content of HCO_3^- in the ECF.

TABLE 4.3   **Clues to Identify the Possible Causes of Metabolic Alkalosis Associated with a Low "Effective" Circulating Volume**

Cause	Diagnostic Features
Recent vomiting	• Unmeasured anion in urine (HCO_3^-) • Urine pH >7, $[Cl^-]$ low, but $[Na^+]$ high • Disturbed body image
Remote vomiting	• Urine $[Na^+]$ and $[Cl^-]$ both low
Recent diuretic	• Urine $[Na^+]$ and $[Cl^-]$ both high
Remote diuretic	• Urine $[Na^+]$ and $[Cl^-]$ both low
Post hypercapnia	• Urine $[Na^+]$ and $[Cl^-]$ both low
Cl^- loss in diarrhea	• Urine pH <6, $[Na^+]$ and $[Cl^-]$ both low; if hypokalemia induces NH_4^+ excretion, urine $[Cl^-]$ will rise
Nonreabsorbable anion	• Urine $[Cl^-]$ low, but $[Na^+]$ high • Unmeasured anion in urine • Urine pH <7

TABLE 4.4 **Conditions in Which Jugular Venous Pressure May Not Accurately Reflect the "Effective" Circulating Volume**

Pulmonary Hypertension

Chronic emphysema
Pulmonary emboli
Idiopathic pulmonary hypertension

Impaired Right Ventricular Emptying

Pulmonary valve stenosis or insufficiency
Cardiomyopathy
Right ventricular infarction
Tricuspid valve insufficiency

Impaired Right Ventricular Filling

Tricuspid valve stenosis
Superior vena cava syndrome
Tamponade

Poor Left Ventricular Output ("Ineffective" Circulating Volume)

Aortic valve stenosis or insufficiency
Myocardial infarction
Mitral valve stenosis or insufficiency
Cardiomyopathy

In diuretic abuse, extra HCO_3^- are generated by the production and excretion of more NH_4^+. For this excretion to occur, hypokalemia must be present (hypokalemia augments renal ammoniagenesis and NH_4^+ excretion). Hypokalemia is also an expected sequela to the actions of aldosterone when the Na^+ salts of nonreabsorbable anions (e.g., carbenicillinates) are given to patients who have a contracted "effective" circulating volume.

In vomiting, the other common clinical cause of metabolic alkalosis in the setting of a low ECF volume, both the contracted ECF volume and HCO_3^- addition are the consequence of the loss of HCl. When HCl is lost, HCO_3^- replace Cl^- in the ECF. The resulting alkalemia leads to the excretion of some $NaHCO_3$ in the urine. The combined loss of HCl via gastric secretion and $NaHCO_3$ in the urine is equivalent to a net loss of NaCl and a tiny loss of $CO_2 + H_2O$:

$$HCl \rightarrow H^+ + Cl^- \rightarrow lost$$
$$NaHCO_3 \rightarrow HCO_3^- + Na^+ \rightarrow lost$$
$$H^+ + HCO_3^- \leftrightarrow CO_2 + H_2O$$

Result: Loss of $Na^+ + Cl^- + CO_2 + H_2O$

A second bout of vomiting will add more HCO_3^- in place of Cl^- (see Figure 4.1), except now the patient will have a mild degree of ECF volume contraction. In this setting, there will be a release of renin, increased formation of angiotensin II, and a release of aldosterone. Although angiotensin II promotes the reabsorption of HCO_3^- in the PCT, some $NaHCO_3$ will escape reabsorption and be delivered distally where it will lead to augmented excretion of K^+ (aldosterone and bicarbonaturia markedly augment kaliuresis).

Summary

Both vomiting and diuretic abuse result in the same findings of metabolic alkalosis, hypokalemia, and ECF volume contraction.

Nevertheless, their routes to this setting differ. Notwithstanding, the therapy (replace the deficits) will be similar once the cause is no longer present (the reason for vomiting or the presence of diuretics).

When treating metabolic alkalosis associated with hypokalemia, one must also consider events in the ICF. In both examples cited previously, the depletion of K^+ leads to a shift of cations Na^+ and H^+ into cells. This shift not only exacerbates the degree of elevation of the $[HCO_3^-]$ in the ECF but also imposes a new demand on therapy: correction of the acidosis and K^+ depletion in the ICF via administration of KCl (see margin note).

Clinical pearls
- The major deficits are Cl^- and K^+.
- A deficit of NaCl is commonly present as well.

ECF Volume Expansion

Patients with a normal or expanded ECF volume (see Table 4.2) form another subgroup of those with metabolic alkalosis (see margin note). They often have hypertension and a modest degree of elevation of their $[HCO_3^-]$. The basis of their disturbance is hyperaldosteronism or enhanced mineralocorticoid actions. Although they are K^+-depleted, simple replacement of electrolyte deficits is not enough. The source of the mineralocorticoids must be addressed.

Assessing the ECF volume in terms of circulating volume is a valuable means of diagnosing the basis of the metabolic alkalosis. The evaluation of the jugular venous pressure (JVP) is an important clue in this regard; however, JVP is a right-sided phenomenon that is used to gain insights into the pressure on the left side of the heart. Do not be misled by events that perturb the relationship between the right- and left-sided cardiac pressures (see Table 4.4).

Note
To maintain an elevated $[HCO_3^-]$ in the plasma, the GFR must be lower and/or reabsorption of HCO_3^- must be higher; both seem to be the result of the deficit of K^+.

Urine Electrolytes

A single random urine sample, or perhaps several random urine samples, can usually unravel the pathophysiology of metabolic alkalosis (see margin note and Table 4.5).

Clinical pearls
- There are no "normal" values for urine electrolytes, just expected values in a given clinical setting.
- In a patient with a contracted ECF volume, the expected values for urine $[Na^+]$ and/or $[Cl^-]$ are close to nil.

TABLE 4.5 **Urine Electrolytes in the Diagnosis of Metabolic Alkalosis**

Values are taken from a random urine sample on presentation. "High" signifies >20 mmol/L and "low" <20 mmol/L. "Remote" means no recent vomiting or drug administration.

Clinical Setting	Urine Values				Comments
	$[Na^+]$	$[K^+]$	$[Cl^-]$	pH	
1. Low ECF volume (excluding edema)					
• Vomiting (recent)	High	High	Low	>7	• If remote, Na^+, Cl^-, and pH will be low
• Diuretic (recent)	High	High	High	<6	• If remote, same as for remote vomiting
					• Values may fluctuate as diuretic action wears off
• Nonreabsorbable anions (recent)	High	High	Low	<6	• If remote, same as for remote vomiting
• Bartter's-like syndromes	High	High	High	6–6.5	• Values are high in each urine sample
2. Normal or expanded ECF volume (see Table 4.2 for list of causes)	High	High	High	5–8	• Hypertension
					• History may change with different underlying diseases

Excretion of a Small Quantity of Na^+ or Cl^-

Metabolic alkalosis, ECF volume contraction, and similar low excretions of Na^+, K^+, and Cl^- could indicate the occurrence of remote vomiting, "yesterday's diuretics," or the prior intake of nonreabsorbable anions. Hence, to make a final diagnosis, one must interpret these urine results in conjunction with other information obtained via the history or repeated urine sampling. Identifying the basis of the ECF volume contraction is usually the key to making the diagnosis.

Excretion of Na$^+$ But Only a Small Quantity of Cl$^-$

Anion revealed by urine net charge:
$[Na^+] + [K^+]$ greatly exceeds $[Cl^-]$.

Some patients with metabolic alkalosis have a low rate of excretion of Cl$^-$, yet the urine contains an abundant quantity of Na$^+$. The reason for the excretion of Na$^+$ is the presence of an anion that was not reabsorbed (this anion is revealed by an increased net charge in the urine; see margin note). If the urine contains a large quantity of HCO$_3$$^-$ (pH > 7), the patient must have a nonrenal source of HCO$_3$$^-$ (the kidneys cannot excrete and generate HCO$_3$$^-$ simultaneously). In this setting, vomiting or nasogastric suction is the most likely diagnosis if the patient is not ingesting HCO$_3$$^-$ or organic anions. A low urine pH suggests the intake or generation of anions that are poorly reabsorbed by the kidneys.

Excretion of Na$^+$ and Cl$^-$

The expected pattern of excretion with a normal ECF volume is excretion of Na$^+$ and Cl$^-$. This same pattern may occur in patients with a contracted ECF volume if there is intrinsic renal disease or the lack of messenger to stimulate Na$^+$ reabsorption (see Chapter 6, pages 253–255). More specifically related to metabolic alkalosis, this pattern of electrolyte excretion suggests diuretic action or Bartter's syndromes.

QUESTION

(Discussion on pages 190–191)

4.13 *How can one distinguish between diuretic abuse and Bartter's-like syndromes using urine electrolytes?*

Plasma Creatinine

Patients with ECF volume contraction will have elevated values for creatinine in plasma corrected for their body mass, especially if the degree of ECF volume contraction is marked. Previous values and the clinical setting make this interpretation relatively simple.

Patients with chronic renal failure usually have a normal or expanded ECF volume and a markedly elevated level of creatinine in plasma. Should such a patient ingest or be given alkali or organic anions, a small quantity of HCO$_3$$^-$ will be filtered, and most HCO$_3$$^-$ will be retained in the body.

QUESTIONS

(Discussions on pages 191–193)

4.14 *A very low GFR plays a prominent role in the metabolic* *alkalosis associated with the milk-alkali syndrome. What is the pathophysiology of this syndrome?*

4.15 *Why does $NaHCO_3$ provide a much larger alkali load to the body than an equivalent dose of $CaCO_3$?*

4.16 *What will increase the alkali load to the body if the amount of $CaCO_3$ ingested remains constant?*

4.17 *What is the pathophysiology of metabolic alkalosis associated with nonreabsorbable alkali and an ion-exchange resin?*

4.18 *What is the pathophysiology of metabolic alkalosis associated with a normal or expanded ECF volume?*

Plasma [K⁺]

Hypokalemia is usually present in most patients with metabolic alkalosis. It may play several roles in the pathophysiology. As mentioned earlier, by augmenting the production and excretion of NH_4^+, it may increase the content of HCO_3^- in the ECF. When intracellular shifts cause the cations Na^+ and H^+ to enter cells, the $[HCO_3^-]$ in the ECF increases because of ECF volume contraction (Na^+ loss from the ECF) and loss of H^+ from the ECF. Hypokalemia also leads to a lower excretion of HCO_3^- because it may decrease the GFR and increase the reabsorption of HCO_3^- by the PCT (intracellular acidosis).

QUESTION

(Discussion on page 194)

4.19 *In what circumstances might metabolic alkalosis be associated with hyperkalemia?*

Clinical Approach

A clinical approach to a patient with metabolic alkalosis is outlined in Figure 4.7. The first step in determining the basis of metabolic alkalosis is to rule out chronic renal insufficiency (GFR < 25% of normal). If renal failure exists, the specific cause of the metabolic alkalosis should be evident from the history.

If a very low GFR plus alkali input are not the cause of metabolic alkalosis (and they usually are not), the ECF volume status is the next critical parameter to assess. The majority of patients have a contracted ECF volume, and the $[Cl^-]$ in their urine is very low (<20 mmol/L). The differential diagnosis in this group with ECF volume contraction is indicated in Figure 4.7. If the history is not available, examine the urine electrolytes in a random urine sample to help identify the possible causes of the metabolic alkalosis (see Table 4.5).

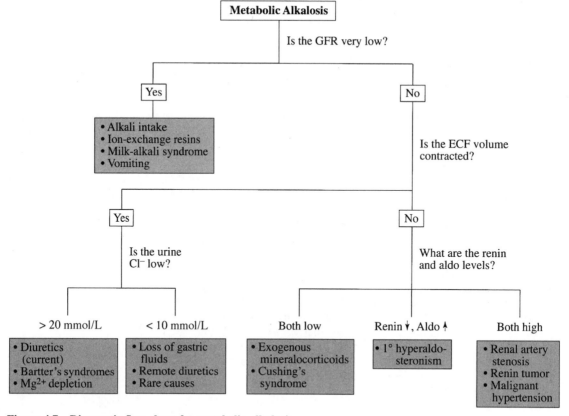

Figure 4.7 Diagnostic flow chart for metabolic alkalosis.
Final diagnoses are shown in the shaded boxes (see the text for details). See Chapter 10 as well.

Examples of Less Common Causes of Chronic Metabolic Alkalosis

Causes Associated with ECF Volume Contraction

The vast majority of patients with metabolic alkalosis will have either diuretic use or loss of gastric content as the basis. The following are the less common causes of metabolic alkalosis.

Nonreabsorbable Anions

Drugs and substances causing metabolic alkalosis
Drugs containing a poorly reabsorbable anion (e.g., carbenicillin), or a substance that can be metabolized to HCO_3^- (e.g., citrate^{3-}), can cause metabolic alkalosis in a patient with high renal avidity for Na^+.

If a patient has a contracted ECF volume and takes an Na^+ salt with an anion that cannot be reabsorbed by the kidney (e.g., Na^+ carbenicillinate), the patient may develop metabolic alkalosis and hypokalemia. ECF volume contraction is usually present for an unrelated reason. Thus, there is a stimulus to Na^+ reabsorption, but all the Na^+ cannot be reabsorbed because of the presence of an anion that cannot be reabsorbed. In the cortical collecting duct, the actions of aldosterone cause Na^+ to be reabsorbed in conjunction with K^+ secretion. The result is hypokalemia, which, in turn, leads to increased production and excretion of NH_4^+ and an increased plasma $[HCO_3^-]$ (a result of renal HCO_3^- generation and ECF volume contraction).

The urine provides the clues to the diagnosis. The findings should be as follows:

1. The $[Cl^-]$ in urine should be low (<20 mmol/L).

2. The $[Na^+]$ in urine will vary (if large, a recent load of nonreabsorbable anion was administered; if the intake of nonreabsorbable anions was discontinued, the $[Na^+]$ in urine may be less than 10 mmol/L).

3. The urine should contain a substantial concentration of unmeasured anion ($[Na^+] + [K^+] > [Cl^-]$). If the urine pH is alkaline, the anion is HCO_3^-; if it is acid, the patient has metabolic alkalosis associated with a nonreabsorbable anion.

Bartter's-Like Syndromes

Patients with these unusual disorders are not hypertensive and have ECF volume depletion, renal NaCl wasting, metabolic alkalosis, hypokalemia, and usually renal Mg^{2+} wasting. The exact basis of the Na^+ and Cl^- wasting is becoming more clear; Bartter's-like syndromes are considered in more detail in Chapter 10, pages 419–422.

Loss of Cl⁻ in the Stool

The loss of Cl^--rich fluid in the stool (e.g., congenital chloridorrhea, a rare disorder) creates a situation identical to the diuretic-induced metabolic alkalosis, except that the urine always has a low $[Na^+]$ and $[Cl^-]$.

Posthypercapnia

In the course of chronic hypercapnia, an increased plasma $[HCO_3^-]$ results in the loss of Cl^- in the urine (i.e., enhanced renal NH_4Cl excretion). If the patient has a contracted ECF volume when the hypercapnia resolves, there will be a stimulus for Na^+ reabsorption and H^+ secretion that results in the reabsorption of luminal HCO_3^-. The increase in the plasma $[HCO_3^-]$ is thus maintained until the ECF volume is reexpanded with NaCl administration.

Causes That are Commonly Associated with a Normal or Expanded ECF Volume

Hyperaldosteronism

When patients with metabolic alkalosis fail to respond to the administration of KCl and NaCl, they are likely to have excessive mineralocorticoid activity of either exogenous or endogenous origin or a process that mimics this pathophysiology (see Table 10.5). The associated hypokalemia is probably of major importance in both the generation and the maintenance of the metabolic alkalosis. Hypokalemia enhances ammoniagenesis, which enables renal new HCO_3^- formation, and it also causes an increased indirect reabsorption of HCO_3^- via the rise in proximal tubular intracellular $[H^+]$. In addition, it reduces the GFR and thereby maintains the elevated blood $[HCO_3^-]$.

Alkali Loading

Under usual circumstances, $NaHCO_3$ loading leads to only a mild elevation in the plasma $[HCO_3^-]$ because most of these HCO_3^- are excreted (see the discussion of Question 4.1). However, in the presence of Na$^+$ depletion or in renal failure, clinically important elevations of plasma [HCO$_3$$^-$] occur with NaHCO$_3$ administration (because of the lack of excretion of HCO$_3$$^-$).

Magnesium Depletion

Patients with Mg^{2+} depletion may have metabolic alkalosis and hypokalemia resembling a high mineralocorticoid state. The hypomagnesemia can be confirmed by plasma analysis. The usual clinical setting for this deficiency includes malabsorption, diarrhea, or the administration of drugs that act on the loop of Henle (e.g., cisplatin, loop diuretics, or aminoglycosides; see margin note). These patients must be distinguished from those with primary hyperaldosteronism who may also have Mg^{2+} deficiency.

Milk-Alkali Syndrome

The milk-alkali syndrome (metabolic alkalosis, hypercalcemia, hypocalciuria, and renal insufficiency; refer to the discussion of Question 4.14) is due to the ingestion of large amounts of milk and absorbable antacids (CaCO$_3$). It has been of mainly historical interest; however, with the current emphasis on preventing osteoporosis by using CaCO$_3$ as a major source of Ca$^+$ supplementation, this syndrome may reappear (see margin note).

Nonreabsorbable Alkali Ingestion with Ion-Exchange Resins

Ion-exchange resins are generally used in patients with renal insufficiency; when combined with nonreabsorbable alkali (aluminum or magnesium hydroxide), their use has resulted in metabolic alkalosis that resolves when either agent is discontinued (refer to the discussion of Question 4.17).

Effect of Metabolic Alkalosis on Ventilation

Because the plasma [H$^+$] is a major determinant of ventilation, metabolic alkalosis depresses ventilation. In fact, there is a linear relationship between the increasing plasma [HCO$_3$$^-$] and the progressive increase in Pa$_{CO_2}$; the slope is approximately 0.7 (see margin note). Thus, when patients present with CO$_2$ retention and metabolic alkalosis, the metabolic alkalosis should be corrected before attributing the CO$_2$ retention to lung disease.

As hypoventilation develops, it is accompanied by hypoxia,

TABLE 4.6 **Impact of Metabolic Alkalosis on Patients with CO$_2$ Retention**

Metabolic Alkalosis	H$^+$ (nmol/L)	HCO$_3$$^-$ (mmol/L)	Pa$_{CO_2}$ (mm Hg)	Pa$_{O_2}$ (mm Hg)
Before correction	40	37	61	52
Partial correction	42	28	48	69

which offsets the degree of respiratory suppression achieved (more severe respiratory suppression is observed in patients receiving O_2 supplementation when hypoxia is prevented). The reduced delivery of O_2 to tissues in metabolic alkalosis is further aggravated by the fact that alkalemia shifts the O_2-hemoglobin dissociation curve to the left; this shift increases the affinity of hemoglobin for O_2 (see Figure 5.3).

Because patients with chronic lung diseases often take diuretics to cope with their Na^+ retention, they may develop metabolic alkalosis. The mixed acid-base disturbance may return their plasma $[H^+]$ to the normal range, but their clinical condition may worsen when they no longer have the acidemic drive to ventilate. These patients need not be alkalemic in order to experience the adverse effects of metabolic alkalosis in chronic respiratory acidosis (see margin note).

Note
Data from eight patients with chronic respiratory acidosis prior to and following the partial correction of the metabolic alkalosis are provided in Table 4.6. The clinical condition (mental function and sense of well-being) was improved in association with the fall in $PaCO_2$ and the increase in PaO_2.

PART C

Treatment of Metabolic Alkalosis

Low ECF or "Effective" Circulating Volume Group

- Identify the basis of the deficits.
- Replace the deficits of Na^+, K^+, and Cl^-.

Patients with ECF volume contraction require Na^+ and Cl^- replacement. When their ECF volume is restored, the $[HCO_3^-]$ will fall somewhat as a result of dilution; bicarbonaturia will occur if the ECF volume is overexpanded. Generally, the $[HCO_3^-]$ in the ECF falls when NaCl is given, even if the K^+ deficits are not completely restored. Up to this point, the large K^+ deficit in cells and the intracellular acidosis have been ignored. Hence, NaCl administration is only partial therapy in these patients because it does not reverse the accompanying intracellular acidosis and K^+ deficit.

Some patients with metabolic alkalosis have little depletion of their ECF volume. Clearly, in these cases, NaCl should not be the linchpin of therapy. To treat the ICF acidosis and K^+ depletion, K^+ must be given with an anion that permits retention of this cation in the ICF. In most cases, KCl is administered because as K^+ enter the ICF, Na^+ and H^+ exit, for the most part. The H^+ titrate the excess HCO_3^- in the ECF and the extra NaCl is retained or excreted depending on the ECF volume status. Obviously, if some of the intracellular K^+ deficit represents loss of K^+ and phosphate, the entire deficit of K^+ cannot be replaced acutely. It must await the synthesis of intracellular phosphate esters, such as DNA, RNA, and phospholipids.

If the metabolic alkalosis is due to a reduction in "effective" circulating volume with ECF volume expansion (e.g., in a patient

Principles of therapy
- NaCl administration is needed only if the ECF volume is contracted.
- K^+ administration is needed in virtually all cases to correct the ICF acidosis and K^+ deficit.
- Cl^- administration is needed to replace the deficit of Cl^-.

Consequences of persisting depletion of K^+
- Intracellular acidosis
- Enhanced ammoniagenesis
- Enhanced reabsorption of HCO_3^- in the PCT
- Persistent metabolic alkalosis

with congestive heart failure who is on diuretics), the patient will require therapy with KCl, and additional Na^+ should not be given (as K^+ enter the ICF, Na^+ leave, adding some Na^+ to the ECF). The patient must excrete the extra Na^+ in the body.

If the patient has been abusing diuretics or inducing vomiting, treatment of the underlying psychopathology will be the greatest challenge.

QUESTION

(Discussion on page 194)

4.20 *How accurate is the term "saline-sensitive metabolic alkalosis"?*

High or Normal ECF Volume Group

- Identify the basis of the deficits.
- Replace K^+ (and possibly Mg^{2+}) deficits.
- Block aldosterone action.

Therapy is generally more difficult in patients with metabolic alkalosis and ECF volume expansion. If they have renal failure and are very alkalemic ($[H^+] < 20$ nmol/L, pH > 7.70) they should receive some H^+ in the form of HCl or NH_4Cl. If these patients are dialyzed, the bath should have the $[HCO_3^-]$ or concentration of acetate reduced to ameliorate the alkalemia.

If the patient has hyperadrenalism, agents that block Na^+ reabsorption in the collecting duct (e.g., amiloride) may play an important role in the therapy, as do mineralocorticoid antagonists (e.g., spirolactone). One must ensure that bowel sounds are present before using K^+ supplements and K^+-sparing diuretics (when the plasma $[K^+]$ rises, bowel motility may increase, and a large quantity of K^+ may be absorbed quickly). Without the capability of renal excretion, a severe degree of hyperkalemia may develop. Even in the absence of an ileus, hyperkalemia may develop if aggressive K^+ replacement is given in conjunction with amiloride or spironolactone. In the acute setting, it is safest to order only 1 day of K^+ therapy at a time, noting the serum $[K^+]$ each day before ordering that day's therapy.

Patients with Mg^{2+} deficiency should have this deficiency corrected, but it is important to follow-up on the effectiveness of the therapy because patients with hyperaldosteronism also have Mg^{2+} deficiency and thus have another basis for the metabolic alkalosis.

Acetazolamide is sometimes used to alleviate the alkalemia quickly (e.g., when weaning from a ventilator), but, because a large load of $NaHCO_3$-rich fluid will be delivered to the collecting duct, this agent often exaggerates K^+ loss. For this reason, the authors prefer an intravenous HCl preparation. An intravenous infusion of HCl also provides better control over the quantitative fall in $[HCO_3^-]$ than does acetazolamide.

If the patient is ventilated and has a fixed alveolar ventilation, the $Paco_2$ may rise with H^+ administration; a small increase in $Paco_2$ may not be detrimental if it is a transient phenomenon.

Review

DISCUSSION OF INTRODUCTORY CASE
Basically, Toby Is Not "OK"
(Case presented on page 158)

What acid-base disturbance is present?

Toby has metabolic alkalosis because the $[HCO_3^-]$ and the pH of plasma are both increased.

Why is the $[Na^+]$ in the urine not lower, given the presence of ECF volume contraction?

For the $[Na^+]$ in urine to be low, all the filtered Na^+ must be reabsorbed. There are two ways in which Na^+ can be reabsorbed: along with Cl^- and in conjunction with the secretion of the cations K^+ and/or H^+. In response to ECF volume contraction, the $[Cl^-]$ in urine is close to 0; this extremely low value indicates appreciable NaCl reabsorption. Some Na^+ were not reabsorbed because they were excreted with an anion other than Cl^- (note the *urine net charge* of 102 mEq/L, as shown in the margin note). The very high urine pH indicates that one of the "nonreabsorbed anions" is HCO_3^-. To the degree that the filtered load of HCO_3^- exceeds the tubular capacity to reabsorb it, HCO_3^- are excreted; this action obligates the coincident excretion of K^+ and/or Na^+. The authors cannot be sure if there is another "nonreabsorbable" anion other than HCO_3^- in the urine at this point. Therefore, bicarbonaturia is at least one cause of the unexpectedly high $[Na^+]$.

Urine net charge

Na^+ (52 mmol/L) + K^+ (50 mmol/L) − Cl^- (0 mmol/L)

Why is Toby hypokalemic?

Toby is hypokalemic because she has ECF volume contraction, which results in the release of renin. Renin, via angiotensin II formation, causes the release of aldosterone, which promotes K^+ secretion and Na^+ reabsorption in the CCD. Adequate delivery of Na^+ to this segment is ensured by the presence of HCO_3^-. Another important effect of HCO_3^- in the CCD is an augmented K^+ secretion, which raises the $[K^+]$ in the lumen (see Chapter 9, pages 385–386).

What is the basis for the acid-base disturbance?

Toby has metabolic alkalosis and coincident renal HCO_3^- excretion. If this condition represents a steady state (continued metabolic alkalosis despite bicarbonaturia), she must have an ongoing supply of HCO_3^- (one cannot lose HCO_3^- and maintain an elevated level in plasma without an ongoing source). If the source were exogenous ingestion of $NaHCO_3$, there would be ECF volume expansion, which is not the case. Hence, there is an endogenous generation of HCO_3^- that is not of renal origin (there is renal HCO_3^- loss, not generation). Therefore, Toby must be vomiting. The alkaline urine pH, the very low $[Cl^-]$ in urine, and the metabolic alkalosis are pathognomonic of metabolic alkalosis secondary to loss of HCl via the GI tract (see Figure 4.1).

Cases for Review

CASE 4.1
Metabolic Alkalosis in the Beautiful People
(Case discussed on pages 181–182)

Farrah, a beautiful person, is concerned about her body image so she diets most of the time. Her food intake is erratic and consists mainly of vegetables and fruits; she consumes little meat or table salt. She jogs 60 km per week and is asymptomatic. When she volunteered for a clinical research project, she was surprised to find that she was hypokalemic (2.7 mmol/L) because she was normokalemic (4.0 mmol/L) 6 months before. She denied vomiting and the use of diuretics or laxatives. Her blood pressure was on the low side (90/55 mm Hg), and she had subtle signs that suggested a contracted ECF volume. Laboratory data are as follows:

		Plasma	Urine
Na^+	mmol/L	138	63
K^+	mmol/L	2.7	34
Cl^-	mmol/L	96	0
HCO_3^-	mmol/L	30	0
Creatinine	μmol/L (mg/dL)	60 (0.7)	—
Osmolality	mOsm/kg H_2O	287	563
pH		7.45	5.6

Do these urine values suggest that Farrah is a surreptitious vomiter or diuretic abuser?

What is the basis for the low urine $[Cl^-]$?

Why isn't her excretion of K^+ lower?

Do you think she has an adrenal tumor?

What advice would you give to Farrah?

CASE 4.2
Solly Has Transient Metabolic Alkalosis
(Case discussed on pages 183–184)

Solly has had abdominal pain and profuse diarrhea for many months. More recently, he has vomited on occasion and has suffered from episodic tingling and weakness. He took antacids to relieve his abdominal pain, but their beneficial effect was transitory. He has been to the hospital on several occasions, each time with a similar story—a set of "laboratory errors" because his condition reverts toward normal without therapy and because there are no physical findings of note. The laboratory values follow.

Plasma		Admission	4 Hours Later
pH		Not done	7.50
Paco$_2$	mm Hg	Not done	48
HCO$_3^-$	mmol/L	62	40
K$^+$	mmol/L	3.1	3.6
Anion gap	mEq/L	15	13
Creatinine	μmol/L (mg/dL)	200 (2.3)	

In the four hours in the emergency room, the urine was alkaline but its volume was small. Why was metabolic alkalosis present?

How did it ameliorate spontaneously?

What is wrong with Solly, and how should he be treated?

CASE 4.3
Mr. Greene Looks Green
(Case discussed on pages 184–185)

Mr. Greene is 42 years old and is a chronic alcoholic. He was brought to the emergency room, obviously intoxicated. He had been lying in the park in a pool of vomitus. On physical examination, he was unkempt and incoherent. He had a markedly contracted ECF volume, was febrile (39°C), and had evidence of pneumonia. Laboratory data are as follows:

Plasma			Plasma		
Na$^+$	mmol/L	130	H$^+$	nmol/L	30
K$^+$	mmol/L	2.9	pH		7.53
Cl$^-$	mmol/L	80	Paco$_2$	mm Hg	25
HCO$_3^-$	mmol/L	20	Pao$_2$	mm Hg	60
Creatinine	μmol/L (mg/dL)	120 (1.4)	Albumin	g/dL	38
Urea	mmol/L (mg/dL)	12 (34)			
Glucose	mmol/L (mg/dL)	15 (270)			
Osmolality	mOsm/kg H$_2$O	320			
Serum ketones		weakly positive (undiluted specimen)			

What are the acid-base diagnoses?

What are the priorities for therapy?

What risks do you anticipate?

Discussion of Cases

DISCUSSION OF CASE 4.1
Metabolic Alkalosis in the Beautiful People
(Case presented on page 180)

It is useful to begin with the diagnostic approach provided in Figure 4.7. The GFR is not very low, and Farrah has a contracted ECF volume. The [Cl^-] in urine now becomes a critical crossroad in the diagnostic flow chart; her [Cl^-] in urine is very low. The differential diagnosis therefore includes loss of gastric fluids, remote diuretic use, and rare causes of metabolic alkalosis.

Do these urine values suggest that Farrah is a surreptitious vomiter or diuretic abuser?

The history could be compatible with vomiting, even if it is denied. The key to the diagnosis is in the random urine sample, because blood tests confirm metabolic alkalosis and hypokalemia. The urine should be "Cl^--free," and it is. As a result of recent vomiting, the urine could have abundant Na^+; if vomiting was remote, however, the urine would be Na^+-free. The urine suggests the possibility of recent vomiting, all except the urine pH, which indicates no bicarbonaturia. Therefore, the urine electrolytes are not typical of vomiting but do suggest a degree of ECF volume contraction and organic anion excretion. The specific nature of the organic anion is unclear. It could be of dietary or metabolic origin.

Using the same type of analysis, because the urine has Na^+ but not Cl^-, recent or remote intake of diuretics is not the best simple answer.

What is the basis for the low urine [Cl^-]?

A low ECF volume is the cause of the low [Cl^-] in urine. Farrah consumes little salt but loses NaCl via sweating.

Why isn't her excretion of K^+ lower?

She should have high levels of aldosterone as a result of the low ECF volume. Given the delivery of Na^+ with a poorly reabsorbed anion to the terminal CCD, kaliuresis should be augmented.

Do you think she has an adrenal tumor?

No. The mineralocorticoid activity is explained by her ECF volume contraction. If she had an adrenal tumor, the Na^+ retention would be a primary event, and she would have ECF volume expansion, hypertension, and her urine would not be Cl^--poor.

What advice would you give to Farrah?

Eating more NaCl and KCl should lead, ultimately, to a normal set of plasma electrolytes. Once Farrah follows these instructions, excessive NaCl retention will not occur, and her results will normalize (see margin note).

Note
When subjects with contracted ECF volumes are given large loads of NaCl, they often have excessive retention of salt, and edema may develop. This phenomenon should be transient (lasting only a few days).

Final Diagnosis. Farrah has a negative NaCl balance because of poor dietary intake and nonrenal loss. She also has an unusual organic anion load that is probably from her diet. These findings mimic vomiting, except for the urine pH. Some physicians may believe that Farrah is a surreptitious vomiter, but Farrah still denies such a practice, and the data available are not characteristic of vomiting (excretion of an unidentified organic anion rather than HCO_3^-).

DISCUSSION OF CASE 4.2
Solly Has Transient Metabolic Alkalosis
(Case presented on pages 180–181)

The diagnostic quandary in this case is that the plasma $[HCO_3^-]$ changes dramatically in a 4-hour period with no obvious external source of HCO_3^- gain or loss.

Why was metabolic alkalosis present?

To have a high plasma $[HCO_3^-]$, either HCO_3^- must be added or the ECF volume must contract. Solly's ECF volume had not been expanded earlier, nor is it very contracted now, so the problem is gain of HCO_3^-.

The HCO_3^- gain was most likely nonrenal because renal HCO_3^- loss, not gain, is present now. He denied any source of exogenous HCO_3^-. The most likely source of endogenous alkali is HCl loss (see Figure 4.1). Perhaps Solly had trapped a large quantity of HCl in the lumen of his stomach, causing severe metabolic alkalosis.

How did metabolic alkalosis ameliorate spontaneously?

Although the urine was alkaline, its volume was small so there was little bicarbonaturia. If bicarbonaturia was the basis for the fall in plasma $[HCO_3^-]$, so much Na^+ and K^+ would be lost that shock and an extreme degree of K^+ depletion would be anticipated. The $[HCO_3^-]$ in the ECF fell by 22 mmol/L, and, if we assume an ECF volume of 15 L, we must account for the loss of almost 330 mmol of HCO_3^-. Because there was no evidence of organic anion accumulation or excretion, the best answer the authors can give is that the HCl that was "hiding" in his stomach was partially reabsorbed 4 hours later; the result was a decrease in the $[HCO_3^-]$ in the ECF with no evidence of external gain or loss of HCO_3^- (the $[Cl^-]$ rose in plasma, and the anion gap did not fall appreciably because Cl^- were reabsorbed from the GI tract).

What is wrong with Solly, and how should he be treated?

Solly suffers from Zollinger-Ellison syndrome with excessive secretion of HCl. The diarrhea is due to HCl-induced damage to the duodenal mucosa plus denaturation of pancreatic enzymes and bile salt precipitation. Gastrin levels should be measured (see margin note).

Final Diagnosis. Solly had excessive gastric HCl secretion; dissociation of the HCO_3^- generation and HCl reabsorption led to a transient severe metabolic alkalosis. This case has implications for the renal handling of HCO_3^-. Little excretion occurs if there is even a minor degree of ECF volume contraction; the low rate of excretion of HCO_3^- was due to a lower filtered load (low GFR, elevated plasma creatinine) and, more importantly, to more reabsorption of HCO_3^- by the kidney. Consider how acidemic, K^+-depleted, and ECF-volume-contracted he would have become if his kidneys had been "fooled" into excreting some of the "excess" HCO_3^- that

Note
Solly's gastrin levels, which were 10-fold higher than the upper limit of normal, confirm the presence of a gastrinoma; the offending tumor was resected, and Solly is now fine.

accumulated in the ECF (see margin note). Finally, this case might help in explaining the wide variation in the normal values for HCO_3^- in plasma in normal individuals.

DISCUSSION OF CASE 4.3
Mr. Greene Looks Green
(Case presented on page 181)

What are the acid-base diagnoses?

Mr. Greene has an increased plasma anion gap and a low [HCO_3^-]; therefore, he has metabolic acidosis. However, the increase in the plasma anion gap is 18 mEq/L (30–12, the normal value, given that his concentration of albumin is normal), but the fall in [HCO_3^-] is only 5 mmol/L. Therefore, a second process is increasing the [HCO_3^-]—metabolic alkalosis. The only other process that could increase the plasma [HCO_3^-] is respiratory acidosis, which was not present (low $PaCO_2$).

With a [HCO_3^-] of 20 mmol/L from metabolic acidosis, one would expect the $PaCO_2$ to be reduced to approximately 35 mm Hg; because it is 25 mm Hg in this case, Mr. Greene also has respiratory alkalosis. The final blood gas abnormality is a low PaO_2 with an increased A-a difference (58 mm Hg) (see Chapter 5, page 203).

Mr. Greene has three acid-base diagnoses: metabolic acidosis with an increased anion gap, metabolic alkalosis (from vomiting), and respiratory alkalosis (from pneumonia). The basis of the metabolic acidosis, given the clinical setting, is most likely alcoholic ketoacidosis. Other diagnostic possibilities to consider are methyl alcohol or ethylene glycol intoxication and L-lactic acidosis resulting from low oxygen delivery, ethanol metabolism, or thiamine deficiency. If he has ketoacidosis, the plasma ketones should be strongly positive in diluted samples (the plasma level would be equal to the increase in anion gap, or 18 mmol/L); his plasma ketones, however, are weakly positive in an undiluted sample. In the setting of alcohol metabolism or hypoxia-induced L-lactic acidosis, there may be a false-negative test for ketones because of the preponderance of β-hydroxybutyrate (see page 101). Also unexpected in ketoacidosis is his hypokalemia; one expects hyperkalemia with ketoacidosis (insulin deficiency).

What are the priorities for therapy?

1. Restore the ECF volume.
2. Replenish the K^+ deficit.
3. Avoid thiamine deficiency.

Mr. Greene has profound contraction of ECF volume because of vomiting and loss of $NaHCO_3$ and $KHCO_3$ in the urine. His deficits are those of NaCl and KCl, and he requires both. Aggressive restoration of ECF volume using nothing but normal saline will run the risk of turning off the catecholamine suppression of insulin release and may aggravate the degree of hypokalemia, because insulin secretion leads to the entry of K^+ into the ICF. A reasonable intravenous (IV) fluid would be 1 L of isotonic saline plus 20 mmol of KCl given during the first 30 minutes. The next IV solution should be isotonic to Mr. Greene and could be 0.45% saline that contains 40–60 mEq/L KCl (depending on the plasma [K$^+$] at that time).

Also send off blood samples to establish the specific diagnosis:

1. β-hydroxybutyrate;

2. methanol, ethanol, and ethylene glycol levels (the high value for the plasma osmolal gap is due in part or entirely to ethanol);

3. L-lactate.

What risks do you anticipate?

The first major risk of acute therapy is thiamine deficiency. Mr. Greene should receive thiamine intravenously. The second danger is overlooking the profound K$^+$ depletion that could cause life-threatening hypokalemia with vigorous ECF volume expansion. This risk would be magnified greatly with the administration or endogenous release of insulin. In this case, there is no immediate need for insulin; probably Mr. Green will secrete endogenous insulin once the ECF volume is restored.

The remaining issue to address is the cause of the wide A-a difference, which is most likely due to aspiration pneumonia; clarification and specific therapy will be necessary.

Summary of Main Points

- Metabolic alkalosis is present when there is a rise in the plasma [HCO$_3^-$] together with a fall in the [H$^+$]. Having an increased [HCO$_3^-$] involves either a source of new HCO$_3^-$ and/or ECF volume contraction.
- Renal mechanisms are necessary to permit a sustained elevation in the [HCO$_3^-$] in plasma.
- Of the important events occurring in the ICF, the principal one is a loss of K$^+$ along with a gain of Na$^+$ and H$^+$. Hence, metabolic alkalosis in the ECF is usually accompanied by intracellular acidosis and K$^+$ depletion.
- Clinically, there are two major subgroups of patients with metabolic alkalosis. The most common group responds to administration of KCl and NaCl and exhibits ECF volume contraction. This form of metabolic alkalosis is caused most often by vomiting or diuretics and is characterized by a very low rate of excretion of Cl$^-$ (when diuretics are not acting). Patients may not admit that they induce vomiting or abuse diuretics.

    The other group does not respond to administration of Cl$^-$ salts and is often hypertensive. This type of metabolic alkalosis occurs most commonly with high aldosterone states. Other diagnoses of persistent metabolic alkalosis after administration of NaCl and KCl include Mg^{2+} depletion, Bartter's syndrome, and renal failure with a NaHCO$_3$ load. Therapy is usually more difficult with these types of metabolic alkalosis and requires that the specific causes be identified and addressed.

- Patients with chronic obstructive pulmonary disease and CO$_2$ retention may also have metabolic alkalosis. Because metabolic alkalosis might have a significant adverse effect on a patient's clinical state, it should be corrected.

Discussion of Questions

4.1 Why will the ingestion of $NaHCO_3$ not lead to the development of chronic metabolic alkalosis?

When the plasma $[HCO_3^-]$ is elevated and the GFR is normal, more HCO_3^- are filtered. Reabsorption of HCO_3^- must be stimulated to retain these extra HCO_3^-. Consider the two components of $NaHCO_3$ separately:

1. Na^+: Intake of $NaHCO_3$ tends to expand the ECF volume, which should lead to a decline in renin and thereby angiotensin II levels. Because angiotensin II normally stimulates the reabsorption of HCO_3^-, fewer, not more, HCO_3^- should be reabsorbed in this setting.

2. HCO_3^-: The alkalemia will lead to a more alkaline proximal cell, which, in turn, will also depress the reabsorption of more HCO_3^- while alkalemia persists.

Hence, taken together, the intake of $NaHCO_3$ does not give the kidney "permission" to reabsorb more HCO_3^- than normal. To do so, one needs a lower GFR or stimulation of the proximal NHE-3 antiporter (high angiotensin II or intracellular acidosis, related to hypokalemia or a high Pa_{CO_2}).

4.2 For net loss of HCl or NH_4Cl to be the sole cause of metabolic alkalosis, what must the mass balance for Na^+, K^+, and Cl^- be?

The net loss of HCl or NH_4Cl requires that the negative balance for Cl^- exceed that for Na^+ plus K^+.

4.3 How many liters of emesis must be lost in order to raise the $[HCO_3^-]$ in plasma by 10 mmol/L in a 70-kg adult?

Assume for simplicity that all the HCO_3^- retained (10 mmol/L) remained in the ECF (15 L in a 70-kg person). Therefore, 150 mmol of HCO_3^- is needed. If the loss of HCl in the stomach was isosmotic (150 mmol of H^+/L and 150 mmol of Cl^-/L), the net loss of emesis would be 1 L. This amount is an underestimate because some HCO_3^- will distribute in the ICF. Hence, this degree of metabolic alkalosis is not due to a single day of vomiting.

4.4 If a patient has gastric drainage, how can the quantity of new HCO_3^- formation be minimized?

Because a patient with gastric drainage can lose large amounts of HCl, metabolic alkalosis may result. The most effective way to reduce the H^+ loss is to administer an H_2-receptor blocker to inhibit secretion of HCl by the gastric mucosa. Although this procedure markedly reduces the HCl loss, some NaCl or $NaHCO_3$ can be lost and must be replaced to avoid ECF volume contraction and a resulting change in plasma $[HCO_3^-]$.

Another way to reduce the acid-base impact of large HCl losses is to keep the patient's ECF volume well expanded with NaCl and replace any K^+ losses with KCl so that the $NaHCO_3$ is excreted (if renal function is adequate). If the renal function is poor, administer H^+ in the form of HCl or NH_4Cl to titrate the excess HCO_3^-, and replace the deficit of Cl^-.

Note
If the patient has severe liver disease, the use of NH_4Cl is not advisable.

4.5 How can the progressive rise in the [HCO₃⁻] in plasma and K⁺ depletion be explained in a patient with metabolic alkalosis due to vomiting?

With vomiting, there is a net loss of Cl^-, which are replaced by HCO_3^- (see Figure 4.1). Given the same ECF volume and GFR, the filtered load of HCO_3^- rises, but proximal H^+ secretion does not rise to the same degree (no depletion of ECF volume or hypokalemia, but alkalemia is present). Hence, because HCO_3^- are less reabsorbable in the distal nephron, this increased filtered load of HCO_3^- results in $NaHCO_3$ excretion, which will lead to a small degree of ECF volume contraction. The urine contains Na^+ despite the ECF volume depletion because Na^+ accompany HCO_3^-, which cannot be reabsorbed. With the next episode of vomiting, the same sequence of events occurs—the [HCO_3^-] rises further in the ECF, and some bicarbonaturia occurs along with some Na^+ loss and more K^+ loss (the low ECF volume leads to aldosterone release and augments the excretion of K^+). This time the [HCO_3^-] in the ECF is slightly higher than previously. The degree of ECF volume depletion depends on the Na^+ intake between episodes of vomiting and the magnitude of the Na^+ losses (both GI and renal). With each episode of vomiting, there is transient bicarbonaturia as the "renal threshold" for HCO_3^- reabsorption is exceeded by the gastric HCO_3^- generation. The [HCO_3^-] in the ECF progressively rises, however, because the bicarbonaturia is not sufficient to excrete all the HCO_3^- generated. The progressive ECF volume depletion limits the amount of HCO_3^- filtered per unit of time (the filtered load), and the stimulation of H^+ secretion by angiotensin II causes an increased reabsorption of HCO_3^-. Therefore, the patient with recurrent vomiting will have chronic metabolic alkalosis, hypokalemia, and ECF volume contraction.

The urine composition varies, depending on when the patient is evaluated. After the patient vomits, the urine contains Na^+, K^+, and HCO_3^- but no Cl^- (as a result of ECF volume contraction and Cl^- depletion, all the Cl^- are reabsorbed); the urine pH is alkaline. Between episodes, the urine contains little Na^+ or Cl^- (from ECF volume contraction) and some K^+ (excreted with SO_4^{2-} and HPO_4^{2-}). The urine pH is close to 6.3 because of an enhanced secretion of H^+ on the one hand and a high NH_3 in the medullary interstitial compartment on the other hand (see margin note).

Note
As K^+ depletion develops, the synthesis of NH_4^+ in cells of the PCT and the [NH_3] in the medullary interstitial compartment increase. The urine pH rises because there is more NH_3 available to bind with H^+ in the lumen of the collecting duct.

4.6 Why might the [HCO₃⁻] in plasma rise in a patient with normovolemia who is undergoing plasmapheresis for rapidly progressive glomerulonephritis and renal failure?

That the patient's [HCO_3^-] in the ECF is increasing with no evidence of ECF volume contraction indicates an increased content of HCO_3^- in the ECF. In the absence of endogenous HCO_3^- generation (no vomiting and no renal HCO_3^- generation resulting from renal failure), the extra HCO_3^- must be due to exogenous bicarbonate,

HCO_3^- mobilized from bone or from a resolving ileus, or the metabolic production of HCO_3^-. Assume that there is no ileus and that the patient is not receiving HCO_3^- per se. Daily plasmapheresis with plasma replacement (and several blood transfusions) will provide a large load of citrate^{3-} with Na^+ (the anticoagulant). The metabolism of citrate^{3-} to CO_2 consumes H^+, yielding HCO_3^-. The renal failure will prevent appreciable $NaHCO_3$ excretion.

4.7 How high might the [HCO_3^-] in plasma rise if a patient has a modest degree of contraction of the ECF volume and no increase in the content of HCO_3^- in the body?

Assume a 10% loss of ECF volume for easy mathematics. With no change in the content of HCO_3^-, the [HCO_3^-] will rise 10% from 25 to 27.5 mmol/L.

4.8 What impact does the loss of 200 mmol of Na^+ and Cl^- from diuretic action have on the content and concentration of HCO_3^- in the ECF? (For simplicity, assume no change in [Na^+], which is 140 mmol/L.)

If it is assumed the patient weighs 70 kg with a [Na^+] in the ECF that equals 140 mmol/L, the total amount of Na^+ in the body is 15 L $\times$ 140 mmol/L, or 2100 mmol. If 200 mmol of Na^+ is lost, the total amount of Na^+ in the body will be 1900 mmol, and if the [Na^+] in the ECF remains at 140 mmol/L, the ECF volume will be 13.6 L (1900/140). The HCO_3^- content, which was 25 mmol/L $\times$ 15 L, or 375 mmol, is now contained in 13.6 L; therefore, the new [HCO_3^-] is 28 mmol/L.

Therefore, it is easy to appreciate that with the loss of NaCl, the [HCO_3^-] in the ECF can rise with no change in the content of HCO_3^- in the ECF, because of a decrease in ECF volume. This process contributes to the metabolic alkalosis that results from diuretic use but is quantitatively small.

Note

Loss of 200 mmol of Na^+ is equivalent to a loss of 1.3 L of ECF, a 10% contraction. A 30% contraction could result in cardiovascular collapse.

4.9 Why do some patients who vomit have a large deficit of Na^+ in the ECF? Hint: In the selective HCl depletion model of metabolic alkalosis, there is no significant deficit of Na^+.

Some patients who vomit profusely have a large deficit of NaCl, but subjects with a selective deficit of HCl did not. Therefore, it is difficult to attribute all the Na^+ loss to renal excretion of Na^+ with HCO_3^-. The authors can think of three other sources of a loss of Na^+. First, there are losses from the GI tract: saliva has an appreciable quantity of Na^+; there is some Na^+ in stomach fluids (minor); if the pyloric sphincter remains patent, fluid from the small intestine, which is Na^+-rich, will mix with stomach contents so now the vomitus will have an appreciable amount of Na^+ and Cl^-. You know this latter admixture occurs because you often see bile-tinged vomitus. Moreover, in children who do not have pyloric stenosis, metabolic acidosis rather than metabolic alkalosis can be the result of vomiting (loss of more $NaHCO_3$ than HCl). The second source of Na^+ loss is via excessive sweating (see Case 4.1 for an example). Third, there is some renal Na^+ loss as $NaHCO_3$ or as Na^+ plus organic anions like citrate before K^+ depletion is evident. Obviously, the intake of a diuretic or a renal defect in Na^+ reabsorption could make renal loss of Na^+ larger.

Overall: Admixture of small-intestinal Na^+-rich fluids and very prolonged continuous HCl loss by which cumulative renal Na^+ loss becomes appreciable are the major reasons for a large degree of NaCl depletion.

4.10 Under what circumstances might vomiting cause metabolic acidosis? How might this be recognized as the pathophysiology?

There are two settings to consider here. The first is due to added acids consequent to a markedly contracted ECF volume or the agent that provoked vomiting. A low delivery of oxygen due to poor hemodynamics will cause L-lactic acidosis. Inhibition of the release of insulin due to the α-adrenergic effect of the adrenergic response can promote ketoacidosis. An example of the causative agent contributing to the ketoacidosis seen with excessive vomiting is ethanol, which permits both a more rapid induction of ketogenesis and a slower oxidation of ketoacids in brain (slow metabolic rate) and the kidney (low GFR). Both of these added acids will be recognized by a very high value for the anion gap in plasma. There may be a positive test result for ketones with ketoacidosis, but beware of the danger of lower than expected values for acetoacetate and acetone (Chapter 12). Either a low level of HCl secretion in the stomach (achlorhydria, drugs blocking HCl secretion such as H_2-blockers or H^+/K^+ antiporter blockers such as omeprazole) or a large admixture of $NaHCO_3$ from small intestine secretions can cause metabolic acidosis with vomiting.

Clinical recognition is from history and finding a lower than expected ECF volume on physical examination. From the point of view of the laboratory, there should be little elevation of the anion gap in plasma. Hypokalemia will be an indicator that this type of scenario may be present.

4.11 What pathophysiologic mechanisms must be involved to have Cl^--depletion metabolic alkalosis? What is the expected mass balance in each case?

Loss of HCl or NH_4Cl. To develop metabolic alkalosis, either the content of HCO_3^- in the ECF must rise or the ECF volume must decline. For the former to occur with a depletion of Cl^-, the pathophysiologic mechanism is loss of Cl^- along with H^+ (e.g., vomiting, nasogastric suction) or with NH_4^+ in the urine (hypokalemia consequent to diuretic actions). The expected mass balance is loss of more Cl^- than $Na^+ + K^+$.

Loss of NaCl. Loss of NaCl will be the pathophysiologic mechanism for alkalosis resulting from contraction of the ECF volume. The mass balance is equimolar loss of Na^+ and Cl^-.

Loss of KCl. Loss of KCl can be the pathophysiologic mechanism for two aspects of Cl^--depletion metabolic alkalosis, depending on which cations entered the ICF in exchange for the K^+ that were lost. If Na^+ entered, there would be contraction of the ECF volume; if H^+ entered, there would be alkalosis of the ECF together with acidosis of the ICF. In either case, the mass balance would be equimolar loss of K^+ and Cl^-.

4.12 Three factors contributed to the degree of intracellular

acidosis in a patient who has vomited on a chronic basis and who has a significant degree of ECF volume contraction. What are they? The pertinent values in plasma are pH 7.48, HCO_3^- 36 mmol/L, K^+ 2.7 mmol/L.

There are three definite factors, and possibly a fourth.

K^+ Depletion. A major component of this picture of metabolic alkalosis is a loss of K^+ from the ICF. Because the loss of K^+ from the ICF is not accompanied by a comparable loss of intracellular anions (phosphate), there was a shift of cations, Na^+ and H^+, into cells. To the extent that H^+ have accumulated, there is an intracellular acidosis.

Higher Arterial P_{CO_2}. When ventilation is suppressed by alkalemia, there is a retention of CO_2 and thereby a rise in the arterial P_{CO_2}. If the arterial P_{CO_2} is high, then the tissue P_{CO_2} must also be high; thereby, there is intracellular respiratory acidosis.

Higher Tissue P_{CO_2}. When the ECF volume declines to a significant degree, the cardiac output declines. With the same rate of production of CO_2, each liter of blood must carry more CO_2 and, of greater importance, at a higher concentration. Therefore, the venous P_{CO_2} will be higher than expected, thereby ensuring an even higher tissue P_{CO_2} (see Figure 1.9).

Formation of Organic Acids. When there is a very poor circulating volume, metabolic acidosis can develop. If the main problem is delivery of oxygen, L-lactic acidosis develops.

The α-adrenergic response to a low ECF volume causes a low level of insulin. In a susceptible individual (diabetic, alcoholic), ketoacidosis can develop.

Overall. Aggressive attempts to restore the deficit of K^+ and reexpand the ECF volume (NaCl) should reverse the important contributions to intracellular acidosis.

4.13 How can one distinguish between diuretic abuse and Bartter's-like syndromes using urine electrolytes?

There are two groups of patients with metabolic alkalosis, ECF volume contraction, and a $[Cl^-]$ in urine that exceeds 20 mmol/L—those who use diuretics and those who have Bartter's-like syndromes.

Diuretic Use. Diuretic use (abuse) is the most likely cause of metabolic alkalosis with ECF volume contraction and a high $[Cl^-]$ in urine. Although a patient may deny using a diuretic, its presence can usually be identified by measuring the electrolytes on serial random urine samples. Some samples will be free of Na^+ and Cl^-, indicating the patient's ability to conserve Na^+ and Cl^- (some time has passed since the diuretic was consumed); other samples will have abundant Na^+ and Cl^- following more recent diuretic ingestion (see Table 4.5; Table 4.7). The patient who has ECF volume contraction and is wasting Na^+ should have excessive K^+ loss in the urine (from the mineralocorticoid secretion that is due to ECF volume contraction); if the $[K^+]$ in urine is not high, suspect the ingestion of a diuretic with "K^+-sparing" qualities. The other clues suggesting the diagnosis of diuretic abuse are access to diuretics (paramedical personnel), patients with distorted body image, ele-

Clinical pearls
With hypokalemia, low ECF volume, and urine $[Cl^-]$ >20 mmol/L, suspect:
• Diuretics (urine $[Na^+]$ may be <20 mmol/L at times);
• Bartter's-like syndromes (urine $[Na^+]$ is not <20 mmol/L).

TABLE 4.7 **Serial Urine Electrolytes in a Patient with
ECF Volume Contraction, Indicating Diuretic Abuse**

		Acting	Diuretics Not Acting	Acting
Na^+	(mmol/L)	30	10	42
K^+	(mmol/L)	43	13	59
Cl^-	(mmol/L)	85	3	108

vated uric acid in serum, and fluctuating body weight. The diagnosis
can be confirmed with a direct assay of the urine for the diuretic
when the $[Na^+]$ and $[Cl^-]$ in the urine are high.

Bartter's-Like Syndromes. Patients with Bartter's-like syndromes
have metabolic alkalosis, ECF volume contraction, and inappropriately high Na^+ and Cl^- excretion via the urine. Serial observations
reveal persistent Na^+ and Cl^- wasting and a relatively constant
body weight, both of which contrast with a diagnosis of diuretic
abuse. In patients with Bartter's-like syndromes, there is a much
more profound degree of K^+ depletion and a much higher transtubular $[K^+]$ gradient (TTKG). Some patients also have hypomagnesemia and persistent renal Mg^{2+} wasting. In these patients, it is
extremely difficult, if not impossible, to return the plasma $[K^+]$ to
normal with K^+ supplements.

4.14 A very low GFR plays a prominent role in the metabolic alkalosis associated with the milk-alkali syndrome. What is the pathophysiology of this syndrome?

The basis of this disorder is the ingestion and absorption of large
amounts of calcium and HCO_3^-. The patients then excrete large
amounts of calcium and HCO_3^- in their urine. This excretion leads
to nephrocalcinosis (calcium salts are less soluble in alkaline urine)
and progressive renal function impairment. As renal function diminishes, the ability to excrete the large calcium load is reduced,
and these patients actually develop hypercalcemia with soft tissue
calcification. Hypercalcemia may, if severe, decrease the rate of
transport via the Na^+, K^+, $2Cl^-$ cotransporter in the thick ascending
limb of the loop of Henle, resulting in NaCl wasting and ECF
volume contraction, thereby promoting the reabsorption of HCO_3^-
in the PCT. The hypercalcemia may also cause vomiting, which
leads to metabolic alkalosis and also stimulates indirect reabsorption
of HCO_3^- in the PCT if there is a contracted ECF volume. The
decreased GFR also causes impaired renal excretion of HCO_3^-.
With the continued ingestion of HCO_3^-, the plasma $[HCO_3^-]$ progressively rises. The metabolic alkalosis and hypercalcemia will
resolve when ingestion of the calcium and alkali ceases.

4.15 Why does $NaHCO_3$ provide a much larger alkali load to the body than an equivalent dose of $CaCO_3$?

The fate of $NaHCO_3$ is easy to follow. In the stomach, HCl is
secreted, converting $NaHCO_3$ to NaCl. The net result is a gain of
HCO_3^- and a loss of Cl^- from the body (see the following figure).
The NaCl enters the small intestine and is reabsorbed. This restores

Cl^- balance and causes a gain of Na^+, which is equimolar to the HCO_3^- gain.

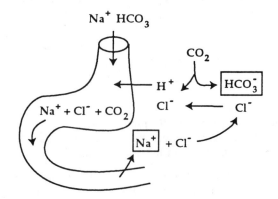

Bottom Line. Gain 1 Na^+ and 1 HCO_3^-.

Following the ingestion of $CaCO_3$, the CO_3^- has the same fate as the HCO_3^- had with $NaHCO_3$ in the stomach. Two H^+ react with CO_3^{2-}, yielding CO_2. In this process $Ca^{2+} + 2\ Cl^-$ is sent to the small intestine.

There is a unique difference between Ca^{2+} and Na^+ when they meet the alkaline pancreatic secretions. The Ca^{2+} will form the insoluble precipitate $CaCO_3$ and be excreted, and the remaining NaCl will be reabsorbed (figure follows). Hence, the net effect is acid-base balance (no alkali load).

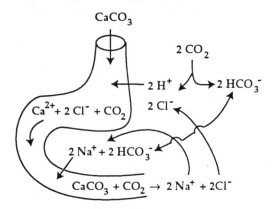

Bottom Line. $CaCO_3$ in and $CaCO_3$ excreted.

4.16 What will increase the alkali load to the body if the amount of $CaCO_3$ ingested remains constant?

To have an absorbed alkali load, the Ca^{2+} formed in the stomach must precipitate with an anion other than CO_3^{2-}. Further, this anion had to be ingested as its Na^+ or K^+ salt, not as a free acid. For example, assume someone ate Na_2HPO_4 and $CaCO_3$ together. In the stomach, there will be precipitation of $Ca_3(PO_4)$. The stoichiometry is shown in the following equations.

$$3\ CaCO_3 \rightarrow 3\ Ca^{2+} + 3\ CO_3^{2-}$$
$$2\ Na_2HPO_4 \rightarrow 2\ PO_4^{3-} + 4\ Na^+ + 2\ H^+$$

Products are: $Ca_3(PO_4)_2 \downarrow + 4\ Na^+ + 2\ HCO_3^- + CO_3^{2-}$

Therefore, if the diet provides a Na^+ or K^+ salt of an anion that will precipitate with Ca^{2+} and prevent the formation of $CaCO_3$ in the small intestine, part of the load of $CaCO_3$ becomes absorbable alkali. This is what happens when $CaCO_3$ is ingested with food as a phosphate binder in patients with impaired renal function.

4.17 What is the pathophysiology of metabolic alkalosis associated with nonreabsorbable alkali and an ion-exchange resin?

The pathophysiology is akin to that in the response to Question 4.13. Ion-exchange resins are given to patients with renal failure to control hyperkalemia (they exchange Na^+ or Ca^{2+} for K^+ in the GI tract). Patients with renal failure also receive nonreabsorbable alkali as phosphate-binding agents (e.g., aluminum hydroxide).

The proposed mechanisms of the metabolic alkalosis are as follows:

- intake of Ca^{2+}, Mg^{2+}, or Al^{3+} salts of organic anions or their hydroxides;
- intake of an ion-exchange resin that is not in a H^+ form (i.e., with Na^+ or Ca^{2+});
- metabolism of organic anions to HCO_3^-;
- formation of a complex of Ca^{2+}, Mg^{2+}, or Al^{3+} with resin in the GI tract, so that there is no GI HCO_3^- loss via carbonate salt formation. In normal circumstances, Ca^{2+}, Mg^{2+}, or Al^{3+} is excreted in the feces as carbonate salts; this process consumes HCO_3^-, so that acid-base balance results. In this case, however, if the patients have a very low GFR, they cannot excrete the absorbed HCO_3^- and could become progressively alkalemic.

Note
The conversion of absorbed OH^- to HCO_3^- is catalyzed by carbonic anhydrase.

$$CO_2 + OH^- \rightarrow HCO_3^-$$

4.18 What is the pathophysiology of metabolic alkalosis associated with a normal or expanded ECF volume?

In all cases of metabolic alkalosis with a normal or expanded ECF volume, Na^+ and Cl^- are delivered to the CCD in the presence of mineralocorticoid activity. The result is the reabsorption of Na^+ along with the excretion of Cl^- and K^+. Because of the K^+ excretion, hypokalemia develops and, as a result, ammoniagenesis and new HCO_3^- generation are stimulated (see margin note). Thereafter, enhanced reabsorption of HCO_3^- and perhaps a lower filtered load (low GFR secondary to the hypokalemia) will lead to a progressive rise in the $[HCO_3^-]$ in plasma. The basis of the mineralocorticoid activity varies, depending on the diagnosis, as outlined in the following table.

Note
Hypokalemia induces a shift of K^+ out of cells together with a shift of H^+ (and Na^+) into cells; this shift of H^+ contributes to a higher plasma $[HCO_3^-]$ and intracellular acidosis.

Diagnosis	Basis of Mineralocorticoid Activity
1° aldosteronism	Autonomous secretion (adenoma, hyperplasia)
Glucocorticoid excess	Autonomous ACTH secretion, drugs mimicking aldosterone actions (see Table 10.5)
Renal-artery stenosis	Secondary to hyperreninemia
Magnesium depletion	Mechanism unclear

**The three components of
metabolic alkalosis**
1. ECF alkalosis
2. ICF acidosis and K^+ depletion
3. Renal "permission" to have a
   high $[HCO_3^-]$ in plasma

4.19 In what circumstances might metabolic alkalosis be associated with hyperkalemia?

In almost all causes of metabolic alkalosis, hypokalemia from renal loss of K^+ is an expected (necessary) finding. If renal failure is present, hyperkalemia could be present; alternatively, look for a sudden shift of K^+ out of cells (e.g., necrosis or lack of insulin).

4.20 How accurate is the term "saline-sensitive metabolic alkalosis"?

Many nephrologists classify metabolic alkalosis as saline-sensitive and saline-resistant, but is this terminology entirely correct? The only times that the ECF, ICF, and renal alterations are "corrected" solely with NaCl are:

1. when the entire deficit is NaCl, a very rare event;

2. when the deficit is HCl (or NH_4Cl), not common in chronic settings of metabolic alkalosis (see Table 4.1).

In these cases, the Cl^- ingested replace the deficit of Cl^-, and the excess Na^+ and HCO_3^- are excreted.

If enough NaCl is given to overexpand the ECF volume (a usual occurrence), the $[HCO_3^-]$ will fall from dilution, and there will be renal excretion of HCO_3^- consequent to the expanded ECF volume. Some view this decrease in the plasma $[HCO_3^-]$ as "correction" of metabolic alkalosis (the plasma $[HCO_3^-]$ is now normal), but the abnormal composition of the ICF persists (low K^+, high H^+, high Na^+). The composition of the ICF will be corrected only when the deficit of K^+ is replaced. It is for this reason that the authors prefer the term "chloride-plus-cation–responsive metabolic alkalosis"; the cation(s) lost along with Cl^- (Na^+ or K^+) must be determined clinically.

Respiratory Acid-Base Disturbances

OBJECTIVES

☐ To provide an understanding of the factors regulating the P_{CO_2} of the blood (arterial and venous) and the impact of a change in P_{CO_2} on the $[H^+]$ in the extracellular fluid (ECF) and intracellular fluid (ICF).

☐ To provide an understanding of the differences in the acid-base status of acute vs chronic respiratory acid-base disturbances. In doing so, the authors present a diagnostic approach that will enable recognition of *respiratory acid-base disturbances*, diagnosis of the underlying disorder, and recognition of coexistent acid-base disorders.

☐ To provide an appreciation of the value and the pitfalls in assessing the difference between the P_{O_2} of alveolar air and that of the arterial blood.

Respiratory acid-base disturbances

Conditions in which an abnormality in the arterial P_{CO_2} is observed. Although the normal Pa_{CO_2} is 40 mm Hg, the Pa_{CO_2} varies with pathophysiologic circumstances (e.g., in a patient with metabolic acidosis and a $[HCO_3^-]$ of 10 mmol/L, the expected Pa_{CO_2} should be 25 mm Hg). Therefore, the Pa_{CO_2} must be evaluated in conjunction with other clinical information.

Outline of Major Principles

1. The arterial P_{CO_2} (Pa_{CO_2}) reflects the concentration of CO_2 in alveolar air required for balance between CO_2 production (metabolism) and CO_2 removal (ventilation).

2. Normal ventilation is mediated by interaction among the central respiratory centers, peripheral chemoreceptors, respiratory muscles, and lung parenchyma.

3. The acid-base status of an acute respiratory acid-base disorder differs greatly from that of a chronic respiratory acid-base disorder because of variations in renal NH_4^+ excretion and/or HCO_3^- reabsorption; these variations influence the plasma $[HCO_3^-]$.

4. Rules:

Acute respiratory acidosis: For every mm Hg increase in Pa_{CO_2} from 40 mm Hg, expect a 0.8 nmol/L increase in the $[H^+]$ from 40 nmol/L. The plasma $[HCO_3^-]$ rises 2.5 mmol/L with a doubling of Pa_{CO_2}.

Chronic respiratory acidosis: For every mm Hg increase in Pa_{CO_2} from 40 mm Hg, expect a 0.3 nmol/L increase in the $[H^+]$ and a 0.3 mmol/L increase in the plasma $[HCO_3^-]$.

Acute respiratory alkalosis: For every mm Hg decrease in Pa_{CO_2} from 40 mm Hg, expect a 0.8 nmol/L decrease in the $[H^+]$ from 40 nmol/L.

Chronic respiratory alkalosis: For every mm Hg decrease in Pa_{CO_2} from 40 mm Hg, expect a 0.2 nmol/L decrease in the $[H^+]$ from 40 nmol/L and a 0.5 mmol/L decrease in the plasma $[HCO_3^-]$ from 25 mmol/L.

INTRODUCTORY CASE
Hack's Future Is Up in Smoke
(Case discussed on pages 214–215)

Hack, a 64-year-old man with a long history of chronic obstructive lung disease, lives at home but requires O_2 therapy. In a 24-hour period, he developed a cough and shortness of breath, became confused, and was taken to the hospital. A diagnosis of pneumonia and acute respiratory failure was made, and he was intubated and ventilated. The results 2 days later are shown in the following table. He was weaned from the ventilator on day 4 of treatment and remained on O_2 by mask.

	Hack's Usual Values	Admission Values	Treatment Day 2	Treatment Day 4
H^+ (nmol/L)	46	63	40	64
pH	7.34	7.20	7.40	7.19
Pa_{CO_2} (mm Hg)	60	80	40	70
Pa_{O_2} (mm Hg)	60	35	180	55

What prompted the changes from the usual values to those seen on admission?

What happened to permit the changes in the blood gases while Hack was on the ventilator on day 2 of therapy?

Why are his postextubation values on day 4 of therapy so different from his original values?

Anatomical dead space
The part of the airway that never takes part in gas exchange (approximately 1 mL/lb body weight).

Alveolar dead space
The part of the alveoli that does not take part in gas exchange because of disease.

Physiologic dead space (PDS)
Anatomical + alveolar dead space.

Tidal volume
The volume of inhaled air.

PART A

Background

Overview of CO_2 Homeostasis

- CO_2 excretion = alveolar ventilation $\times$ [CO_2] in alveolar air.

	CO_2 Excretion	Alveolar Ventilation	[CO_2] in Alveolar Air
Normal	10 mmol/min	5 L/min	2 mmol/L
Chronic respiratory acidosis	10 mmol/min	3 L/min	3.3 mmol/L

Alveolar ventilation
Tidal volume − PDS $\times$ respiration rate.

The major end-product of oxidative metabolism is CO_2. When carbohydrates are oxidized, 1 mmol of CO_2 is produced for every mmol of O_2 consumed (the respiratory quotient (RQ) is 1.0). In contrast, less CO_2 is formed per O_2 consumed when fat is oxidized; in this case, the RQ is 0.7. On a typical Western diet, the usual RQ is close to 0.8. To place these numbers in a quantitative perspective, normal adults consume 12 mmol of O_2 per minute and produce 10 mmol of CO_2 per minute. The concentrations of O_2 and CO_2 in alveolar air are close to 6 and 2 mmol/L, respectively, and O_2 consumption and CO_2 production occur in close to a 1:1 ratio. Therefore, because the supply of O_2 at the level of the alveolus markedly exceeds demand, control of the rate of ventilation is via changes in the $[CO_2]$ rather than in the $[O_2]$. Hence, the authors focus on CO_2 in this chapter.

Normal metabolism results in the production of 10 mmol of CO_2 per minute at rest. This CO_2 leaves cells and enters venous capillary blood for transport to the lungs. Because cardiac output is 5 L/min at rest, venous blood must carry an extra 2 mmol of CO_2 per liter (10 mmol/min ÷ 5 L/min) as compared with arterial blood. This 10 mmol of CO_2 is exhaled in 5 L of alveolar ventilation per minute. If the alveolar ventilation is doubled to 10 L/min for any reason (e.g., metabolic acidosis or salicylate ingestion) with no change in production of CO_2, the $P{CO_2}$ of alveolar air and arterial blood will fall by 50%. Thus, with twice the alveolar ventilation rate, the same amount of CO_2 can be exhaled, but at half the concentration in each liter of alveolar air. Conversely, as alveolar ventilation falls, the concentration of CO_2 in alveolar air must rise (as will the $Pa{CO_2}$) to remove the CO_2 produced daily (compare with serum creatinine and the glomerular filtration rate (GFR); when the GFR halves, the concentration of creatinine in plasma will double).

QUESTIONS

(Discussions on pages 219–220)

5.1 *Assume that the consumption of O_2 is 12 mmol/min, that alveolar ventilation is 5 L/min, and that 21% of air is O_2. Why is the $P{O_2}$ of alveolar air 100 mm Hg and not 150 mm Hg, as it is in room air? How many mmol of O_2 are in 1 L of alveolar air? What percentage of the O_2 delivered to the alveoli is extracted?*

5.2 *Fish exchange gases through gills by taking up the O_2 dissolved in water and adding CO_2 to that water. CO_2 is 30-fold (for easy mathematics) more soluble in water than O_2. What does this solubility imply for the $Pa{CO_2}$ and the pH of blood in fish in steady state?*

5.3 *By what proportion must alveolar ventilatory capacity decline to have a $Pa{CO_2}$ of 50 vs the expected 40 mm Hg?*

In addition to alveolar ventilation, the other major factor determining the $Pa{CO_2}$ is the rate of CO_2 production, which is determined by the following:

TABLE 5.1 **Clinical Settings Resulting
in Altered CO$_2$ Production**

State	Organ	Usual CO$_2$ Production Rate	Altered CO$_2$ Production
Coma/anesthesia	Brain	3	1.5
Low GFR	Kidney	2	<1
Cachexia/paralysis	Muscle	2.4	<1
Vigorous exercise	Muscle	2.4	160
Ketogenesis	Liver	2.4	0

Legend for Table 5.1
The values for the production of CO$_2$ are shown as mmol/min and are representative values for a 70-kg adult. The values for altered rates are rough estimates and are for illustrative purposes only. (*Nephron* 64:514–517, 1993.)

1. Metabolic work (the need to regenerate adenosine triphosphate [ATP]; see Tables 5.1 and 5.2);

2. Mechanical work (patients who are cachectic may produce less CO$_2$ and have a lower Pa$_{CO_2}$ when hyperventilating);

3. Fuels being utilized (oxidation of carbohydrates yields more CO$_2$ relative to ATP production than does the oxidation of fat-derived fuels; see Table 5.2).

TABLE 5.2 **Importance of the Metabolic Fuel Utilized
in Determining the Rate of CO$_2$ Production**

Fuel	mmol CO$_2$/100 mmol ATP	Products
Carbohydrate	16.7	CO$_2$ + H$_2$O
Fatty acids	12.2	CO$_2$ + H$_2$O
Fatty acids	0	Ketoacids
Ethanol	11.1	CO$_2$ + H$_2$O
Ethanol	0	Ketoacids
Ethanol	0	Acetic acid

Legend for Table 5.2
The oxidation of carbohydrates produces more CO$_2$ than does the oxidation of fat-derived fuels when viewed in terms of the yield of ATP. (*Nephron* 64:514–517, 1993.)

Physiology of O$_2$ and CO$_2$ Transport

Oxygen Transport

Oxygen is transported bound to hemoglobin, with four molecules of O$_2$ bound per molecule of hemoglobin. Normally there are 2.25 mmol (140 g) of hemoglobin per liter of blood. The affinity of hemoglobin for O$_2$ is high but can be reduced by elevated concentrations of H$^+$, CO$_2$, and 2,3-diphosphoglycerate (2,3-DPG).

Effect of H$^+$ (Bohr Effect)

An increase in the [H$^+$] in plasma enhances the discharge of O$_2$ from hemoglobin because H$^+$ bind to hemoglobin and lessen hemoglobin's affinity for O$_2$. This effect is important during exercise because when L-lactic acid is produced, the [H$^+$] rises and facilitates the release of O$_2$ at the tissue level (Figure 5.1).

O$_2$ transport and concentration of hemoglobin
Blood can carry close to 9 mmol of O$_2$ per liter. Even if the hemoglobin is decreased by a factor of 12, delivery of O$_2$ to organs can still be maintained because the extraction of O$_2$ from each liter of blood can increase threefold and the cardiac output can increase fourfold. Therefore, anemia per se will never be the sole cause of hypoxia-induced lactic acidosis at rest.

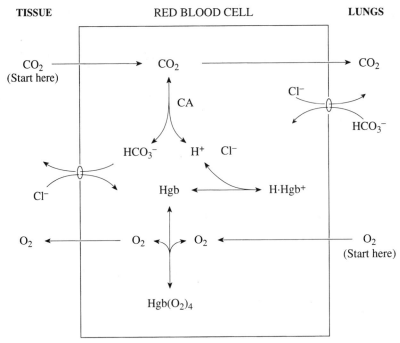

Figure 5.1 Interplay of CO_2 and O_2 transport. For CO_2 transport, begin at the upper left. CO_2 diffuses from the tissues into the red blood cells (RBC) where, under the influence of carbonic anhydrase (CA), HCO_3^- and H^+ are formed. The H^+ bind to hemoglobin (Hgb) and promote the unloading of O_2, which diffuses into tissues.

For O_2 transport, begin at the lower right. O_2 diffuses from the alveoli into the RBC. Binding of O_2 to hemoglobin releases H^+, which promote the exit of CO_2 from the blood. See the text for additional details.

Carbamates

When CO_2 is exposed to an R-NH$_2$ group, but not an R-NH$_3^+$ group, (e.g., the terminal amino group on globin molecules), a spontaneous reaction occurs that yields an anionic carbamate (see Chapter 9, page 398).

Effect of CO_2

An increase in the P_{CO_2} in tissue facilitates release of O_2 from hemoglobin by two mechanisms: a rise in $[H^+]$ and the formation of carbamates.

Effect of 2,3-DPG

When 2,3-DPG binds to hemoglobin, the affinity of hemoglobin for O_2 is reduced. Increases in 2,3-DPG in red blood cells result in increased delivery of O_2 at any given P_{O_2}. The signal for a rise in 2,3-DPG is the alkalemia that results from hyperventilation (e.g., high altitude, exercise, anemia). These effects require many hours to take place.

Effect of Temperature

When the temperature rises, the affinity of hemoglobin for O_2 falls. This lower affinity aids the downloading of O_2 at a higher P_{O_2} in muscle capillaries during vigorous exercise, because there is a large rise in the temperature of contracting muscles.

Transport of CO_2

At the tissue level, 10 mmol of CO_2 per minute diffuses into red blood cells. The carbonic anhydrase in these cells converts the CO_2 to H^+ and HCO_3^- (see Figure 5.1). Maintenance of a low P_{CO_2} in the red blood cell aids further diffusion of CO_2. The HCO_3^- formed

(8.5 mmol/min) is transported into the plasma in exchange for Cl^- ("chloride shift"), and the H^+ bind to hemoglobin.

Once at the lung, the process is reversed (see margin note). The lower Pco_2 of alveolar air aids in the diffusion of CO_2 from blood to the alveolus. The high Po_2 of alveolar air promotes the binding of O_2 to hemoglobin, which leads to the dissociation of H^+ bound to hemoglobin. These H^+ combine with the HCO_3^- that were in plasma (reversal of the "chloride shift"), and the resultant CO_2 diffuses into the alveoli. The net result is oxygenation in concert with CO_2 unloading in the lung.

Note
CO_2 diffuses between blood and the alveolar space much more rapidly than does O_2.

Arterial or Venous Blood for Analysis?

Mixed venous Pco_2
The Pco_2 of central venous blood.

> • The mixed venous Pco_2 reflects the tissue Pco_2 and, hence, the metabolic and/or circulatory status. The arterial Pco_2, on the other hand, reflects the alveolar Pco_2 and, hence, largely the ventilating function of the lungs.

Although it is "traditional" to use arterial blood for blood gas analysis, the sample used should depend on the information required. The venous Pco_2 reflects the tissue Pco_2; it is determined by the rate of production of CO_2 and the rate of blood flow. Thus, the Pco_2 of the venous blood from a specific limb can reflect local rather than systemic conditions. A high mixed venous Pco_2 can occur in three circumstances:

1. a high rate of aerobic metabolism (e.g., exercise);
2. a very high rate of H^+ formation (formation of CO_2 as a result of buffering of H^+ by HCO_3^-, e.g., during a sprint);
3. a reduced cardiac output, in which case the same amount of CO_2 is formed by an organ but is added to a smaller volume of blood flowing through that organ.

Note
Refer to Chapter 1, page 22, for the effect of a high venous Pco_2 on the buffering of H^+ on proteins in the ICF.

QUESTIONS

(Discussion on page 220)

5.4 *Why is the venous Pco_2 much higher than the arterial Pco_2 in each of the following: exercise, a convulsion, and diabetic ketoacidosis (DKA)?*

5.5 *Why might the rate of production of CO_2 be lower than normal in a patient with DKA?*

Pulmonary Physiology

To maintain a constant $Paco_2$, the lungs must remove the 10 mmol of CO_2 produced per minute by normal metabolism. The body produces a huge amount of CO_2—more than 14,000 mmol/day. Furthermore, with CO_2 accumulation, H^+ and HCO_3^- are produced in equimolar amounts (Figure 5.2) even though the $[HCO_3^-]$ normally exceeds the $[H^+]$ by 10^6-fold. The lungs therefore have a critical role in the maintenance of acid-base balance. Failure to remove this CO_2 leads to the generation of H^+ by displacement of

Point of emphasis
H^+ and HCO_3^- are produced in a 1:1 ratio from CO_2, but their relative concentrations are close to $1:10^6$, respectively.

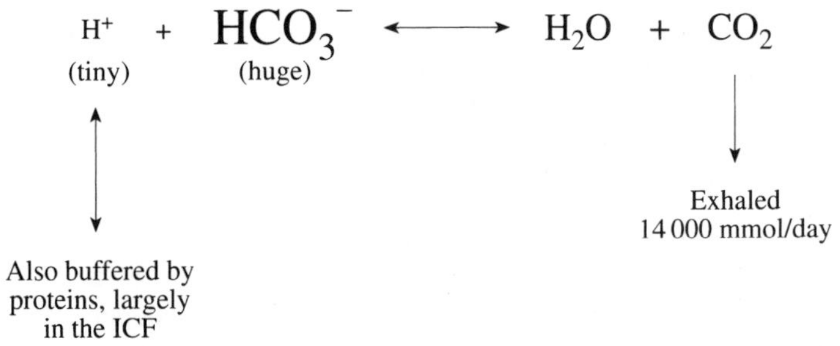

$$H^+ \quad + \quad HCO_3^- \quad \longleftrightarrow \quad H_2O \quad + \quad CO_2$$

(tiny)   (huge)

Exhaled
14 000 mmol/day

Also buffered by
proteins, largely
in the ICF

Figure 5.2 Bicarbonate buffer system (BBS) and respiratory acid-base disorders. The key principle is that the $[H^+]$ is tiny, and the $[HCO_3^-]$ is 10^6-fold larger. Shifting this equilibrium requires a 1:1 stoichiometry that results in an enormous H^+ load relative to the basal level of H^+.

the bicarbonate buffer system equilibrium to the left; acidemia (respiratory acidosis) then ensues. Excessive removal of CO_2 results in alkalemia (respiratory alkalosis) via displacement of the equilibrium to the right (see Figure 5.2).

The three components of pulmonary function that regulate gas exchange are ventilation, diffusion, and perfusion. Abnormalities of CO_2 homeostasis are generally related to derangement of ventilation. The authors therefore focus on the physiology and control of ventilation (see margin note for comments concerning a patient with fixed volume ventilation).

Control of Ventilation

Although the normal $Paco_2$ is 38–42 mm Hg, in states of metabolic acidosis and hypoxia, one expects to see a lower $[CO_2]$ or Pco_2 in arterial blood. Similarly, in association with metabolic alkalosis, there should be a modest rise in the $Paco_2$. Therefore, the $Paco_2$ must be assessed in the context of the pathophysiologic state of the patient with consideration of the existing stimulators and suppressors of ventilation.

The three components of the control of ventilation are central control, receptors for CO_2 and O_2, and the respiratory muscles and their workload.

The Central Control of Ventilation

Several centers in the medulla and in the pons, which are often referred to as the "central respiratory centers," control the rhythmic nature of ventilation. In addition, voluntary control of breathing is mediated via the cerebral cortex and is capable of overriding the brain stem, within limits.

Receptors

- There are both central and peripheral chemoreceptors that play an important role in the control of ventilation.

The central chemoreceptors, located on the ventral surface of the medulla, stimulate ventilation primarily in response to increases in

---

$Paco_2$ change resulting from change in CO_2 production

In patients with fixed alveolar ventilation (on ventilator without patient triggering), the $Paco_2$ will increase:

1. When a patient with metabolic acidosis produces more CO_2 in response to treatment with $NaHCO_3$;
2. When a patient who has fasted (metabolizing fatty acids) is fed and begins to oxidize carbohydrates.

Note

There are also numerous receptors in the lung parenchyma (pulmonary capillary, or "J" receptors) that respond to a variety of stimuli, such as inflammation or edema, by leading to an increase in the central ventilatory drive. Thus, patients with lung disease characteristically hyperventilate and have a reduced $Paco_2$, at least until the disease becomes quite severe.

the $[H^+]$ of the cerebrospinal fluid and also in response to increases in P_{CO_2} (thought to be mediated by a rise in the $[H^+]$). Ventilation is inhibited when the $[H^+]$ falls.

The peripheral chemoreceptors, found primarily in the carotid bodies, are responsible for the ventilatory response to a low Pa_{O_2}. These receptors also play a less important role in the ventilatory response to increased Pa_{CO_2} and acidemia.

QUESTIONS

(Discussion on pages 220–221)

5.6 *How might peripheral chemoreceptors detect a lower Pa_{O_2}?*

5.7 *Can respiratory alkalosis and respiratory acidosis occur in the same patient at the same time?*

Note
These questions are for the more curious.

Respiratory Muscles and Their Workload

The final determinants of ventilation, given the appropriate signals, are the respiratory muscles, their innervation, and the magnitude of the resistance they must overcome. A severe catabolic state, muscle disease, or metabolic disorder such as hypokalemia or hypophosphatemia may reduce the function of the respiratory muscles. Nerve damage (e.g., phrenic nerve) or changes in either the elastic load (lung and chest wall compliance, e.g., pulmonary fibrosis) or the resistive load (airway resistance, e.g., chronic bronchitis) may also increase the work of ventilation. Therefore, for any given level of central stimulation, the respiratory muscles may not be able to respond adequately. Ventilation will then decrease and lead to a rise in the Pa_{CO_2}.

The Alveolar-Arterial Po_2 Difference

> - Using the alveolar-arterial P_{O_2} difference (P_{O_2} in alveolar air–P_{O_2} in arterial blood) to evaluate the exchange of O_2 between alveolar air and blood enables assessment of the causes of hypoxemia. Alveolar P_{O_2} is calculated as inspired $P_{O_2} - 1.25 \times$ arterial P_{CO_2}. The normal value, which depends on age, is up to 15 mm Hg.
> - The major difficulties with this approach are that the content of O_2 and P_{O_2} are related in a sigmoid fashion, not a linear fashion, and that the calculation is affected by several nonpulmonary parameters.

Alveolar-arterial Po_2 difference
1. The difference in P_{O_2} between the alveolar air and arterial blood is referred to as the *A-a gradient*. In truth, this calculation should be a "difference" rather than a "gradient" because diffusion of nonelectrolytes is involved.
2. There is a problem with the A-a P_{O_2} difference, because the relationship between P_{O_2} and O_2 content of blood is not linear (Figure 5.3).

Although respiratory acid-base disorders are defined by changes in the Pa_{CO_2}, important clinical information can also be derived by interpreting the Pa_{O_2}. The arterial P_{O_2} is a function of both the P_{O_2} of alveolar air and the diffusion of O_2 across the alveolar capillary membrane.

Air is approximately 79% nitrogen and 21% O_2. In the lungs, CO_2 and water vapor are part of the "nonnitrogen" gases. Therefore, if one is breathing room air, as the P_{CO_2} of alveolar air rises, the P_{O_2}

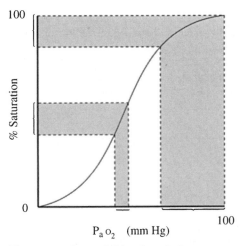

Figure 5.3 The oxygen-hemoglobin dissociation curve. Note that the shape of this curve is not linear, so a given absolute change in % saturation (shaded areas from the y-axis) leads to a very different change in P_aO_2 in the two examples illustrated in this figure.

must fall. Similarly, for any given inspired O_2 tension, a reduction in alveolar P_{CO_2} (hyperventilation) leads to an increase in alveolar and, hence, arterial P_{O_2}.

One can calculate the alveolar P_{O_2} using the abbreviated alveolar gas equation (equation follows). Thereafter, examining the difference between the alveolar P_{O_2} and the arterial P_{O_2} (A-a P_{O_2} difference) becomes a useful diagnostic tool. However, this approach has several pitfalls; they are discussed in the following paragraphs.

$$\text{Alveolar air } P_{O_2} = \text{Inspired air } P_{O_2} - (Pa_{CO_2})/RQ$$
$$= \text{Inspired air } P_{O_2} - (Pa_{CO_2})/0.8$$

Note
Dividing by 0.8 is the same as multiplying by 1.25.

Utility of the A-a P_{O_2} Difference

The calculation of the A-a P_{O_2} difference allows an estimation of how much of the derangement in arterial P_{O_2} is due to a change in alveolar P_{O_2} (ventilation) and how much is due to reduced transfer of O_2 from alveolus to blood (intrinsic lung disease). One must have an accurate estimate of the P_{O_2} of the inspired air to calculate the A-a difference. If air is 21% O_2, barometric pressure is 760 mm Hg, and water vapor pressure is 47 mm Hg, the P_{O_2} of inspired air is 0.21 (760 − 47), or 150 mm Hg. The alveolar P_{O_2} can be estimated from the abbreviated alveolar gas equation.

There are two major types of pulmonary lesions that cause the Pa_{O_2} to be substantially lower than that of alveolar air:

1. Blood could pass from the pulmonary artery to the pulmonary vein without perfusing alveoli that have a high P_{O_2} (i.e., a shunt that prevents a good exchange of air). In reality, most lung diseases that cause hypoxemia have numerous small areas of shunting as well as areas of nonventilated, nonperfused lung; together, these lesions lead to ventilation-perfusion mismatch.

2. There might be a barrier to diffusion of O_2 from alveolar air to the capillaries in lungs. The magnitude of the A-a difference is a parameter to be evaluated when trying to decide if a pulmonary

condition is improving or worsening. The A-a difference can also clarify whether hypoxemia is due to lung disease or central suppression of ventilation. In the latter case, the A-a difference should be normal (corrected for the sigmoid vs linear relationship; see Figure 5.3).

Pitfalls to Recognize in the Use of the A-a Difference

The difference between the alveolar and the arterial P_{O_2} is normally less than 15 mm Hg, but this value increases with age. While the A-a difference is widely used clinically, there are several pitfalls that must be kept in mind:

1. The A-a difference utilizes the P_{O_2} instead of reflecting the content of O_2 (O_2 saturation). Thus, the same reduction in O_2 content will have a different impact on the P_{O_2} at different sites on the oxygen-hemoglobin dissociation curve because this function is sigmoid rather than linear (see Figure 5.3).

2. In a fixed volume of shunt from pulmonary artery to pulmonary vein, the arterial P_{O_2} is strongly influenced by the content of O_2 in the blood in the pulmonary artery (see margin note).

3. The cardiac output is important in determining the extent to which a fixed shunt from pulmonary artery to pulmonary vein has affected the arterial P_{O_2} (see Question 5.8).

4. The P_{O_2} of inspired air must be known. When patients are receiving O_2 by mask or nasal prongs, the inspired P_{O_2} may not be known with sufficient accuracy. Therefore, the A-a difference is most useful when patients are breathing room air or are on ventilators with a measured content of inspired P_{O_2}.

5. In the calculation of the alveolar P_{O_2}, one must estimate the amount of O_2 removed and replaced by CO_2. To do so, one uses the arterial P_{CO_2} and assumes an RQ of 0.8. The RQ could be 1 if carbohydrate is the only type of fuel being metabolized (see margin note for an example).

6. The determination of the alveolar P_{O_2} assumes a steady state, so if an acute event has occurred (a sudden change in alveolar ventilation or an acute production of CO_2 from the administration of $NaHCO_3$ in L-lactic acidosis), an error will be introduced.

7. The normal A-a O_2 difference is increased with increasing F_iO_2 (percentage of inspired air that is O_2), even in patients on a ventilator.

Impact of the content of O_2 in shunted blood on the A-a difference

Assume that arterial blood has 9 mmol of O_2 per liter and that 10% of the blood in the pulmonary artery bypasses aerated alveoli via a shunt into the pulmonary vein. The content of O_2 in the blood in the pulmonary artery is 6 mmol/L. After this 10% shunt, arterial blood would contain 8.7 mmol of O_2 per liter (0.9 L with 9 mmol/L + 0.1 L with 6 mmol/L). In a second example, assume that blood in the pulmonary artery contains 3 mmol of O_2 per liter. After the 10% shunt, the arterial blood would have 8.4 mmol of O_2 per liter instead of 9 mmol. Assume that the new Pa_{O_2} in the first instance would be 95 mm Hg and that it would be 65 mm Hg in the second example. The corresponding A-a differences would be 5 and 35 mm Hg.

Effect of the RQ on the A-a difference

1. Assume an RQ of 0.8:
   Alveolar O_2 = 150 − (40/0.8)
   = 100 mm Hg
2. Assume an RQ of 1:
   Alveolar O_2 = 150 − (40/1)
   = 110 mm Hg

Therefore, the A-a differs by 10 mm Hg.

Note

These questions illustrate the clinical application and value of the A-a difference.

QUESTIONS

(Discussions on pages 221–222)

5.8 *A patient has a 0.1 L/min shunt from pulmonary artery to pulmonary vein. Would the A-a difference be different if the cardiac output was 5 vs 2 L/min? (Assume no other abnormality.)*

5.9 *A patient, comatose from a drug overdose, has the following blood gases. The basis of the hypoxia is thought to be aspiration. Is this diagnosis correct?*

pH		7.24	Pco$_2$	mm Hg	64
H$^+$	nmol/L	58	Pao$_2$	mm Hg	66

5.10 *Two days later the patient in Question 5.9 is awake but coughing. The following blood gases are obtained. Because his Pao$_2$ has improved, he is declared ready for discharge. Is this decision appropriate?*

pH		7.60	Paco$_2$	mm Hg	24
H$^+$	nmol/L	25	Pao$_2$	mm Hg	70

Clinical pearls

1. It is too difficult to assess the Paco$_2$ simply by clinical examination. Therefore, blood gas analysis is the key to the diagnosis of respiratory acid-base disorders.

2. In a patient who is breathing room air, adding the Po$_2$ and Paco$_2$ and subtracting the total from 150 will give a quick estimate of the A-a difference.

Renal response to chronic respiratory acid-base change

Acidemia from respiratory acidosis increases NH$_4$$^+$ excretion on a transient basis. This increase leads to a higher [HCO$_3$$^-$] in plasma. As a result, the filtered load of HCO$_3$$^-$ rises, as does the amount that is indirectly reabsorbed. Therefore, the plasma [HCO$_3$$^-$] is higher than normal in chronic respiratory acidosis. The opposite occurs in chronic respiratory alkalosis.

Respiratory Acid-Base Disorders

- Respiratory acidosis is an increased Paco$_2$ and [H$^+$] in plasma.
- Respiratory alkalosis is a decreased Paco$_2$ and [H$^+$] in plasma.
- Chronic respiratory disorders have a renal response that causes:
  -increased plasma [HCO$_3$$^-$] in acidosis;
  -decreased plasma [HCO$_3$$^-$] in alkalosis.

Respiratory acid-base disorders arise from primary changes in Paco$_2$. There is a very large flux of CO$_2$ relative to the [CO$_2$] in the plasma (i.e., 10 mmol of CO$_2$ is produced per minute, yet the Paco$_2$ and H$_2$CO$_3$ are only 1.2 mmol of CO$_2$ per liter of blood and usually vary by less than 10% on a moment-to-moment basis). If a discrepancy develops transiently between production and removal of CO$_2$, the resultant change in Paco$_2$ will then displace the BBS equilibrium (see Figure 5.2). Accumulation of CO$_2$ results in an increased [H$^+$] (respiratory acidosis). A fall in Paco$_2$ displaces the equilibrium and results in a fall in the [H$^+$] (respiratory alkalosis).

In chronic respiratory acidosis, an increase in the indirect reabsorption of HCO$_3$$^-$ by the proximal convoluted tubule permits an increase in the plasma [HCO$_3$$^-$]; in contrast, a fall in the plasma [HCO$_3$$^-$] occurs during chronic respiratory alkalosis. Thus, chronic respiratory acid-base disturbances have a different steady-state plasma [HCO$_3$$^-$], and hence [H$^+$], than do the acute respiratory acid-base disorders. It is therefore important for the clinician to clarify, on clinical grounds, whether the acid-base disturbance is acute or chronic in origin.

Buffering of H$^+$ in Respiratory Acidosis

Buffering in the ICF

The BBS is the major buffer in the ECF, and its effectiveness is compromised with a defect in CO$_2$ removal (it cannot adjust the [CO$_2$], as shown in Figure 5.2).

The ICF buffers consist of approximately equal proportions of bicarbonate and nonbicarbonate buffers; only the latter are effective buffers of H_2CO_3. A rise in $Paco_2$ leads to binding of H^+ in the ICF and to formation of HCO_3^- (in the equations below, B° represents the histidine buffers in intracellular proteins; see Chapter 1, pages 19–22, for complete discussion of ECF and ICF buffers). When H_2CO_3 is buffered in cells, HCO_3^- are formed in the ICF. Because some HCO_3^- are exported into the ECF, a small rise in the $[HCO_3^-]$ occurs in the ECF.

$$CO_2 + H_2O \leftrightarrow H^+ + HCO_3^-$$
$$H^+ + B^\circ \leftrightarrow H \cdot B^+$$

Sum (equations above): $CO_2 + H_2O + B^\circ \leftrightarrow H \cdot B^+ + HCO_3^-$

Quantitative Analysis

Given that the ICF buffer capacity is large, the quantity of H^+ buffered in the ICF depends on the rise in the $[H^+]$ in cells, which is proportional to the rise in the tissue Pco_2. Therefore, the rise in the $[HCO_3^-]$ in the ICF (and hence in the ECF) that accompanies a rise in Pco_2 is proportional to the relative increment in Pco_2 rather than the absolute increment. In the example in the margin note, with different original values for the Pco_2, a 20 mm Hg increase in Pco_2 has a different impact on the $[H^+]$ in cells; therefore, the larger the percentage change in Pco_2, the larger the generation of HCO_3^- from nonbicarbonate buffers in cells.

Example
Consider a 20 mm Hg rise in Pco_2 in two circumstances:
1. If the Pco_2 rises from 20 to 40 mm Hg, there is a 100% change.
2. If the Pco_2 rises from 60 to 80 mm Hg, there is a 33% change.

Empiric Observations

The patient with acute retention of CO_2 has acidemia, an elevated $Paco_2$, and a slight rise in the plasma $[HCO_3^-]$; in contrast, the rise in plasma $[HCO_3^-]$ is greater, and the rise in $[H^+]$ is smaller in chronic respiratory acid-base disorders (Figure 5.4).

PART B

Respiratory Acidosis

Clinical Approach

Respiratory acidosis is the result of alveolar hypoventilation. The clinician's problem is to establish the basis of the hypoventilation. Patients who hypoventilate can be divided into two groups: those who will not breathe (defective stimulus) and those who cannot breathe (defective equipment). In addition, patients with a fixed alveolar ventilation (i.e., those on ventilators) develop increased $Paco_2$ if they have an increased rate of production of CO_2 or an increase in dead space (e.g., pulmonary embolus).

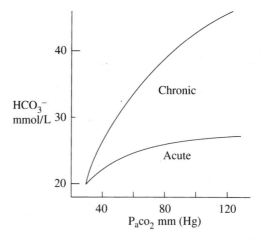

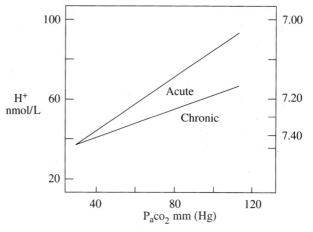

Figure 5.4 Empiric relationship of the P_{aCO_2} and the $[HCO_3^-]$ or $[H^+]$ in plasma. Note the different relationships with acute vs chronic changes in P_{aCO_2}. The flatter slope of the H^+ vs P_{CO_2} regression line in chronic respiratory acidosis reflects the renal generation and retention of HCO_3^-.

Patients Who Will Not Breathe Because of Defects in Neurologic Input

Some patients may hypoventilate because they lack the normal respiratory neurologic input at one of three levels: first, cerebral nonrhythmic neurons; second, brain stem rhythmic function; third, upper airway reflexes (Table 5.3).

Patients Who Cannot Breathe Because of Respiratory or Muscular Disorders

The causes of inability to breathe fall into three categories (Table 5.4): first, primary muscle disorders; second, increased elastic work (restrictive disease); and third, increased resistance to flow (obstructive disease).

TABLE 5.3 **Patients Who Will Not Breathe**

Category	Cause	Diagnostic Test Results
Cerebral nonrhythmic neurons	• Posthypoxic brain damage • Cerebral trauma • Intracranial disease • Psychotropic drugs	• Inability to cough, talk, or hold breath
Brain stem rhythmic function	• Brain stem herniation • Encephalitis • Central sleep apnea • Metabolic alkalosis (severe) • Drugs (sedatives, narcotics)	• Abnormal ventilatory response to changes in inhaled CO_2 and O_2
Upper airway reflexes	• Bulbar palsy • Anterior horn cell lesions • Disruption of airway	• Inability to swallow • Absent nasal, tracheal, and pharyngeal reflexes

TABLE 5.4 **Patients Who Cannot Breathe**

Category	Cause	Diagnostic Test Results
Respiratory muscle disease	• Myasthenia • Relaxant drugs • Muscular dystrophy • Muscle fatigue or paralysis	• Reduced maximum inspiratory and expiratory pressures
Increased elastic work	• Interstitial lung disease • Pulmonary fibrosis	• Reduced lung volumes • Reduced lung compliance • Normal flow rates
Increased resistance to flow	• Asthma • Bronchitis • Emphysema • Upper airway obstruction	• Reduced flow rates • Increased airway resistance • Increased lung compliance • Abnormal flow-volume loop

Acid-Base Aspects

Respiratory acidosis occurs when ventilation transiently fails to remove the CO_2 produced by normal metabolism. As a result, the alveolar PCO_2 rises and increases the $PaCO_2$. At this new arterial and alveolar PCO_2, the CO_2 produced can now be removed despite the reduced ventilation.

Clinical pearl
Make the diagnosis of acute or chronic disease on a clinical basis, not on laboratory values.

Diagnostic Approach

The diagnostic approach to respiratory acidosis is outlined in Figure 5.5. First, decide if the patient has chronic lung disease by the history, physical examination, and available past records. Then, compare the acid-base status with that expected for that acid-base disorder. If a discrepancy exists, a mixed disorder is present.

In acute and chronic respiratory acidosis in patients who were previously normal, an empirical linear relationship has been found between the $[H^+]$ and the $PaCO_2$ (see Figure 5.4 and the margin note). In patients who do not begin with a normal acid-base state (e.g., they have coexisting metabolic acidosis or alkalosis), the plasma $[HCO_3^-]$ rises 2.5 mmol/L for a twofold change in $PaCO_2$.

Acute respiratory acidosis
For every mm Hg increase in $PaCO_2$ from 40 mm Hg, expect a 0.8 nmol/L increase in $[H^+]$ from 40 nmol/L.

Chronic respiratory acidosis
For every mm Hg increase in $PaCO_2$ from 40 mm Hg, expect a 0.3 nmol/L increase in $[H^+]$; for every mm Hg increase in $PaCO_2$, expect a 0.3 mmol/L increase in the plasma $[HCO_3^-]$.

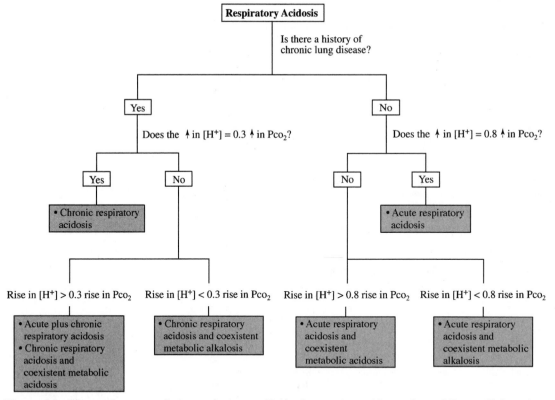

Figure 5.5   Diagnostic approach to respiratory acidosis. In a patient with an elevated $Paco_2$, if there is no evidence of chronic lung disease or a chronic central reason for hypoventilation, assume that the patient has acute respiratory acidosis. The final diagnoses are shown in the shaded boxes.

QUESTIONS

(Discussions on pages 222–223)

Note
Question 5.11 is for the more curious.

5.11 *When cold-blooded animals live at 37°C, their $Paco_2$ is close to 40 mm Hg, and their pH is close to 7.4. At colder temperatures, their pH rises, and their $[HCO_3^-]$ in plasma remains constant. What might these values imply for regulation of ventilation and pH?*

5.12 *Three patients all experience an acute increase in $Paco_2$ to 80 mm Hg. Each has a different $[H^+]$. What is the acid-base status in each case?*

Patient	[H+]	pH
A	96 nmol/L	7.02
B	70 nmol/L	7.25
C	50 nmol/L	7.30

5.13 *A patient with chronic stable obstructive lung disease ($Paco_2$ = 60 mm Hg, plasma $[HCO_3^-]$ = 31 mmol/L) developed shortness of breath and was admitted with a diagnosis of congestive heart failure. During treatment with diuretics and*

O₂, he vomited a few times, but his chest x-ray film showed improvement. The following blood gases were obtained after therapy: [H⁺] = 38 nmol/L, Paco₂ = 80 mm Hg, Pao₂ = 70 mm Hg. What is the basis of the increased CO₂ retention? What therapy would be appropriate?

PART C

Respiratory Alkalosis

Clinical Approach

Respiratory alkalosis is a common abnormality that is often ignored. Its mortality rate in the hospital, which may well be greater than that for respiratory acidosis, reflects the importance of the underlying disease process. Hypocapnia is often difficult to recognize clinically, and the diagnosis is often made only by determination of blood gases.

Respiratory alkalosis occurs when the ventilatory removal of CO_2 transiently exceeds its rate of production: thus, the alveolar and arterial P_{CO_2} fall. At this lower level of Pa_{CO_2}, the daily production of CO_2 is then removed by the increased ventilation, which leads to a new steady state.

A fall in tissue P_{CO_2} has an important impact on the $[H^+]$ in the ICF in moderate metabolic acidosis. The associated decrease in $[H^+]$ results in back-titration of the protonated ICF proteins and shifts the majority of the ICF buffering to HCO_3^-. This action may preserve the structure and function of the ICF proteins. In the alkalemic patient, hyperventilation is likely to make these intracellular proteins less positively charged than normal, a change that could lead to altered function.

Respiratory alkalosis may result from stimulation of the peripheral chemoreceptors (hypoxia or hypotension), the afferent pulmonary reflexes (intrinsic pulmonary disease), or central stimulation by a host of stimuli (Table 5.5).

TABLE 5.5 **Causes of Respiratory Alkalosis**

Hypoxia

Intrinsic pulmonary disease, high altitude, congestive heart failure, congenital heart disease (cyanotic)

Pulmonary Receptor Stimulation

Pneumonia, pulmonary embolism, asthma, pulmonary fibrosis, pulmonary edema

Drugs

Salicylates (the most common), nikethamide, catecholamines, theophylline, progesterone

CNS Disorders

Subarachnoid hemorrhage, Cheyne-Stokes respiration, primary hyperventilation syndrome

Miscellaneous

Psychogenic hyperventilation, cirrhosis, fever, gram-negative sepsis, recovery from metabolic acidosis, pregnancy

Acid-Base Aspects

The acid-base impact of respiratory alkalosis is analogous to that of respiratory acidosis in that the acute and chronic states differ because of the role of the kidneys in altering the concentration of HCO_3^- in the body.

Acute Respiratory Alkalosis

Acute respiratory alkalosis
For every mm Hg reduction in $Paco_2$ from 40 mm Hg, expect a 0.8 nmol/L decrease in $[H^+]$ from 40 nmol/L.

In acute respiratory alkalosis, displacement of the BBS to the right leads to a reduction in both the $[H^+]$ and the $[HCO_3^-]$ (see Figure 5.2). The impact on the $[H^+]$ in the ECF in acute respiratory alkalosis is virtually identical to that in acute respiratory acidosis (although opposite in direction).

Chronic Respiratory Alkalosis

Chronic respiratory alkalosis
For every mm Hg reduction in $Paco_2$ from 40 mm Hg, expect a 0.2 nmol/L fall in $[H^+]$ from 40 nmol/L and a 0.5 mmol/L fall in $[HCO_3^-]$ from 25 mmol/L.

In chronic respiratory alkalosis, there is a temporary small suppression of renal NH_4^+ production and excretion, and the $[HCO_3^-]$ in the ECF falls (H^+ of dietary origin continue to consume HCO_3^- without equivalent renal formation of new HCO_3^-) until the plasma $[H^+]$ approaches normal. This acid-base disorder is the only one in which a normal plasma $[H^+]$ might be expected.

Diagnostic Approach

The diagnostic approach to respiratory alkalosis is detailed in Figure 5.6. One begins by deciding on clinical grounds whether there is a disease process associated with chronic respiratory alkalosis; if not, the patient is presumed to have acute respiratory alkalosis.

PART D

Paco$_2$ in Metabolic Acid-Base Disorders

The normal $Paco_2$ at a $[HCO_3^-]$ of 25 mmol/L is 40 mm Hg; in contrast, the expected $Paco_2$ in metabolic acidosis at a plasma $[HCO_3^-]$ of 10 mmol/L is 25 rather than 40 mm Hg (see Chapter 2, page 62). Therefore, at a $[HCO_3^-]$ of 10 mmol/L, a patient with a $Paco_2$ of 40 mm Hg has respiratory acidosis in addition to metabolic acidosis.

A failure to hyperventilate appropriately in metabolic acidosis has a dramatic impact on the plasma $[H^+]$. A patient with a plasma $[HCO_3^-]$ of 10 mmol/L has a $[H^+]$ of 60 nmol/L (pH 7.22) with a

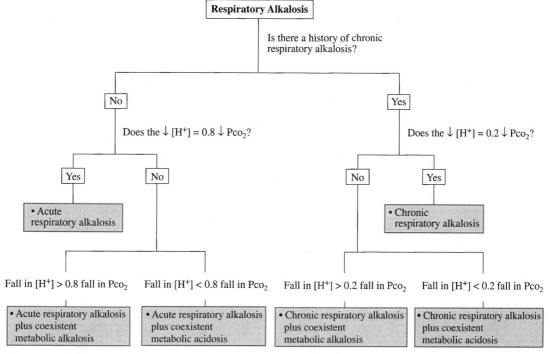

Figure 5.6   Diagnostic approach to respiratory alkalosis. In a patient with a reduced $PaCO_2$, decide whether a disease process that is associated with chronic respiratory alkalosis is present; if not, assume that the patient has acute respiratory alkalosis. The final diagnoses are shown in the shaded boxes.

$PaCO_2$ of 25 (see margin note); with a $PaCO_2$ of 40 mm Hg, the $[H^+]$ is 96 nmol/L (pH 7.02). The impact on the ICF buffering, however, may be much more important both physiologically and clinically than the impact on the plasma $[H^+]$. Hyperventilation in metabolic acidosis transfers the H^+ burden from the ICF protein buffers to the BBS (see Chapter 1, pages 19–22, for more details). Because ICF buffering on histidine may change the structure and function of ICF proteins, it is most desirable for the BBS to buffer as great a quantity of H^+ as possible.

Patients with chronic obstructive pulmonary disease are often on diuretics and may have a coexistent metabolic alkalosis. Because H^+ stimulate ventilation, a lower $[H^+]$ can make the hypoventilation more severe. Interestingly, correction of the metabolic alkalosis in these patients does not result in a large change in their $[H^+]$; instead, there is a significant fall in both the $[HCO_3^-]$ and $PaCO_2$, coupled with an increase in PaO_2. These changes are associated with a dramatic clinical improvement. It is tempting to speculate that the clinical improvement is due, in part, to the reduction in H^+ buffering on the ICF proteins.

Calculations

$$[H^+] = \frac{24}{[HCO_3^-]} \times PCO_2$$

$$60 = \frac{24}{10} \times 25$$

$$96 = \frac{24}{10} \times 40$$

Net charge on ICF proteins in metabolic alkalosis
The $[H^+]$ in the ICF may be elevated as a result of hypokalemia, a higher $PaCO_2$, and the lower blood flow rate (higher venous PCO_2). If, in addition, respiratory acidosis is present, these proteins could bear an even greater positive net charge.

QUESTIONS

(Discussions on page 224)

5.14 *A 30-year-old businessman had just returned from Europe when he suddenly developed a severe left-sided pleuritic chest pain and hemoptysis. He had no history of chest disease and* *exercised regularly. He was cyanotic, he had an elevated jugular venous pressure (8 cm above the sternal angle), and his blood pressure was 80/50 mm Hg. The blood gases were $[H^+] = 40$ nmol/L (pH 7.40), $Paco_2 = 25$ mm Hg, and $Pao_2 = 50$ mm Hg. What is the most likely diagnosis?*

5.15 *A patient with cirrhosis of the liver was found in a confused state by his landlady. His physical examination results were normal except for a low blood pressure and the stigmata of chronic liver disease. His laboratory results were as follows:*

Na^+	mmol/L	133	H^+	nmol/L	36	pH 7.44
K^+	mmol/L	3.3	$Paco_2$	mm Hg	20	
Cl^-	mmol/L	115	HCO_3^-	mmol/L	13	

The initial diagnosis was L-lactic acidosis secondary to severe hepatic insufficiency. Is this diagnosis appropriate? If not, why, and what is the most likely diagnosis?

P A R T   E

Review

DISCUSSION OF INTRODUCTORY CASE
Hack's Future Is Up in Smoke
(Case presented on page 197)

What prompted the changes from the usual values to those seen on admission?

Note

$$[H^+] = \frac{24}{[HCO_3^-]} \times Pco_2$$

$$46 = \frac{24}{[HCO_3^-]} \times 60$$

$$[HCO_3^-] = 31 \text{ mmol/L}$$

Hack's usual plasma $[HCO_3^-]$ can be calculated as shown in the margin note. His usual $[H^+]$ in simple chronic respiratory acidosis with a $Paco_2$ of 60 mm Hg is 46 mmol/L because the rise in Pco_2 of 20 mm Hg $\times$ 0.3 results in the addition of 6 nmol/L to the normal value of H^+ (40 nmol/L).

When Hack was admitted, he had an acute increase in $Paco_2$ to 80 mm Hg with profound hypoxia. The $[HCO_3^-]$, calculated as above, was still 31 mmol/L. Therefore, the severe acidemia was due largely to the presence of acute respiratory acidosis combined with chronic respiratory acidosis. There may have been an added element of metabolic acidosis that could be confirmed by evaluating the plasma anion gap. The acute respiratory acidosis was due to pneumonia.

What happened to permit the changes in the blood gases while Hack was on the ventilator on day 2 of therapy?

While Hack was ventilated on day 2 of therapy, his acid-base values returned to normal: $[H^+] = 40$ nmol/L, $[HCO_3^-] = 24$ mmol/L, $Paco_2 = 40$ mm Hg. Although one can achieve a normal acid-base status with artificial ventilation, Hack has severe lung disease and will not be able to maintain a $Paco_2$ of 40 mm Hg once he is extubated. Therefore, it is inappropriate to ventilate him to this level; he should be maintained with a $Paco_2$ of 60 mm Hg (his chronic steady-state value) to preserve his renal adaptation to chronic respiratory acidosis. In this case, his kidneys were "fooled" into thinking that his lungs were normal. He therefore excreted the extra HCO_3^-, and his plasma $[HCO_3^-]$ fell to 24 mmol/L instead of the 31 mmol/L that was present before the acute illness.

Why are his postextubation values on day 4 of therapy so different from his original values?

With extubation on day 4 of therapy, Hack went from a normal acid-base state to acute respiratory acidosis with a $Paco_2$ of 70 mm Hg. The $[H^+]$ was appropriate for acute respiratory acidosis: the rise in $[H^+]$ was 30 mm Hg $\times$ 0.8, or 24 nmol/L, which is a $[H^+]$ of 64 nmol/L. His plasma $[HCO_3^-]$ was $24 \times 70/64$, or 26 mmol/L, which rose appropriately for acute respiratory acidosis.

On day 4 of therapy, his $Paco_2$ was slightly higher than his chronic steady state (70 vs 60 mm Hg). This increase may represent an incomplete resolution of the pneumonia or may indicate permanent destruction of lung tissue. Time will tell.

Cases for Review

CASE 5.1
Annie-Abigale Has Chronic Lung Disease
(Case discussed on pages 216–217)

An 87-year-old lady with chronic obstructive lung disease and congestive heart failure with marked edema was treated with a diuretic and lost 5 L of ECF. Her mental state deteriorated following treatment. Physical examination revealed that she was obtunded; she had all her previous lung findings except that her edema disappeared. A summary of results follows. Note that she developed an extremely high $Paco_2$ breathing room air. The diuresis caused little rise in net acid excretion (data not shown).

Parameter		Steady State	Postdiuretic
H^+	nmol/L	51	44
pH		7.29	7.34
$Paco_2$	mm Hg	60	85
Pao_2	mm Hg	50	39
A-a	mm Hg	25	5
HCO_3^-	mmol/L	28	44
K^+	mmol/L	4.1	3.1
Anion gap	mEq/L	11	16
Creatinine	μmol/L (mg/dL)	57 (0.7)	66 (0.8)

What are the acid-base disorders after diuresis?
Why did the $[HCO_3^-]$ and $Paco_2$ rise so markedly?
Why did the A-a difference fall?
What should the therapy be?

CASE 5.2
Is Doreen a "Blowhard"?
(Case discussed on pages 217–218)

Doreen, age 84 years, was transferred from a nursing home for evaluation of chest pain. She has Alzheimer's disease and end-stage renal disease that requires chronic ambulatory peritoneal dialysis (CAPD) and the oral intake of calcium carbonate. She does not take other drugs. All investigations, including her physical examination, have yielded negative results so far. She is afebrile, and there is no evidence of deep and/or extremely rapid respirations.

Laboratory results reveal an incidental finding of an extreme degree of alkalemia (pH 7.70). The remainder of the pertinent values are shown as follows.

$[H^+]$	nmol/L	20	pH		7.70
HCO_3^-	mmol/L	26	Anion gap	mEq/L	14
Pa_{CO_2}	mm Hg	22	Albumin	g/L	32
Pa_{O_2}	mm Hg	107			

What is (are) the acid-base disorder(s)?

What is the basis of the acid-base disorder(s)?

What other investigations are in order to clarify the basis of respiratory alkalosis?

Discussion of Cases

DISCUSSION OF CASE 5.1
Annie-Abigale Has Chronic Lung Disease
(Case presented on page 215)

What are the acid-base disorders after diuresis?

The acid-base disturbance before therapy was chronic respiratory acidosis. Two major changes occurred with diuresis: there was a large rise in the $[HCO_3^-]$ in plasma (metabolic alkalosis) and in the Pa_{CO_2} (coexistent acute and chronic respiratory acidosis). There could have been a minor component of metabolic acidosis as well because the plasma anion gap also rose.

Why did the $[HCO_3^-]$ and Pa_{CO_2} rise so markedly?

The elevation in the $[HCO_3^-]$ was not due to intake of the HCO_3^- or excretion of net acid. Therefore, it may have been due to an internal shift of H^+ when K^+ exited from cells (minor) or to a loss of ECF volume (i.e., the same content of HCO_3^- in a smaller ECF volume, a major effect that causes a "contraction" metabolic alkalosis; see margin note).

The rise in Pa_{CO_2} would also have led to a modest rise in the $[HCO_3^-]$ (2.5 mmol/L per doubling of the Pa_{CO_2}). This rise in Pa_{CO_2} was probably the result of suppressed ventilation caused by reduction in the stimulus of acidemia and was possibly also due to weakness of respiratory muscles (hypokalemia).

Calculation
- Assume her normal ECF volume is 12 L.
- She had 5 L of edema fluid that was lost, so her original ECF volume was 17 L.
- Her initial content of HCO_3^- was 476 mmol (17 L × 28 mmol of HCO_3^-).
- After the diuresis, the 476 mmol of HCO_3^- would have distributed in 12 L, and her new $[HCO_3^-]$ would have been 40 mmol/L.

Why did the A-a difference fall?

The major problem here is the use of the PO_2 scale vs the oxygen content (or saturation of hemoglobin) scale. The difference between alveolar and arterial PO_2 was greater before therapy (75–50 mm Hg) than after diuresis (44–39 mm Hg)—a misleading A-a difference. If one recalculates the A-a difference values using O_2 content rather than PO_2, they are 8.4–7.2 mmol/L (1.2 mmol/L difference) before therapy and 6.7–5.8 mmol/L (0.9 mmol/L difference) after therapy. Therefore, because of the shape of the oxygen-hemoglobin dissociation curve, what appeared to be a large difference between the pre- and posttreatment values when the PO_2 was measured is actually very small when the O_2 content is used.

What should the therapy be?

The aim of therapy is to lower the $PaCO_2$ and $[HCO_3^-]$ in arterial blood. The first step is to replace the deficit of K^+ to see if ventilation will improve (it did not).

The next step is to administer 250 mg acetazolamide, a carbonic anhydrase inhibitor diuretic, to induce a degree of bicarbonaturia; losses of K^+ in the urine should be replaced. With bicarbonaturia, the PCO_2 and $[HCO_3^-]$ in arterial blood returned to her steady-state values within 24 hours. The patient then felt better.

Another option would have been to administer HCl (NH_4Cl) to titrate HCO_3^-, but, because CO_2 production will rise transiently, this mode of therapy is possibly less desirable.

DISCUSSION OF CASE 5.2
Is Doreen a "Blowhard"?
(Case presented on page 216)

What is (are) the acid-base disorder(s)?

The pH of blood is very alkaline and the $PaCO_2$ is very low, so the most important acid-base diagnosis is respiratory alkalosis. Her plasma $[HCO_3^-]$ is higher than one might expect for acute or chronic respiratory alkalosis, so she has a coexistent metabolic alkalosis.

What is the basis of the acid-base disorder(s)?

1. Respiratory alkalosis may have resulted from increased ventilation and a low production of CO_2.

   Increased Ventilation. A low $PaCO_2$ indicates an abnormal drive to respiration. Organic diseases to consider are pulmonary diseases (pulmonary embolism is a good bet, but any intrinsic pulmonary, central nervous system, or liver disease is possible). The A-a difference is slightly increased (15 mm Hg; see margin note) but is in keeping with her advanced age.

   The other considerations are her anxiousness about her health and the possibility of "occult" sepsis, brain disease, or lung disease. Her plasma levels of Ca^{2+}, Mg^{2+}, phosphate, Na^+, and glucose are all normal, so a specific lesion is not identified.

Calculation
A-a PO_2 = 150 − (107 + (22/0.8))
         = 15 mm Hg

Low Production of CO$_2$. The quandary for the clinician is that she has a very low Pa$_{CO_2}$ yet shows little clinical evidence of an extreme degree of hyperventilation. The next step is to determine if she has a low rate of production of CO$_2$.

On a general basis, she is not hypothermic, so hypothyroidism should be considered. With respect to specific organs, her Alzheimer's disease may decrease CO$_2$ production in her brain. Her renal failure limits CO$_2$ production by her kidneys. She is very inactive (lies in bed), so her muscles produce little CO$_2$. Therefore, one basis for her low Pa$_{CO_2}$ is low production of CO$_2$.

Summary. Her respiratory alkalosis is very severe because she has a pathologic drive to ventilation in the setting of very low production of CO$_2$.

2. Her metabolic alkalosis probably reflects the intake of alkali (calcium carbonate) in the presence of renal failure, as well as the metabolism of the D- and L-lactate anions from the CAPD fluid.

What other investigations are in order to clarify the basis of respiratory alkalosis?

First, one should seek a possible basis of the abnormal drive to respiration (e.g., if sepsis and pulmonary embolism are present). She should also be investigated for occult hypothyroidism. Confirm that her rate of production of CO$_2$ is really low by measuring her rates of O$_2$ consumption and CO$_2$ production.

Summary of Main Points

- Alterations in Pa$_{CO_2}$ have a major impact on the BBS; a Pa$_{CO_2}$ that is too high renders the BBS ineffective and increases buffering by intracellular proteins (the converse applies to a low Pa$_{CO_2}$). Both may have significant clinical impact.
- Examining the arterial blood P$_{CO_2}$ permits one to assess the ventilation function of the lungs; the venous P$_{CO_2}$ reflects the tissue P$_{CO_2}$ and thereby provides information about the metabolic rate, blood flow rate, and/or buffering of a H$^+$ load.
- In chronic respiratory acidosis and alkalosis, the kidneys return the [H$^+$] toward normal by transiently increasing or decreasing the rate of NH$_4^+$ excretion and thereby increasing the plasma [HCO$_3^-$] in chronic respiratory acidosis or decreasing the plasma [HCO$_3^-$] in chronic respiratory alkalosis.
- In both acute and chronic respiratory acidosis and alkalosis, there are predictable physiologic responses in the [H$^+$] and [HCO$_3^-$] that enable the clinical detection of mixed acid-base disorders.
- Metabolic alkalosis may coexist with chronic respiratory acidosis (because of the use of diuretics) and may have a significant deleterious impact on the clinical status of the patient.

Discussion of Questions

5.1 Assume that the consumption of O_2 is 12 mmol/min, that alveolar ventilation is 5 L/min, and that 21% of air is O_2.

Why is the Po_2 of alveolar air 100 mm Hg and not 150 mm Hg, as it is in room air?

The usual Po_2 in humidified inspired air is $(760 - 47)$ mm Hg $\times$ 0.21, or 150 mm Hg. In the alveoli, nitrogen gas is still 79% of total air, but CO_2 occupies some of the space left for O_2. If the RQ is 0.8 (see margin note), a Pco_2 of 40 mm Hg is derived from 50 mm Hg O_2. Therefore, alveolar air has two-thirds the content of O_2 vs inspired air (100 vs 150 mm Hg).

Note
RQ = CO_2 produced/O_2 consumed. Therefore, with an RQ of 0.8, 40 mm Hg of CO_2 is derived from 50 mm Hg of O_2.

How many mmol of O_2 are in 1 L of alveolar air?

Calculate the mmol of O_2 provided by 100 mm Hg Po_2:
- 1L of air contains 210 mL of O_2 (21%), but alveolar air has two-thirds this volume (or concentration) of O_2 (Po_2 is 100 vs 150 mm Hg). Therefore, 1 L of alveolar air contains 140 mL of O_2 (2/3 $\times$ 210 mL).
- For every 22.4 mL of gas at standard temperature and pressure, there is 1 mmol of that gas. Accordingly, 1 L of air contains close to 9 mmol of O_2, and 1 L of alveolar air contains close to 6 mmol of O_2.

What percentage of the O_2 delivered to the alveoli is extracted?

Because alveolar ventilation is 5 L/min, close to 45 mmol of O_2 enters alveoli each minute, but only 12 mmol is "extracted." Therefore, there is a large reserve, and 27% of O_2 (100 $\times$ 12/45) is extracted.

5.2 Fish exchange gases through gills by taking up the O_2 dissolved in water and adding CO_2 to that water. CO_2 is 30-fold (for easy mathematics) more soluble in water than O_2. What does this solubility imply for the $Paco_2$ and the pH of blood in fish in steady state?

If the concentrations of O_2 and CO_2 are equal in the capillary blood of the gills, the solution bathing the gills (lake water) will wash away 30-fold more CO_2 than the amount of O_2 that it will supply. Accordingly, because the amounts of CO_2 produced and O_2 consumed are roughly equal (RQ = 1), the $[CO_2]$ must be 1/30 that of O_2. This relationship requires a very low $[CO_2]$ (Pco_2) in the arterial blood of fish (values close to several mm Hg).

Given the $Paco_2$, either the fish will have a very alkaline blood (Henderson equation) or a very low $[HCO_3^-]$ in plasma. The fish usually has a very low $[HCO_3^-]$. In acid-base terms, it does not have an important BBS.

Henderson equation

$$[H^+] = \frac{24}{[HCO_3^-]} \times Pco_2$$

5.3 By what proportion must alveolar ventilatory capacity decline to have a $Paco_2$ of 50 vs the expected 40 mm Hg?

A simple answer, but one the authors believe to be less correct, is to assume that there is only a 20% reduction in alveolar ventilation

Note
- CO_2 excretion can be 160 mmol/min.
- Each liter of alveolar air contains 2 mmol of CO_2 (at a Pco_2 of 40 mm Hg).
- Therefore, alveolar ventilation is 80 L/min.

$(5 - 1)$ L/min/5 L/min. Consider the following analogy: normal individuals excrete 40 mmol of NH_4^+ per day but can increase this excretion to 200 mmol/day with chronic metabolic acidosis. If, during chronic metabolic acidosis, the kidneys excrete only 30 mmol of NH_4^+ per day, a loss of more than 80% of the capacity to excrete NH_4^+ has occurred.

Because a rise in $Paco_2$ should stimulate alveolar ventilation, the authors suggest that in our analogy the entire capacity for enhanced alveolar ventilation has been inhibited. If the expected alveolar ventilation was as high as possible (80 L/min; see margin note and Table 5.1), the percent decline in potential alveolar ventilation was $(160 - 4)$ L/min/160 L/min, or close to 97.5%. Thus, the answer depends on what you think the denominator of the observed vs expected alveolar ventilation should be.

5.4 Why is the venous Pco_2 much higher than the arterial Pco_2 in each of the following: exercise, a convulsion, and diabetic ketoacidosis (DKA)?

Exercise: In essence, because the athlete is hyperventilating, the arterial Pco_2 is not high. The muscle mass, which is actively burning glucose and glycogen, generates CO_2 to meet the need to regenerate ATP. Therefore, the Pco_2 in tissues is high; because this CO_2 must diffuse into venous blood, the Pco_2 remains very high in venous blood.

Convulsion. With a convulsion, there is vigorous muscle activity associated with insufficient O_2 to meet the body's needs. Anaerobic glycolysis ensues and generates L-lactic acid. Burning glucose to L-lactate anions generates ATP and H^+ without consuming O_2. Because H^+ react with HCO_3^-, the production of CO_2 is very high from both aerobic and anaerobic metabolism and results in a high venous Pco_2.

Note
Ventilatory alkalosis (a very low $Paco_2$) and respiratory acidosis (high tissue Pco_2) can occur simultaneously in DKA.

DKA. In DKA, the arterial Pco_2 is low because of the hyperventilation that results from the acidemia. At the tissue level, the flow of blood is very slow because of the contracted ECF volume, so each liter must carry more CO_2. The venous Pco_2 can therefore be very high.

5.5 Why might the rate of production of CO_2 be lower than normal in a patient with DKA?

Patients with ketoacidosis have a lower rate of CO_2 production. Their use of fatty acids as a fuel produces less CO_2/ATP than would the use of proteins or carbohydrates (see Table 5.2). Also, ketogenesis from fatty acids is not a CO_2-producing reaction. In addition, renal and cerebral ATP needs may be markedly reduced (decreased GFR and coma), so the kidneys and the brain may produce much less CO_2 than normal.

Note
Question 5.6 is for the more curious.

5.6 How might peripheral chemoreceptors detect a lower Pao_2?

The detection of Pao_2 is an important function of the carotid body. The authors find the following hypothesis attractive: to detect a lower Pao_2, unique cells in the carotid body have a change in their mitochondria. The last step in the electron transport system (the conversion of O_2 to H_2O) is the rate-limiting step in the regeneration of ATP; it is dependent on the activity of cytochrome oxidase. This enzyme in the carotid body has a unique property: a low affinity for O_2 (in all other cells, this enzyme has a very high affinity for O_2 because it is saturated with O_2 at very low PO_2 values). When the PaO_2 falls below 70 mm Hg or so, cytochrome oxidase in these unique cells is no longer saturated with O_2. As a result, less ATP is regenerated, and Ca^{2+} leak out of their mitochondria and signal a drive to ventilation (see margin note).

Another hypothesis
Cells of the carotid body have a K^+ channel that is regulated by the PO_2. Therefore, a low PO_2 can induce an electrical signal to indicate a low PaO_2.

5.7 Can respiratory alkalosis and respiratory acidosis occur in the same patient at the same time?

On the surface, the obvious answer is no because one cannot have a high and a low PCO_2 at the same time. Nevertheless, when considered in more depth, and defining events at the cellular level, the better answer becomes yes (see Figure 1.9).

Think of ventilation controlling the arterial PCO_2 in a patient with diabetic ketoacidosis who is hyperventilating excessively due to aspiration pneumonitis (respiratory alkalosis is present).

In response to the low ECF volume, the cardiac output is very low. Now the venous PCO_2 is high and therefore the tissue PCO_2 is high, so the patient has respiratory acidosis at the cellular level (respiratory acidosis is present). This is more than a play on words because the emergency therapy to help the ICF composition is rapid reexpansion of the ECF volume.

5.8 A patient has a 0.1 L/min shunt from pulmonary artery to pulmonary vein. Would the A-a difference be different if the cardiac output was 5 vs 2 L/min? (Assume no other abnormality.)

Yes. Because the volume of the shunt is 0.1 L/min, mixing it with 5 L of cardiac output would create a shunt that is 2% by volume. In contrast, with a very low cardiac output of 2 L/min, the same shunt would be 5% by volume. The net effect of the A-a difference would be much larger with the lower cardiac output.

5.9 A patient, comatose from a drug overdose, has the following blood gases. The basis of the hypoxia is thought to be aspiration. Is this diagnosis correct?

pH		7.24	PCO_2	mm Hg	64
H^+	nmol/L	58	PaO_2	mm Hg	66

The PO_2 of inspired air is $(760 - 47)$ mm Hg $\times$ 0.21, or 150 mm Hg, when 47 mm Hg is the water vapor pressure. The alveolar PO_2 is $150 - (1.25 \times 66)$, or 68 mm Hg. The arterial PO_2 is 66 mm Hg; therefore, the A-a difference is 2 mm Hg $(68 - 66)$—a normal value (the A-a difference is low as a result of the sigmoid shape of the oxygen-hemoglobin dissociation curve).

Note
Multiplying by 1.25 is equivalent to dividing by 0.8.

With respect to the acid-base disturbance, the plasma $[HCO_3^-]$ is $24 \times 64/58$, or 26 mmol/L, and the $[H^+]$ is 58 nmol/L; both are expected values for acute respiratory acidosis. Together, acute CO_2

Henderson equation

$$[H^+] = \frac{24}{[HCO_3^-]} \times P_{CO_2}$$

$$58 = \frac{24}{[HCO_3^-]} \times 64$$

$$[HCO_3^-] = 26.5 \text{ mmol/L}$$

Alveolar P_{O_2} = 150 − (24/0.8)
= 150 − 30
= 120 mm Hg
Measured arterial P_{O_2} = 70 mm Hg

Note
Question 5.11 is for the more curious.

retention and hypoxia with a normal A-a difference suggest that the patient has decreased ventilation because of central respiratory suppression from drug overdose. Because intrinsic lung disease is not the problem, it is incorrect to postulate aspiration pneumonitis based on these values.

5.10 Two days later the patient in Question 5.9 is awake but coughing. The following blood gases are obtained. Because the P_{aO_2} has improved, the patient is declared ready for discharge. Is this decision appropriate?

pH		7.60	P_{aCO_2}	mm Hg	24
H^+	nmol/L	25	P_{aO_2}	mm Hg	70

The alveolar P_{O_2} in the second set of blood gases is 150 − 30, or 120 mm Hg. Therefore the A-a difference is 120 − 70, or 50 mm Hg. On this occasion, the patient has a frankly increased A-a difference, which indicates the presence of a disease that impairs O_2 exchange between alveoli and blood. The hypoxia is less evident because of hyperventilation (if the patient had a normal P_{aCO_2} and an A-a difference of 50 mm Hg, the P_{aO_2} would have been 50 mm Hg). Therefore, significant lung disease is now present and its basis must be established. Discharge without a diagnosis is clearly inappropriate.

5.11 When cold-blooded animals live at 37°C, their P_{aCO_2} is close to 40 mm Hg, and their pH is close to 7.4. At colder temperatures, their pH rises, and their $[HCO_3^-]$ in plasma remains constant. What might these values imply for regulation of ventilation and pH?

It appears that warm-blooded species behave as if they choose to defend their pH. It is equally valid to say that they defend the net charge on their proteins (governed by pH at a constant pK of the major buffer, the imidazole group on histidines). When the temperature falls, there is a considerable rise in the pK of the imidazole group (with a lower temperature, these groups behave as if they were weaker acids). Hence, to keep the same net charge on imidazole groups at different temperatures, the pH must change; the pH must rise with decreasing strength of acid (higher pK) to keep the same net charge on imidazoles.

Cold-blooded animals do not defend a specific intracellular pH. Rather, they behave as if they choose to defend the same net charge on their proteins by adjusting ventilation (called the *aminostat hypothesis*).

5.12 Three patients all experience an acute increase in P_{aCO_2} to 80 mm Hg. Each has a different $[H^+]$. What is the acid-base status in each case?

Patient	$[H^+]$	pH
A	96 nmol/L	7.02
B	70 nmol/L	7.25
C	50 nmol/L	7.30

The $[HCO_3^-]$ can be calculated in each case from the Henderson equation (see margin note). The $[HCO_3^-]$ for patients A, B, and C are 20, 27, and 38 mmol/L, respectively. Because each patient has acute respiratory acidosis, the authors expect the plasma $[HCO_3^-]$ to increase 2.5 mmol/L in association with the acute doubling of the Pa_{CO_2}.

In fact, patient A has a $[HCO_3^-]$ that is below normal rather than increased; therefore, patient A has metabolic acidosis in addition to the acute respiratory acidosis.

In patient B, the rise in plasma $[HCO_3^-]$ is close to 2.5 mmol/L, so this case could be simple acute respiratory acidosis.

In patient C, the plasma $[HCO_3^-]$ is 38 mmol/L. Thus, patient C has metabolic alkalosis in addition to the acute respiratory acidosis (see Chapter 4).

Alternatively, the expected $[H^+]$ for a patient with an acute increase in blood P_{CO_2} can be calculated from 40 to 80 mm Hg on the basis of the $[H^+]$ equaling the original P_{CO_2} plus ($0.8 \times$ the rise in Pa_{CO_2}). The expected $[H^+]$ is 40 + 32, or 72 nmol/L, and the $[HCO_3^-]$ is $24 \times 80/72$, or 27 mmol/L—virtually identical to the values in patient B. Thus, patient B indeed has blood gas values compatible with acute respiratory acidosis. Both approaches are consistent.

5.13 A patient with chronic stable obstructive lung disease (Pa_{CO_2} = 60 mm Hg, plasma $[HCO_3^-]$ = 31 mmol/L) developed shortness of breath and was admitted with a diagnosis of congestive heart failure. During treatment with diuretics and O_2, he vomited a few times, but his chest x-ray film showed improvement. The following blood gases were obtained after therapy: $[H^+]$ = 38 nmol/L, Pa_{CO_2} = 80 mm Hg, Pa_{O_2} = 70 mm Hg. What is the basis of the increased CO_2 retention? What therapy would be appropriate?

The patient's chronic steady-state $[H^+]$ is $24 \times 60/30$, or 46 nmol/L, which is appropriate for chronic respiratory acidosis (rise in $[H^+]$ = 6 nmol/L = 0.3×20). In response to therapy, his Pa_{CO_2} has risen, but his $[H^+]$ has fallen to 38 nmol/L, and the $[HCO_3^-]$ is thus $24 \times 80/38$, or 50 mmol/L. This $[HCO_3^-]$ is much higher than it should be for chronic respiratory acidosis. Thus, the patient has a mixed disorder: chronic respiratory acidosis and metabolic alkalosis. The patient has developed metabolic alkalosis subsequent to the diuretic therapy and vomiting. This alkalosis has resulted in some suppression of ventilation. If his previous A-a difference were known, one could ensure that it had not changed and therefore be more certain that all of his CO_2 retention was due to the alkalosis and none was subsequent to aspiration. The O_2 administration has allowed hypoventilation to occur without increasing hypoxia (hypoxia might have provided an additional stimulus to ventilate).

The goal of therapy is to correct the metabolic alkalosis. The patient will require KCl therapy and a careful assessment of his ECF volume. If the diuretic therapy has been excessive and the patient has developed ECF volume contraction, he will require NaCl therapy; one must be cautious in view of the recent congestive heart failure.

Henderson equation

$$[H^+] = \frac{24}{[HCO_3^-]} \times P_{CO_2}$$

$\text{nmol/L} \qquad \text{mmol/L} \qquad \text{mm Hg}$

Hemoptysis
Coughing up blood.

Henderson equation

$$[H^+] = \frac{24}{[HCO_3^-]} \times P_{CO_2}$$

$$40 = \frac{24}{[HCO_3^-]} \times 25$$

$$[HCO_3^-] = 15 \text{ mmol/L}$$

5.14 A 30-year-old businessman had just returned from Europe when he suddenly developed a severe left-sided pleuritic chest pain and hemoptysis. He had no history of chest disease and exercised regularly. He was cyanotic, he had an elevated jugular venous pressure (8 cm above the sternal angle), and his blood pressure was 80/50 mm Hg. The blood gases were [H+] = 40 nmol/L (pH 7.40), P_{aCO_2} = 25 mm Hg, and P_{aO_2} = 50 mm Hg. What is the most likely diagnosis?

From the patient's history, there was no obvious chronic stimulus for hyperventilation, so he probably had acute respiratory alkalosis. The plasma [HCO_3^-] was 15 mmol/L (see margin note). Therefore, if the patient had acute respiratory alkalosis with a P_{aCO_2} of 25 mm Hg, his plasma [H^+] should have been 28 nmol/L (40 − [0.8 × 15]), not 40 nmol/L. His higher plasma [H^+] and lower plasma [HCO_3^-] indicate that he had metabolic acidosis (L-lactic acidosis caused by low oxygen delivery to tissues). Thus, the combination of respiratory alkalosis and metabolic acidosis resulted in a normal plasma [H^+]. The L-lactic acidosis would be substantiated by finding an increased anion gap in plasma.

This patient's history and physical findings strongly suggest a pulmonary embolism, with severe hemodynamic compromise (right-sided heart failure). His blood gases demonstrate hyperventilation and hypoxia and indicate a wide A-a difference (50 mm Hg); these findings are also in keeping with a large shunt resulting from pulmonary embolism.

5.15 A patient with cirrhosis of the liver was found in a confused state by his landlady. His physical examination results were normal except for a low blood pressure and the stigmata of chronic liver disease. His laboratory results were as follows:

Na$^+$	mmol/L	133	H$^+$	nmol/L	36	pH 7.44
K$^+$	mmol/L	3.3	P_{aCO_2}	mm Hg	20	
Cl$^-$	mmol/L	115	HCO$_3^-$	mmol/L	13	

The initial diagnosis was L-lactic acidosis secondary to severe hepatic insufficiency. Is this diagnosis appropriate? If not, why, and what is the most likely diagnosis?

Although the low [HCO_3^-] might initially suggest the presence of L-lactic acidosis, the anion gap is only 5 mEq/L. If this were L-lactic acidosis, the anion gap would be increased by 10 mEq/L, so the diagnosis is not correct.

Chronic liver disease is associated with chronic respiratory alkalosis. In chronic respiratory alkalosis, for every mm Hg decrease in P_{aCO_2}, one should see a 0.2 nmol/L decrease in plasma [H^+]. In this case, the plasma [H^+] would be 40 nmol/L − (0.2 × 20), or 36 nmol/L. Therefore, this patient's acid-base status is consistent with chronic respiratory alkalosis. The reason for the low plasma anion gap may be hypoalbuminemia.

Sodium and Water

6

Sodium and Water Physiology

- Concepts in Sodium and Water Physiology
  1. Water moves to osmotic equilibrium across cell membranes. Because Na^+ are restricted primarily to the ECF, the content of Na^+ determines the ECF volume.
  2. An ultrafiltrate moves between the vascular and interstitial spaces. This movement is controlled by the hydrostatic pressure and colloid osmotic pressure (largely due to albumin).
  3. The body regulates the content of Na^+ and H_2O in an independent fashion.
  4. Water balance is the result of the interplay of thirst and renal actions of ADH.
  5. The kidney controls the content of Na^+ in the body. Changes in "effective" circulating volume lead to the retention or excretion of Na^+.

"Effective" osmolality (tonicity)
Osmolality refers to the number of particles dissolved in water. Water moves across cell membranes to ensure equal osmolalities in the ECF and ICF. Some particles determine the volume in a single compartment because they are restricted to that compartment (e.g., Na^+ in the ECF); these particles are called "effective osmoles." Other particles exist at equal concentrations in both the ECF and the ICF and do not influence water movement (e.g., urea); these particles are called "ineffective osmoles." A term used to describe the concentration of effective osmoles is "tonicity."

ECF volume
The volume of water held outside cells by the osmotic force created by Na^+ and its attendant anions Cl^- and HCO_3^-.

Ultrafiltrate
All the small constituents of plasma (water and solutes) that readily cross the capillary membrane (larger proteins do not readily cross the capillary membrane).

Albumin
The protein in plasma that is the principal determinant of colloid osmotic pressure.

OBJECTIVES

☐ To explain the forces that regulate the movement of water across cell membranes:
Water moves across cell membranes in response to a change in *"effective" osmolality;* only those particles that are restricted to the extracellular fluid (ECF) or the intracellular fluid (ICF) determine these volumes. Because there are twice as many particles in the ICF (primarily K^+ salts of macromolecular anions) as in the ECF (primarily Na^+ salts), the *ICF volume* is twofold larger than the *ECF volume.*

☐ To explain the distribution of the ECF volume:
The content of Na^+ determines the ECF volume, for the most part.
The major factor promoting the movement of *ultrafiltrate* from the intravascular to the interstitial space is the capillary hydrostatic pressure. The colloid osmotic pressure (largely the result of *albumin*) and lymphatic flow cause the ultrafiltrate to reenter the intravascular volume.
The most important principle concerning Na^+ and water in the body is that control of the "effective" ECF volume takes precedence over the control of water balance (i.e., the body "hates" shock).

☐ To explain the regulation of water balance:
Water intake is stimulated primarily by a high effective plasma osmolality and to a lesser degree by a fall in ECF volume. Notwithstanding, a positive stimulus of a low ECF volume will lead to thirst and the release of antidiuretic hormone (ADH) even if the "effective" osmolality is low.
The renal excretion of water depends for the most part on the level of ADH: a high level diminishes the excretion of pure water, and a low level of ADH enhances its excretion.

☐ To explain the relationship between Na⁺ balance and control of the ECF volume:

Na⁺ intake is stimulated by a low effective ECF volume, but this stimulus is weak.

Control over the excretion of Na⁺ is the primary means of defending the ECF volume. The signal is the "effective" circulating volume, and control is exerted by a number of factors (hormones, neuronal activity) that influence the quantity of Na⁺ reabsorbed by the nephron.

Outline of Major Principles

1. Consider Na⁺ and water separately because they are regulated independently.

2. The principal particle retained in the ECF is Na⁺. The **content** of Na⁺ in the ECF determines the ECF volume. The concentration of albumin and, to a lesser extent, its valence determine the movement of fluid from the interstitial to the intravascular space. Many hormones, renal nerves, and hemodynamic factors act in concert to regulate Na⁺ balance and thereby the ECF volume.

3. The **concentration** of Na⁺ in the ECF reflects the *tonicity* of body fluids and thus the ICF volume because there is little change in the number of particles in the ICF of most cells; *hyponatremia* implies swollen cells and *hypernatremia* reflects shrunken cells. The [Na⁺] in plasma does not indicate whether the ECF volume is normal, high, or low.

4. Thirst and release of ADH are stimulated by shrunken cells and by ECF volume contraction. ADH is the major hormone controlling the excretion of water.

Clinical pearl
Note the different implications of the content and the concentration of Na⁺.

Hyponatremia
A decreased [Na⁺] in plasma (<136 mmol/L) can be due to Na⁺ loss or water gain. The most important defense that guards against hyponatremia is the renal excretion of electrolyte-free water.

Hypernatremia
An elevated [Na⁺] in plasma (>144 mmol/L) can be due to Na⁺ gain or water loss. The most important defense that guards against hypernatremia is thirst.

INTRODUCTORY CASE
Lee Is Sweet and Not Salty
(Case discussed on page 256)

Lee, the patient with diabetes mellitus in poor control, returns (see pages 4, 50, 75). She complains of excessive urination and thirst. The points to focus on with respect to Na⁺ and water pathophysiology are as follows:

1. Her ECF volume is contracted;

2. She has hyponatremia (126 mmol/L) and hyperglycemia (50 mmol/L, 900 mg/dL);

3. Her urine has a high [Na⁺] (46 mmol/L, [K⁺] is 20 mmol/L; see margin note), given her ECF volume contraction (see margin note); the urine osmolality is 525 mOsm/kg H₂O, and the flow rate is 3 mL/min.

Why is her ECF volume contracted?
How did her physician know?
Why is she hyponatremic, given the composition of her urine?
What stimulated her thirst?
Why is her urine volume so high?

Note
When the ECF volume is contracted, the "expected" renal response is the excretion of as small a quantity of Na⁺ as possible.

P A R T   A

Composition of Body Fluids

Concept

1. Water moves to osmotic equilibrium across cell membranes. Because Na$^+$ are restricted primarily to the ECF, the content of Na$^+$ determines the ECF volume.

- Water is 60% of body mass; two-thirds of body water is located in the ICF and one-third in the ECF.
- As the proportion of muscle to body weight declines, the percentage of water declines as well (muscle usually contains 50% of body water).

Notes for the expert

- The volume of the ICF is usually considered to be twice that of the ECF, but the data to support this claim are not clear. It is equally possible that just over half of body water (55%) is intracellular, and 45% is extracellular.

- The ECF volume cannot be predicted apriori from the change in [Na$^+$] in plasma (see text).
- During pregnancy, plasma osmolality is reduced by 10 mOsm/kg H$_2$O and [Na$^+$] by 5 mmol/L, on average. This reduction seems to be associated with a resetting of the "osmostat."

The most abundant constituent of the body is water (see margin note); it accounts for approximately 60% of the body mass (Tables 6.1 and 6.2). This water is divided into two main compartments, ECF and ICF (Figure 6.1). In relating total body water to body weight, the assumption has been made that the relative proportion of fat is constant. Obviously, this assumption is not true, as judged from a simple inspection of people in a shopping center. Therefore, a correction must be made for body composition because neutral fat does not dissolve in water. Females tend to have a lower water content per body mass (50% body weight vs 60% for males). Older people also tend to have a relatively smaller water content because of their relatively small proportion of muscle mass. Infants, however, store less adipose tissue and therefore have a higher proportion of water (70%).

TABLE 6.1 **Composition of the Body**

Values are approximations for a 70-kg person. The amount of water present depends on the mass of adipose tissue. There is a large percentage of water in infants (70%) and smaller in obese people, in females, and in the elderly, largely because of a lower proportion of muscle vs adipose tissue.

	Water (L)	Protein (kg)	Na$^+$ (mmol)	K$^+$ (mmol)
Total body	45	6	2550	4560
ECF	15	0.3	2250	60
ICF	30	5.7	300	4500

TABLE 6.2 **Composition of the ECF**

Values are approximations in a 70-kg adult.

Compartment	Water (L)	Other Constituents
Total ECF	15	• Contains 230 g of albumin and 2250 mmol of Na$^+$
Interstitial volume	12	• Contains one-fourth of the concentration of albumin in plasma, close to 50% of total albumin
Plasma volume	3	• Contains 120 g of albumin; exists with 2 L of red blood cells in blood volume

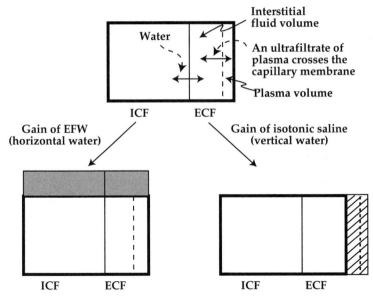

Figure 6.1   Body fluid compartments. The normal distribution of the ECF and ICF is shown in the top rectangle. Note that an ultrafiltrate of plasma moves across the capillary membrane, and water moves across cell membranes. During hypernatremia, the ICF volume is contracted; the converse occurs during hyponatremia. When there is a *gain of electrolyte-free water* (bottom left), this water distributes in the ICF and ECF in proportion to their existing volumes (depicted by the horizontal rectangle above the normal compartment sizes). This water expands both volumes, and therefore it leads to hyponatremia and an increased ICF volume. In contrast, when there is a *gain of isotonic saline,* only the ECF volume expands (bottom right); this is depicted by the vertical, hatched rectangle. There is no change in the plasma [Na⁺] or the ICF volume.

The ECF consists of plasma fluid (4% body weight) and interstitial fluid (i.e., water in tissues between the cells, 16% body weight). Water in the abdominal cavity *(ascites)* or thoracic cavity *(pleural effusion)* is a component of the interstitial space. In certain disease states, fluid accumulates in the interstitial space of the ECF to an appreciable degree and is called *edema,* ascites, or pleural effusion.

Composition of Fluid in Compartments

> - Particles restricted to a compartment determine its volume.
>   1. Na^+ (and Cl^- plus HCO_3^-) determine ECF volume.
>   2. K^+ (held in cells by large *macromolecular* anions) largely determine the ICF volume.

Water crosses cell membranes rapidly (through pores or channels) to achieve osmotic equilibrium; however, not all materials dissolved in water disperse equally in the ICF and ECF because there are differences in permeability, transporters, and active pumps that regulate their distribution (Table 6.3).

Ascites
Accumulation of an ultrafiltrate of plasma plus some albumin in the abdominal cavity.

Pleural effusion
Accumulation of an ultrafiltrate of plasma with or without albumin in the pleural cavity.

Edema
Accumulation of an ultrafiltrate of plasma in the interstitial space (usually the dependent area via gravity).

Macromolecular
Referring to a compound that has many charged groups (phosphate in DNA, RNA, etc.) but only a few particles.

TABLE 6.3
(A) Composition of the ECF and ICF

The data are expressed as mmol/kg of water (approximate values of ICF of skeletal muscle).

	ECF	ICF
Na^+	141	10
K^+	4.1	120–150
Cl^-	113	3
HCO_3^-	26	10
Phosphate	2.0	140 (organic phosphates)

(B) Distribution and composition of the ICF

Values are approximations for a 70-kg adult.

	Water (L)	K^+ mmol	Na^+ mmol
Muscle	22	3300	220
Brain, liver, and kidneys	2.5	375	25
Other	5.5	825	55
Total	30	4500	300

(C) Size of Various Body Fluid Compartments

Values are reported for a 70-kg normal male. The authors arbitrarily selected ECF and ICF volumes of 15 and 30 L respectively.

Compartment	% Body Weight	Volume (L)
Body	60	45
ICF	40	30
ECF	20	15
Interstitial	16	12
Plasma	4	3
Blood	7	5

Distribution of Water Across Cell Membranes

- Water (without Na^+) crosses cell membranes until the osmolality (particle/H_2O ratio) is equal on both sides of that membrane.
- Tonicity ("effective" osmolality) = total osmolality − (urea + alcohol, both in mmol/L).
- The total number of particles in the ICF in most cells rarely changes, but changes do occur in brain cells during chronic shrinking or swelling.
- Bottom line: the *content* of Na^+ determines the ECF volume, and the *concentration* of Na^+ ([Na^+]) in the ECF reflects the ICF volume.

[Na^+]
The ratio of Na^+ to water reflects the ICF volume; conceptually, it is the only time that the denominator of a ratio is the most important of the components of that ratio.

Water distribution depends on the number of particles restricted to the ICF or to the ECF (Figure 6.2). These particles account for the "effective" osmolality, or tonicity, in these compartments (see

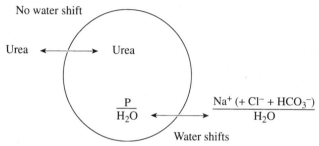

Figure 6.2   Factors regulating water distribution across cell membranes. The circle represents the cell membrane. Water crosses this membrane rapidly to achieve osmotic equilibrium. Particles such as urea (and alcohol) also cross this membrane rapidly, and their concentrations are equal in the ICF and the ECF; hence, they play no role in water distribution. The major particles restricted largely to the ECF are Na^+ and the anions Cl^- plus HCO_3; the particles (P) restricted primarily to the ICF are predominantly the K^+ (salts of organic phosphates).

margin note). The particles restricted to the ECF (which thereby control the ECF volume) are Na^+ and its attendant anions (Cl^- plus HCO_3^-). It is not that Na^+ cannot cross the cell membrane, although permeability of cell membranes to Na^+ is relatively low compared with permeability to K^+); rather, any additional Na^+ that enter the ICF are actively transported out of the cell by the membrane enzyme $Na^+K^+ATPase$. In normal conditions, it is believed that there are roughly twice as many particles in the ICF as in the ECF; it therefore follows that the ICF volume is twice as large as that of the ECF.

The particles that attract water into cells differ from one cell type to another. The major factor responsible for water movement into the cell is the retention of large macromolecular anions (organic phosphates) inside the cell. Although the macromolecules do not exert a large osmotic pressure (there are not a large number of particles), they bear a large anionic net charge and, as a result, have a large number of cations associated with them (primarily K^+) that not only provide electroneutrality but also account for the majority of the osmoles in the ICF (see Table 6.3). Because the ICF macromolecules are largely organic phosphate esters (adenosine triphosphate (ATP), creatine phosphate, RNA, DNA, phospholipids, etc.) and are essential for cell function, only small net changes in their content occur. Thus, it follows that the total number of ICF particles is relatively "fixed" in number and charge; hence, changes in the ratio of particles to water in the ICF usually come about only by a change in the water content of the ICF.

Clinical points
- Particles like urea or alcohol cross cell membranes rapidly so that their concentrations are equal in the ICF and ECF; thus, they do not change the "effective" osmolality or tonicity and do not induce water movement between the ECF and ICF (Figure 6.2). Nevertheless, they do change the osmolality of the ICF and ECF compartments.
- Brain cells are virtually the only ones that regulate their volume by changing the number of intracellular particles.

QUESTION

(Discussion on page 264)

6.1 *How might an osmolality of 285 mOsm/kg H_2O in the ICF be reconciled with a [K^+] in the ICF that is only 150 mmol/L (i.e., what constitutes the osmolality of 285 mOsm/kg H_2O in the ICF)?*

Idiogenic osmoles
Some clinicians use this term to describe how certain cells of the brain may defend their ICF volume. The authors do not find this term "attractive" because it is deliberately ambiguous, the particles are not completely identified, the measurements of osmolality are somewhat inexact, and the normal particles that constitute the ICF osmoles are not defined (see the discussion of Question 6.1).

Chronic hypernatremia and hyponatremia
Disorders that are associated with regulation of cerebral cell volume. Rapid corrections (or overcorrection) may be associated with irreversible cell damage (osmotic demyelination; see Chapter 7).

It is not certain whether the concentration of glucose rises in all types of brain cells during hyperglycemia (see Chapter 12 for more discussion).

Note
The Na^+, K^+, ATPase either must have a lower affinity for Na^+ or there must be less active pump units to permit a rise in the $[Na^+]$ in the ICF.

Defense of Cell Volume

The number of particles in the ICF is relatively constant for the majority of cells; however, brain cells can specifically defend against a large water shift by varying the number of their intracellular particles. This defense is advantageous because the brain is contained in a rigid box (the skull); if brain cells were to increase markedly in size, they might occupy too large a space in the skull. The increased pressure would cause herniation and diminished cerebral blood supply. In contrast, diminishing the ICF volume in the brain would shrink the brain, stretch vascular connections to the skull, and ultimately lead to an intracranial hemorrhage. Recall that the large intracellular macromolecular anions are essential compounds and are not expendable; hence, defense of a cell volume occurs only if there are a sufficient number of ions or nonelectrolytes that can be translocated across cell membranes. A "loose" term used for these particles that change in the ICF of the brain is *idiogenic osmoles.*

Regulatory Decrease in Brain Cell Volume

One mechanism used in the controlled return of swollen cells toward their original volume is the extrusion of electrolytes (see margin note). Typically, it involves a decrease in the content of K^+ in the ICF. Cl^- is the major anion to be lost with K^+ if this loss is to shrink the ICF volume. The $[Cl^-]$ in the ICF varies widely between 3 mmol/L in muscle and 70 mmol/L in red blood cells. In addition, the time for this effect varies greatly among species and cell types. Amino acids or small peptides, if present in large enough concentrations, may be extruded from cells as part of the regulatory decrease in volume. Alternatively, it is possible that a decrease in ICF volume could occur without ion extrusion if ions were bound and thus made "osmotically inactive" (see the margin note regarding idiogenic osmoles).

Regulatory Increase in Brain Cell Volume

The mechanism for a gain in ICF volume during hypernatremia also varies among species and cell types. Typically, controlled return of shrunken cells toward their original volume involves an influx of Na^+ (see margin note). In certain cases, the furosemide-sensitive Na^+, K^+, 2 Cl^- cotransporter is involved, but, in others, the amiloride-sensitive Na^+/H^+ antiporter works with the Cl^-/HCO_3^- antiporter. It is also possible to change the number of organic compounds (e.g., amino acids or taurine, among others).

Distribution of an Ultrafiltrate Across Capillary Membranes

- Movement of an ultrafiltrate of plasma across capillary membranes does not cause water to shift between the ECF and ICF.
- Hydrostatic pressure is the major force moving fluid out of the capillary lumen, and the colloid osmotic pressure (COP) (largely the result of albumin) is the major force moving fluid into the capillary lumen.

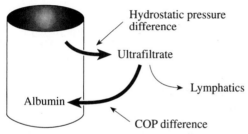

Figure 6.3   Review of factors controlling distribution of ultrafiltrate across the capillary membrane. There are two major forces to consider: a higher hydrostatic pressure causes fluid to leave the vascular space, and the colloid osmotic pressure (COP) causes fluid to enter the vascular space. Because the interstitial fluid volume is so much larger than the vascular volume, any time expansion (edema) of the interstitial space is detected, the patient will always have ECF volume expansion, even if the vascular volume is reduced (i.e., chronic hypoalbuminemia).

The factors controlling ultrafiltrate movement across the capillary membrane are shown in Figure 6.3; the major outward driving force is the hydrostatic pressure difference. When this pressure difference increases, more ultrafiltrate exits. The hydrostatic pressure at the venous end of the capillary increases with venous hypertension (e.g., with venous obstruction, congestive heart failure).

The major inward (interstitial to vascular) flow of fluid is driven by the COP difference, which is ultimately due to the higher concentration of albumin in the vascular fluid as compared with that in interstitial fluid. Interstitial fluid is also returned to the venous system via the lymphatics.

Because not all capillary pores are smaller than the diameter of plasma proteins, albumin leaks into the interstitial space. The concentration of albumin in the interstitial space is close to 10 g/L, and it exerts a COP of close to 5 mm Hg. Interestingly, the content of albumin in the interstitial space (10 g/L $\times$ 12 L) is equal to that in vascular volume (40 g/L $\times$ 3 L).

Donnan Equilibrium

In the Donnan equilibrium, there is a difference in the concentrations of impermeant ions (largely anionic albumin) located in the vascular and interstitial compartments. The negative net charge on albumin causes ions to redistribute between the vascular and interstitial spaces. Albumin attracts cations (largely Na^+) into the vascular compartment and repels anions (largely Cl^- plus HCO_3^-) out. Because the $[Na^+]$ exceeds the $[Cl^- + HCO_3^-]$, the vascular space ultimately has a larger number of ionic species due to the Donnan effect (Figure 6.4). Although small in number relative to the plasma $[Na^+ + Cl^- + HCO_3^-]$ (0.2 mmol/L vs 280 mmol/L), the difference in ion concentrations is large relative to the concentration of albumin in plasma (0.6 mmol/L).

Concept

2. An ultrafiltrate moves between the vascular and interstitial spaces. This movement is controlled by the hydrostatic pressure and colloid osmotic pressure (due largely to albumin).

Colloid osmotic pressure (COP)
This force is due principally to the concentration of albumin in plasma; however, the quantitative relationships are interesting. The total COP is 25 mm Hg, 19 mm of which is due to dissolved protein and 6 mm of which is due to attracted Na^+ (the Donnan effect). The other plasma proteins account for 50% of the weight of proteins, but only 25% of the COP.

- In edematous states resulting from a low COP, one may increase the tissue hydrostatic pressure with support stockings and thereby diminish the degree of edema.

CASE 6.1
Donnie Is All Charged Up
(Case discussed on page 257)

Donnie, age 62 years, has three long-term medical problems— hypertension (high blood pressure), a congenital malformation in

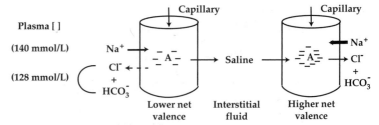

Figure 6.4 Valence of albumin and the Donnan distribution. The barrel-shaped structure is a capillary. On the left, plasma proteins (A) have a smaller net valence so they "attract" less Na^+ and "repel" less Cl^- and HCO_3^- than usual; the net effect is a lower Donnan force and a lower COP in the vascular space. Hence, the distribution of saline is outward into the interstitial fluid. The converse is true for the figure to the right, in which the net anionic valence of plasma proteins is greater, and the vascular volume increases.

her brain that had led to difficulty emptying her urinary bladder, and a questionable history of diabetes mellitus (her most recent glucose tolerance test result was normal). She stated that she vomited on several occasions and drank regular soft drinks because of thirst.

Physical examination revealed there was only a modest degree of contraction of her ECF volume.

Her laboratory data are summarized as follows:

		Plasma	Urine	Plasma (24h)
Glucose	mg/dL	2016	—	190
	mmol/L	112	300	16
Anion gap	mEq/L	41	2	15
Lactate	mmol/L	3	0	2
β-HB	mmol/L	1	0	1
HCO_3	mmol/L	17	0	22

What would happen to the vascular volume if the charge on her plasma proteins became more anionic?

For defense of the vascular volume, should a greater anionic valence occur when the vascular volume was expanded or contracted?

How would the properties of an anionic charge on albumin differ from that on a similar number of small organic anions like lactate$^-$ in plasma?

What data would help establish that the high value for the anion gap was due to an increased negative valence on plasma proteins?

QUESTIONS

(Discussions on pages 264–266)

6.2 *What intravenous (IV) solution would you give if you wanted all of it to stay in the ECF? What IV solution would you give to expand the ECF volume but contract the ICF volume?*

6.3 *What proportion of a liter of dextrose in water (D_5W) ends up in the ICF once glucose is metabolized?*

6.4 *How can more of this infused water enter cells?*

6.5 *A 70-kg person perspires and loses 4 L of a NaCl solution; the $[Na^+]$ in this fluid is one-half that in the ECF. What changes should occur in ICF and ECF volumes, and what will the resultant $[Na^+]$ be? (For this calculation, assume that the starting $[Na^+]$ is 150 mmol/kg H_2O and that the ECF and ICF volumes are 15 and 30 L, respectively.)*

6.6 *Will exchanging a K^+ in the ICF for a Na^+ in the ECF have a direct effect on the ICF and ECF volumes?*

6.7 *What is the effect of hyperglycemia on a water shift between the ICF and the ECF? For simplicity, assume that no insulin is present and that no excretions occur.*

6.8 *What would happen acutely to the ICF volume if the permeability of capillary membranes to albumin were to increase?*

D_5W

A commonly infused solution that contains 5 g of glucose per 100 mL of water, or 50 g/L. The concentration of glucose is close to isosmolal, or 276 mmol/L.

Water Physiology

PART B

- Defense of tonicity involves thirst and excretion or conservation of *electrolyte-free water* (EFW).
- The controls of tonicity are remarkably sensitive, responding to 1–2% changes.
- Change of tonicity is virtually synonymous with change in the $[Na^+]$ in plasma. An increased tonicity results in thirst and a reduction in EFW excretion. Reduction of tonicity diminishes thirst and increases excretion of *osmole-free* water.

Electrolyte-free water (EFW)

A term used to describe water that is gained into or lost from total body water instead of from either the ECF or ICF. The solution can be electrolyte-free but can have a high osmolality if it contains a considerable amount of urea.

Osmole-free water

A term used to describe water that is excreted without solutes. It is not the best term for describing the influence of urinary excretion on body water distribution; the use of *electrolyte-free water* is better for this purpose).

Overview

Assume a normal subject consumes 1 L of EFW and that this liter mixes with all body fluids. To excrete this liter of EFW, it must be sensed, a message must be sent to the kidney, and then this liter of EFW must be segregated from the electrolytes (Na^+ salts) dissolved in it so that this excess EFW can be excreted.

Pure water per se cannot be excreted by the kidney because there must always be some dissolved particles such as electrolytes and/or urea (the minimum urine osmolality is 20–50 mOsm/kg H_2O).

Mechanisms of Excretion

Sensor

The addition of EFW dilutes body constituents. In the ECF, this dilution is recognized clinically as hyponatremia. In contrast, in the ICF, the important compartment, this dilution is recognized as swelling of cells. The sensor (a cell that is sensitive to its volume) is located in the CNS and is a "tonicity receptor" linked to both the thirst center and the antidiuretic hormone (ADH) release center.

Tonicity receptor
This is called an "osmo-receptor" in most texts. Because this receptor senses changes in cell volume, and because osmolality is also composed of components that do not affect the cell volume such as urea, the authors believe that *tonicity receptor* is a superior term.

Antidiuretic hormone (ADH)
A hormone that the brain synthesizes, stores, and releases. ADH acts on the collecting duct, making it permeable to water.

Concept
3. The body regulates the content of the Na^+ and H_2O in an independent fashion.

Concept
4. Water balance is the result of the interplay of thirst and renal actions of ADH.

Angiotensin II
The vasoconstrictor formed when renin is produced (in response to ECF volume contraction). It also causes aldosterone to be released, more $NaHCO_3$ to be reabsorbed by the proximal tubule, and thirst to be stimulated.
   Renin acts on angiotensinogen from the liver, forming angiotensin I, which is cleaved to angiotensin II by angiotensin-converting enzyme.
1. When assessing a conscious patient with hypernatremia, first ask if the patient is thirsty to evaluate the intake component of water regulation.
2. If the ECF volume is contracted, thirst will be stimulated even if the tonicity of body fluids is low.

Messages

Swelling of *tonicity-receptor* cells sends a message to the thirst center to diminish water intake and to the kidneys to excrete as much osmole-free water as possible. The message to the kidneys is the absence of *ADH*. With a surplus of water, there is little if any release of ADH, and its level in plasma declines markedly and rapidly.

Renal Events

In the kidney, saline is filtered, and some Na^+ and Cl^- are reabsorbed without water in the thick ascending limb of the loop of Henle and the distal nephron. The water remaining is excreted because the luminal membrane of the distal nephron has a low permeability to water when there is no action of ADH. The basis for the low permeability for water will be considered later.

Control of Water Intake

Thirst is stimulated by an increased tonicity. Particles like urea are not involved in tonicity and are not sensed by the hypothalamic centers because they have similar concentrations in the ICF and ECF.
   Contraction of the ECF volume is also a weak stimulus to thirst. In this regard, elevated levels of *angiotensin II* might operate as a signal. Other factors unrelated to a need for water may also stimulate water intake (e.g., dryness of the mouth, habit, culture, psyche, etc.). The major inhibitors of thirst are hypotonicity and ECF volume expansion.

Control of Water Excretion

Excretion of a Dilute Urine

- Excretion of a dilute urine requires three steps:
  1. delivery of Na^+, Cl^-, and water to the diluting sites (delivery);
  2. reabsorption of solutes without water (separation or desalination);
  3. excretion of this electrolyte-free water (maintenance of separation).

   When water is ingested without electrolytes, for balance EFW must be excreted in the urine. There are several nephron sites where Na^+ and Cl^- are reabsorbed but water is not. The most important of these sites is the thick ascending limb of the loop of Henle. Other segments are the early distal convoluted tubule (not sensitive to ADH), the late distal convoluted tubule, and the collecting ducts (the latter require absence of ADH to maintain impermeability to water). To excrete a dilute urine, three processes must occur. They are considered in quantitative terms in Figure 6.5.

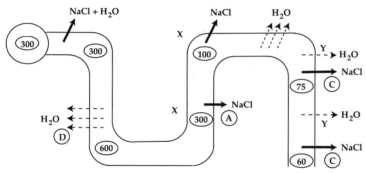

Figure 6.5   The excretion of a dilute urine. A stylized nephron is shown. The numbers in the ovals represent the osmolality of the fluid in the lumen of the specific nephron segments. Isosmolal fluid is reabsorbed in the PCT so that the osmolality remains similar to plasma. EFW is reabsorbed passively from the descending limb of the loop of Henle (D) because it is permeable to water, and the osmolality is higher in the medullary interstitial fluid. This water dilutes the interstitial fluid and raises the osmolality of luminal fluid. The most important active step is the reabsorption of NaCl from the ascending limb of the loop of Henle (A). Part of this NaCl can be thought of as maintaining an unchanged interstitial and luminal fluid osmolality (not directly useful for EFW excretion or conservation). In contrast, it is the additional NaCl that is reabsorbed here that is the physiologically relevant reabsorption because it lowers the osmolality of luminal fluid in the loop of Henle, which is useful for EFW excretion. Because more Na^+ than water may be reabsorbed in the CCD (C), the final urine may be even more hypoosmolal and hypotonic than the fluid delivered from the loop of Henle. The detailed steps in the nephron segments involved are provided in Figure 6.6.

1. **Delivery of saline to the thick ascending limb of the loop of Henle:**
   One-third of the GFR (60 L/day) is delivered to diluting sites of the nephron (i.e., 40 times more than is needed to excrete the usual daily water load of 1.5 liters). Therefore, only a very major reduction in glomerular filtration rate can reduce delivery sufficiently to be the sole cause of a limited excretion of EFW.

2. **Separation of salt and water (reabsorption of NaCl without water):**
   This separation begins in the thick ascending limb of the loop of Henle; there is a net reabsorption of Na^+ and Cl^- without water. This net transport of Na^+ and Cl^- is inhibited by *furosemide,* a diuretic that binds to the luminal Na^+, K^+, 2 Cl^- cotransporter. In the distal convoluted tubule and the collecting ducts, the urine can be diluted further when NaCl is reabsorbed to a greater degree than water; ADH must be absent for this dilution to occur.

3. **Maintenance of separation:**
   The hypotonic fluid that exits from the loop of Henle must not equilibrate with the isosmolar and hyperosmolar fluid surrounding the remainder of the nephron. These membranes must remain relatively water-impermeable; therefore, ADH secretion must cease when osmole-free water is to be excreted (Table 6.4, Figure 6.6).

   It is important to note that ADH can also be released for a variety of reasons unrelated to tonicity of plasma (see Chapter

Furosemide
A loop diuretic that inhibits the reabsorption of Na^+ and Cl^- in the thick ascending limb of the loop of Henle. Because an electrical gradient develops (lumen positive), furosemide also inhibits the reabsorption of Mg^{2+} and Ca^{2+} here (Figure 6.6). For the luminal concentration of furosemide to be high, it must be secreted in the proximal convoluted tubule; in renal insufficiency or with drugs inhibiting proximal secretion, this diuretic is less potent. By inhibiting Na^+ and Cl^- reabsorption in the loop, loop diuretics can compromise the ability to dilute and to concentrate the urine.

TABLE 6.4 **Effect of Water Reabsorption on Volume and Osmolality**

These representative values do not include the reabsorption of isotonic saline. ADH makes the cortical and medullary collecting ducts permeable to water (Figures 6.5, 6.6). The osmolality of the urine rises threefold in the cortex and a further fourfold in the medulla; however, the bulk (67%) of the water is reabsorbed in the cortex so that solutes are not "washed out" in the hypertonic medulla.

Nephron site	Volume exiting (L)	Volume reabsorbed (L)	Osmolality (mOsm/kg H$_2$O)	Rise in osmolality
End—loop of Henle	12	—	100	—
End—cortical collecting duct	4	8	300	Threefold
End—medullary collecting duct	1	3	1200	Fourfold

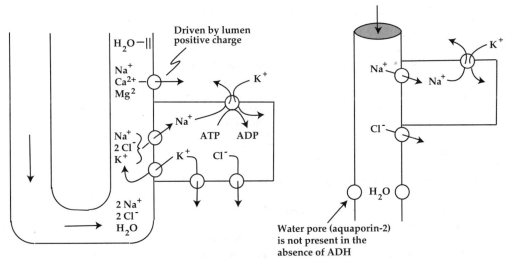

Figure 6.6   Formation of a dilute urine; events in the medulla. The events in the thick ascending limb of the loop of Henle are shown on the left, and events in the CCD are shown on the right. At the molecular level, note the importance of two luminal and three basolateral membrane transporters or channels in the loop of Henle. **Luminal:** (i) Electroneutral Na$^+$, K$^+$, 2 Cl$^-$ (NKCC) cotransporter. (ii) A K$^+$ ion channel that is responsible for the entry of a positive charge into the lumen. This positive charge "pushes" Na$^+$, Ca^{2+}, and Mg^{2+} between cells in the thick ascending limb of the loop of Henle. **Basolateral:** (i) Na$^+$, K$^+$, ATPase. This is responsible for creating a low [Na$^+$] in the ICF, the driving force for the reabsorption of NaCl by the NKCC contransporter. (ii) Cl$^-$ ion channel. (iii) K$^+$ ion channel. These latter two channels permit all the ion fluxes to occur. In the excretion of a dilute urine, there is little secretion of ADH so aquaporin-2 water channels are not inserted into the luminal membranes of the late distal nephron (see right-hand portion of the figure).

7, pages 298–299, for more discussion). Thus, a hyperosmolar urine can be excreted during a hypoosmolar state, even though one would expect a dilute urine.

Bottom Lines:
- To assess medullary hyperosmolality, measure urine osmolality after ADH acts. The expected value is 1200 mOsm/kg H_2O.
- To assess ADH action, you must know the medullary osmolality.
- To assess whether a given urine will lead to a rise or fall in the plasma $[Na^+]$, examine the $[Na^+] + [K^+]$ in the urine, not the urine osmolality. Compare this sum of electrolyte concentrations with that in plasma (see margin note).

Note
If the K^+ in urine came from the ICF, and Na^+ entered the ICF as K^+ exited, excretion of these K^+ in the urine would represent loss of Na^+ from the ECF.

QUESTIONS

(Discussions on pages 266–268)

6.9 *What mechanisms are responsible for the excretion of more water when furosemide is given?*

6.10 *What can limit the renal excretion of "osmole-free water" in a person who drinks a large amount of water?*

6.11 *The plasma $[Na^+]$ was 160 mmol/L in a patient who was otherwise unaware of the problem. What aspect of the history should catch your attention?*

6.12 *Several days after a car accident, a patient has hypernatremia and a marked degree of ECF volume contraction. Three to four liters of urine is passed each day (osmolality = 420 mOsm/kg H_2O). What is the most likely cause of polyuria?*

6.13 *How would you know that the failure to excrete "osmole-free water" was not due to an inadequate delivery of filtrate to the loop of Henle?*

6.14 *Two normal 70-kg persons excrete the following urine during the same period. Both subjects have 40 L of body water before the urine losses. If neither has any fluid intake, who will have the greater fall in plasma $[Na^+]$ in this period?*

	Volume (L)	$[Na^+]$ mmol/L	$[K^+]$ mmol/L	$[Na^+ + K^+]$ mmol/L
A	1	210	90	300
B	4	140	45	185

Excretion of Concentrated Urine

- ADH is required for excretion of a concentrated urine.

In the absence of water intake, the tonicity of body fluids rises because there is ongoing water loss via the skin, respiratory system, and gastrointestinal tract. This rise in tonicity leads to cell shrinkage

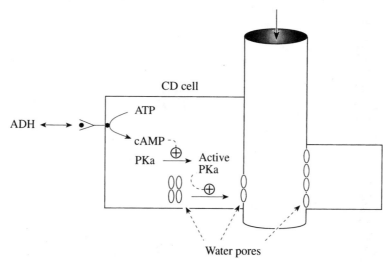

Figure 6.7 ADH actions on the distal nephron. The binding of ADH to its V_2 receptor on the basolateral membrane leads to activation of adenylate cyclase in these cells and thereby to a rise in cyclic AMP (cAMP). The next step in the cascade is to activate a cAMP-dependent protein kinase (PKa = protein kinase a) and phosphorylate intracellular elements favoring the insertion of open water pores (called aquaporin-2) into the luminal membrane (open circles). In the medullary collecting duct, ADH also leads to the insertion of a pore that permits urea to diffuse across the luminal membrane (not shown).

V_2 Receptor

There are two ADH receptors: V_1 receptors are vascular and lead to an increase in blood pressure in response to ADH (vasopressin); V_2 receptors are in the distal nephron and lead to increased permeability for water and urea.

and thereby stimulates the release of ADH from the posterior pituitary gland. Binding of ADH to V_2 *receptors* on the basolateral membrane of late distal convoluted tubular cells, as well as on cells of the cortical and medullary collecting duct, results in the formation of cyclic AMP (cAMP), which ultimately increases the permeability of the collecting duct to water by the insertion of aquaporin-2 water channels (AQP-2) into the luminal membrane (Figure 6.7). Therefore, water is reabsorbed passively down an osmotic difference from the collecting duct lumen to the hyperosmolar renal medullary interstitium; as a result, a hyperosmolal urine is excreted, and osmole-free water is conserved.

Molecular Advances

- Regulation of the permeability of water in the kidney is by the hormone ADH, which causes AQP-2 (active water channels) to be inserted into the luminal membrane of the distal nephron.

Dysnatremia

An abnormal value for the plasma $[Na^+]$.

There have been a number of advances at the molecular level that have clarified understanding of the basis for *dysnatremias*. Water does not cross a lipid barrier readily by simple diffusion. A special pathway, called a channel or a pore, is needed in a lipid membrane through which water can move (Table 6.5). In the distal nephron, AQP-2 is the important water channel; it is active in the luminal membrane of the late distal nephron when ADH acts. The driving force for water movement is a difference in "effective" osmolality (i.e., tonicity) across that membrane—water moves from the less concentrated (lower tonicity) to the more concentrated (higher tonicity) solution.

TABLE 6.5 **Channels Influenced by ADH in the Nephron**

The water channels are called aquaporins (AQP). The urea transporters are either responsive to vasopressin (VRUT) or not (UT).

I. Water Channels	Most Important Location	Regulation by ADH
AQP-1 (also called CHIP-28)	Many cells; e.g., proximal convoluted tubular cells	None
AQP-2	Luminal or vesicle membranes of late distal nephron cells	Activated, inserted, and synthesis increased
AQP-3	Basolateral membrane of late distal nephron cells	None
AQP-4	Basolateral membrane of late distal nephron cells	None
II. Urea Transporters		
UT	Permit urea to cross cell membranes of the descending thin limb of the LOH (DTL) and the descending vasa recta	None
VRUT	Luminal membrane of late IMCD cells. Descending limb loop of Henle of short loop nephrons	Active if ADH

Activation of AQP-2 Channels. When ADH binds to the basolateral aspect of late distal nephron cells, cAMP is formed and, as a result, protein kinase A is activated. This leads to phosphorylation of AQP-2 (more insertion of AQP-2 and/or more active transporters in the luminal membrane), and the transport of water is enhanced. AQP-2 is located in vesicles in the cytosol. When ADH acts on the kidney (see Figure 6.7), these vesicles ultimately fuse to the cell membrane, and this results in more AQP-2 channels to permit water movement down the activity difference for water.

Diseases in Which AQP-2 is Not Inserted Properly in the Luminal Membrane of the MCD. There are a number of disorders characterized by too few AQP-2 channels in the terminal distal nephron membranes.

• Lack of ADH
Obviously, if ADH is needed to insert AQP-2 in the luminal membrane, a lack of ADH (central DI) will cause too few of them to reside in the luminal membrane of the late distal nephron. The disorder is reversed by giving ADH or a compound that mimics the V_2 receptor activity of ADH (e.g., DDAVP). ADH can also be destroyed by a protease in the circulation (called a vasopressinase).

• ADH Does Not Act Properly
ADH activates its receptor on the blood side of distal nephron cells. If there is a failure of ADH to bind to its receptor, activate the protein kinase and insert active water channels into the luminal membrane; if something else removes or inactivates these water channels, the disease process is called nephrogenic DI.

DI = Diabetes insipidus

Vasopressinase
Whereas vasopressinase destroys ADH, it does not remove DDAVP.

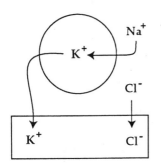

Renal impact on body tonicity
To analyze the impact of a given urine excretion on body tonicity, ignore the urine osmolality and consider only the osmoles critical for water distribution across cell membranes—Na^+ and possibly K^+ (plus accompanying anions)—and the water itself.

Clinical note
High vasa recta flow rates (renal vasodilation), lack of ADH, and inhibition of the NKCC cotransporter all compromise the ability to generate a hyperosmolal outer medullary interstitium. In addition, diseases involving this area also limit the ability to excrete a concentrated urine.

Components Required for a Concentrated Urine

> • Urine osmolality = medullary function plus ADH action.
> • Urine $[Na^+] + [K^+]$ = *renal impact on body tonicity.*

The following processes generate a hyperosmolal medullary interstitium. Two areas are considered separately because they carry out two different functions.

1. Outer Medulla

(a) Process
Single effect. To excrete a concentrated urine, there must be a hyperosmolal medullary interstitium (up to 800 mOsm/kg H_2O in humans). This hyperosmolality is the result of a "single effect"—the active transport of NaCl in the loop of Henle (via the NKCC cotransporter—see Figure 6.6). Flow along the nephron as one proceeds deeper into the medulla permits a progressive rise in absolute osmolality (see discussion of Question 6.15).

Selective Permeabilities. Different permeabilities of the descending and ascending limbs of the loop of Henle help generate a very hyperosmolal medullary interstitium in the outer medulla. The descending limb is permeable to water and somewhat permeable to Na^+. Hence, its luminal $[Na^+]$ and osmolality rise while the interstitial fluid osmolality declines (Figure 6.8).

In contrast, the ascending limb is not permeable to water. Active reabsorption of NaCl adds solute to the interstitial fluid and leads to an overall decline in osmolality of luminal fluid in the loop of Henle (see Figure 6.8; see margin note); this is useful for EFW excretion and/or conservation (see Figure 6.5).

The vasa recta act as a countercurrent exchanger to preserve this hyperosmolality (see discussion of Question 6.15).

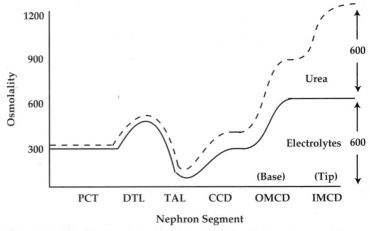

Figure 6.8   Osmolality throughout the nephron during maximum water conservation. The dashed line represents values for total osmolality in the lumen in each of the nephron segments; the solid line represents values for the osmolality due to electrolytes. The distance between the solid and dashed lines represents the contribution of urea.

(b) Function

By having a high interstitial osmolality, EFW can be reabsorbed from the medullary collecting duct (MCD), and this results in EFW conservation (see margin note). A second function of reabsorption of water from the MCD is to raise the concentration of urea in its lumen. Raising this urea concentration is essential for the function of the inner medulla.

2. Inner Medulla

This is a site where the interstitial osmolality rises further. The function of this rise in osmolality and the compounds responsible for it are different than in the outer medulla. The physiology is explored in more depth in the appendix to this chapter.

(a) Process

The osmolality due to electrolytes is close to 600 mOsm/kg H_2O at both the base and the tip of the inner medullary interstitial fluid (see Figure 6.8). In contrast, the concentration of urea is much lower at the junction between the inner and outer medulla (200 mmol/L) than at the tip of the inner medulla (600 mmol/L).

Bottom Line. The major effect of events in the inner medulla is to raise the concentration of urea from the inner medulla's base to its tip.

(b) Function of the Inner Medulla

It is sometimes necessary to excrete a large amount of urea, but to avoid a large volume of urine. At this time, the function of the inner medulla is to permit the inner medullary collecting duct (IMCD) to have a high concentration of urea without having that urea obligate the excretion of water. Because urea is permeable and achieves a nearly equal concentration on both sides of this nephron segment, this means that a considerable amount of urea can be excreted as a "passenger" in the urine (not obligating water to stay in the lumen—Figure 6.9).

Unique Aspects of Blood Vessels in the Inner Medulla. The vessels function as countercurrent exchangers as in the outer me-

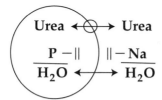

Urea ←⊗→ Urea

$\dfrac{P-\|}{H_2O}$ ← ⊗ → $\dfrac{\|-Na}{H_2O}$

Figure 6.9 Urea and fluid movement in the IMCD. First consider the circle as a cell membrane. Because urea crosses this cell membrane fast enough to have an equal concentration in the ECF and ICF, urea does not obligate water movement. Now consider the circle as the IMCD and its center as the lumen. Because ADH makes urea a permeable compound here, think in non–urea osmolality terms to determine the distribution of water here. In other words, when ADH acts in the IMCD, permeability for urea rises, making the concentration of urea similar in its lumen and the inner medullary interstitial fluid. This means that urea will not have a direct influence on the movement of water here (i.e., excrete a more concentrated urine; there will be a higher concentration of urea but the same amount of EFW).

More information
Most Na⁺ reabsorption occurs in the medullary thick ascending limb of the loop of Henle.
- Adds most NaCl deep in the medulla.
- It is presented with the highest luminal [Na⁺] due to water removal from, and Na⁺ addition into, the descending thin limb (DTL).
- Useful to have Na⁺ enter the DTL because this brings NaCl deeper into the medulla.
- Most water is reabsorbed early from the DTL (half by the time the osmolality is 600 mOsm/kg H_2O. See Appendix at end of chapter.)

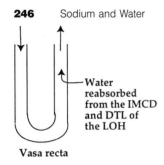

Water reabsorbed from the IMCD and DTL of the LOH

Vasa recta

dulla. The major solute recycled is urea, whereas Na$^+$ ions were the major solute recycled in the outer medulla.

The main reason solutes are removed from the inner medulla is that the volume of fluid in the ascending limbs of vasa recta is larger than in its descending limb due to water reabsorbed from the descending thin limb of the loop of Henle and the IMCD. Because there are no lymphatics in the inner medulla, all fluid reabsorbed from the nephron here returns to the body via the ascending vasa recta.

CASE 6.2
Ted Is Truly Number One
(Case discussed on page 258)

Ted, an accountant, is now 24 years old. He is distressed because he must void every 30–60 minutes; he must catheterize his bladder to void, a potentially dangerous situation. This polyuria has been a life-long problem. He excretes 24 L of urine per day.

Ted is thirsty if he does not drink.

Ted has never had a brain injury or defect. No members of his family suffer from a similar problem. He eats a typical Western diet.

Laboratory results reveal normal values for all parameters except for his plasma urea level, which is 2 mmol/L (5 mg/dL); his plasma [Na$^+$] is 139 mmol/L.

How will you confirm that his polyuria is a water diuresis? What is the predicted numerical value for this test?

How would you be sure that his excessive urine output is a renal problem?

What could his lesion be at the molecular level?

What therapy might be of benefit? Organize your answer into two categories: enhance water reabsorption in the distal nephron, or decrease distal delivery of filtrate. Think about his plasma [Na$^+$] of 139 mmol/L.

If you use a natriuretic agent, which one(s) would you choose, and which should you avoid?

QUESTIONS

(Discussions on pages 268–270)

6.15 *Why does a penguin standing on a block of ice not freeze itself or melt that ice?*

6.16 *A patient has a contracted ECF volume and the following values in plasma and urine:*

		Plasma	Urine
[Na$^+$]	mmol/L	130	60
[K$^+$]	mmol/L	5.0	20
Osmolality	mOsm/kg H$_2$O	270	520

Why is hyponatremia present? Is the plasma ADH high, low, or normal in this patient?

6.17 *Patients A and B both start with a plasma [Na$^+$] of 140 mmol/ L. Patient A just excreted 1 L of urine with a [Na$^+$ + K$^+$] of 300 mmol/L and an osmolality of 600 mOsm/kg H$_2$O. Patient B* *just excreted 1 L of urine with the same osmolality of 600 mOsm/kg H₂O, but now the sole urine osmole was urea. Will the plasma [Na⁺] be the same or different in these two patients? What changes do you expect in their ECF volumes?*

Calculation of a Water Deficit or Surplus

In calculating a loss or gain of water, the simplest approach is to obtain quantitative estimates of ECF and ICF volume deficits. Consider this example. The plasma [Na⁺] in a 70-kg patient rose to 160 mmol/L from the normal value of 140 mmol/L because of a loss of water; his ECF volume, however, was normal on physical examination. His normal values were an ICF volume of 30 L and an ECF volume of 15 L.

Calculation of a Change in Water Balance

Change in ICF Volume. The total number of particles in the ICF that affect water movement is 2 (plasma [Na⁺]) × ICF volume (30 L), or 8400 mOsm. The new "effective" osmolality is 320 mOsm/kg H₂O (2 × new plasma [Na⁺] of 160 mmol/L). Dividing 8400 by 320 yields the new ICF volume of 26.25 L, a fall of 3.75 L (see margin note).

Change in ECF Volume. This change is a clinical impression and cannot be calculated (see margin note); it is not directly influenced by the plasma [Na⁺].

Change in Total Body Water. Add the new volumes of the ICF and ECF; this patient needs a positive balance of 3.75 L of water for the ICF; to provide 3.75 L of water for the ICF, 5.6 L of pure water must be retained.

Calculation of a Change in Na⁺ Balance

Change in Content of Na⁺ in the ECF. This calculation is simply the product of the [Na⁺] in plasma and the estimated ECF volume on clinical grounds. One can ignore the Donnan distribution. In a normal 70-kg adult, the ECF volume is 15 L and the plasma [Na⁺] is 140 mmol/L; hence, the ECF contains 2100 mmol of Na⁺. In the preceding example, the ECF now contains 2400 mmol of Na⁺ (15 L × 160 mmol/L). Hence, this patient needs to lose a net of 300 mmol of Na⁺ to achieve a balance for Na⁺.

Note
1. Total effective osmoles in the ICF: 2 (140 mmol/L × 30 L = 8400 mOsm.
2. Assumption: After the water loss, there is no change in number of particles in the ICF.
3. New ICF volume: total osmoles in the ICF divided by osmolality equals new ICF volume.

$$\frac{8400 \text{ mOsm}}{320 \text{ mOsm/kg H}_2\text{O}} = 26.25 \text{ L}$$

$$30 \text{ L} - 26.25 \text{ L} = 3.75 \text{ L}$$

Clinical estimate of ECF volume
Although clinicians attempt to estimate the ECF volume at the bedside, this is at best a very crude approximation.

PART C

Sodium Physiology

- The content of Na⁺ determines the ECF volume because Na⁺ are restricted to the ECF; Na⁺ and the accompanying anions account for more than 90% of the ECF osmoles.
- Control of renal excretion of Na⁺ is the major way to regulate the content of Na⁺ in the body.

Concept
5. The kidney controls the content of Na⁺ in the body. Changes in "effective" circulating volume signal the retention or excretion of Na⁺.

Overview

People on a typical Western diet consume close to 150 mmol of NaCl each day (see margin note). To remain in NaCl balance, 150 mmol of NaCl must be excreted daily. To do so, the extra Na^+ must be sensed, and a message must be sent to the kidney so that this extra NaCl can be excreted with or without water (depending on the independent controls of water balance). Three components are involved: a sensor of the "effective" arterial volume, the messengers to the kidney, and the intrarenal events.

Sensor

When NaCl is retained, the ECF volume expands; the most important component of the ECF is the effective arterial volume. Therefore, it is not surprising that the sensors to detect important changes in the ECF volume are located in the arterial and central venous vessels. Once stimulated by hypervolemia, these sensors send messages to the kidney via renal nerves, circulating messengers, and by direct means (physical factors) to promote the excretion of NaCl, largely by decreasing its reabsorption.

Normal ECF Volume in More Detail

> • The ECF volume is not a constant value in normal physiology.

It is obvious that the ECF volume should not be a simple static value as described for a 70-kg adult (15 L total, with 12 L of interstitial volume and 3 L of plasma volume). For example, people who eat a high-salt diet have a larger ECF volume and maintain this volume (remain in Na^+ balance) as long as NaCl intake is high. The converse applies to a person consuming a low-salt diet.

The ECF Volume in an Elite Athlete

A more dynamic way to think of the ECF volume is to consider an elite athlete who is in training. This athlete retains extra NaCl and water so that the ECF volume will be larger than normal. This larger ECF volume is retained, day in and day out, as long as training persists, even though exercise is performed over less than 10% of the day. A part of this ECF volume is retained in the venous system (in the vascular bed). A lower venous tone permits this blood to remain and not influence hemodynamics at rest. When exercise is anticipated, venoconstriction causes this blood to enter the "effective" vascular volume. Physicians may recognize this condition as *sports anemia;* the runner might recognize it by the weight loss that occurs along with a diuresis several days after exercise stops.

QUESTION

(Discussion on page 270)

6.18 *Sports anemia is puzzling. Assume athletes are perfectly nor-*

Control of Na^+ intake
There is some evidence of stimulation of Na^+ intake when the ECF volume is low (craving salt).

Sports anemia
A lower hematocrit level resulting from a normal red blood cell pool size within an increased plasma volume.

mal (at least from the point of view of their bone marrow and kidneys). Why might sports anemia (low hematocrit level) be tolerated without an apparent erythropoetin-induced drive to synthesize red blood cells to correct the anemia? This differs from the expected response to blood loss, for example, where there is evidence of accelerated synthesis of new red blood cells. Please speculate, because the authors do not know a definitive answer.

Hint
Erythropoietin, the hormone that stimulates the bone marrow to make new red blood cells, is synthesized in the kidneys. The renal site is interesting; erythropoietin is made in the corticomedullary junction, a site with a relatively low amount of oxygen. Consider why this site, for its synthesis, makes sense from an evolutionary perspective.

Messages

Expansion of the "effective" arterial volume sends messages to the kidneys to excrete the extra NaCl (150 mmol in our example) and no more. Part of the message is delivered by renal nerves, part by hemodynamic or physical factors, and part by hormones. Because delivery of this message is such an important factor to regulate, it is not surprising to find many forms of regulation and, indeed, many regulators acting in concert to achieve this task. Only hormones are listed in this section but an example of other possible factors is illustrated in the following case. The major hormones and their sites of action are summarized in Table 6.6. Their more detailed renal actions will be considered after the normal renal physiology of Na^+ handling has been discussed.

TABLE 6.6 **Hormones and Renal Reabsorption of NaCl**

Only the major hormones are presented. Other hormones, such as an ouabain-like factor or dopamine from the CNS, are not included because their physiologic role has yet to be established.

Hormone	Major Stimulus	Major Nephron Site	Major Effect
Angiotensin II or β-adrenergics via renin release	Low ECF volume	Proximal convoluted tubule	Enhanced reabsorption of $NaHCO_3$ and thereby NaCl
Aldosterone	Angiotensin II Hyperkalemia	Cortical distal nephron	Reabsorption of NaCl Secretion of K^+
Atrial natriuretic peptide	Vascular volume expansion	GFR Medullary collecting duct	Increased GFR Reduced reabsorption of NaCl

CASE 6.3
Brain Tumor With an "Assault"
(Case discussed on page 261)

Mary, age 43 years and weighing 50 kg, had a large tumor in her brain. In her steady state, she had a contracted ECF volume and hyponatremia (128 mmol/L). To avoid symptoms of a low ECF volume, she required a very high intake of NaCl (15 g or close to 300 mmol/day). To determine her absolute requirement for NaCl, she was given a very low Na intake (2.5 mmol/day). With this treatment, she proceeded to lose 626 mmol of Na over 9 days, her jugular venous pressure was markedly decreased, but surprisingly she did not have an appreciable decline in her blood pressure and her periphery remained warm.

What change should occur in her ECF volume and blood pressure? Be quantitative.

How was her blood pressure maintained?

Given the well-maintained blood pressure despite a low venous volume, what did her brain release?

Control of Na⁺ Excretion

In the kidney, NaCl and water are filtered, but their reabsorptions are regulated independently. The regulation of Na^+ excretion is the most important factor in maintaining Na^+ balance. In a normal adult, close to 27000 mmol of Na^+ is filtered each day. In our example, only 150 mmol need be excreted; therefore, more than 99% of these filtered Na^+ must be reabsorbed. Control of reabsorption is the key to regulation of balance for Na^+. Filtration and reabsorption of Na^+ are linked so that the right amount is excreted no matter what the GFR is (within reason); the phenomenon whereby changes in GFR are accompanied by parallel changes in tubular Na^+ reabsorption is known as glomerular tubular balance. In the paragraphs to follow, the authors first consider the nephron sites where Na^+ are reabsorbed and then the role of hormones in modulating this segmental Na^+ reabsorption. Before dealing with the specific nephron segments, the overall strategy for the reabsorption of Na^+ is considered. The authors identify three steps for this function.

Creation of the Driving Force

> • The main driving force is a low $[Na^+]$ in the ICF of tubular cells; a second driving force is the negative voltage of the ICF.

The important first step is to have a low $[Na^+]$ in the ICF. This is achieved by the Na^+, K^+, ATPase. This ion pump consumes energy (ATP) and pumps three Na^+ ions out while transporting two K^+ ions into cells; hence it also helps create a net negative voltage inside cells. This negative voltage becomes even greater when K^+ diffuse through their ion-specific channels on the basolateral aspect of these cells (see Figure 9.1).

Use of the Low $[Na^+]$ and Negative Voltage of the ICF

> • Transport of Na^+ occurs if there is a transporter in the luminal membrane that binds Na^+ and another ligand.

Having the $[Na^+]$ in the lumen of 150 mmol/L (same as the plasma Na^+:water ratio) and a $[Na^+]$ of 15 mmol/L in the ICF leads to a driving force for Na^+ to cross the luminal membrane, but this membrane is impermeable to Na^+. Specific transporters are inserted into the luminal membrane, and they are capable of transporting Na^+ only if another ligand is bound to it (Figure 6.10). Examples of these ligands in the lumen are glucose, amino acids, phosphate, and organic anions. In contrast, another ligand is H^+; in this case, the H^+ bind to an intracellular site and are transported from the cell to the lumen when Na^+ move in the opposite direction. In this latter case, the transporter is a special Na^+:H^+ exchanger called NHE-3; its function is to reabsorb filtered $NaHCO_3$ in a rather complicated fashion (see Figure 1.10).

Reabsorption of Filtered Glucose

- Coordination of glucose movement across the luminal and basolateral membranes is needed. The former is Na^+-linked, and the latter is independent of Na^+.

The overall process is summarized in Figure 6.10. At the luminal membrane, one wants to reabsorb all filtered glucose. Simple diffusion is too slow. Hence, using the concentration difference for Na^+ and the negative intracellular voltage drives glucose entry along with Na^+ into cells via a Na^+-linked glucose transporter (see margin note).

Transfer of Glucose to Plasma

- Transporters are needed to have glucose diffuse into plasma.

Because the Na^+ concentration is higher in plasma than in the ICF, a Na^+ independent transport system is needed to carry glucose across the basolateral membrane. This is achieved by a glucose transporter called GLUT-2; it is different from the insulin-sensitive glucose transporter (GLUT-4).

Note:
If this transporter is defective, glucose will appear in the urine in the absence of hyperglycemia. This is called renal glucosuria if it is an isolated lesion, or the Fanconi syndrome if there are other defects of reabsorption in the proximal convoluted tubule.

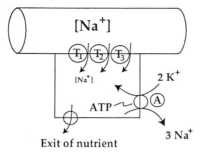

Figure 6.10 Driving force for the reabsorption of Na^+. The most important point in this figure is that the $[Na^+]$ inside cells is very low (10–15 mmol/L) because Na^+ are pumped out by the Na^+, K^+, ATPase (A) on the basolateral membrane. This low $[Na^+]$ in the ICF permits Na^+ to enter from the lumen down a favorable electrochemical gradient on a number of different transporters (T_1, T_2, T_3). For example, glucose, phosphate, and amino acids are cotransported with Na^+, whereas H^+ are transported in the opposite direction to Na^+ by the NHE-3.

TABLE 6.7 **Water and Na⁺ Reabsorption in the Kidney**

Assuming a normal GFR (180 L/day), 27000 mmol of Na⁺ is filtered per day. This table indicates the events involved in the excretion of 150 mmol of Na⁺ in 1 L of urine.

Nephron Site	Na⁺ Reabsorbed (mmol)	Na⁺ remaining (mmol)	[Na⁺] (mmol/l)
Proximal convoluted tubule	18 000	9 000	150
Loop of Henle	6 000	3 000	45
Distal convoluted tubule	2 000	1 000	100*
Cortical collecting duct	700	300	100*
Medullary collecting duct	150	150	150*

*The concentration of Na⁺ in the luminal fluid depends on whether water was reabsorbed as well. When ADH acts, the osmolality in the CCD is equal to that in plasma. Given the concentrations of urea and K⁺ in the luminal fluid, these values are reasonable guesses. The [Na⁺] in the urine requires a urine volume of 1 L.

Nephron Sites Involved in the Transport of Na⁺

The renal handling of Na⁺ is best considered by examining the nephron segments individually (see also Tables 6.7, 6.8).

Na⁺ Handling in the Proximal Tubule

Note
CAI = carbonic anhydrase inhibitors. These drugs do not block the Na⁺/H⁺ antiporter but inhibit indirect reabsorption of HCO₃⁻ by blocking the luminal carbonic anhydrase (see page 25 for details).

Osmotic diuresis
See the discussion of Question 6.19.

Close to two-thirds of the Na⁺ that are filtered are reabsorbed in the proximal tubule, and electroneutrality is maintained by either Cl⁻ reabsorption (majority) or by H⁺ secretion (minority). The epithelium of the proximal tubule is permeable to water, and the osmolality of the fluid leaving this tubule is the same as that of the ECF. The proximal tubular luminal membrane cannot generate a large transtubular [Na⁺] gradient; in fact, the maximum [Na⁺] gradient here is 33% and is generated during an *osmotic diuresis*. Na⁺ reabsorption occurs down the [Na⁺] gradient between the lumen and the ICF, which is produced by the Na⁺K⁺ATPase on the

TABLE 6.8 **Summary of Transporters in the Nephron and the Diuretics That Inhibit Them**

Nephron Site	Luminal Transporter	Function	Diuretic
Proximal convoluted tubule	NHE-3 Na⁺-nutrient NaCl	Reabsorption of NaHCO₃ Reabsorption of nutrients ECF volume regulation	CAI for NaHCO₃ reabsorption
Loop of Henle	Na⁺, K⁺, 2 Cl⁻	NaCl Mg²⁺, Ca²⁺ reabsorption Concentration and dilution	Furosemide
Distal convoluted tubule	NaCl	NaCl Ca²⁺ reabsorption Dilution	Thiazide class
Cortical collecting duct	Na⁺ channel NaCl reabsorption H⁺ATPase	K⁺ secretion NH₄⁺ excretion	Amiloride Triamterene Spironolactone None in use
Medullary collecting duct	NaCl Na⁺ channel H⁺ ATPase K⁺/H⁺ATPase	Na⁺ balance Na⁺ balance NH₄⁺ excretion K⁺ reabsorption	ANF Amiloride None in use None in use

basolateral membrane of these cells. This lower intracellular [Na$^+$] provides the driving force for nutrient and HCO$_3^-$ reabsorption by Na$^+$-dependent transporters (see Table 6.8).

Na$^+$ Handling in the Loop of Henle

NaCl reabsorption in the loop of Henle enables the excretion of a concentrated or dilute urine (see Figures 6.5 and 6.6). NaCl is actively transported in the thick ascending limb via the luminal electroneutral Na$^+$, K$^+$, 2 Cl$^-$ cotransporter. Again, the driving force is provided by the basolateral Na$^+$K$^+$ATPase, but only half of the Na$^+$ use the transcellular route. Absolute Na$^+$ reabsorption in the loop of Henle varies directly with delivery. Net NaCl reabsorption is stimulated by ADH in the medullary thick ascending limb and is inhibited by loop diuretics. Water is not reabsorbed to an appreciable degree in the ascending limb of this nephron segment.

Na$^+$ Handling in the Distal Convoluted Tubule

The major function of this segment of the nephron is Na$^+$ balance and formation of electrolyte-free water. Na$^+$ are actively reabsorbed in this nephron segment along with Cl$^-$; high transepithelial [Na$^+$] gradients can be maintained. Because this nephron site is sparingly permeable to water, the *thiazide class of diuretics,* which acts on this site, leads to a compromised ability to excrete a load of EFW.

> **Thiazide class of diuretics**
> Diuretics that inhibit the reabsorption of Na$^+$ via the Na$^+$, Cl$^-$ cotransporter in the distal convoluted tubule.

Na$^+$ Handling in the Collecting Ducts

The major functions of the cortical collecting duct are NaCl reabsorption and secretion of K$^+$ and H$^+$. *Quantitative aspects* are provided in the margin note. The major step is Na$^+$ transport through an Na$^+$-specific channel. This channel is inhibited by the diuretic amiloride, a K$^+$-sparing type of diuretic. Mineralocorticoids play an important role here by leading to a greater *"open probability"* of this Na$^+$ channel. The medullary collecting duct is the site where final decisions are made about the excretion of NaCl. The medullary collecting duct is capable of maintaining a large [Na$^+$] gradient across its epithelium. During ECF volume contraction, virtually all the Na$^+$ delivered are reabsorbed—a process that requires the absence of *atrial natriuretic peptide (ANP)*. In contrast, with ECF volume expansion, only a small quantity of the Na$^+$ delivered are reabsorbed because ANP is acting. The other major functions of the medulla are concentration of the urine and NH$_4^+$ excretion.

> **Quantitative aspects of Na$^+$** handling in the cortical collecting duct
> In a 24-hour period, 1 000 mmol of NaCl is delivered to the cortical collecting duct:
> • reabsorbs 700 mmol of NaCl;
> • permits the excretion of 60 mmol of K$^+$;
> • secretes 20 mmol of NH$_4^+$, but this amount can rise to 200 mmol in chronic metabolic acidosis.

> **Open probability**
> A term used to imply that more channels and/or channels with greater conductivity are open.

> **Atrial natriuretic peptide (ANP)**
> A hormone released from the right atrium of the heart when the central venous volume is high. It causes a fall in vascular resistance and promotes the excretion of NaCl.

QUESTION

(Discussion on page 271)

6.19 *Why does glucosuria cause enhanced excretion of Na$^+$ and Cl$^-$?*

Regulation of Na$^+$ Excretion

ECF Volume

When examining Na$^+$ excretion within the context of the ECF volume, expect to see urine that is virtually free of Na$^+$ (and/or

Cl^-) when the ECF volume is contracted (see margin note and Table 6.9). Also, expect to see Na^+ excretion when the ECF volume is expanded. During euvolemia, the kidney excretes the dietary NaCl load. Hence, there are no normal values for urine Na^+ and Cl^-; these values must be interpreted relative to the physiologic state and dietary intake of the patient.

TABLE 6.9 **Urine Electrolytes in a Patient with ECF Volume Contraction**

All values are in mmol/L; these numbers will be lower in a polyuric state.

Condition	Electrolyte in the Urine		
	Na^+	K^+	Cl^-
Nonrenal or previous renal loss of NaCl	0–15	Variable	0–15
Vomiting			
Recent	>20	>50	0–15
Remote	0–15	Variable	0–15
Diuretics			
Recent	>20	>20	>20
Remote	0–15	Variable	0–15
Renal disorders involving wasting of salt	>20	Variable	>20

Anions in the Urine

Na^+ (and K^+) excretion can be influenced by the anion composition of the filtrate. For example, a patient who vomits will deliver more HCO_3^- to the collecting duct than can be reabsorbed; the urine should contain Na^+ (and K^+) in conjunction with the HCO_3^- that are not reabsorbed even though the ECF volume may be contracted. The effect of ECF volume contraction is evident from the fact that the urine contains at most a small quantity of Cl^-.

Need to Excrete NH_4^+

During chronic metabolic acidosis resulting from laxative abuse, the 24 hr urine may contain 200 mmol of NH_4^+. If the patient has a contracted ECF volume, the urine will not contain Na^+. Nevertheless, electroneutrality in the urine must be maintained and usually requires that Cl^- accompany the NH_4^+ in the urine. Hence, the urine contains an abundant amount of Cl^- despite ECF volume contraction in this setting.

Role of Hormones

The major hormones acting in the kidney to preserve Na^+ homeostasis are listed in Table 6.6.

Angiotensin II

Angiotensin II is produced when renin is released from the juxtaglomerular apparatus. A low renal perfusion pressure leads to renin release, as does a rise in β_1-adrenergic agonists; both reflect a low

ECF volume. The major renal effect of angiotensin II is to stimulate the reabsorption of $NaHCO_3$ in the proximal convoluted tubule (PCT). Because fluid must remain isosmotic here, water is reabsorbed, and the $[Cl^-]$ in the luminal fluid rises. This increase then creates a concentration difference for Cl^- and drives the passive reabsorption of Cl^- (dragging Na^+ for electroneutrality and water for isosmolality). The effects of this hormone are also discussed in Chapters 4 and 9 in the context of metabolic alkalosis and K^+ physiology. Angiotensin II is also a potent vasoconstrictor and selectively constricts efferent arterioles. Thus, angiotensin II leads to an increase in the filtration fraction and alters proximal reabsorption secondary to changes in physical factors.

Aldosterone

Aldosterone has an important influence on renal Na^+ reabsorption in the distal nephron; it is responsible for 5% of the total Na^+ reabsorption. The secretion of aldosterone is stimulated by contraction of the "effective" circulating volume via angiotensin II and by hyperkalemia; the converse is also true. Quantitatively, the most important action of aldosterone is to lead to the reabsorption of NaCl. It also promotes the net secretion of K^+ and stimulates H^+ secretion.

Aldosterone
A hormone released by the adrenal cortex that leads to reabsorption of NaCl and secretion of K^+ in the cortical distal nephron.

Atrial Natriuretic Peptide (ANP)

ANP leads to a natriuresis when the ECF volume is expanded. ANP acts by increasing the GFR and decreasing Na^+ reabsorption in the medullary collecting duct.

In addition to the GFR, ANP, and aldosterone, other factors can influence renal Na^+ reabsorption. Peritubular capillary colloid osmotic pressure and renal perfusion pressure both may modulate Na^+ reabsorption.

QUESTIONS

(Discussions on pages 272–274)

6.20 *What is the volume of distribution of the common IV solutions?*

6.21 *What are the purposes for administration of the various IV solutions?*

6.22 *When should hypertonic NaCl be infused? How much should be given?*

6.23 *The ECF volume is expanded chronically in trained athletes. Why might this expansion be advantageous?*

6.24 *A person was in Na^+ balance on two occasions, eating and excreting 150 mmol of Na^+ each day. On the first occasion, he had two kidneys (the GFR was 200 L/day), and on the second, he had one kidney (the GFR was 100 L/day). What was his fractional excretion of Na^+ on each occasion?*

PART D

Review

DISCUSSION OF INTRODUCTORY CASE
Lee Is Sweet and Not Salty
(Case presented on page 229)

Why is her ECF volume contracted?

Because of hyperglycemia, Lee has a glucose-induced osmotic diuresis, which results in an increased delivery of more volume and Na^+ out of the loop of Henle. If all of these Na^+ are not reabsorbed in the collecting duct, some will be excreted (note that her urine $[Na^+]$ is 46 mmol/L despite ECF volume depletion; see the discussion of Question 6.19).

How did her physician know?

She had the following physical signs of ECF volume depletion: low blood pressure, a postural fall in blood pressure, tachycardia, and a low jugular venous pressure along with the absence of edema or ascites (see margin note).

Why is she hyponatremic, given the composition of her urine?

Her urine contains only 46 mmol/L Na^+ and 20 mmol/L K^+; therefore, this urine is removing more water than Na^+ and would tend to make her hypernatremic if there was no entry of water into her ECF. There are two reasons why she has hyponatremia (see margin note). First, she has an impermeant osmole (glucose) in her ECF that has raised the tonicity of the ECF. Movement of water from the ICF of those cells (muscle) requiring insulin for the entry of glucose has caused hyponatremia. The $[Na^+]$ will fall close to 1.5 mmol/L for every 5.5 mmol/L (100 mg/dL) above the normal concentration of glucose. Therefore, her $[Na^+]$ has fallen 11 mmol/L as a result of the hyperglycemia, close to the observed value of 126 mmol/L. The second reason for hyponatremia is that she is thirsty and is drinking a large quantity of water. The low ECF volume has led to the release of ADH, which prevents excretion of the ingested water (see margin note).

What stimulated thirst?

Thirst was stimulated primarily by the contracted ECF volume. It is not clear whether hyperosmolality resulting from hyperglycemia stimulates thirst on a chronic basis.

Why is her urine volume so high?

The glucose excreted in her urine led to the high urine volume (see margin note and question 6.19).

Clinical steps
1. Assess the vascular volume first.
   - Arterial signs.
   - Venous signs.
2. Assess the interstitial fluid volume.
   - Not sensitive or specific unless changes are marked.

Tonicity balance
Calculate input and output
- Water
- $Na^+ + K^+$

Hyponatremia
1. Source of EFW.
2. Reason not to excrete EFW (ADH).

Urine volume = # osmoles/Uosm
She has a large number of "non-urea" osmoles (or tonomoles) in her urine (Uosm = urine osmolality).

DISCUSSION OF CASE 6.1
Donnie Is All Charged Up
(Case presented on page 235)

What would happen to the vascular volume if the charge on her plasma proteins became more anionic?

If the net valence on plasma proteins became more anionic, this would attract more Na^+ (140 mmol/L) into the vascular space than the number of $Cl^- + HCO_3^-$ molecules (103 + 25 mmol/L); the net valence would repel from the vascular compartment. Having more solutes in the vascular volume causes a shift of interstitial fluid into the vascular space (the Donnan effect; see Figure 6.4); the vascular volume would increase.

For defense of the vascular volume, should a greater anionic valence occur when the vascular volume was expanded or contracted?

If the major aim is to reexpand the vascular volume, interstitial fluid should enter capillaries. Apply these data to Donnie's case and the contracted ECF volume. Note the much higher anion gap in her plasma; this could help defend her vascular volume by an increase in Donnan force.

Can these data be applied to the patient who had a contracted ECF volume? A rise in anionic valence in plasma occurs in other settings in which the ECF volume is contracted, such as in metabolic alkalosis; the converse is seen when the ECF volume is expanded, as in the syndrome of inappropriate antidiuretic hormone. The change in anionic charge is far too large to be explained simply by changes in the plasma albumin level or the plasma pH.

How would the properties of an anionic charge on albumin differ from that on a similar number of small organic anions like lactate⁻ in plasma?

There are two major differences.

1. In contrast to small organic anions, because albumin is not filtered by the kidney, these unmeasured anions will not appear in the urine. Moreover, they are distributed primarily in the vascular volume.

2. Being in a small compartment only (plasma), the total number of anions (plus H^+) added are far fewer if a protein like albumin was the sole added new anion. In contrast, because lactate (plus H^+) distributes in the entire ECF volume and much of the ICF volume, many more lactate anions (plus H^+) must have been added to have the same high value for the anion gap in plasma (see margin note).

What data would help establish that the high value for the anion gap was due to an increased negative valence on plasma proteins?

The major difference between the negative charge due to the valence of plasma proteins and that due to the anion of an organic acid (e.g., lactate⁻) is the volume of distribution. Organic anions and

Change in HCO_3^- balance:
Notice the minor changes in the $[HCO_3^-]$ in plasma when the anion gap was high and again when it was low in Donnie. This, together with the absence of extra unmeasured anions in the urine, led the authors to speculate about an albumin-like rather than a lactate-like origin of these added anions.

HCO_3^- generally have the same volume of distribution; therefore the H^+ that accompanies the organic anion will lower the plasma $[HCO_3^-]$ to the same degree as the increase in the anion gap. On the other hand, the volume of distribution of the plasma proteins is only 20–25% of the ECF. Because the anion gap is measured in plasma, the increase in the magnitude of the anion gap due to an increase in the negative valence of plasma protein will greatly exceed the fall in the plasma $[HCO_3^-]$ because HCO_3^- are distributed in a volume exceeding the ECF.

In this case, the increase in anion gap $(41 - 12 = 29 \text{ mEq/L})$ far exceeds the fall in $[HCO_3^-]$ $(25 - 17 = 8 \text{ mmol/L})$. Therefore the differential diagnosis should include:

1. Mixed metabolic alkalosis and metabolic acidosis.

2. Increased anion gap due to increased negative valence on protein. The following points are helpful in the differential diagnosis: first, the discrepancy between the increase in anion gap and fall in $[HCO_3^-]$ is too great to be explained by coexistent metabolic alkalosis. Second, the presence of hypokalemia might be more supportive of the diagnosis of preexisting metabolic alkalosis. Third, the fact that the plasma anion gap is so high yet the unmeasured anion does not appear in the urine suggests that the unmeasured anion is not filtered by the glomerulus (plasma protein) or is completely reabsorbed (e.g., L^- lactate$^-$), yet the plasma L^- lactate$^-$ is only 2 mmol/L. Additional support for the cause of the high value for the plasma anion gap being the negative charge on plasma protein will come with therapy and ECF volume restoration (the assumption being that the increased negative valence is a compensatory response to maintain circulating volume). Therapy with NaCl will cause a fall in the anion gap to normal, but the plasma $[HCO_3^-]$ will not rise by a similar amount. It will be important to collect the urine and prove that there has been excretion of neither unmeasured anions nor HCO_3^-. Thus, the unmeasured anion has disappeared with only modest HCO_3^- generation and no renal excretion. The authors speculate that this situation is best explained by the titration of the anions on plasma proteins.

DISCUSSION OF CASE 6.2
Ted Is Truly Number One
(Case presented on page 246)

How will you confirm that his polyuria is a water diuresis? What is the predicted numerical value for this test?

In a water diuresis, the urine osmolality will be very low. Just how low it will be depends on the osmole load Ted excretes. For easy mathematics, if his osmole excretion rate is 720 mOsm/day, his urine osmolality will be 30 mOsm/kg H_2O with a urine volume of 24 L/day.

How would you be sure that his excessive urine output is a renal problem?

To decide whether this is a renal problem, give ADH. The dose should be a physiologically relevant one because a defect in the

Note

$$\frac{720 \text{ mOsm}}{24 \text{ L}} = 30 \text{ mOsm/L}$$

receptor (low affinity to ADH) might respond to very high ADH levels. He did not respond to ADH—there was no change in the urine flow rate or osmolality. He did not respond to a high (supraphysiologic) dose of ADH, either. Therefore, he has nephrogenic DI.

What could his renal lesion be at the molecular level?

As shown in Figure 6.7, the lesion could be anywhere between the V_2 receptor for ADH and the properly inserted activated AQP-2 water channels. Ted has a V_2 receptor defect.

What therapy might be of benefit?

Enhance Water Reabsorption in the Distal Nephron
All of the following strategies failed here. The authors used very high ADH levels, phosphodiesterase inhibitors, and drugs that can activate adenylate cyclase.

Decrease Distal Delivery of Filtrate
All nephron segments before the bend of the loop of Henle are permeable to water, and this permeability is insensitive to ADH, so the goal is to have more filtrate reabsorbed here.

There are three methods of leverage: lower the GFR, increase the reabsorption of filtrate in the PCT, or increase the reabsorption of filtrate in the descending thin limb (DTL) of the loop of Henle (the ascending thin limb is not sufficiently permeable to water).

Summary. When the $[Na^+]$ is lower in the medullary interstitial fluid, more of the filtrate is transferred from an ADH-insensitive (DTL) to an ADH-sensitive (distal nephron) location, and as a result, the urine volume rises. Thus, a vicious cycle is established—as more filtrate is delivered distally, more EFW is reabsorbed in the MCD, and this further decreases the interstitial $[Na^+]$.

Consideration of His Plasma $[Na^+]$ of 139 mmol/L
Thirst is a very powerful urge and is unrelenting, so the patient does everything he can to avoid thirst. By habit, he knows that drinking a large volume of water removes this unpleasant feeling.

There must be a stimulus for thirst—that stimulus is hypernatremia. In general, patients like Ted with diabetes insipidus who have the largest daily urine volumes will have the greatest stimulus to drink (highest plasma $[Na^+]$). The plasma $[Na^+]$ of 139 mmol/L rather than a value in the high 140 range suggests that part of Ted's polyuria is due to excessive water intake; this can be tested by having him drink *only* when thirsty. If this results in less water delivery to the distal nephron and thereby less addition of EFW to the medullary interstitial fluid, the $[Na^+]$ may rise here and, as a result, more filtrate may be reabsorbed in the DTL and thereby lead to a much lower urine volume.

If you use a natriuretic agent, which one(s) would you choose, and which should you avoid?

The authors want to create a negative balance for Na^+. This requires both a low NaCl intake and the use of a natriuretic agent (see margin note). This latter drug should not compromise the outer medullary concentrating mechanism; therefore, a natriuretic that

Note
The choice of which natriuretic agent is considered in the discussion of Question 6.9.

acts on the distal convoluted tubule (thiazide class) and not a loop diuretic should be used. To avoid hypokalemia and enhance the loss of Na$^+$, add a K$^+$-sparing diuretic to the regimen (amiloride).

The natriuretic agents act by binding to a specific transporter in the lumen, the Na$^+$:Cl$^-$ cotransporter for thiazides, and the epithelial Na$^+$ channel in the cortical collecting duct for amiloride. The concentration of these agents must achieve a therapeutic concentration in the luminal fluid (see margin note). Because the volume of fluid in the lumen of Ted's distal convoluted tubule is at least twofold higher than normal, Ted will need at least a twofold larger dose of these drugs to achieve the same biologic effect as in normal individuals.

Lower GFR. This in essence means to contract the ECF volume by inducing a negative balance for NaCl. This requires a low salt intake in conjunction with a natriuretic agent. There is little opportunity for a major effect here without causing undue ECF volume contraction.

More Reabsorption of NaCl (and Water) in the Proximal Convoluted Tubule (PCT). A lower ECF volume will accomplish this aim, but to have a large impact on the delivery of water to the distal convoluted tubule, a major decrease in ECF volume is also required.

Increased Reabsorption of Water in the DTL of the Loop of Henle. Normally, more than 30 of the 60 L of pure water delivered out of the PCT each day is reabsorbed in the DTL in a passive fashion because water is permeable and the interstitial fluid has a higher osmolality (see Figure 6.8). There are three major points about this reabsorption of water:

1. The water channels in the DTL (and in the PCT) are not AQP-2 and are insensitive to ADH actions. Hence, it is critical to reabsorb as much water as possible in these nephron segments where reabsorption is possible rather than send water distally where its reabsorption is compromised in Ted.

2. A high osmolality in the interstitial fluid, the result of active transport of Na$^+$ in the ascending thin limb, is required to reabsorb water from the DTL. Therefore, do *not* give a loop diuretic because this class of drugs will block this reabsorption of Na$^+$ and thereby prevent the reabsorption of water from the DTL. In fact, low reabsorption of water in the DTL is a major reason for a higher delivery of water to the distal convoluted tubule.

3. Creation of a higher interstitial osmolality: There are two factors that are needed to have a high interstitial [Na$^+$]: reabsorption of Na$^+$ in the thick ascending limb (TAL) of the loop of Henle (LOH) and low addition of EFW from the medullary collecting duct (MCD) (see margin figure).

TAL. Reabsorption of Na$^+$ is load-dependent here. This means that a relatively fixed proportion of the delivered Na$^+$ (85%) is reabsorbed. Nevertheless, there are some control mechanisms operating. ADH normally augments this reabsorption so there will be somewhat less reabsorption of Na$^+$ in Ted's loop of Henle.

Reabsorption of Na$^+$ in the loop of Henle is diminished if there is a limiting supply of K$^+$, or when prostaglandins act. A trial with an inhibitor of prostaglandin synthesis (nonsteroidal antiinflamma-

Concentration

Amount
Volume

TAL

High Na$^+$
reabsorption

$\dfrac{Na^+}{H_2O}$

Low EFW
reabsorbed

LOH

EFW

Low EFW
reabsorbed

MCD

tory drugs) did not have an effect on urine volume, so they were discontinued as they are nephrotoxic agents.

Inner MCD. This nephron structure has a degree of permeability to water even in the absence of ADH. In fact, ADH only increases water permeability severalfold. Hence, the more water delivered at an osmolality less than that in the interstitial fluid, the greater the amount of water reabsorbed, and thereby the lower the interstitial $[Na^+]$ will be.

DISCUSSION OF CASE 6.3
Brain Tumor With an "Assault"
(Case presented on page 249)

What change should occur in her ECF volume and blood pressure? Be quantitative.

Because Na^+ is in the body to keep water out of cells (defend the ECF volume), a large loss of Na^+ should contract her ECF volume (see margin figure).

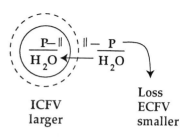

ICFV larger

Loss ECFV smaller

Quantities. If 50–60% of her body weight (52 kg) is water, for easy calculation, assign a body water of 30 L. If her ECF volume is one-third of total body water, she should have 10 L of ECF and a total of 1400 mmol Na^+ in her ECF (plasma $[Na^+]$ is 140 mmol/L). This negative balance of 700 mmol Na^+ would contract her ECF volume by 50%, and she should be in shock and not be able to survive, but she did. Why?

How was her blood pressure maintained?

The blood pressure is a function of cardiac output and peripheral resistance. Simply increasing vasoconstriction is one possibility, but this will lower the GFR and resemble shock. Her warm skin and ability to function suggest a major impact on her heart—a myocardial stimulant was probably present (Figure 6.11).

Given the well-maintained blood pressure despite a low venous volume, what did her brain release?

The simplest answer is something that increased the force of cardiac muscle contraction. This means a substance with β-adrenergic activity. Moreover, to maintain the GFR, having a selective renal vasodilatation is important. A substance with these properties is dopamine.

Speculation. The authors assume that the following sequence of events could have occurred. The large intracerebral tumor caused a massive sympathetic discharge, including the release of dopamine. The inotropic action on the heart caused a pressure natriuresis, and dopamine itself inhibits Na^+ reabsorption, too. ANP could continue to cause a natriuresis because there is no major fall in the blood pressure despite a large decline in the ECF and venous blood volumes. This will be explored in Part 2 of this case in Chapter 7.

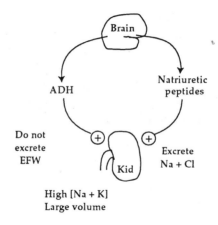

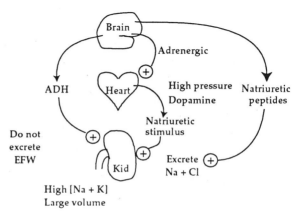

Figure 6.11 Possible models to explain cerebral salt wasting. In the top portion of the figure, the brain releases ADH to conserve water and an "ANP-like" agent to cause Na$^+$ wasting. In the bottom portion of the figure, there is an additional release of substance(s) (probably a large adrenergic stimulus) to stimulate the heart and possibly help the natriuresis. This could account for the well-preserved GFR and blood pressure despite the large deficit of Na$^+$.

Summary of Main Points

Body Compartments

Note
In a 70-kg person, total body water is 45 L, with 30 L in the ICF and 15 L in the ECF.

Particles to be ignored
Because urea and ethanol cross cell membranes readily, they have no impact on water distribution between the ECF and ICF.

- Approximately 60% of body weight is water; two-thirds is ICF and one-third is ECF (see margin note).
- Water crosses cell membranes rapidly; therefore, the osmolality in the ECF equals that in the ICF.
- Particles that readily cross the cell membrane and achieve an equal concentration in the ECF and the ICF can be ignored with respect to the distribution of water during steady state (see margin note).
- A major function of Na$^+$ (and Cl$^-$ and HCO$_3^-$) is to keep water out of cells, thereby maintaining ECF volume (glucose acts like Na$^+$ for some cells only).
- The particles that determine ICF volume are large macromolecular anions and their attendant cations (K$^+$); these anions rarely leave the ICF.

- The [Na^+] in the ECF (Na^+/H_2O) reflects the ICF volume of most cells; hypernatremia signals ICF contraction, and hyponatremia signals ICF expansion, except during hyperglycemia.
- The total Na^+ content (not the Na^+/H_2O) determines the ECF volume.
- An ultrafiltrate (not just water) crosses the capillary wall. A hydrostatic force (capillary pressure) is the major outward-driving force, and vascular colloid osmotic pressure (albumin:saline ratio) is the major inward-driving force.

Water Physiology

- There is an *obligatory loss of 0.8 L of water each day;* therefore, mechanisms are needed to ensure this minimum water intake and to excrete any excess water.
- Adequate water intake is ensured by the CNS thirst center. A rise in tonicity of only 1–2% provides a powerful urge to drink.
- ADH is the hormone that limits water excretion. A rise in tonicity or a fall in the "effective" blood volume causes ADH release from the posterior pituitary.
  –For dilute urine to be excreted, ADH must be absent. The presence of ADH results in the excretion of a concentrated urine.
  –Assess ADH action on the kidney by two parameters—urine osmolality and volume. ADH produces a urine with maximum osmolality and usually a minimum volume. Conversely, in the absence of ADH, the urine has a minimum osmolality and maximum volume.

Obligatory loss of water
Water is lost by evaporation from sweat (a hypotonic solution) and from the upper respiratory tract. The former losses increase with a rise in temperature (fever) or a need for loss of heat (exercise). The loss via the respiratory tract is enhanced with more rapid breathing and by a less humid environment.

Na^+ Physiology

- Na^+ content determines the ECF volume. With ECF volume expansion, there is an excess of total body Na^+; with ECF volume contraction, there is a Na^+ deficit.
- The renal response to ECF volume contraction is the excretion of a urine with a low Na^+ and/or Cl^- content; failure to conserve Na^+ and/or Cl^- points toward a renal problem (see margin note).
- When the ECF volume is low, the major renal mechanisms preventing Na^+ excretion are enhanced proximal Na^+ reabsorption, aldosterone-stimulated Na^+ reabsorption, and increased Na^+ reabsorption in the medullary collecting duct.
- When a Na^+ load is ingested, renal mechanisms are called into play to cause a natriuresis; these mechanisms include an increased GFR, a relatively diminished proximal Na^+ reabsorption (low angiotensin II), suppression of aldosterone release, and the release of ANP.
- Heart failure and hypoalbuminemia are associated with excessive Na^+ retention.
- Water and Na^+ are regulated independently.

Low ECF volume
The most important changes for Na^+ balance focus on renal Na^+ reabsorption (99.5% of the filtered load of Na^+ is reabsorbed normally; this can rise to almost 100%). There is also a lower GFR when the ECF volume declines.

Clinical Applications

> • Four distinct primary clinical abnormalities can be recognized, two regarding Na$^+$ and two regarding water.
>
> 1. **Excess Na$^+$.** The cardinal feature will be ECF volume expansion. Two prerequisites are required: an intake of Na$^+$ and "renal permission" to have an expanded ECF volume, which often means a low "effective" circulating volume (e.g., heart failure, hypoalbuminemia, or renal insufficiency) and thereby the kidneys fail to excrete the "extra" Na$^+$.
>
> 2. **Deficit of Na$^+$.** The cardinal feature will be a contracted ECF volume. Two major aspects should be identified: low intake of NaCl and/or excessive loss of Na$^+$ by renal or nonrenal routes. An examination of the urine electrolytes, plasma [K$^+$], and acid-base status will help identify the basis of this deficit.
>
> 3. **Excess water.** The cardinal features are water intake and "renal permission," usually via ADH, to retain this extra water. Excess water implies swelling of cells and is recognized clinically by finding hyponatremia and hypo-osmolality.
>
> 4. **Deficit of water.** The cardinal features are a problem with water intake (lack of thirst, communication, and/or access to water) and loss of water by renal or nonrenal routes; urine osmolality, volume, and osmole excretion rates help in the differential diagnosis. A deficit of water implies cell shrinking and is recognized clinically by hypernatremia and hyperosmolality (not necessarily hyperosmolality alone if urea or alcohols have led to the high plasma osmolality).

Discussion of Questions

6.1   How might an osmolality of 285 mOsm/kg H$_2$O in the ICF be reconciled with a [K$^+$] in the ICF that is only 150 mmol/L (i.e., what constitutes the osmolality of 285 mOsm/kg H$_2$O in the ICF)?

Structural water
Water that is bound to ionic groups or compounds in cells and is not able to dissolve materials in cells. For example, when magnesium sulfate (MgSO$_4$) is isolated in dry form, each crystal rapidly picks up water so that its natural form has bound water which accounts for half of its weight (MgSO$_4$ · 7 H$_2$O). Consult reference list for more details.

Because water moves to osmotic equilibrium, the osmolality of the ICF is also 285 mOsm/kg H$_2$O. The basis of the problem is that the anions in the ICF are largely macromolecular and will not make a large direct contribution to the osmolality of the ICF. Although K$^+$ may account for 150 of these milliosmoles in a liter of ICF, we are unable to identify all 135 milliosmoles of other intracellular particles. Other uncharged compounds might exist, or much of the water in cells may be structural instead of solvent water, and the osmotic contribution of K$^+$ could be much higher (see margin note).

6.2   What IV solution would you give if you wanted all of it to stay in the ECF?

Isotonic saline is the solution to give to keep the entire volume in the ECF. If a patient has a severe degree of hyponatremia (e.g., 105 mmol/L), give a solution containing 105 mmol/L

NaCl to expand the ECF quickly; this solution will stay in the ECF and not change the ICF volume.

What IV solution would you give to expand the ECF volume but contract the ICF volume?

To contract the ICF volume but expand the ECF volume, give saline that is hypertonic to the patient.

6.3　What proportion of a liter of dextrose in water (D_5W) ends up in the ICF once glucose is metabolized?

Water moves to achieve osmotic equilibrium between the ICF and ECF. Once the glucose is metabolized, it no longer requires consideration. Water will distribute in proportion to the existing ICF and ECF volumes. Therefore, two-thirds of the volume enters the ICF.

6.4　How can more of this infused water enter cells?

If something is done in addition, such as decreasing the number of ECF particles (Na^+, Cl^-) or increasing the number of ICF particles, a larger proportion of infused water can enter cells. The converse is true for a loss of ICF particles (K salts) causing hyponatremia (see discussion of Question 7.25.)

6.5　A 70-kg person perspires and loses 4 L of a NaCl solution; the [Na^+] in this fluid is one-half that in the ECF. What changes should occur in ICF and ECF volumes, and what will the resultant [Na^+] be? (For this calculation, assume that the starting [Na^+] is 150 mmol/kg H_2O and that the ECF and ICF volumes are 15 and 30 L, respectively.)

Each rectangle represents a 1-L volume.

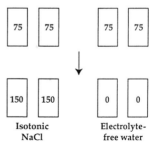

Isotonic NaCl

(ECF only)

Electrolyte-free water

(Total body water)

Divide the fluid loss into two components: isotonic saline and pure water (see margin illustration). Because the [Na^+] is one-half of normal in this example, the 4 L could be thought of as 2 L of EFW and 2 L of isotonic saline. The EFW loss occurs from the ICF and ECF in direct proportion to their existing volumes; thus, two-thirds of the 2 L of EFW is lost from the ICF (1.33 L) and one-third from the ECF (0.67 L). In contrast, the 2 L of isotonic saline is lost exclusively from the ECF (no change in the Na^+/H_2O, the driving force for a water shift). Thus, the ECF is 15 − 0.67 L − 2 L, or 12.33 L. Although we ignored the fact that the ECF volume was no longer half that of the ICF volume (a small error), we prefer this form of deductive calculation to the application of a formula. The final [Na^+] is the Na^+/water ratio in the ECF. The ECF volume is known (12.33 L). The original [Na^+] is 150 mmol/L × 15 L, or 2250 mmol, from which the patient lost 300 mmol of Na^+; therefore, the total Na^+ content is now 2250 − 300, or 1950 mmol. The resulting [Na^+] is 1950 mmol/12.33 L, or almost 159 mmol/L. Hypernatremia signals a loss of ICF volume in virtually every case.

6.6　Will exchanging a K^+ in the ICF for a Na^+ in the ECF have a direct effect on the ICF and ECF volumes?

To change compartment volumes, one must either change the

ratio of water to "particles that count" or lose particles and water in their existing ratios in body compartments. Because no K^+ are excreted in this example, there is simply an exchange of particles, both of which are not bound in the ICF, so no change in ECF or ICF volume should occur. If K^+ are excreted (with Cl^-), the ECF will lose two particles and become contracted. In contrast, if K^+ exit and H^+ enter the ICF, the osmolality of the ICF will fall, and water will move from the ICF to the ECF because H^+ are largely bound to proteins or remove HCO_3^- in the ICF.

6.7 What is the effect of hyperglycemia on a water shift between the ICF and ECF? For simplicity, assume that no insulin is present and that no excretions occur.

With hyperglycemia, the gain of particles is restricted to the ECF for the most part. Therefore, hyperglycemia causes a shift of water from the ICF (cells that have a low concentration of glucose) to the ECF and into cells where the concentration of glucose is the same as that in the ECF. As discussed in Chapter 12, pages 494–495, only those cells that depend on insulin for the transport of glucose and always have a very low concentration of glucose (e.g., muscle cells) are important in this regard.

6.8 What would happen acutely to the ICF volume if the permeability of capillary membranes to albumin were to increase?

Nothing would happen because the Na^+/H_2O ratio would not change. The distribution of ECF would change—more interstitial volume and less vascular volume.

6.9 What mechanisms are responsible for the excretion of more water when furosemide is given?

The effects are indirect. The most important action of furosemide is to block the reabsorption of NaCl in the thick ascending limb of the loop of Henle, a segment with low permeability to water. Because Na^+ are normally reabsorbed, and water is not, hypoosmolal fluid is created in the loop of Henle. This fluid normally enters the cortex. Under the influence of ADH, water is reabsorbed in the late distal convoluted tubule and collecting ducts, providing that the luminal fluid is hypoosmolal. Furosemide prevents the creation of desalinated, hypoosmolal fluid in the lumen and, as a result, prevents subsequent water reabsorption by this mechanism (see Table 6.4). There will also be less water reabsorbed in the descending thin limb of the loop of Henle because of a lower medullary interstitial osmolality.

6.10 What can limit the renal excretion of "osmole-free water" in a person who drinks a large amount of water?

Osmole-free water excretion may be limited by a marked reduction in GFR (decreased delivery to diluting sites);

blocking Na^+ reabsorption in diluting sites (loop diuretics); and actions of ADH (failure to maintain separation).

6.11 The plasma [Na^+] was 160 mmol/L in a patient who was otherwise unaware of the problem. What aspect of the history should catch your attention?

No normal patient will permit hypernatremia to develop because thirst is such a powerful stimulus. Therefore, you would suspect a deficit in the thirst mechanism (local or general central nervous system problem). In cases where the thirst mechanism is intact, you may see hypernatremia if there is either a communication problem or restricted access to water.

6.12 Several days after a car accident, a patient has hypernatremia and a marked degree of ECF volume contraction. Three to four liters of urine is passed each day (osmolality = 420 mOsm/kg H_2O). What is the most likely cause of polyuria?

The patient is undergoing an osmotic diuresis (excreting 1680 mOsm/day, whereas the expected value is less than half this amount). Therefore, one would suspect an osmotic diuresis induced by glucose, urea, or mannitol. Look at the glucose and urea in blood and urine; check to see if mannitol was given.

6.13 How would you know that the failure to excrete "osmole-free water" was not due to an inadequate delivery of filtrate to the loop of Henle?

Look at the GFR. Normally less than one-third of the filtrate is delivered to the thick ascending limb of the loop of Henle. If the GFR is not markedly reduced, the lesion is due to something else or is in addition to a lower delivery of filtrate to the loop of Henle.

6.14 Two normal 70-kg persons excrete the following urine during the same period. Both subjects have 40 L of body water before the urine losses. If neither has any fluid intake, who will have the greater fall in plasma [Na^+] in this period?

	Volume (L)	[Na^+] mmol/L	[K^+] mmol/L	[$Na^+ + K^+$] mmol/L
A	1	210	90	300
B	4	140	45	185

Patient A. Divide the urine into two components: isotonic saline (1 L containing 150 mmol $Na^+ + K^+$) and the residual, which is 150 mmol $Na^+ + K^+$ without water. This "desalinates" 1 L of body water (see Figure 7.2) so the body will have an extra liter of EFW. The plasma [Na^+] will decline by 1/TBW (total body water) in liters times the original plasma [Na^+]. Because the TBW is now 39 L, the decline in plasma [Na^+] is close to 4 mmol/L.

Note
A water load expands the ECF and ICF volumes temporarily. In response to an expanded ECF volume, a natriuresis occurs. If NaCl is not ingested, the natriuresis and subsequent ECF volume contraction will prevent the complete excretion of the water load (because of the release of ADH), resulting in hyponatremia.

There is a loss of 1 L of ECF volume due to the excretion of 1 L of isotonic fluid. Moreover, there is a shift of water from the ECF into the ICF because of the loss of electrolytes without water from the ECF; this amounts to close to two-thirds of 1 L because 1 L of ECF was desalinated, and the net loss of ECF volume is 1.67 L (i.e., in proportion to the existing distribution of water between the ECF and the ICF).

Patient B. In this example, the urine is again divided into two components, isotonic saline (4 L) and an additional almost 150 mmol of $Na^+ + K^+$ as in Patient A. Because the TBW is now 36 L, the deficit of 1 L of EFW will also cause the plasma $[Na^+]$ to rise by close to 4 mmol/L. The net loss of 150 mmol of $Na^+ + K^+$ as in Patient A will cause a similar shift of water from the ECF to the ICF (not exactly the same because of the lower ECF volume, but close enough).

Therefore, both patients have the same new plasma $[Na^+]$. This calculation points out the need to know both the $[Na^+ + K^+]$ and the volume of urine in order to understand the contribution of renal excretion to body tonicity.

6.15 Why does a penguin standing on a block of ice not freeze itself or melt that ice?

Countercurrent exchanger
The essential feature is to have a blood vessel flow in one direction (descending limb), bend back on itself, and flow in the opposite direction (ascending limb) right beside the descending limb. In this way, important constituents can flow between the descending and ascending limbs horizontally, avoiding the loss of important substances from an area. This in turn avoids a large change in composition over the area the blood traverses.

The main reason a large amount of heat is not transferred to the ice is that the blood vessels in the penguin's leg act as a countercurrent exchanger (see margin note). For the leg of the penguin, the commodity transferred is heat (figure on the left). The critical issue here is anatomy of the blood vessels in which the vessels that descend into the limb lie in close proximity to the vessels that ascend out of the limb. By transferring heat, blood in the vessels that descend into the limb is cooled in conjunction with rewarming of the blood in the vessels that ascend out of the limb.

Applying this same logic to the outer medulla, the Na^+ reabsorbed from the thick ascending limb of the loop of Henle is added to the vasa recta deep in the outer medulla. This Na^+

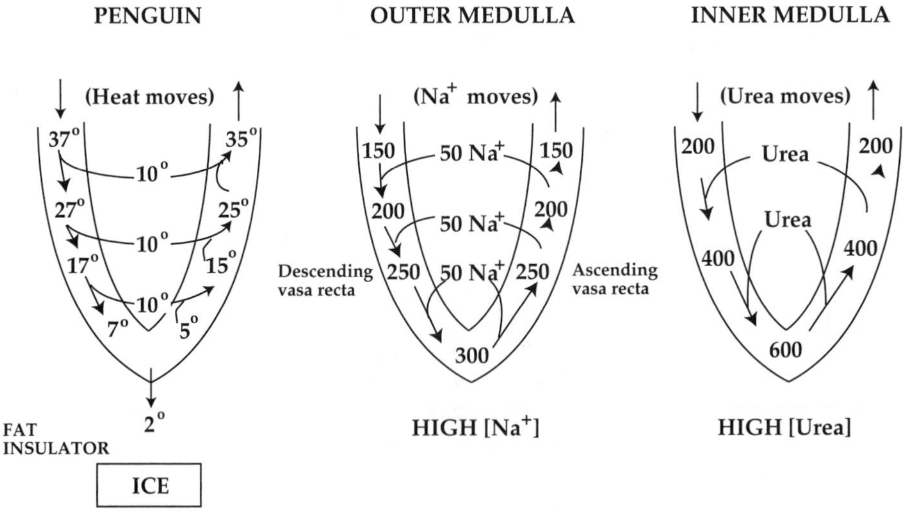

PENGUIN

↓ (Heat moves) ↑

37° ⟍ 35°
10°
27° ⟍ 25°
10°
17° 15°
10°
7° 5°

2°
FAT
INSULATOR

ICE

OUTER MEDULLA

↓ (Na^+ moves) ↑

150 ⟍ 50 Na^+ ⟍ 150
200 50 Na^+ 200
Descending 250 50 Na^+ 250 Ascending
vasa recta vasa recta
300

HIGH $[Na^+]$

INNER MEDULLA

↓ (Urea moves) ↑

200 Urea 200
Urea
400 400
600

HIGH [Urea]

recycles as shown in the figure so it is not quickly washed out of the interstitial fluid of the outer medulla.

A similar story occurs in the inner medulla, but now the main commodity recycled is urea. Urea enters the interstitial fluid from the IMCD.

The exit of urea from the medulla has another "twist." Urea exits the inner medulla via the ascending vasa recta because of its larger volume (blood from the descending limb + reabsorbed fluid); however, these vasa recta "give back" most of this urea to nephrons in the outer medulla. They surround the descending thin limbs of the loop of Henle in the outer medulla, and urea diffuses from the ascending vasa recta to these descending thin limbs and the descending vasa recta (see Figure 6.14 in the discussion of Question 6.34).

6.16 A patient has a contracted ECF volume and the following values in plasma and urine:

		Plasma	Urine
[Na$^+$]	mmol/L	130	60
[K$^+$]	mmol/L	5	20
Osmolality	mOsm/kg H$_2$O	270	520

Why is hyponatremia present?

Hyponatremia can be present if there is a deficit of Na$^+$ and/or a gain of water (see margin note).

Deficit of Na$^+$. The contracted ECF volume implies a deficit of Na$^+$. With ECF volume contraction, the urine should be free of Na$^+$, but it is not. Therefore, there is a renal cause for the deficit of Na$^+$; the clue to its basis is revealed by examining the [K$^+$] in plasma and urine. A contracted ECF volume should cause aldosterone release and a high urine [K$^+$]. The high plasma [K$^+$] and the relatively low urine [K$^+$] suggest that aldosterone activity is deficient and is a cause for the renal Na$^+$ loss. One underlying diagnosis in this patient is aldosterone deficiency.

Gain of Water. The ECF volume contraction also causes ADH release, which accounts for the failure to excrete free water.

Is the plasma ADH high, low, or normal in this patient?

Because the urine osmolality is 10-fold greater than minimum values, ADH is acting. Therefore, plasma ADH levels should be high.

Note

In a patient who has a deficit of Na$^+$, there may be some water loss; if this loss is relatively small, hyponatremia can still be present.

6.17 Patient A and B both start with a plasma [Na$^+$] of 140 mmol/L. Patient A just excreted 1 L of urine with a [Na$^+$ + K$^+$] of 300 mmol/L. Patient B just excreted 1 L of urine with the same osmolality of 600 mOsm/L, but now the sole urine osmole was urea. Will the plasma [Na$^+$] be the same or different in these two patients? What changes do you expect in their ECF volumes?

This question illustrates the difference between osmole-free water and electrolyte-free water.

Patient A. Dividing the urine into isotonic saline (1 L) and residual component (150 mmol Na^+ + K^+), there is a desalination of 1 L of body water. The latter will lower the plasma [Na^+] by close to 4 mmol/L as discussed in Question 6.14. The ECF volume will decline by 1.67 L, 1 L of isotonic saline loss, plus a shift of 0.67 L of EFW into the ICF.

Patient B. The urine contains 1 L of EFW so the plasma [Na^+] will rise by close to 1/40 × the plasma [Na^+] or 4 mmol/L. The ECF volume will decline by 0.33 L (one-third of the liter of negative EFW balance).

6.18 Sports anemia is puzzling. Assume athletes are perfectly normal (at least from the point of view of their bone marrow and kidneys). Why might sports anemia (low hematocrit level) be tolerated without an apparent erythropoietin-induced drive to synthesize red blood cells to correct the anemia? This differs from the expected response to blood loss, for example, where there is evidence of accelerated synthesis of new red blood cells. Please speculate, because the authors do not know a definitive answer.

The authors speculate in the following three areas to develop our answer.

(i) Difference in the Anemias. Because red blood cells normally constitute 2 of the 5 L of blood, a loss of red blood cell mass will cause a decrease in the blood volume. The response is to increase renal retention of NaCl to expand the plasma component of the blood volume. Part of this response is mediated by a rise in renin and angiotensin II and thereby aldosterone.

In contrast, with sports anemia there is a primary gain of NaCl and a dilution of the red blood cell mass. This expansion of the circulating volume could depress the levels of renin and angiotensin II at rest or certainly avoid markedly increased levels.

(ii) The local Po_2. The PO_2 depends on supply vs demand. Supply of blood is poised so that it is relatively limited in the area of the corticomedullary junction. Demand depends on the rate of Na^+ reabsorption here. If Na^+ reabsorption was stimulated in this region, the Po_2 would fall.

(iii) Effect of Angiotensin II in the Kidney. Angiotensin II stimulates the reabsorption of Na^+ in the proximal convoluted tubule. With more Na^+ reabsorption, the consumption of O_2 increases, and this should lower the Po_2 in this region. A low Po_2 is needed here to stimulate the release of erythropoietin.

Bottom Line. Sports anemia may be "tolerated" because the lower local angiotensin II levels do not result in more localized O_2 consumption. This could have a biologic advantage because the athlete will lose ECF volume during strenuous exercise (sweat loss, shift of water into cells when intracellular osmolality rises) without raising hematocrit values dangerously high, at which time the viscosity of blood could rise too much, compromising maximal O_2 delivery and increasing the likelihood of blood coagulation.

6.19 Why does glucosuria cause enhanced excretion of Na^+ and Cl^-?

There are two answers to this question, a short one that is not really correct and a longer one that is better. The short answer is that glucose prevents the reabsorption of water in the earlier nephron segments because fluid here must remain isosmolal to plasma, and more glucose is filtered than can be reabsorbed in the proximal convoluted tubule (PCT). This extra volume drags Na^+ and Cl^- to distal sites at a rate that exceeds their reabsorptive capacity.

The longer answer requires more specificity. In the PCT, if the degree of hyperglycemia is less than 50 mmol/L (900 mg/dL), there will be no change in proximal Na^+ reabsorption. When the fluid leaves the PCT, however, the composition differs; total osmolality is 300 mOsm/L; of this, 100 mOsm/L is glucose, so the $[Na^+]$ is half of the remainder (i.e., 100 mmol/L). Hence, the $[Na^+]$ is lower (100 vs the usual 150 mmol/L), and a larger volume will be delivered to the loop of Henle (see margin illustration). Fewer Na^+ can be reabsorbed in the loop of Henle because the $[Na^+]$ in each liter of fluid delivered to the loop is now smaller (100 vs the usual 150 mmol/L), and reabsorption in the loop proceeds to a limiting $[Na^+]$ of close to 50 mmol/L. Hence, there is a lower osmolality in the interstitial fluid so less water was reabsorbed in the water-permeable descending thin limb. Thus, there is a larger volume and increased number of osmoles (glucose) that cannot be reabsorbed in the loop of Henle, leading to a larger volume of fluid with a higher osmolality being delivered to the distal nephron. Even when ADH acts, less water will be reabsorbed distally because the osmolality of fluid entering the distal convoluted tubule is higher than normal (see Table 6.4). As a result, a much larger volume is delivered to the collecting duct and might compromise complete reabsorption of Na^+ and Cl^- in these final nephron segments.

Fluid delivery to the LOH

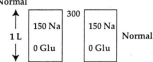

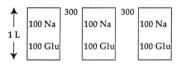

TABLE 6.10 **Changes Following the Infusion of 1 L of Commonly Used Intravenous Solutions**

Solution	Composition	Volume Change (L)	
		ECF	**ICF**
Saline			
0.9%	150 mmol Na^+, Cl^-	1	0
0.45%	75 mmol Na^+, Cl^-	0.67	0.33
3.0%	512 mmol Na^+, Cl^-	2.6	−1.6
D_5W	276 mmol glucose	0.33	0.67
⅔ D_5W, ⅓ Saline	183 mmol glucose 50 mmol Na^+, Cl^-	0.55	0.45

Sample calculation

Assume that all the glucose infused in D_5W was metabolized.
1. Calculate the total osmoles in the body and in the ECF (osmolality × total body water, one-third in the ECF).
2. Add osmoles added (Na^+ and Cl^-) to total body osmoles, then divide by new total body water (original and infused volumes).
3. Divide new total osmoles by new total volume to obtain new osmolality.
4. Divide total ECF osmoles (original osmoles plus added Na^+ and Cl^-) by new osmolality to obtain new ECF volume.
5. Subtract new ECF volume from new total body water to deduce new ICF volume.

6.20 What is the volume of distribution of the common IV solutions?

The major premise is that isotonic saline remains entirely in the ECF, and EFW distributes in proportion to the ICF and ECF volumes (two-thirds in the ICF and one-third in the ECF). Accordingly, the distribution of infusates can be calculated by dividing each solution into equivalent volumes of isotonic NaCl and EFW (i.e., 1 L of 75 mmol/L saline is 0.5 L of isotonic saline and 0.5 L of EFW; see Table 6.10).

6.21 What are the purposes for administration of the various IV solutions?

There are four different impacts that IV infusions have on body fluid compartments.

1. Expand the ECF only.

Isotonic saline is the solution to infuse in patients with ECF volume contraction; the tonicity should be isotonic to the patient, not the clinician. Even if there is a coexistent abnormality in the ICF volume, the ECF volume might need re-expansion rapidly at a time when the ICF volume should be normalized slowly.

2. Expand the ICF with as little fluid to the ECF as possible.

Infuse water with a particle that prevents osmotic lysis of blood cells but disappears promptly. The water disperses, with two-thirds going to the ICF. Glucose is the most commonly used particle, but beware—not all patients can metabolize large quantities of glucose rapidly (see margin note). This technique is used in patients with ICF volume contraction (hypernatremia).

Rate of metabolism of glucose
Glucose can be metabolized at a rate of only 0.2 g/kg body weight per hour in an ill or stressed patient, equivalent to 14 g in a 70-kg patient. Because 14 g is close to 30% of 50 g, do not infuse more than 300 mL of D_5W per hour in this setting; less should be infused if the patient is already hyperglycemic.

3. Expand both the ICF and ECF volumes.

With salt and water deficits, a dilute saline is infused. The first option is half-normal saline (75 mmol/L, 0.45%), two-thirds of which is distributed in the ECF; the second option, a solution of two-thirds D_5W and one-third NaCl, distributes close to 50% in each compartment (see Table 6.10). This latter solution requires removal of glucose and expands the ICF volume to a greater extent than half-isotonic saline for a given degree of expansion of the ECF volume.

4. Remove water from cells.

Hypertonic saline (3%, 5%) causes a water shift from cells. However, a necessary concomitant event is expansion of the ECF volume. This therapy is used in patients with symptomatic hyponatremia (see margin note).

Use of diuretics to minimize ECF volume expansion
To avoid excessive expansion of the ECF volume when using hypertonic saline, give a potent diuretic (e.g., furosemide), and replace the unwanted water and K^+ losses.

6.22 When should hypertonic NaCl be infused?

Hypertonic saline is used to draw water out of cells (especially brain cells) in patients with symptomatic hyponatremia (e.g., convulsions). The driving force for this water shift is a rise of tonicity in the ECF (a rise in the Na^+/H_2O ratio). This therapy has the major disadvantage of expanding the ECF volume (see Chapter 7, pages 316–317).

How much should be given?

The answer is: enough to stop the symptoms (i.e., the convulsion). Usually such an amount will be sufficient to raise the $[Na^+]$ in plasma to the level that it was before the convulsion (3–5 mmol/L). A little caution is needed here because the convulsion increases the number of particles in the ICF, and this increase raises the plasma $[Na^+]$ (see margin note).

6.23 The ECF volume is expanded chronically in trained athletes. Why might this expansion be advantageous?

During exercise, the heart needs a large stroke volume; blood must fill the expanded capillary beds of exercising muscle to deliver O_2 and to dissipate heat via the skin. Also, there must be sufficient volume in the ECF to permit a shift of water into cells because vigorous exercise promotes a rise in particles in cells. In addition, because exercise generates excessive heat, the body loses water and some Na^+ via sweat. To accommodate all of these demands, trained athletes maintain much of their extra ECF volume in the venous capacitance vessels. The bottom line is that the ECF volume varies in normal physiology.

6.24 A person was in Na^+ balance on two occasions, eating and excreting 150 mmol of Na^+ each day. On the first occasion, he had two kidneys (the GFR was 200 L/day), and on the second, he had one kidney (the GFR was 100 L/day). What was his fractional excretion of Na^+ on each occasion?

The fractional excretion of an electrolyte is used to analyze how the kidneys handle that ion. It is calculated by dividing the quantity excreted by the quantity filtered. Because it is usually expressed as a percent, the value is multiplied by 100.

1. **Fractional excretion when GFR was 200 L/day:** GFR (200 L/day) $\times$ $[Na^+]$ in plasma (140 mmol/L) = 28000 mmol.
   Excretion of Na^+ = 150 mmol.
   Therefore, fractional excretion was 0.50% (i.e., he was excreting .5% of the filtered load of 30000 mmol of Na^+).
2. **Fractional excretion when GFR was 100 L/day.** In this setting, the excretion of Na^+ was identical, but the filtered load was halved. Therefore, the fractional excretion was double, or 1%.

Interpretation of the Fractional Excretion of Na^+ in Chronic Renal Insufficiency. Assume that the fall in the GFR is now 10-fold but that the intake and excretion of Na^+ are the same. For balance, the fractional excretion will have to be 10-fold higher than normal, or 5%. This increase in fractional excretion means that a much smaller quantity of Na^+ was reabsorbed compared with the

Study by Welt:
Blood was drawn immediately following a convulsion and later in steady state. The $[Na^+]$ in plasma was 154 mmol/L during the convulsion and 140 mmol/L in steady state. The reason for the water shift was the creation of new particles in the ICF of muscle (50% of body water). The new particles are largely inorganic phosphate (Pi):

$$ATP \rightarrow AMP + 2\ Pi$$
$$Creatinine - phosphate \rightarrow$$
$$Creatinine + Pi$$

In addition, lactic acid is formed during anaerobic oxidation from the macromolecule glycogen. If the H^+ are buffered by proteins rather than HCO_3^- and lactate anions remain in the ICF, there will be a shift of EFW from the ECF to the ICF because of the new particles (lactate anions) retained in the ICF. In contrast, if the H^+ reacted with HCO_3^-, there would be no change in the number of particles (gain of lactate = loss of HCO_3^-).

filtered load (rather than with intake of Na^+) and that changes in reabsorption of Na^+ are induced in the kidney without necessarily being due to a change in the ECF volume or external stimuli to the kidney. These adaptations, in turn, say something about flow rates per nephron and tubuloglomerular signals.

Appendix

Detailed Analysis of Events in the Inner Medulla

- In the inner medulla, the concentration of urea in the interstitial compartment becomes progressively higher toward the papillary tip.
- The interstitial $[Na^+]$ is virtually identical at all levels of the inner medulla.

The $[Na^+]$ remains close to 300 mmol/L in the interstitial fluid at all levels of the inner medulla despite the fact that hyponatric fluids are added to this compartment from the IMCD and the DTL of the LOH. Moreover, there is no active transport of Na^+ from the ATL of the LOH. To understand how this might operate, a series of unique permeabilities of the medullary structures are summarized in Table 6.11. As shown in Figure 6.8, the concentration of urea rises dramatically in the interstitial fluid toward the papillary tip. Nevertheless, by answering the following questions, it should become clear what accounts for the rise in the concentration of urea in the inner medulla.

PCT = Proximal convoluted tubule.

LOH = Loop of Henle

DTL = Descending thin limb of the loop of Henle

ATL = Ascending thin limb of the loop of Henle

DCT = Distal convoluted tubule

CCD = Cortical collecting duct

MCD = Medullary collecting duct

IMCD = Inner medullary collecting duct

QUESTIONS

(Discussions on pages 275–276)

6.25 *What process leads to a rise in the osmolality of the interstitial fluid?*

TABLE 6.11 **Unique Permeabilities in the Inner Medulla**

For this analysis, assume ADH has led to the insertion of a water (AQP-2) and urea (VRUT) transporter in the luminal membrane of the IMCD permitting water and urea to reach virtual diffusion equilibirum.

	Permeability		
Structure	**Water**	**NaCl**	**Urea**
Loop of Henle			
Descending thin limb	Yes	Modest	Modest
Ascending thin limb	Modest	Yes	Modest
Outer medullary collecting duct	Yes*	No	No
Inner medullary collecting duct	Yes*	No	Yes (at tip)*

*If ADH is present

6.26 *How can a nephron segment add solute without water to the interstitial fluid?*

6.27 *What solutes are added from the ATL of the LOH?*

6.28 *How will the [Na⁺] and [Cl⁻] in the interstitial fluid be lowered given the permeabilities outlined in Table 6.11?*

6.29 *What is the impact of the higher interstitial osmolality on water movement in the DTL and the IMCD?*

Discussion of Questions

6.25 What process leads to a rise in the osmolality of the interstitial fluid?

To raise the osmolality, one must either add solute and/or remove water. Because the purpose of the inner medulla is to cause water to move from the IMCD into the interstitial fluid, the way to raise the osmolality is to add solute *without* water to the interstitial fluid (see margin note).

Note
The force that causes water to move from the IMCD to the interstitial fluid is the higher osmolality in the interstitial compartment.

6.26 How can a nephron segment add solute without water to interstitial fluid?

Solute must be added from a water-impermeable nephron segment. This addition can come from only the ATL of the LOH (see Table 6.11).

6.27 What solutes are added from the ATL of the LOH?

The major solutes added from the ATL are Na⁺ and Cl⁻. Because these ions must enter by passive diffusion, the [Na⁺] and [Cl⁻] must be higher in the lumen than in the interstitial fluid. This can occur in two ways; either the [Na⁺] and/or [Cl⁻] in the interstitial compartment falls, or one or both of their concentrations in the lumen of the ATL rise. The traditional explanation is that a higher osmolality in interstitial fluid draws water out of the DTL, and this raises its luminal [Na⁺]. Notwithstanding, this conclusion cannot be correct because the rise in osmolality in the interstitial fluid in the inner medulla has not occurred yet. Therefore, the first step is to lower the [Na⁺] and [Cl⁻] in the interstitial fluid.

6.28 How will the [Na⁺] and [Cl⁻] in the interstitial fluid be lowered given the permeabilities outlined in Table 6.11?

The answer is: reabsorb urea plus water from the IMCD because both are permeable here. The fluid absorbed from the IMCD has the same osmolality as that of the interstitial fluid, but it is Na⁺ and Cl⁻–poor; the osmoles are urea. The net result is a larger volume in the interstitial fluid, a lower [Na⁺] and [Cl⁻], a higher concentration of urea, and the *same* total osmolality (Figure 6.12). A lower interstitial [Na⁺] favors diffusion of Na⁺ and Cl⁻ but not of water from the ATL (impermeable to water). Now the osmolality of the interstitial fluid rises (and that in the lumen of the ATL declines).

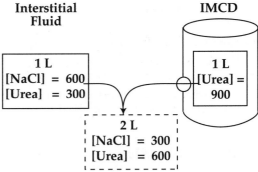

Figure 6.12 Effect of reabsorbing isosmolar urea from the IMCD.
Urea and water are permeable deep in the IMCD (the barrel-shaped structure). For illustrative purposes, the solid rectangles represent 1 L volumes of 900 mOsm/L solutions. When the 900 mOsm/L urea solution is added to the isosmolar interstitial fluid (also 1 L), the net result will be an interstitial fluid with 300 mOsm/L NaCl and 600 mOsm/L urea and a total volume of 2L (dashed rectangle). This lower [NaCl] creates the favorable concentration difference for Na^+ and Cl^- to diffuse from the ATL into the interstitial fluid and raise the osmolality in the interstitial fluid.

6.29 What is the impact of a higher interstitial osmolality on water movement in the DTL and the IMCD?

The DTL. This segment is more permeable to water than urea, so water will diffuse from its lumen into the medullary interstitial fluid where the osmolality is higher; as a result, the luminal $[Na^+]$ and $[Cl^-]$ rise. This secondary rise in luminal $[Na^+]$ and $[Cl^-]$ aids passive diffusion of $Na^+ + Cl^-$ out of the ATL after this fluid traverses the bend of the thin LOH.

The IMCD. In the IMCD, the higher osmolality in the interstitial fluid (as a result of the addition of $Na^+ + Cl^-$ from the ATL) permits more solute-free water to diffuse into the interstitial fluid, and this causes the concentration of urea to rise even further in the lumen as fluid descends deeper into the IMCD. Urea is an impermeable compound across the more proximal IMCD when this structure first enters the inner medulla, but it becomes permeable near the end of the nephron. Accordingly, both the high luminal concentration of urea in the IMCD and the ADH-induced permeability for urea here permit urea to enter the medullary interstitial compartment at the papillary tip.

Conclusions

1. The main change in interstitial fluid composition in the inner medulla is a higher concentration of urea.

2. Having a higher concentration of urea in the medullary interstitium permits a similar high concentration of urea in the lumen of the IMCD without obligating extra water to excrete it.

3. Having a high concentration of urea in the medullary interstitium leads to a higher urine osmolality, but as discussed in the following illustrative case examples, not necessarily to a better opportunity to conserve water.

Illustrative Examples

1. Criteria to assess renal concentrating ability at the bedside.

> - The minimum urine flow rate depends on the rate of excretion of "effective" osmoles.
> - The maximum value for urine osmolality is strongly influenced by the filtered load of urea (see margin note).

Clinical pearl
There are no normal values for urinary parameters, just "expected" values for a given clinical setting. If the blood urea nitrogen is very low, there will be a lower urine osmolality but not a lower urine tonicity when ADH acts.

Consider two people who must conserve water maximally; ADH acts, and they have "perfect" kidneys. One is eating a typical Western diet (high urea), and the other has ketoacid accumulation because of lack of food and water for 1 week (low urea). The composition of their urines is shown in Table 6.12.

TABLE 6.12 **Composition of the Urine During Water Deprivation**

Nutritional State	Volume L/Day	Urea mOsm/day	Urea mmol/L	Electrolytes mOsm/day	Osmolality mOsm/kg H_2O	Electrolytes
Fed	0.67	400	600	400	1200	$Na^+ + Cl^-$
Starved	0.5	75	150	300	750	$NH_4 + \beta\text{-HB}^-$

QUESTIONS

(Discussions on pages 278–279)

6.30 *What should be used as a "normal" value in the urine for the maximum urine osmolality?*

6.31 *Must the urine volume be lower if its osmolality is higher?*

6.32 *What are the determinants of the urine volume when ADH acts?*

6.33 *If urea is permeable across the IMCD, should it be included in an analysis of the control of the urine flow rate?*

2. Ensuring a small, but not too small, urine volume:

> - When ADH acts, the number of effective osmoles excreted ensures a minimum (but not absent) flow rate.
> - Oliguria without renal stone formation is the goal.

When there is a deficit of water, renal mechanisms are called into play to minimize a further loss of water. This response depends on ADH actions to increase the permeability of water and urea in the distal nephron and the renal events described earlier to have a maximum tonicity of the interstitial compartment of the medulla.

There is a second consideration for this response. On the one hand, the urine volume must be small to avoid increasing the deficit

Note
• Urine volume =

$$\frac{\#\ \text{"effective" osmoles}}{[\text{"Effective" osmoles}]}$$

• Substitute "non-urea" osmoles for "effective" osmoles in most circumstances. The non-urea osmolality is the urine osmolality minus [urea] in mmol/L.
• In states with a deficit of Na^+ and Cl^-, urea is virtually the sole osmole in the urine, and it becomes an effective osmole (see discussion of Question 6.35).

of water. On the other hand, the urine volume must be large enough to avoid stone formation. How excessive oliguria is avoided becomes evident from the equation in the margin note. When the osmolality (or, more properly, tonicity) of the urine is at its highest level, the only way to increase the volume is to have more "effective" urinary osmoles (tonomoles). Examples of the important tonomoles in the urine are shown in Table 6.13.

TABLE 6.13   **Urinary Solutes During Water Deprivation**

Setting	Tonomoles	Others
Normal diet	Na, Cl, K, NH_4^+	Urea
Prolonged fasting	NH_4^+, β-HB	Urea
NaCl deficit	Urea	None

QUESTIONS

(Discussions on pages 279–281)

6.34 *Given the information in Table 6.13, what effect would an infusion of 150 mmol of urea have on the urine flow rate and composition of normal persons who are water-deprived?*

6.35 *Given the information in Table 6.13, what effect would an infusion of urea have on the urine flow rate and composition of persons who have a deficit of Na^+, Cl^-, and water?*

6.36 *What ensures that the urine volume is not too low in persons who have fasted for a prolonged period?*

6.37 *Why might a high rate of excretion of glucose cause an increase in urine flow rate in normal, water-deprived persons?*

Discussion of Questions

6.30 What should be used as a "normal" value in the urine for the maximum urine osmolality?

The maximum value for the urine osmolality when ADH acts is determined in large part by what is eaten. In people on a typical Western diet, the value would be 1200 mOsm/kg H_2O, whereas it would be 750 mOsm/kg H_2O in people on a very low protein diet.

The nature of the "non-urea" osmoles may differ in the fed and fasted state; fed, they are Na^+ and Cl^-; fasted, they are NH_4^+ and ketoacid anions, for the most part.

6.31 Must the urine volume be lower if its osmolality is higher?

No. Note the starved person who has a lower urine volume despite a lower urine osmolality. Hence, another factor is important in addition to the urine osmolality. The other factor is the number of "effective" osmoles excreted (see discussion of Question 6.32).

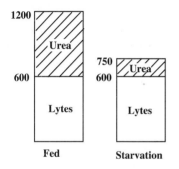

Figure 6.13 Urine osmolality during prolonged fasting. The height of each rectangle is the maximum urine osmolality; in normal subjects, the value was 1200 mOsm/kg H_2O, whereas it was only 750 mOsm/kg H_2O in fasted subjects. Nevertheless, the "nonurea" osmolalities are similar (clear areas marked "Lytes"); all that differs is the concentration of urea in the urine (hatched area).

6.32 What are the determinants of the urine volume when ADH acts?

When ADH acts, the urine volume is a function of its non-urea osmolality and the rate of excretion of non-urea osmoles (usually electrolytes). The major property of non-urea osmoles is that they are impermeable enough to maintain a concentration difference across the terminal IMCD. The non-urea osmolality in the urine and in the interstitial compartment was 600 mOsm/kg H_2O in both the fed and the chronically fasted persons (1200–600 and 750–150 mOsm/kg H_2O, respectively; Figure 6.13). Hence, the urine osmolality did not reveal why the urine flow rate was low because of the differences in the rate of excretion of urea. To interpret the urine osmolality when ADH acts, the best clue is to examine the plasma level of urea as well.

6.33 If urea is permeable across the IMCD, should it be included in an analysis of the control of the urine flow rate?

In the simplest form, the answer is: do not include urea as a determinant of urine flow. Nevertheless, urea may influence the urine flow rate because it led to a lower $[Na^+]$ and $[Cl^-]$ in the medullary interstitial fluid. To understand how this comes about, the handling of urea in the distal nephron will be reviewed. In the late DCT and CCD, water is reabsorbed under the influence of ADH. However, ADH does not induce urea permeability here. Thus, the concentration of urea in the luminal fluid rises progressively (same amount of urea but less water). As fluid descends in the MCD, the concentration of urea becomes higher than in the medullary interstitium. Uniquely in the IMCD, ADH induces urea permeability. Hence, some urea diffuses into the medullary interstitium, adding EFW to this area, and thereby lowering the $[Na^+]$ and $[Cl^-]$ here. There is also recycling of urea in the kidney, and this also contributes to the amount of urea + EFW added to the interstitial fluid near the papillary tip (Figure 6.14).

6.34 Given the information in Table 6.13, what effect would an infusion of 150 mmol of urea have on the urine flow rate and composition of normal persons who are water-deprived?

If urea is a permeable solute in the IMCD, excreting a little more urea should increase only the concentration of urea in

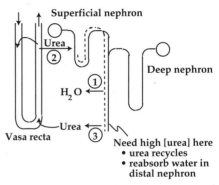

Figure 6.14 Urea recycling in the medulla. Urea recycles within the kidney so its concentration can be high in the inner medullary interstitium (and thereby in the urine without obligating extra water excretion). Absorption of water from the collecting duct (1) raises the concentration of urea in the lumen of the collecting duct. Adding urea to the DTL of superficial nephrons (2) also raises the concentration of urea in the lumen of the collecting duct. To complete this cycle, urea diffuses from the lumen of the IMCD (3) to the interstitial compartment, down its concentration difference. The net effect is to have a high concentration of urea in the interstitial fluid of the inner medulla; urea is "trapped" here by countercurrent exchange in the vasa recta.

the urine and not affect urine flow rate because urea is not an "effective" osmole in this setting. Data to substantiate this are provided in the following table from rats treated with ADH with and without the supplement of urea.

		Urine	
Urea Given	*Flow Rate μL/min*	*Urea mmol/L*	*Osmolality mOsm/L*
No	7	500	1500
Yes	7	1500	2500

6.35 Given the information in Table 6.13, what effect would an infusion of urea have on the urine flow rate and composition of persons who have a deficit of Na^+, Cl^-, and water?

An "effective" osmole is one that has a concentration difference across a membrane; "effective" osmoles also obligate water movement. When there is both water deprivation and a deficit of Na^+ and Cl^-, the urine contains few electrolytes, and urea is virtually its sole solute. Because the interstitial compartment at that horizontal plane has the same osmolality but contains an appreciable concentration of electrolytes, its concentration of urea must be lower than that in the lumen of the IMCD. Accordingly there is now a concentration difference for urea, higher in the IMCD than in the papillary interstitial compartment. Thus, urea seems to be an "effective" osmole when the urine is electrolyte-poor. Now excreting more urea obligates the excretion of more water or causes a much higher urine flow rate.

Urea Given	Urine		
	Flow Rate *μL/min*	*Urea* *mmol/L*	*Osmolality* *mOsm/L*
No	7	500	1500
Yes	21	500	1500

In contrast, when the urine contained many electrolytes, urea moved quickly enough to avoid a concentration difference between the lumen of the IMCD and the papillary interstitial compartment when ADH was present (urea is an "ineffective" osmole at this time). Hence, urea did not obligate the excretion of more water in the normal subjects (see discussion of Question 6.34).

6.36 What ensures that the urine volume is not too low in persons who have fasted for a prolonged period?

To have a urine flow rate, one needs "effective" osmoles in the urine; in prolonged fasting, these "effective" osmoles are NH_4^+ and β-HB (see Table 6.12). Hence, excreting NH_4^+ and β-HB protects against having too low a urine flow rate when ADH acts in prolonged fasting. This minimum urine volume will allow excretion of relatively insoluble solutes, such as uric acid, without kidney stones being formed.

6.37 Why might a high rate of excretion of glucose cause an increase in urine flow rate in normal, water-deprived persons?

There are two factors to consider in an osmotic diuresis. The first factor is the number of "effective" osmoles in the urine. With glucosuria, their number increases markedly. The second factor is the concentration of "effective" osmoles in the interstitial fluids. A high rate of excretion of glucose influences the $[Na^+]$ in interstitial fluid in two ways. First, when more glucose is delivered to the ATL of the LOH, it leads to less reabsorption of Na^+ here (it ensures a higher volume in the

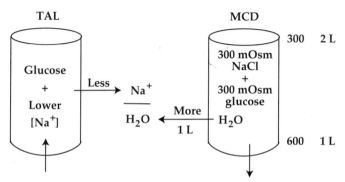

Figure 6.15　How an osmotic diuresis develops. There are two major effects: less reabsorption of Na^+ in the loop of Henle and more reabsorption of water from the MCD, both lowering the interstitial osmolality.

lumen and thereby a lower [Na^+] at any given osmolality). Second, when more "effective" osmoles are delivered to the MCD, more EFW will be reabsorbed for any given rise in osmolality. This in turn will lower the "effective osmolality" in the interstitial fluid, so the urine volume will be higher for any given rate of excretion of effective osmoles (Figure 6.15).

Bottom Line. There are two major reasons for an osmotic diuresis with glucosuria when ADH acts—more "effective" osmoles in the urine and a lower interstitial osmolality. The latter is due to a limited addition of Na^+ and an increased addition of EFW from the MCD.

OBJECTIVES

☐ To emphasize that *hyponatremia* indicates an increase in water relative to Na⁺ and implies expansion of the intracellular fluid (ICF) volume (unless the hyponatremia is due to hyperglycemia).

☐ To emphasize that two components are needed to develop hyponatremia: a source of electrolyte-free water (EFW) and antidiuretic hormone (ADH) to prevent the excretion of EFW. In acute hyponatremia, the clinical emphasis is on the source of EFW; in chronic hyponatremia, the clinical emphasis is on the reason ADH is present, both from a diagnostic and a therapeutic point of view.

☐ To provide a therapeutic approach to hyponatremia, emphasizing the important differences between acute and chronic hyponatremia and the risk of inappropriately aggressive therapy in the latter.

☐ To highlight the importance of tonicity balance for deciding why hyponatremia developed and where leverage can be exerted in therapy. This approach is facilitated by thinking in terms of EFW and isotonic solutions.

Hyponatremia
- Definition: [Na⁺] less than 136 mmol/L.
- Causes: Na⁺ loss and/or water gain.
- Hyponatremia without cell swelling indicates the presence of hyperglycemia or a laboratory error caused by hyperlipidemia or hyperproteinemia.
- When hyponatremia is present during hyperglycemia, some cells swell and others shrink.

Outline of Major Principles

1. With the exceptions of *pseudohyponatremia*, hyperglycemia, and a loss of certain K⁺ salts, hyponatremia indicates a net water shift into cells and swelling of cells. This shift is especially important in the central nervous system (CNS) because the brain is enclosed in a fixed space, and swelling may cause symptoms.

2. Hyponatremia is divided clinically into acute and chronic subtypes. This provides the rationale for anticipating dangers and selecting the correct plan for therapy.

   Acute Hyponatremia. The duration must be less than 48 hours (documented). The diagnostic issue is to identify the source of electrolyte-free water (EFW). The main danger is brain swelling. Treatment should be aggressive, with its aim being rapid reduction of the brain cell volume with hypertonic saline for the symptomatic patient who has a plasma [Na⁺] of less than 125 mmol/L. The classic example is hyponatremia that occurs in the first 48 hours after surgery.

   Chronic Hyponatremia. The diagnostic issue is to identify why antidiuretic hormone (ADH) is present. The main danger is overly aggressive therapy as brain cells have reduced their osmoles and thereby their volume. The goal is to raise the plasma [Na⁺] by up to 8 mmol/L per 24 hours. The physician can be more aggressive temporarily only if the patient is having a convulsion or is in a comatose state.

3. In virtually every patient with chronic hyponatremia, evidence of Na⁺ depletion and water gain can be found. A clinical aim is to find out which of these processes is the primary one. Excessive EFW intake alone is virtually never the primary cause of hypona-

Pseudohyponatremia
A condition in which the Na⁺-to-water ratio in plasma is normal, but the laboratory reports hyponatremia because the nonaqueous phase of plasma (protein or lipids) is increased, and Na⁺ are distributed only in the aqueous phase (discussed in detail later).

Notes
- The [Na⁺] is the Na⁺-to-H₂O ratio.
- Hyponatremia indicates swelling of cells. This is virtually the only time in clinical medicine that the *denominator* of the ratio is more important than the *numerator* in providing critical information (e.g., glucose concentration).
- A Na⁺ deficit means ECF volume contraction, and a Na⁺ excess means ECF volume expansion.

Note
The therapeutic aggressiveness for the correction of hyponatremia is determined by its acuteness and/or the presence of serious symptoms (seizure, coma)—not by the plasma [Na⁺].

tremia because normal kidneys can excrete close to 12 L of EFW/day. Nevertheless, the amount of water intake in relation to the rate of excretion of EFW is a critical factor that contributes to the development of hyponatremia. Reduced EFW excretion is usually due to ADH. In some patients with chronic hyponatremia, a negative balance for Na^+ is the primary event; the resultant extracellular fluid (ECF) volume contraction leads to ADH release. Treatment is now primarily Na^+ replacement (isotonic to the patient) if the ECF volume is low. Beware of a rapid excretion of water once the ECF volume is reexpanded (ADH level falls).

4. There can be no specific therapy for hyponatremia because it can be associated with different diseases and clinical settings. The emphasis for therapy can be to create either a negative balance for EFW and/or a positive balance for Na^+, depending on the ECF volume. The underlying disorder will require specific treatment.

INTRODUCTORY CASE
Water, Water, Everywhere, So Not a Drop to Drink
(Case discussed on page 306)

Five days ago, a previously healthy young man developed aseptic meningitis accompanied by frequent vomiting. He had taken no medications. Physical examination revealed ECF volume contraction on day 3, but the volume was normal on day 5. Laboratory results are summarized as follows.

		Day 3	Day 5
Plasma			
Na^+	mmol/L	130	117
K^+	mmol/L	3.1	4.0
Cl^-	mmol/L	87	83
HCO_3^-	mmol/L	33	24
Osmolality	mOsm/kg H_2O	270	245
Glucose	mmol/L (mg/dL)	5.0 (90)	3.0 (54)
Creatinine	mmol/L (mg/dL)	200 (2.3)	90 (1.0)
Urine			
Na^+	mmol/L	60	50
Cl^-	mmol/L	6	48
Osmolality	mosm/kg H_2O	450	407

Note
To use the urine electrolytes in a more sophisticated way to determine the basis for a contracted ECF volume, see Table 4.5.

Could Na^+ loss have caused the hyponatremia on day 3?
   Why was the ADH level elevated on day 3?
   Why was the plasma [Na^+] lower on day 5?
   Was the ADH level higher on day 5?
   What are the best urine electrolytes to indicate whether the ECF volume is contracted?
   Would your answer change if the patient had vomiting or diarrhea?

PART A

PART A

Clinical Approach

Background

Plasma [Na⁺] Reflects ICF Volume

Note
A "Na⁺-like" particle is one that is largely restricted to the ECF.

The intracellular fluid (ICF) volume, which can be deduced from the plasma [Na⁺], is contracted in hypernatremia and expanded in hyponatremia. There are several exceptions to this rule, such as pseudohyponatremia and the addition of a "Na⁺-like" particle to the ECF, such as glucose or mannitol (*translocational hyponatremia*; see margin note).

In the presence of pseudohyponatremia, the *"effective" plasma osmolality* (Na⁺-to-plasma water ratio) and the ICF volume are normal, but the Na⁺-to-total volume of plasma is low because of a gain of nonaqueous volume of plasma (protein and/or lipid). The problem is that the laboratory uses plasma volume, not plasma water, as the denominator of this ratio (see the discussion of Question 7.1).

Note
A "Na⁺-like" particle is one that is largely restricted to the ECF.

Translocational hyponatremia
This is due to a shift of water from the ICF to the ECF. There are two subtypes:
• Addition of particles to the ECF that are obligated to remain in the ECF (the best example is hyperglycemia);
• Loss of particles from the ICF (K⁺ salts).

"Effective" osmolality of plasma
The aspect of osmolality that causes the movement of water across cell membranes. When determining the "effective" osmolality of plasma, ignore the contribution of urea and ethanol because they do not influence water shifts across cell membranes.

Na⁺ Content Reflects ECF Volume

Sodium, an osmole that is largely restricted to the ECF, keeps water out of cells; thus, the Na⁺ content determines the ECF volume because Na⁺ (and attending anions) are the principal solutes of the ECF.

Renal Response to Na⁺ Loss

The appropriate renal response to a Na⁺ deficit (ECF volume contraction) is to avoid additional excretion of Na⁺, Cl⁻, or water in the urine. Check for these responses: the urine should have a very low [Na⁺] and [Cl⁻], and the urine osmolality should be high (a reduced "effective" vascular volume leads to ADH release).

Renal Response to Water Excess

Note
Compare urine osmolality to the "expected" value, not to plasma osmolality.

The appropriate renal response to water excess is to excrete the maximum volume of maximally dilute urine (20–80 mOsm/kg H₂O) (see margin note). If this response is not observed, suspect that ADH is acting (seek the cause) or that the kidneys are abnormal.

QUESTIONS

(Discussions on pages 317–318)

7.1 *What laboratory methods to measure the [Na⁺] in plasma will provide a lower value if hyperlipidemia is present?*

7.2 *A diabetic patient has renal failure. His blood sugar is 1000 mg/dL (55 mmol/L), [Na⁺] is 127 mmol/L, and blood urea nitrogen is 70 mg/dL (urea is 25 mmol/L). What is his calcu-*

lated plasma osmolality? Has hyperglycemia changed his ECF and/or ICF volumes?

7.3 *In what circumstances will the plasma osmolality help or be misleading with respect to diagnosis in a patient with hyponatremia?*

7.4 *Three patients have hyponatremia (120 mmol/L). In case A, it is due to water gain; in case B, Na⁺ loss; in case C, hyperglycemia. Which patient(s) will have swelling of brain cells? Give reasons for your answer.*

Classification of Hyponatremia

- Separate into acute and chronic hyponatremia (see margin note).
- In acute hyponatremia, the critical question is, "What is the source of EFW?"
- In chronic hyponatremia, the critical question is, "Why is ADH present?"
- Treat acute hyponatremia aggressively to reduce brain cell swelling; raise the plasma [Na⁺] to 130–135 mmol/L.
- Treat chronic hyponatremia slowly to avoid osmotic demyelination; raise the plasma [Na⁺] by <8 mmol/L/day. Beware: A water diuresis may occur after correcting ECF volume contraction.

Basis for the different approach to acute and chronic hyponatremia
Acute: There was insufficient time for brain cells to lose important intracellular particles. Hence, brain cells are swollen, and the danger is from an acute rise in intracranial pressure.
Chronic: The brain has undergone cell volume regulation by losing osmoles. Brain cells are now near-normal in size, and these cells are at risk of shrinkage with overaggressive therapy, inducing osmotic demyelination.

When faced with a patient with hyponatremia, the most critical decision to make is whether the problem is an acute or chronic one (see margin note). These two entities represent very different pathophysiologic conditions, pose different risks, and require a very different therapeutic approach (Figure 7.1, Table 7.1).

Basis for hyponatremia
1. Source of EFW.
2. ADH to prevent the excretion of EFW.
Seek the reason for each of these components of hyponatremia.

Acute Hyponatremia

- The major risk is a rise in intracranial pressure and herniation of the brain.

TABLE 7.1 **Time Frame Classification of Hyponatremia**

	Duration	**Common Setting**	**Risk**	**Therapy**
Acute	<48 h	• Post-operative	• Brain-cell swelling	• Hypertonic saline; raise plasma [Na⁺] by up to 5 mmol/L
Chronic	Unknown or >48 h	• Many	• Osmotic demyelination	• Raise plasma [Na⁺] <8 mmol/L/day

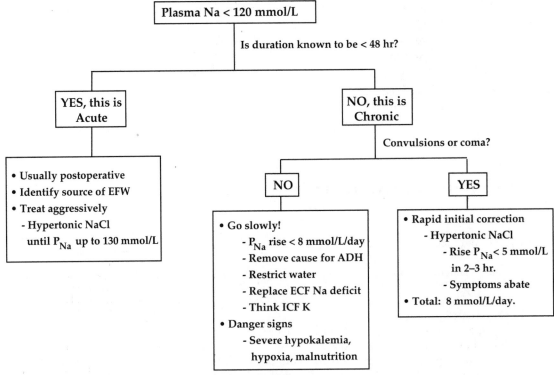

Figure 7.1   First steps in a patient with hyponatremia. First identify whether this is acute hyponatremia. Aggressive therapy is recommended only for acute or severely symptomatic hyponatremia. (1997. *The Acid Truth and Basic Facts,* 4th ed., ML Halperin, RossMark Medical Publishers, Stirling, Ontario, Canada.)

Response to brain-cell swelling
The initial defense is a lower cerebrospinal fluid volume, but this provides only a limited capacity to deal with brain-cell swelling.

Acute hyponatremia develops in less than 48 hours, so there is insufficient time for swollen brain cells to shrink their volume. Due to the physical restriction imposed by the cranial vault, there is a rise in intracranial pressure causing central nervous symptoms that may become serious (seizures, coma, and ultimately respiratory arrest and irreversible brain damage).

TABLE 7.2   **Classification of Hyponatremia**

Acute Hyponatremia (<48-h Duration)
1. Source of EFW:
   • Exogenous (intravenous or oral)
   • Endogenous = desalination of intravenous or body fluids
     • Acute postoperative period
     • Cerebral salt wasting
     • Thiazide diuretics in an edematous patient (see margin note)
     • Giving isotonic saline to a patient with SIADH
2. Reason for ADH being present (see Table 7.3)

Thiazides and acute hyponatremia
Thiazides in this setting lead to a large excretion of Na^+, but ADH prevents the excretion of EFW (see Figure 7.2).

Chronic Hyponatremia
1. Source of EFW is always needed, but usually is not the most important component of the problem.
2. Reason for ADH:
   • Low "effective" ECF volume
   • Pain, anxiety, nausea, psychosis
   • Endocrine reasons (adrenal, thyroid, pituitary)
   • Metabolic disorder (e.g., porphyria)
   • Drugs
   • None of the above (see Table 7.3)

> • In acute hyponatremia, the emphasis is on the source of EFW; the cause for ADH release is usually obvious.

The most common setting for acute and potentially life-threatening hyponatremia is in the intra- and postoperative setting, and thus most of these cases occur in hospital (Table 7.2). There are three obvious sources of EFW:

1. The most common is the administration of glucose in water (D_5W) or hypotonic saline as intravenous (IV) fluids (virtually always a mistake in the perioperative period).

2. The "kindly administered" ice chips or sips of water (also a mistake in the perioperative period).

3. The generation of EFW by *desalination* when isotonic or hypotonic saline is administered. For the latter to occur, the kidney must excrete urine that is hypertonic to the infusate (or to body fluids in the absence of polyuria) (Figure 7.2).

There are four settings in which desalination can cause acute hyponatremia. These are summarized in Table 7.2.

D_5W
A solution of glucose in water with close to the same osmolality as body fluids but not the same tonicity once glucose is metabolized. It contains 5 g of glucose per 100 mL, or 50 g of glucose per liter.

QUESTIONS

(Discussions on pages 319–320)

7.5 *How can the kidney generate 1 L of EFW if isotonic saline is the only fluid administered?*

7.6 *If a person on a low-salt diet has surgery, what features might be present in the postoperative period to minimize the degree of hyponatremia in the acute postoperative period?*

7.7 *A patient had surgery. Although the plasma [Na^+] was in the range of 139–141 mmol/L 1 week before surgery, the preoperative plasma [Na^+] was 136 mmol/L. Why? The plasma [Na^+] was 128 mmol/L 36 hours after surgery. Why?*

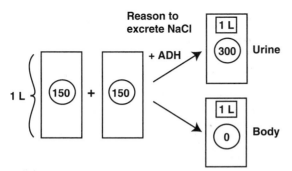

Desalination
Overgenerous administration of isotonic fluids during the pre- and postoperative period may be dangerous in the face of ADH release.

Figure 7.2 Generation of EFW by desalination. The rectangles represent 1 L volumes, and the [Na^+] in each liter is shown inside the rectangle. The two rectangles on the left represent intravenous infusion of isotonic saline. The top rectangle on the right represents 1 L of hypertonic urine, and the bottom rectangle on the right represents 1 L of EFW generated and retained in the body due to ADH actions. (1997. *The Acid Truth and Basic Facts,* 4th ed., ML Halperin, RossMark Medical Publishers, Stirling, Ontario, Canada.)

7.8 *What volume of an IV solution containing 856 mmol/L Na$^+$ (5% saline) must be infused to raise the plasma [Na$^+$] by 1 mmol/L in a 70-kg patient? (Ignore the water infused, for simplicity.)*

Prevention

Tonicity balance
• Consider both input and output. By calculating a tonicity balance, one can understand why hyponatremia develops and devise a more rational plan for its therapy.
1. Input of Na$^+$, K$^+$, and water
2. Output of Na$^+$, K$^+$, and water

• Apply the principles of a tonicity balance:
1. Input message: Do not give EFW.
2. Output message: A "good" urine output is a danger sign for acute hyponatremia if that urine is hypertonic.

The general principles of fluid management in these conditions can now be appreciated; for example, the best way to avoid postoperative hyponatremia is:

1. Do not give solutions that are hypotonic to the urine if polyuria is present; do not give solutions that are hypotonic to body fluids in the oliguric patient.

2. Give isotonic fluids only to replace losses and to maintain hemodynamics.

3. Be very suspicious of a "good" urine output because this might be hypertonic to the infused solutions and generate EFW (see Figure 7.2). In this regard, monitor the plasma [Na$^+$] in settings associated with ADH release (Table 7.3), particularly in patients who excrete more than 1–2 L of urine per day.

TABLE 7.3 **Causes of High ADH Levels in Patients with Hyponatremia**

ADH Release in Response to Physiologic Stimuli

Low "effective" circulating volume:
  ECF volume depletion
  Blood loss
  Hypoalbuminemia
  Low cardiac output
Excessive pain, nausea, vomiting, or anxiety.

ADH Release Without a Physiologic Stimulus

Prostaglandins
Prostaglandins antagonize ADH action by inhibiting the formation of cyclic AMP. The synthesis of prostaglandin, stimulated by ADH, diminishes the ADH-induced cyclic AMP rise. In addition, the vasodilator action of prostaglandin increases medullary flow, which lowers medullary hyperosmolality. These actions of prostaglandins promote the excretion of a less concentrated urine.

CNS or lung lesions
Neoplasms and granulomas such as tuberculosis
Metabolic lesions such as acute intermittent porphyria
Administration of agents that simulate ADH:
  DDAVP (e.g., treatment for diabetes insipidus or urinary incontinence)
  Oxytocin for labor induction
Drugs that augment or stimulate ADH release:
  Examples include nicotine, morphine, clofibrate, tricyclic antidepressants, and antineoplastic agents (probably via nausea and emesis)
Drugs that promote the actions of ADH on the kidney by increasing cyclic AMP levels or its bioactivity:
  Examples include oral hypoglycemics (e.g., chlorpropamide), methylxanthines (e.g., caffeine, aminophylline), analgesics that inhibit prostaglandin synthesis (e.g., aspirin, nonsteroidal anti-inflammatory drugs; see margin note)

4. Be extremely cautious with the volume given to a smaller patient; this is especially important in females, because acute hyponatremia may be more dangerous in menstruant females (see margin note).

Therapy for Acute Hyponatremia

> • Shrink the size of brain cells with hypertonic saline.

The immediate goal is to shrink the expanded ICF volume of the brain sufficiently to curtail the serious CNS symptoms (see margin note). Administer hypertonic saline until the plasma $[Na^+]$ is close to 130 mmol/L. When calculating the amount of Na^+ required, assume that the volume "behaves" as if the Na^+ is dissolved in total body water, because the cell membrane is permeable to water and not Na^+.

Example: Emergency Treatment for a Patient with a Seizure Due to Acute Hyponatremia

A 50-kg person with acute postoperative hyponatremia (plasma $[Na^+]$ is 120 mmol/L) is having a seizure 24 hours after surgery. The aim is to shrink the size of brain cells acutely to a level before seizures occurred. A reasonable target is to raise the plasma $[Na^+]$ by 5 mmol/L during the next hour. To raise the plasma $[Na^+]$ by 5 mmol/L, 150 mmol of Na^+ must be administered because the total body water is 30 L (60% of body weight). Because 1 L of 5% saline contains 856 mmol of Na^+, 175 mL will be required to achieve this aim (see margin note). After the seizure is controlled, slow the rate of infusion, raising the $[Na^+]$ to 130 mmol/L at the rate of 1–2 mmol/L/h.

Prevention of a Further Fall in Natremia

Once the plasma $[Na^+]$ has reached 130 mmol/L, maintain it at this level until the reason for ADH release has abated. Using a tonicity balance approach, there are two general strategies to prevent a further fall in natremia in a patient who is excreting a large volume of hypertonic urine.

Strategy Focusing on Input. If the input is equal to the output with respect to Na^+, K^+ and water, there will be no change in the plasma $[Na^+]$. For example, if hypertonic urine is being excreted, the same volume and same composition of hypertonic saline must be administered.

Strategies Focusing on Output. The aim is to lower the $[Na^+ + K^+]$ in the urine so that isotonic fluids can be administered. If the patient's urine excretion is hypertonic, it can be rendered isotonic with a loop or osmotic (urea) diuretic, and isotonic IV fluids can be administered at the same rate as the urine output. Once the reason for the ADH release is no longer present, this therapy will not be required—the patient will begin to excrete dilute urine, and hence the plasma $[Na^+]$ will rise.

Impact of body size
• Larger patient (70 kg, 40 L total body water)
  —Deficit 400 mmoles $Na^+ + K^+$
  ∴ Fall in plasma $[Na^+]$ = 400 mmol/40 L = 10 mmol/L
• Smaller patient (35 kg, 20 L total body water)
  —Same deficit
  ∴ Fall in plasma $[Na^+]$ = 400 mmol/20 L = 20 mmol/L

Clinical pearl
Use hypertonic saline to avoid desalination of isotonic saline and worsening of acute hyponatremia.

Volume of distribution of Na^+
As the $[Na^+]$ in the ECF rises, water leaves the ICF, raising its osmolality to equal that in the ECF. Therefore, calculate the volume of distribution as if total body water were the actual denominator.

Dose of Na^+
• To raise the plasma $[Na^+]$ by 5 mmol/L in a 50-kg person (total body water 30 L), administer 150 mmol Na^+. Because hypertonic saline (5%) has 856 mmol Na^+/L, 150 mmol of Na^+ is found in 175 mL (150/856 × 1000 mL).
• In addition, replace ongoing renal losses.

Hypertonic saline
• Some physicians hesitate to give hypertonic saline, fearing the risk of osmotic demyelination syndrome (ODS) (not a problem in acute hyponatremia) or acute ECF volume expansion. Often, isotonic saline is given because it is still hypertonic to the patient. This logic is incorrect because one must match the tonicity of infused solutions to that of the urine in polyuric states (a tonicity balance).
• The risk of isotonic saline is that in the presence of ADH the patient may "desalinate" it and make hyponatremia worse (see Figure 7.2).
• The risk to the ECF volume stems from the absolute number of mmol of Na^+ administered, not its concentration.

Gender Issues in Acute Hyponatremia

- Hyponatremia has different implications in females and males.
- Examine the basis for the hyponatremia.

Acute Hyponatremia in Females

Most commonly, this follows otherwise uneventful gynecologic surgery, which leads to the sustained release of ADH. The ill-advised infusion of D_5W completes the picture (source of EFW). The severity of hyponatremia may become a major problem because the volumes given are not scaled down to body size.

Bottom Line. This form of acute hyponatremia leads to brain-cell swelling; rarely, intracranial pressure is so high that certain patients die.

Acute Hyponatremia in Males

The list of causes is short and determined by which males frequently undergo surgery. The most common setting for males is prostate gland resection. Obviously, this population is different from females in gender and age, but let us examine the basis for, and impact of, this type of hyponatremia on brain-cell volume before drawing conclusions about gender and age.

Basis for Hyponatremia. The main reason for hyponatremia in this setting is that half-isotonic solutions of organic compounds were used to lavage the prostatic bed, and many liters may be absorbed (see Question 7.10). Hence, there are now two reasons to develop hyponatremia; they become obvious after dividing the absorbed fluid into its two constituent parts (see margin note).

1. Osmole-free (and electrolyte-free) water. This is simple EFW gain that causes cells to swell. It has the same impact as the infused hypotonic fluid in females, but it is not the major cause for the hyponatremia (see Question 7.10).

2. Isosmolar fluid. Solutes such as mannitol, glycerol, and glycine do not cross cell membranes at an appreciable rate. Hence, they remain in the ECF and because they are Na^+-free, they cause hyponatremia. This form of hyponatremia is not associated with brain-cell swelling nor will it pose a threat of brain herniation. One needs to be somewhat more cautious interpreting events with glycine (see Question 7.10).

Calculation 1: Gain of EFW
For illustrative purposes, there is a 10% expansion of total body water (30 L) with EFW (3 L).
Intracellular fluid volume (ICFV) rises from 20 to 22 L.
Extracellular fluid volume (ECFV) rises from 10 to 11 L.
Plasma $[Na^+]$ declines from 140 to 127 mmol/L.

Calculation 2: Gain of mannitol
For illustrative purposes, there is a 10% expansion of total body water (30 L) as a half-isosmotic solution (3 L).
ICFV rises from 20 to 21 L.
ECFV rises from 10 to 12 L.
Plasma $[Na^+]$ declines from 140 to 116 mmol/L (see Figure 7.6).

Lavage fluid and gender
This lavage fluid hyponatremia also occurs in females who have conditions such as endometriosis in which nonelectrolyte lavage solutions are instilled into the peritoneal cavity so that cautery can be used during the surgical procedure.

QUESTIONS

(Discussions on pages 320–321)

7.9 *Why do surgeons use solutions that are electrolyte-free to lavage the prostatic bed during a transurethral prostatic resection? (Hint: There is considerable bleeding in this procedure.)*

7.10 *A 50-kg patient (total body water 30 L) absorbed and retained 3 L of a half–iso-osmotic solution of mannitol during his transurethral resection of the prostate (TURP). What is the*

*quantitative role of mannitol and EFW in causing his hypona-
tremia (plasma [Na$^+$] fell from 140 mmol/L to 113 mmol/L)?
What happens to the ICF volume and plasma [Na$^+$] once the
mannitol is excreted as a 300 mOsm/kg H$_2$O solution?*

7.11 *Should hyponatremia in patients who undergo a TURP be
classified as a form of translocational hyponatremia similar to
that of hyperglycemia?*

7.12 *What properties of glycine make this compound unique in the
pathogenesis of the post-TURP hyponatremia syndrome?*

Hyponatremia with Primary Polydipsia

Normally, one cannot become hyponatremic simply from drinking
EFW because ADH will not be present. In the absence of ADH,
normal kidneys can excrete close to 1 L of EFW per hour, more
than almost anyone can drink. Nevertheless, if there is a reason for
ADH release such as a low ECF volume, anxiety, or psychosis,
ingestion of EFW will result in hyponatremia. A discussion of
hyponatremia in an infant follows, and a second example is provided
in Case 7.3.

QUESTION

(Discussion on page 322)

7.13 *How much water must a normal person drink to produce
hyponatremia? Would it matter if this person is on a low-
salt diet?*

Hyponatremia in an Infant

Apart from unique disorders such as inborn errors, hyponatremia in
this setting is most commonly due to a loss of Na$^+$ (e.g., in
diarrhea). ADH is released in response to the contracted ECF
volume and leads to the retention of the water that is ingested. If a
hyponatremic infant is fed sugar water to "rest the GI tract" and
avoid dehydration, this EFW will be retained. Thus, hyponatremia
has two components—Na$^+$ loss and water gain—and its degree may
be very severe. The primary aims during therapy are to reexpand the
ECF rapidly and to return the ICF to normal more slowly. The
problem to be aware of is that ADH levels might fall precipitously
once the ECF volume is reexpanded and may therefore yield a very
rapid water diuresis. If the plasma [Na$^+$] rises too rapidly, ODS
could occur; to avoid this problem, a fast-acting ADH preparation
should be available for use.

Dehydration
The authors dislike this term
because it is ambiguous. To some,
it means a lack of water, but to
others it means a deficit of ECF
volume.

Chronic Hyponatremia

* The danger is that too rapid a rise in the plasma [Na$^+$] will
  lead to osmotic demyelination.

Osmotic demyelination syndrome (ODS)

A symmetrical demyelination commonly involving the base of the pons. Clinically, there is a wide spectrum of presentations, ranging from the absence of symptoms to a devastating disorder characterized by confusion, agitation, and, eventually, flaccid or spastic quadriparesis. This disorder may be accompanied by bulbar involvement. It is usually observed after therapy for hyponatremia, and the incidence rises sharply if the hyponatremia is corrected too rapidly. Hyponatremic patients with a poor nutritional condition or those with hypokalemia seem more likely to develop ODS. ODS may occur in patients with disorders other than hyponatremia. The diagnosis can be confirmed by magnetic resonance imaging scanning, including coronal views. There is no known treatment, and the mortality and morbidity rates are high.

Why a malnourished patient may have a greater risk during therapy

The malnourished patient requires exogenous organic osmolytes to replace those lost when hyponatremia developed. Failure to supply these can result in brain-cell shrinkage when hyponatremia is corrected; this might help explain the susceptibility of these patients to ODS following even slow correction of hyponatremia.

Chronic hyponatremia is the most common electrolyte abnormality in hospitalized patients, but these patients rarely have significant symptoms specifically related to this electrolyte disorder. The patient with chronic hyponatremia is often identified by the determination of "routine" electrolytes; the duration of the disorder is unknown. The fundamental issue is that adaptive responses have had time to occur, the most important of which are in the brain. Brain cells have returned their ICF volume virtually to normal. In this latter regard, the mechanism in the first day or so is the export of ions (K^+ and Cl^-). During the next few days, organic molecules such as *myo*-inositol, amino acids, and alcohols are exported. This latter information provides the rationale for deciding the rate of correction of hyponatremia (see margin note). The critical issue is that these volume-regulated cells are at risk of actual contraction if the plasma [Na^+] is raised too rapidly, because these cells do not have available organic osmolytes to reestablish their normal ICF osmole composition. A patient with poor nutrition may take an even longer time to obtain these intracellular organic osmolytes (see margin note). If correction is too rapid, this can lead to the devastating neurological syndrome ODS (see margin note).

Diagnostic Issues

To develop hyponatremia, a source of EFW (usually the ingestion of water) coupled with a limitation to its excretion (release of ADH) must be present. Virtually everyone drinks EFW so one need not dwell on this for diagnostic purposes unless the intake is very large. The issue is why the rate of excretion of EFW is so low. The diagnostic challenge to the physician is to identify the basis for the release of ADH (see Table 7.3; Figure 7.3).

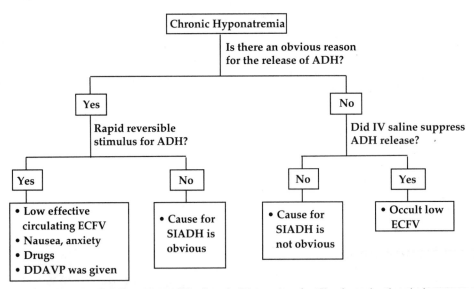

Figure 7.3   Steps to take in the patient with chronic hyponatremia. The focus in chronic hyponatremia is to determine why ADH is present. If the reason for the release of ADH is reversible, a patient might be at risk of having a water diuresis when the release of ADH is suppressed—e.g., when the ECF volume is reexpanded.

QUESTIONS

(Discussions on pages 322–323)

7.14 *Match the four separate causes of hyponatremia with the critical parameter for diagnosis.*

Etiology	Critical Parameter Measured
(1) Chronic diuretic intake	(a) Normal plasma osmolality
(2) Hyperlipidemia	(b) Normal ECF volume and low urine osmolality
(3) Excess ADH	(c) ECF volume contraction and hypokalemia
(4) Compulsive water consumption	(d) Low plasma and high urine osmolality

7.15 *What is the average urine osmolality in a 24-hour urine sample from a normal subject? Is the urine composition in a patient with SIADH different? If so, in what way?*

7.16 *What conclusions can be drawn when the urine osmolality is high?*

Seek Reason for ADH (see Figure 7.3)

> • Is the effective circulating volume adequate?
> • Not always easy to answer with confidence.

When a low "effective" vascular volume is sensed, ADH is released even if hyponatremia is present (see margin note). Because thirst is also stimulated by a low ECF volume, both a source of EFW and ADH to prevent its excretion are present. The problem is that a clinician may have great difficulty in deciding whether the "effective" ECF volume is contracted unless the changes are marked.

Deducing Whether the "Effective" ECF Volume is Contracted

One can use clues from the clinical story to suggest that there is a contracted "effective" ECF volume. First, there may be a loss of Na^+. The most common renal cause is the ingestion of a diuretic; less often, renal salt wasting and/or an osmotic diuretic (glucose, urea) may cause Na^+ loss. At this point, one should examine the rate of K^+ excretion. A low $[K^+]$ in urine in the face of renal Na^+ loss and ECF volume contraction should suggest low aldosterone bioactivity (see Chapter 9 for details). In contrast, a high $[K^+]$ in urine with renal Na^+ wasting suggests that the abnormal loss of Na^+ occurred in the proximal convoluted tubule, loop of Henle, or early distal convoluted tubule.

Loss of Na^+ can occur via nonrenal and renal mechanisms. The nonrenal sources are usually obvious (gastrointestinal tract, skin) and should be suspected when the urine is virtually Na^+- and/or Cl^+-free all the time.

Pathophysiology
• Na^+ maintain the ECF volume.
• Loss of Na^+ (ECF volume) stimulates ADH release.
• ADH prevents the excretion of EFW.

Problem for diagnosis
The patient who poses the major problem for diagnosis is one in whom the clinician cannot be sure whether the "effective" ECF volume is contracted.

> - A patient need not have a reduced ECF volume to release ADH on a "volume basis."

Even if the total ECF volume is normal or high, the arterial blood may not be "pumped in an optimum fashion" by the heart. The "effective" circulating volume is decreased either when the overall ECF volume is reduced or when the ECF volume is maldistributed such that there is insufficient volume in the "effective" vascular compartment (edema states, e.g., hypoalbuminemia). A second type of maldistribution occurs when the arterial volume is low and the venous volume is high (when there is a primary decrease in cardiac function; see Table 7.3).

Clinical Clues Concerning the ECF Volume

"Effective" circulating volume
The term refers to the critical component of the ECF required for adequate tissue perfusion (notice the vague terms in this description).

There are four laboratory tests that may suggest that the "effective" circulating volume is contracted.

1. Plasma [K$^+$]

> - In the syndrome of inappropriate ADH secretion (SIADH), the plasma [K$^+$] is usually normal.

SIADH
A syndrome in which ADH is present and acting but the two primary stimuli for its release (hypernatremia and low "effective" circulating volume) are absent.

When the ECF volume is low, release of aldosterone results in renal K$^+$ loss. This loss is especially high when volume and HCO$_3^-$ delivery to the cortical collecting duct are high. Therefore, diuretic-induced or vomiting-induced hyponatremia should be suspected if hypokalemia is present. In contrast to the above, suspect states with low levels of aldosterone if hyponatremia is accompanied by hyperkalemia.

2. Plasma [HCO$_3^-$]

> - In SIADH, the plasma [HCO$_3^-$] is usually normal.

The plasma HCO$_3^-$ may be high in vomiting or in diuretic-induced hyponatremia (metabolic alkalosis). In contrast, hyponatremia of hypoaldosteronism is generally accompanied by a mild fall in the plasma [HCO$_3^-$] (to close to 20 mmol/L) because of a low excretion of NH$_4^+$ consequent to renal actions of hyperkalemia (see Question 1.24).

3. Plasma [Urea] and Its Fractional Excretion

> - In SIADH, the blood urea nitrogen (BUN) is often low.

In patients with SIADH, urea clearance increases, probably as a result of ECF volume expansion. This occurrence, together with dilution due to water retention and possibly a low protein intake, results in a fall in the concentration of urea in plasma (BUN).

In hyponatremia associated with a low "effective" circulating volume, there is a higher plasma urea level because the stimulus to ADH release (ECF volume contraction) leads to a fall in the glomerular filtration rate and an enhanced rate of reabsorption of filtered urea in the proximal convoluted tubule in response to a contracted ECF volume.

Urea:creatinine ratio
Because the changes in the concentration of creatinine in plasma are less pronounced, the ratio of urea to creatinine in plasma is likely to be low in SIADH and high with ECF volume contraction. The fractional excretion of urea is elevated in SIADH.

4. Plasma Urate and Its Fractional Excretion

> • In SIADH, the plasma [urate] is low.

Note
The fractional excretion of urate is elevated in SIADH.

The urate level may be quite low in the patient with hyponatremia caused by SIADH. The mechanism is thought to be due to the expanded ECF volume in this condition. If the ECF volume is contracted, more urate is reabsorbed, and its level in plasma could rise.

Importance of Examining a Tonicity Balance

When ADH acts, the urine will contain little EFW in patients who maintain their usual intake of salt. Nevertheless, to deduce what the anticipated changes are likely to be, the clinician must examine the input and output—perform a tonicity balance (see the following).

Example 1
Subjects on a normal Western diet consume 150 mmol of NaCl and 50 mmol K^+ and excrete 1.5 L of urine a day. They remain in balance, and their 24-hour urine [Na^+ + K^+] is 133 mmol/L. Because the urine [Na^+ + K^+] can rise to only twice this value because of a limit set by medullary tonicity, positive EFW balance can be only 0.75 L/day (see margin note). Stated another way, it is difficult to have a large daily positive EFW balance unless EFW intake increases appreciably.

Calculation 1
If the urine [Na^+ + K^+] can rise twofold from 133 mmol/L, the positive EFW balance will be only 0.75 L/day (1/2 × 1.5 L).

Example 2
An elderly woman consumes tea and toast (see Case 10.1). Her intake of EFW is high because she eats so little Na^+ + K^+. To stay in balance, she must excrete urine with a very low [Na^+ + K^+]. If ADH is present, her urine [Na^+ + K^+] can rise precipitously, and hyponatremia can develop quickly (see margin note). Hence, both the electrolyte and EFW intake plus the capacity to have a high urine [Na^+ + K^+] impact on the likelihood of developing hyponatremia and contributing to its severity.

Calculation 2
With the same intake of 1.5 L of water but only 75 mmol Na^+ + K^+, the urine [Na^+ + K^+] is 50 mmol/L (75 mmol/1.5 L). When ADH acts, if her urine [Na^+ + K^+] rose to, say, 225 mmol/L, the urine volume would be only 0.33 L (75 mmol/0.33 L = 225 mmol/L), so the positive EFW balance is 1.2 L/day.

Clinical Settings for Chronic Hyponatremia

1. Patients with an "effective" circulating volume that is obviously contracted.

Clinical pearl
A patient with SIADH may also have ECF volume contraction for other reasons. In this case, the urine [Na$^+$] should be very low unless there is a renal basis for the Na$^+$ loss. In this setting, however, hyponatremia will not be corrected by a large water diuresis after the Na$^+$ deficit is replaced.

Source of ADH
ADH release in SIADH may be from the posterior pituitary or from a nonphysiologic source (e.g., a neoplasm).

Conditions with chronic but reversible release of ADH
Examples include chronic nausea or vomiting (chemotherapy), chronic pain, and/or a low "effective" circulating volume (diuretics, hypoalbuminemia, or chronic heart failure).

2. Patients taking medications or who have a condition that is very likely to cause the release of ADH (Figure 7.4; Table 7.4).

3. Patients in whom the cause for ADH release is not obvious. Here, the major clinical diagnoses are a more subtle contraction of the ECF volume, causing ADH release, or those patients with SIADH. In this group, a trial of isotonic saline could help. The key endpoint is the excretion of dilute urine (suppress the release of ADH) when the ECF volume is reexpanded (do not give too much isotonic saline as this can cause the hyponatremia to become more severe in a patient with SIADH; see discussion of Question 7.16).

SIADH: Hyponatremia Associated with Autonomous Release of ADH

> • If a low "effective" circulating volume is not present, ADH release is not under the usual physiologic control in a patient with hyponatremia; this is called the *syndrome of inappropriate ADH secretion* (SIADH).

The consequence of a persistently elevated ADH level is to limit the excretion of EFW (see margin note). When EFW is ingested, much is retained and causes hyponatremia with initial ECF volume expansion (see margin note). In response to this ECF volume expansion, Na$^+$ are excreted in the urine. Hence, the characteristic findings in steady state are hyponatremia and the absence of ECF volume contraction (Figure 7.5). The urine has an osmolality that exceeds the minimum value of 20–80 mOsm/kg H$_2$O and contains an appreciable quantity of Na$^+$. After attaining a steady state, the rate of excretion of Na$^+$ and water matches their dietary intake (see Question 7.15).

Before confirming the diagnosis of SIADH in a patient with chronic hyponatremia, be sure that there is no reduction of the "effective" circulating volume; this could require an infusion of isotonic saline (see Figure 7.4). Patients with SIADH can be classified into four subcategories, depending on why ADH is present (see Figure 7.4).

TABLE 7.4 **Drugs That May Cause High ADH Activity**

This table is only a partial listing because the list continues to grow.

Central Stimulation of ADH Release

Drugs include nicotine, morphine, clofibrate, tricyclic antidepressants, antineoplastic agents such as vincristine, cyclophosphamide (probably acting via nausea and emesis)

"ADH-Like" Agents such as Oxytocin

Drugs that Promote the Actions of ADH on the Kidney by Increasing Cyclic AMP Levels or Bioactivity

Oral hypoglycemics (e.g., chlorpropamide), methylxanthines (e.g., caffeine, aminophylline), analgesics that inhibit prostaglandin synthesis (e.g., aspirin, indomethacin)

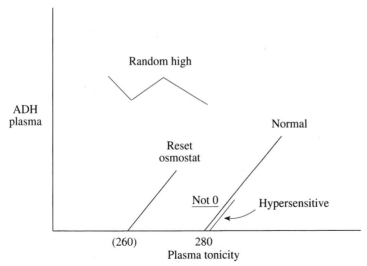

Figure 7.4 Subclassification of patients with SIADH (modified from the original by G. L. Robertson).

There are four subgroups of SIADH:

1. Random high autonomous ADH release (e.g., carcinoma of the lung). These patients represent 35–40% of those with SIADH.
2. Reset osmostat. These patients have normal regulation of ADH release, but it is focused around a hypotonic setting. About 33% of patients with SIADH are in this subcategory.
3. Failure to suppress ADH totally with hypotonicity. About 15% of patients have this disorder, in which ADH release is normal at high tonicity but is not 0 at low tonicity.
4. About 15% of patients with SIADH have no problem with ADH secretion, but their kidneys are either overly sensitive to it, there is an ADH-like material present, or if there is a very low distal delivery of solutes.

QUESTION

(Discussion on pages 323–324)

7.17 *A patient with hyponatremia (127 mmol/L) excretes urine with an osmolality of 176 mOsm/kg H_2O. How would you know if this excretion was due to a reset osmostat type of SIADH?*

Therapy for SIADH

> - The acute discovery of a chronic condition does not make it an acute condition.
> - Beware of the patient with chronic hyponatremia and a contracted ECF volume.
> - Deal with the underlying disorder (see margin note).

Prevention. Certain clinical situations are associated with chronic but reversible release of ADH (see margin note). These patients will be exposed to a more severe degree of hyponatremia if they

Conditions with chronic but reversible release of ADH
Examples include chronic nausea or vomiting (due to chemotherapy), chronic pain and/or a low "effective" circulating volume (due to diuretics, hypoalbuminemia, or chronic heart failure). Do not neglect to establish the underlying diagnosis. There are no prizes for an excellent slow correction of the patient's hyponatremia but leaving the tuberculosis untreated.

receive EFW, and they are in danger of "spontaneous" excessively rapid correction of their hyponatremia.

Active Treatment. Although the physician must not forget about the underlying illness, the authors focus here on dealing with the *rate* of correction of hyponatremia. In only rare circumstances should this rate of correction be rapid; nevertheless, we start with rapid correction because it may be necessary in the case of a medical emergency.

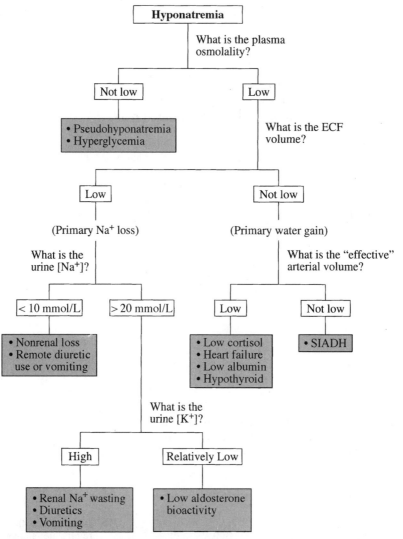

Figure 7.5   Approach to hyponatremia. The final diagnoses are shown in the shaded boxes (see the text for details).

Rapid Correction

> • Use aggressive treatment only for patients whose symptoms are very serious (coma, seizures).

1. Give hypertonic saline to raise the plasma [Na$^+$] to a level at which the seizure was not present (usually a rise in natremia of up to 5 mmol/L).

2. Do not let the rise in plasma [Na$^+$] exceed an overall 24-hour rate of 8 mmol/L/day.

Caution. With an acute seizure, the plasma [Na$^+$] may rise by 10–15 mmol/L because of an acute shift of water into muscles, so the plasma [Na$^+$] at the time of the seizure may be artificially high (see Chapter 6).

Slow Correction

> • Brain-cell size is currently nearly normal—do not permit it to change rapidly. Limit rise in [Na$^+$] to 8 mmol/L/day.

Note
This represents the vast majority of patients.

1. Choose a rate of correction at which virtually no patient developed the ODS (<8 mmol/L/day).

2. Make the rate of correction even slower if the patient could have difficulty with the availability of K$^+$ and/or organic osmolytes (malnutrition, catabolic state such as in a burn victim).

Specific Emphasis for Therapy. The authors can identify three areas, each with its specific therapy. These will be applied to three patients in the next section.

1. The ICF volume

> • Create a negative balance for EFW.

Cells have an excess of EFW, so they must lose EFW at a slow rate; this requires a negative balance for EFW. Therefore, EFW input should be limited, and strategies should be employed to increase its loss (Table 7.5). The degree of loss of ICF volume will be indicated by the rise in the plasma [Na$^+$].

TABLE 7.5 **Treatment of a Water Surplus**

Restrict water intake.

Promote water loss independent of ADH.
Give diuretics and replace electrolytes but not water.
Give osmoles (urea) to increase the volume of EFW in the urine.

Reduce ADH levels.
Correct the low "effective" circulating volume.
• Give NaCl if the total ECF volume is low.
• Give albumin if its concentration is very low.
• Improve myocardial function (inotropic agents, afterload reduction, chronotropic agents).
• Replace hormone deficiencies (glucocorticoids, thyroid hormone).
• Remove drugs that promote ADH release or potentiate ADH action.

Administer antagonists to ADH.
Give receptor blockers (new), lithium, demeclocycline.

2. Return the Composition of the ECF to Normal

> • Virtually every patient will require a positive balance for Na^+.

Calculation
- Normal
  —ECFV 10 L
  —$[Na^+]$ = 140 mmol/L
  ∴ Na^+ content is 1400 mmol.
- Hyponatremia
  —ECFV 10 L
  —$[Na^+]$ = 120 mmol/L
  ∴ Na^+ content is 1200 mmol, a deficit of 200 mmol.

Most patients with SIADH have a near-normal ECF volume. Nevertheless, the content of Na^+ in each liter of ECF is lower than normal. Therefore, to maintain a normal ECF volume, as the EFW is lost, there must be a positive balance for Na^+. By examining the quantitative changes in Question 7.21, one can appreciate the importance of the deficit for Na^+ (see Figure 7.7).

QUESTIONS

(Discussions on pages 324–326)

7.18 *The brain has an acute (1–3 h) and a chronic (1–3 days) mechanism to avoid too great a degree of increase in its overall volume when hyponatremia develops. What is the acute mechanism? What is the chronic mechanism?*

7.19 *When a 60-kg patient with hyponatremia (100 mmol/L) and a near-normal ECF volume received 150 mmol of hypertonic NaCl, the plasma $[Na^+]$ rose to 115 mmol/L. Why did it rise: Na^+ gain or water loss?*

7.20 *Could Na^+ loss have occurred via the renal route if the urine is now Na^+-free?*

7.21 *A 50-kg person (30 L total body water) is in a positive balance of 3 L of EFW in steady state; the plasma $[Na^+]$ is 127 mmol/L. Moreover, the ECF volume is normal. What are the total body and ECF balances, and what should be done about this? Consider three parts for your answer: first, the positive balance of EFW only; second, how the ECF volume returns to normal; third, your therapy.*

7.22 *Why do patients with adrenal insufficiency commonly present with hyponatremia?*

3. Return the composition of the ICF to normal

> • Replace the deficit of K^+ in the ICF.

As EFW in the ICF was considered earlier, we are now concerned with two issues: restoring a deficit of K^+ if a deficit was present, and restoring organic osmoles to the ICF of the brain. Focusing first on K^+, if a deficit was present, it should be replaced with KCl. In balance terms for the ICF, KCl creates a positive balance for K^+ and a negative balance for Na^+ and H^+. In the ECF, there is a positive balance for Na^+ and Cl^- that draws EFW out of cells.

Because the KCl is usually given in a hypertonic form, there will be a net gain of hypertonic NaCl in the ECF, a rise in natremia, and an expanded ECF volume. If the ECF volume was normal initially, the final step is to obligate the excretion of the extra ECF volume as "isotonic to the patient" NaCl.

The time needed to restore intracellular organic compounds that were lost in the development of hyponatremia is an important consideration. In this regard, an even slower rate of correction of hyponatremia is prudent when there is a large deficit of K^+ (hypokalemia), a malnourished or an intensely catabolic state (as in burn victims), and/or hypoxia.

Cautions

1. Do not let the plasma $[Na^+]$ rise by more than 8 mmol/L/day.
2. Watch out for a water diuresis.
3. Do not give KCl quickly once the plasma $[K^+]$ rises above 3.0 mmol/L.

> **Slower correction of hyponatremia in malnourished or catabolic patients**
> To replace the organic osmoles extruded from brain cells in response to swelling, patients are dependent in large part on their dietary intake. Accordingly, if they are deficient of these compounds (as are malnourished patients), correction of hyponatremia should be slower.

QUESTIONS

(Discussions on pages 326–328)

7.23 *If a 60-kg woman has a plasma $[Na^+]$ of 110 mmol/L, how quickly will her $[Na^+]$ rise due to water loss with a restriction of water intake to 1 L/day in fluids and food? (Assume that the urine osmolality is 600 mOsm/kg H_2O and that she has 600 mOsm to excrete.)*

7.24 *What role might K^+ depletion play in determining the severity of hyponatremia?*

7.25 *If K^+ is lost from the ICF with an accompanying ICF anion, hyponatremia will develop. Will this type of hyponatremia be accompanied by a rise or fall in the ICF volume?*

Case Examples

The following four cases are provided to emphasize that the first step in therapy might differ in individual patients with chronic hyponatremia.

CASE 7.1
Focus Solely on ICF Volume

A 50-kg person has SIADH due to a tumor; the plasma $[Na^+]$ is in steady state and 120 mmol/L, and the plasma $[K^+]$ is 4.0 mmol/L. There are no symptoms attributable to hyponatremia. Assume that the ECF volume is normal and that the patient is consuming a usual diet (150 mmol NaCl per day).

What is your therapy?

DISCUSSION OF CASE 7.1

> **Note**
> 50 kg patient has:
> TBW = 30 L
> ICF = 20 L
> Total ICF osmoles normally = 20 L × 2 × 140 = 5600
> Assume ICF osmoles unchanged; therefore ICF volume = 5600/(2 × 120) = 23.2 L

- There is no urgency here.

This patient will need to lose 3 L of EFW and gain 191 mmol NaCl (see discussion of Question 7.21 and Figure 7.7). The course for this therapy will be 2–3 days. The simplest approach is to reduce the intake of EFW. Empirically, the authors recommend water restriction to 0.5 L/day and observation.

1. The deficit of NaCl in the ECF can be restored without supplement as the diet has abundant NaCl.

2. If this therapy does not work, we would add leverage to increase the excretion of EFW in the urine.

When one considers output, one must enhance the excretion of EFW. This type of therapy becomes more important when water restriction fails to raise the plasma $[Na^+]$ sufficiently. The best way to increase the excretion of EFW is to add osmoles such as urea to obligate the excretion of water at a given high urine osmolality (see margin note). In general, the addition of 400 mmol of urea (24 g) will cause the excretion of 1 L of EFW. Another strategy is to use a loop diuretic to cause the excretion of isotonic saline. In this case, replacing all the ions excreted without water will cause a loss of EFW (see Table 7.5 and the figure in the margin).

Use a loop diuretic to cause a negative balance for water:

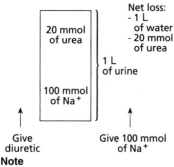

Note
The mechanism of action of urea in lowering the urine $[Na^+ + K^+]$ is discussed in this chapter.

CASE 7.2
Focus on the ECF Volume

A 50-kg person consumed a low-salt diet and took a thiazide diuretic for hypertension. The only symptoms are weakness, a lack of energy, and a feeling of lightheadedness on standing. The ECF volume was contracted on physical examination (blood pressure is now 135/70 mm Hg—it was 160/90 mm Hg—and there is a 20 mm Hg postural drop in blood pressure). Hyponatremia (115 mmol/L) and a slightly low plasma $[K^+]$ (3.6 mmol/L) are present. Urine output is close to 1 L/day with diuretic use.

What is your therapy?

DISCUSSION OF CASE 7.2

- Restore the low "effective" circulating volume promptly.

For now, it is safe to ignore the ICF volume and its composition. The aim of therapy is to administer 1–2 L of saline "isotonic to the patient" to achieve this aim (see margin note).

Caution. A major risk in these patients is if the ADH release was due to ECF volume contraction. Now when the ECF volume is reexpanded, ADH secretion may stop, and a large water diuresis will occur. If therapy is not changed, the plasma $[Na^+]$ could rise too rapidly, making ODS a more likely event. Therefore, have an ADH preparation available should the patient excrete enough dilute urine to raise the plasma $[Na^+]$ by more than 8 mmol/L/day.

One other point merits emphasis. Because the patient is consuming a low-salt diet and has a large deficit of Na^+ in the ECF (see Question 7.21), add NaCl to the intake until hyponatremia is corrected.

Clinical note
If 1 L of isotonic saline plus 0.5 L of half-isotonic saline is administered, this is close to saline isotonic to the patient (125 mmol/L).

Once the ECF volume is near normal, the design of therapy reverts to that described for Case 7.1.

CASE 7.3
Hyponatremia Accompanied by a Severe Degree of Hypokalemia

A 50-kg person was placed on a low-salt diet and a thiazide diuretic for hypertension. The clinical condition of the patient has deteriorated throughout the past month. The person has a poor attention span, a general lack of interest in events, profound weakness, and depression. There are no seizures or coma. On physical examination, the ECF volume appears normal (but it could be low). On laboratory examination, there is a profound degree of both hyponatremia (103 mmol/L) and hypokalemia (1.8 mmol/L). The electrocardiogram reveals changes associated with the profound hypokalemia.

What is your therapy?

* Hypokalemia has three major implications:
  1. a danger of a cardiac arrhythmia.
  2. a need to treat with K^+ rather than Na^+ salts.
  3. a much greater risk of developing ODS.

DISCUSSION OF CASE 7.3

There are several issues here for acute therapy. First, the degree of hypokalemia must be reduced to decrease the risk of a cardiac arrhythmia. One cannot tell in advance how much K^+ will be required. Having the plasma $[K^+]$ rise to 3 mmol/L as an initial target would be a reasonable choice. If the load of KCl expands the ECF volume too much, administer a loop diuretic to restore a normal ECF volume, and give DDAVP if there is a large water diuresis. The overall rate of correction of hyponatremia should not exceed 8 mmol/L/day. There is also a greater danger of developing ODS in patients with hypokalemia.

This problem concerning the ICF osmole deficit might help explain the poorer prognosis with therapy in this setting. Accordingly, the authors attempt to correct the hyponatremia in this setting at an even slower rate if dietary intake remains poor ($\sim$ 5–6 mmol/L/day).

As in Case 7.2, NaCl has to be added to the diet to repair the deficit of NaCl in the ECF.

CASE 7.4
Hyponatremia in a Patient with an Expanded ECF Volume

An elderly person has a long-standing history of congestive heart failure. With the usual treatment, hyponatremia commonly develops.

Note
The physician must also try to
improve cardiac function.

Hence we have to deal with it in conjunction with edema and a
low-salt diet (see margin note).

DISCUSSION OF CASE 7.4

The major problems in this setting are a surplus of Na^+ and an
even larger surplus of water. Therefore, the aim of therapy is to
create a negative balance for both Na^+ and water. The speed with
which Na^+ should be lost depends on clinical features; it should be
very rapid if there is acute pulmonary edema.

The intake of Na^+ and water should be close to nil. Urinary
losses of Na^+ and water may have to be augmented with a loop
diuretic, and part of the loss of Na^+ and/or water may have to be
replaced to have the desired rate of rise in the plasma $[Na^+]$ in
plasma (8 mmol/L/day). Losses of K^+ will have to be replaced as
well. The $[Na^+ + K^+]$ in the urine should be lower than that of
intake to cause a rise in the plasma $[Na^+]$. Adjust the negative
balances for Na^+ and/or water to produce the desired slow rise in
the plasma $[Na^+]$.

PART B

Review

DISCUSSION OF INTRODUCTORY CASE
Water, Water, Everywhere,
So Not a Drop to Drink
(Case presented on page 285)

Could Na^+ loss have caused the hyponatremia on day 3?

Yes. Not only does Na^+ loss directly cause hyponatermia, it also
leads to ECF volume contraction. In response to ECF volume
contraction, ADH is released; the result—water retention—contributes to a greater degree of hyponatremia.

The physical examination revealed ECF volume contraction.
Laboratory evidence to support this clinical impression was the
elevated plasma creatinine, low plasma $[K^+]$, and elevated plasma
$[HCO_3^-]$. The urine $[Na^+]$ of 60 mmol/L is not usual for ECF
volume contraction, but the low urine $[Cl^-]$ is. Perhaps the Na^+
excretion is obligated by the presence of a nonreabsorbable anion
(HCO_3^-) that appears as a result of recent vomiting (see margin
note).

Note
The difference between the urine
$[Na^+]$ and $[Cl^-]$ indicates that there
is an unmeasured anion in the
urine. If the urine pH is alkaline,
some or all of these anions are
HCO_3^-; otherwise they will usually
be organic anions.

Why was the ADH level elevated on day 3?

The ADH level was elevated because the urine osmolality was 450
mOsm/kg H_2O. A low ECF volume causes ADH release and thereby
prevents free water loss in the urine.

Patients with meningitis can have ADH release independent of
their tonicity and ECF volume status. Hence, there are at least two
causes of a high ADH level: ECF volume contraction and a CNS
lesion. Other causes could include drugs, vomiting, or the stress of

the illness. EFW intake or infusion in this situation would lead to more water retention and a more severe degree of hyponatremia.

Why was the plasma [Na⁺] lower on day 5?

The lower plasma [Na⁺] on day 5 occurred because the patient either lost more Na⁺ and/or had a net EFW gain in the face of continuing actions of ADH. The improved ECF volume suggests that EFW gain is the basis—most likely the result of EFW intake or the infusion of a hypotonic solution.

Was the ADH level higher on day 5?

The absolute ADH level cannot be deduced from the plasma [Na⁺], but it was high enough to have prevented sufficient renal excretion of EFW.

What are the best urine electrolytes to indicate whether the ECF volume is contracted?

Following NaCl loss, the urine should contain minimal quantities of Na⁺ and Cl⁻ (usually less than 10 mmol/L if the kidney is functioning normally).

Would your answer change if the patient had vomiting or diarrhea?

Vomiting. Vomiting results in the loss of Cl⁻ and a commensurate rise in the [HCO_3^-] in the ECF. The filtered load of HCO_3^- should rise, and some of this excess may be excreted; for electroneutrality, Na⁺ and K⁺ will also be lost in the urine. The resultant Na⁺ loss will lead to ECF volume contraction, renin release, angiotensin II formation, and, thereby, aldosterone release. Aldosterone causes the K⁺ loss in the urine. Hence, a very low [Cl⁻] in urine is expected at all times, but the [Na⁺] may not be low if bicarbonaturia persists (as it was on day 3).

Note
The very low urine [Cl⁻] is the best indicator of ECF volume contraction in a patient who vomits.

Diarrhea. A different urine electrolyte pattern occurs with diarrhea and ECF volume contraction. $NaHCO_3$ loss with diarrhea can also produce ECF volume contraction, but in this case there is a low plasma [HCO_3^-]. The kidneys respond to acidemia by excreting a large quantity of NH_4^+ (with Cl⁻). Thus, the urine should have a very low [Na⁺], which indicates the ECF volume contraction, but not a very low [Cl⁻] because of the electroneutrality required for NH_4^+ excretion.

Note
A very low urine [Na⁺] is the best indicator of ECF volume contraction in a patient with diarrhea.

Cases for Review

CASE 7.5
Jerry, the Executive
(Case discussed on page 310)

Jerry is an entrepreneur. Because his mother, Emily of Case 10.1, was recently diagnosed as having hypertension, Jerry had his blood pressure checked, and he had a similar degree of hypertension (160/

110 mm Hg). Like his mother, he was started on a thiazide diuretic and asked to eat a diet without added salt. While on this regimen, his blood pressure was normalized, but routine electrolytes revealed two new abnormalities, a mild degree of hyponatremia (133 mmol/L) and hypokalemia (3.3 mmol/L). There were no obvious clinical findings of a contracted ECF volume. Other laboratory data follow.

Plasma		Usual Values	Present Values
Na^+	mmol/L	140	133
K^+	mmol/L	4.0	3.3
Cl^-	mmol/L	103	90
HCO_3^-	mmol/L	25	28
Creatinine	μmol/L (mg/dL)	88 (1.0)	110 (1.2)
Osmolality	mOsm/kg H_2O	288	276

Is Jerry's ECF volume contracted?

Does Jerry now maintain mass balance for Na^+? If so, how?

Is the hyponatremia due to Na^+ loss, water gain, or both?

Why is Jerry's hyponatremia less severe than Emily's (Case 10.1)?

Why is Jerry's hypokalemia much less severe than Emily's (Case 10.1)?

CASE 7.6
Hyponatremia and Hypo-osmolal Urine
(Case discussed on pages 311–312)

Cindy had surgery to remove a tumor of her pituitary many years ago. She did reasonably well during the ensuing years by taking the appropriate hormonal replacements for her anterior pituitary deficits. Although she drank and eliminated large volumes daily, this aspect of her problem was never investigated further or treated.

More recently, she developed inflammatory bowel disease, had a colectomy, and lost many liters of fluid daily via her ileostomy. On many occasions, she was admitted for episodes that are best characterized by profound contraction of her ECF volume. The most recent one was typical. She had marked ECF volume contraction, hyponatremia (134 mmol/L), a large urine volume (0.2 L/h), and a low urine osmolality (160 mOsm/kg H_2O). She was given many liters of isotonic saline intravenously, and the following changes were observed in these parameters: the ECF volume was normal, the plasma [Na^+] was 138 mmol/L, the urine flow rate doubled, and the urine osmolality fell to 80 mOsm/kg H_2O.

Does Cindy have central diabetes insipidus (DI), nephrogenic DI, or primary polydipsia?

CASE 7.7
Hyponatremia and the Guru
(Case discussed on page 312)

In order to "cleanse her soul," Tracy's guru recommended that she "wash away evil spirits" by consuming nothing but water. Tracy followed this advice enthusiastically. She drank approximately 1 L of water per hour, hour after hour while awake. Urine output came close to matching input initially but then fell off considerably. This procedure was repeated daily for many days. Because of other aspects of a behavior problem, Tracy was brought to the emergency room. Physical examination revealed no abnormalities apart from confusion and paranoid delusions. Laboratory results follow.

		Plasma	Urine
Na$^+$	mmol/L	107	46
K$^+$	mmol/L	3.6	10
Cl$^-$	mmol/L	75	30
HCO$_3$$^-$	mmol/L	21	0
Urea	mmol/L (mg/dL)	1.0 (2.8)	34
Creatinine	μmol/L (mg/dL)	60 (0.7)	3000 (35)
Glucose	mmol/L (mg/dL)	3.3 (60)	0
Osmolality	mOsm/kg H$_2$O	220	160

Is ADH acting now?

What limits free water excretion?

What role did the fasting play, and how did it affect the urine osmolality?

What is the differential diagnosis of hyponatremia and a urine osmolality of 160 mOsm/kg H$_2$O?

Supplemental Information

Another random urine sample revealed a urine with an osmolality of 50 mOsm/kg H$_2$O; the plasma [Na$^+$] was 110 mmol/L.

How does this information help in the differential diagnosis?

What treatment should Tracy receive?

CASE 7.8
The Post–Transurethral Resection of the Prostate (TURP) Syndrome
(Case discussed on page 314)

Barry underwent a TURP for a very large prostate. The large prostatic bed was exposed to the irrigating solution; blood loss was higher than usual. The irrigating solution was 6 L of an equal mixture of sorbitol and mannitol; final osmolality was 150 mOsm/kg H$_2$O. Barry's plasma [Na$^+$] was 138 before surgery and 93 mmol/L 6 hours after surgery. His cerebral function did not change markedly, and his ECF volume was not greatly changed.

What is the basis of the hyponatremia?

What simple laboratory test will help in confirming the diagnosis?

What treatment should be ordered?

CASE 7.9
Hyponatremia: A Swell Way to Think
(Case discussed on page 315)

A 42-year-old previously healthy person had neurosurgery to stop a subarachnoid hemorrhage; an uneventful recovery was anticipated. Because of the presence of polyuria (flow rate 10 mL/min), the following were measured:

Urine osmolality 400 mOsm/kg H_2O.
Urine Na^+ 175 mmol/L, K^+ 14 mmol/L.
Plasma $[Na^+]$ 133 mmol/L.
Plasma glucose 5 mmol/L (90 mg/dL).
Your assessment of the ECF volume was low. Therapy was isotonic saline at a rate equal to urine output.

Has ADH acted?

Why is the urine flow rate so high?

The plasma $[Na^+]$ decreased during this time. Why?

Was there a physiologic stimulus for the excretion of Na^+?

Why was so much Na^+ excreted?

Discussion of Cases

DISCUSSION OF CASE 7.5
Jerry, the Executive
(Case presented on page 307)

Is Jerry's ECF volume contracted?

Yes. Given the history of a low-salt diet and the thiazides, he was probably in negative Na^+ balance intially, and his total body Na^+ content is lower than when he began this regimen. Each liter of ECF has lost 7 mmol of Na^+, so he has lost at least 100 mmol of Na^+ from his ECF plus all the Na^+ lost in each liter of ECF lost (see margin note). Because one cannot detect a mild degree of ECF volume contraction on physical examination, other data are needed to support this impression. In the laboratory data, the hyponatremia (ADH action), hypokalemia (aldosterone action), and the higher values for creatinine and HCO_3^- in plasma support this impression.

Calculation
- The fall in $[Na^+]$ is 7 mmol/L (140 − 133 mmol/L).
- His ECF volume is normally 15 L. Therefore, Na^+ loss is 7 L × 15 mmol/L, or 105 mmol.
- If his ECF volume is now 14 L, he lost an additional 133 mmol of Na^+.

Does Jerry now maintain mass balance for Na^+? If so, how?

Yes. In a chronic situation, one achieves a new steady state or mass balance. Two opposing forces are in operation. When the diuretic is not working, Jerry's kidneys, stimulated by the contracted ECF volume, actively reabsorb all filtered Na^+, so he retains all dietary Na^+ at this time. In contrast, he is in negative balance for Na^+ when the diuretic acts.

Is the hyponatremia due to Na^+ loss, water gain, or both?

Both. The diuretic and diet modification (see preceding) induced the Na^+ loss. Water gain is present because the contracted ECF volume has stimulated thirst and release of ADH.

Why is Jerry's hyponatremia less severe than Emily's (Case 10.1)?

To answer this question, consider the factors that influence Na^+ and water.

Na^+. Both Jerry and Emily have a mild degree of ECF volume contraction, but Emily has a much greater deficit of Na^+ in her ECF. This deficit reflects the much greater negative mass balance for K^+ because she has shifted some Na^+ into her ICF (see following).

H₂O. Emily may or may not have a larger water intake (tea) relative to body mass, but this intake cannot be assessed. She probably has a much lower excretion of water. Two factors must be assessed: urine osmolality and the osmole excretion rate.

1. **Urine osmolality:** Emily should excrete more water because her urine osmolality is lower than Jerry's. In more detail, water excretion depends on the urine osmolality and the osmole excretion rate. Older people cannot excrete as concentrated a urine as do younger people (urine osmolality was 402 mOsm/kg H₂O in Emily and 850 mOsm/kg H₂O in Jerry). For the same rate of osmole excretion, Emily excretes more water, but she has many fewer osmoles to excrete.

2. **Osmole excretion rate:** Emily eats tea and toast (little urea produced) so she has far fewer osmoles for excretion and thus excretes a decreased amount of EFW. Quantitatively, if Jerry excretes 850 mOsm/day, he will excrete 1 L of urine. Emily, on the other hand, excretes only 300 mOsm, so she excretes 0.75 L of water daily at her usual urine osmolality.

$$\text{Urine volume} = \frac{\text{osmole excretion rate}}{\text{urine osmolality}}$$

Why is Jerry's hypokalemia much less severe than Emily's (Case 10.1)?

Intake of K⁺. Again, consider mass balance. Jerry eats more K⁺ than Emily does.

Excretion of K⁺. With respect to excretion, aldosterone may lead to similar concentrations of K⁺ in their cortical collecting ducts (CCD), but Emily should have a lower volume delivered to the CCD (excretion = [K⁺] × volume). The basis of this statement is as follows: volume delivery to the CCD depends on the number of osmoles excreted when ADH acts because the osmolality of luminal fluid approaches that of plasma. Although Emily has a lower plasma osmolality, she has a much, much lower rate of osmole excretion because of her dietary intake.

Overall. Up to this point, it appears that Jerry should have a greater K⁺ deficit. Nevertheless, when the diuretic acts, Emily and Jerry both deliver high volumes of fluid to the CCD. Thus, Emily will excrete almost as much K⁺, but the low dietary K⁺ may account for her greater negative K⁺ balance. Hence, the much lower dietary K⁺ in Emily is probably the most important reason for her larger deficit of K⁺.

DISCUSSION OF CASE 7.6
Hyponatremia and Hypo-osmolal Urine
(Case presented on page 308)

Does Cindy have central DI, nephrogenic DI, or primary poly-dipsia?

The issue here is to explain the presence of hypo-osmolal urine (160 mOsm/kg H₂O) when Cindy was hyponatremic. Consider the following three diagnoses:

Central DI. This diagnosis can be established by finding a urine with a very low osmolality and large volume when ADH should be acting. The two major stimuli to ADH release are hypernatremia (not present) and marked ECF volume contraction (present on admission). Thus, it appears that ADH release was abnormally low, given her ECF volume status. This view is supported by two pieces of evidence: first, she had a decrease in urine osmolality when the ECF volume was reexpanded (80 mOsm/kg H_2O); this decline in urine osmolality was accompanied by a doubling of her urine output. Second, by history, she had a pituitary tumor resected. Hence, the authors believe she had partial central DI. This view was confirmed later when ADH was given, and the urine osmolality rose acutely to 456 mOsm/kg H_2O (this value is not her maximum attainable urine osmolality because several days of protein intake plus avoidance of polyuria are needed to reestablish medullary hyperosmolality).

Nephrogenic DI. The diagnosis of nephrogenic DI is possible, but, given the preceding renal response to ADH, it is no longer tenable.

Primary polydipsia. Patients with central DI usually have polyuria caused by a water diuresis. If they can gain access to water, they usually have a slightly elevated plasma [Na^+]; without adequate water intake, frank hypernatremia is expected. Cindy was accustomed to drinking large quantities of water, independent of thirst. When water output was curtailed somewhat (50%) by the release of ADH (which causes a rise in urine osmolality) and by the lower glomerular filtration rate (GFR) (which lowers the delivery of hypotonic fluid to the distal nephron), she went into positive water balance and became hyponatremic. Therefore, in this setting, she also has polydipsia that is due in part to ECF volume contraction.

DISCUSSION OF CASE 7.7
Hyponatremia and the Guru
(Case presented on page 308)

Is ADH acting now?

Yes. The urine osmolality exceeds the expected value of 20–80 mOsm/kg H_2O.

What limits free water excretion?

Free water excretion can be as high as 10% of the GFR. Because the minimum urine osmolality is 20–30 mOsm/kg H_2O, each of the following might limit free water excretion:

1. low GFR;
2. number of osmoles available for excretion;
3. ADH or ADH-like drugs.

What role did the fasting play, and how did it affect the urine osmolality?

There are two factors to consider: ADH levels and available osmoles to excrete.

ADH Levels. With a positive balance of EFW, the ECF volume expands, and this causes a natriuresis that will ultimately cause the

ECF volume to return toward normal (see Figure 7.7). Because of her low-salt diet, Tracy does not replace her deficit of Na$^+$. Therefore, an ECF volume that is high enough to permit suppression of the release of ADH due to hyponatremia is entirely dependent on continued drinking. Nevertheless, Tracy must sleep at times (stop drinking). When this occurs, excretion of EFW will continue because ADH is suppressed; nevertheless, ultimately the ECF volume will decline. As a result, ADH is released, and less water can now be excreted, and the urine osmolality will rise. Next day, when water is ingested and retained, the ECF volume reexpands, ADH is suppressed, and the urine osmolality declines again until the cycle repeats itself. Hence, the urine osmolality may be very low or surprisingly high in the various stages of this clinical story.

Osmoles to Excrete. Tracy eats little protein, so she will have little urea to excrete. Moreover, the previous water diuresis washed out much endogenous urea. Therefore, each liter of dilute urine excreted now has little urea and thereby a very low urine osmolality.

What is the differential diagnosis of hyponatremia and a urine osmolality of 160 mOsm/kg H$_2$O?

With this osmolality, ADH is present and acting. The differential diagnosis is summarized in Table 7.6 and includes polydipsia and a mild degree of contraction of her ECF volume or some other stimulus for ADH release (e.g., drugs, vomiting). Alternatively, Tracy could have SIADH of the reset osmostat type. Finally, Tracy could conceivably have central DI and be treated with an ADH preparation. She may drink in response to nonosmotic stimuli.

Supplemental Information
Another random urine sample revealed a urine with an osmolality of 50 mOsm/kg H$_2$O; the plasma [Na$^+$] was 110 mmol/L.

How does this information help in the differential diagnosis?

Because the urine osmolality declined when the plasma [Na$^+$] rose, the data suggest that ADH was suppressed at this time. The data are most compatible with the input of NaCl in a patient with psychogenic polydipsia. The data are not consistent with reset osmostat, but it still could be possible if another stimulus for the release of ADH is being removed (psychosis) or if the effects of the exogenous ADH preparation wore off.

TABLE 7.6 **Differential Diagnosis of Hyponatremia with a Urine Osmolality of Approximately 160 mOsm/kg H$_2$O**

Polydipsia in the face of mild ADH actions

- A mild degree of ECF volume contraction (usually psychogenic polydipsia)
- Psychosis, which causes ADH release that wanes in degree
- Intermittent vomiting and nausea
- Drugs that are taken intermittently or are weak stimulators of ADH release

Exogenous ADH given to a patient who either:

- Is accustomed to drinking large quantities of water
- Has a fall in the GFR but did not decrease the intake of water

Reset osmostat type of SIADH

- Loss of osmoles from the ICF
- Afferent overload via the vagus nerve

What treatment should Tracy receive?

Tracy needs negative water and positive Na$^+$ balance. Water intake must be curtailed. It is best to give judicious amounts of NaCl. The danger to anticipate is excessive water loss when endogenous ADH is suppressed by ECF volume reexpansion (see margin note). Slow down this rapid water loss with small amounts of ADH. The rate of rise of the plasma [Na$^+$] should be 8 mmol/L/day. Do not give large amounts of hypertonic saline without observing Tracy for a rapid water diuresis.

DISCUSSION OF CASE 7.8
The Post–Transurethral Resection of the Prostate (TURP) Syndrome
(Case presented on page 309)

What is the basis of the hyponatremia?

Hyponatremia implies a loss of Na$^+$ or a gain of water in the ECF.

Loss of Na$^+$. Because Barry's ECF volume is not greatly changed and he is very hyponatremic, there was a large loss of Na$^+$ (675 mmol; see margin note). His ECF volume is being maintained by the presence of a particle that has a distribution similar to Na$^+$ and keeps water from shifting from his ECF to his ICF.

Gain of water in the ECF. Although a gain of water is the primary reason for hyponatremia, several points need to be explained:

1. Acute hyponatremia to this degree should have caused his brain to occupy "four-thirds" of his skull (impossible). Therefore, the basis of his hyponatremia is not just water gain. Barry's normal mentation despite such a severe and acute degree of hyponatremia is a clue of critical importance.

    The volume of EFW needed to lower his plasma [Na$^+$] from 138 to 93 mmol/L is close to 15 L (see margin note). Because he was given only 6 L of dilute solution, there is more to the answer.

2. Given the preceding, Barry must have retained (formed and/or was given) an osmole that remained in his ECF (like glucose) and drew water out of cells. This particle was the mannitol and sorbitol used in the irrigating solution for his prostate. It was given as hypo-osmolal lavage solution (150 mOsm/kg H$_2$O). Much of this fluid was probably absorbed via the exposed veins in his prostatic bed (see margin note).

What simple laboratory test will help in confirming the diagnosis?

The *plasma osmolality* should be much greater than twice the plasma [Na$^+$] + urea + glucose, all in mmol/L. It was.

What treatment should be ordered?

Barry is asymptomatic; he should be allowed to correct his hyponatremia himself by excreting the offending osmoles and the extra water load. The deficit of Na$^+$ that is present plus the additional loss of Na$^+$ induced by the ongoing osmotic diuresis must be replaced; to do so, simply maintain his ECF volume. This instance is one in which rapid correction of the plasma [Na$^+$] can occur and not be harmful. (To be sure that the authors made a correct analysis, the plasma [Na$^+$], osmolality, urinary excretions, and Barry's clinical state were observed closely. Barry's numbers moved in the appropriate direction and at the expected rate; Barry did not suffer a change in cerebral function.)

DISCUSSION OF CASE 7.9
Hyponatremia: A Swell Way to Think
(Case presented on page 309)

Has ADH acted?

Yes, because the urine osmolality is so much higher than the minimum value of 50 mOsm/kg H$_2$O. Of even more importance, the [Na$^+$ + K$^+$] in the urine was higher than that of plasma.

Why is the urine flow rate so high?

The urine flow is dependent on both the urine "effective" osmolality and the rate of excretion of "effective" osmoles (see margin). In this case, given the high urine non-urea osmolality, the high urine flow rate was due to the high rate of excretion of Na$^+$ + K$^+$ salts.

The plasma [Na$^+$] decreased during this time. Why?

Calculate a tonicity balance. The [Na$^+$ + K$^+$] infused was 154 mmol/L. The urine volume is large, and the excretion is hypertonic to the fluid given, so hyponatremia must develop (and it did). The source of EFW was desalination of body fluids (excretion of Na$^+$ + K$^+$ with little water; see Figure 7.2).

Was there a physiologic stimulus for the excretion of Na$^+$?

No. Given the low ECF volume, there was no apparent physiologic stimulus for continued excretion of NaCl (see next question).

Why was so much Na$^+$ excreted?

The authors do not know but offer the following ideas.
1. A way to think about an unexpected natriuresis is that there is the presence of an inhibitor of Na$^+$ reabsorption (a diuretic) or the absence of a stimulator (like aldosterone) (see margin note). In general, the kidney has so many mechanisms to control the excretion of Na$^+$ that it excretes Na$^+$ very slowly when the ECF volume declines even if the clinician continues to give diuretics or there is a lack of aldosterone. This was not the case in our example.
2. The ECF volume depletion was large as judged by the balance for Na$^+$, yet the blood pressure was well maintained. This suggests that the kidney was seeing a high enough blood pressure to drive the excretion of Na$^+$.
3. The two models for cerebral salt wasting are presented below. We favor the one at the bottom. Do you agree?

Plasma osmolal gap (POG)
The POG was defined in Chapter 2. It is used to detect missing osmoles (usually small alcohols like ethanol and methanol, or ethylene glycol). In this case, it is used to quantitate the contribution of osmoles such as mannitol absorbed from the lavage fluid.

Urine volume = $\dfrac{\text{No. "effective" osmoles}}{[\text{"Effective" osmoles}]}$

Note
Changes in the GFR do not exert an important control on the rate of excretion of Na$^+$.

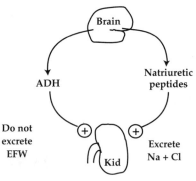

High [Na + K]
Large volume

Note

Two models of Cerebral Salt Wasting are presented. In both, natriuretic peptides are present. In the bottom portion, hemodynamic changes help these peptides to be effective.

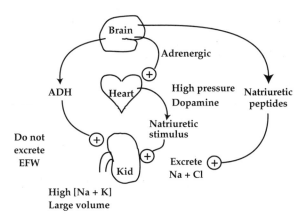

High [Na + K]
Large volume

Summary of Main Points

Incidence
- Hyponatremia is a very common fluid and electrolyte disorder. The approach the authors recommend is as follows:

Concepts
- Plasma [Na^+] reveals the ICF volume.
- Amount of Na^+ reflects the ECF volume.

Tools
- Divide solutions into components:
  Isotonic saline, EFW plus $Na^+ + K^+$ without water.
- Calculate tonicity balance:
  Consider input *and* output.

Approach to Hyponatremia
- Identify source of EFW and reason for ADH.
- Decide whether it is acute or chronic.

Acute Hyponatremia
- **Issue for diagnosis:**
  Identify the source of EFW.
  The reason for ADH is usually obvious.

- **Settings and the gender issue:**
  - Usually postoperative:
    - EFW for females.
    - Hypo-osmolal fluid for males.
- **Issues for therapy:**
  - Emergency: Plasma [Na$^+$] <125 mmol/L:
    - Raise the plasma [Na$^+$] rapidly with hypertonic saline (1 mmol Na$^+$ positive balance for every liter of total body water raises the plasma [Na$^+$] by 1 mmol/L); raise the plasma [Na$^+$] 5 mmol/L during 1–2 hours.
  - Prevention: Do *not* give EFW.
  - Stop the kidney from desalinating administered fluid:
    - Use hypertonic infusion.
    - Loop diuretic or osmotic diuretic.

Chronic Hyponatremia
- **Issues for diagnosis:**
  - Identify why ADH is present. The difficulty is that the most common cause for ADH release is a low ECF volume; this may be difficult to ascertain at the bedside.
  - The source of EFW is not usually a concern.
  - The most important issue here is the [Na$^+$ + K$^+$] in the input because the urine [Na$^+$ + K$^+$] can rise only to 300 mmol/L.
- **Issues for therapy:**
  - Osmotic demyelination is a danger if correction too rapid (>8 mmol/L/day).
  - Risk is greater (and correction rate should be slower) if there is a K$^+$ deficit, malnutrition, and/or a catabolic state.
  - Options for therapy; the emphasis depends on the clinical setting:
    - Create a negative balance for EFW.
    - Create a positive balance for Na$^+$.
    - Replace any deficit for K$^+$.
  - Dangers to anticipate:
    - Removing ADH if its basis was a low ECF volume:
      - Give ADH to stop the large water diuresis.
    - If the patient has severe symptoms (seizure, coma), raise the plasma [Na$^+$] by up to 5 mmol/L over 2 hours with hypertonic saline:
      - Maintain 24-hour rate of correction of only 8 mmol/L/24 h.

Discussion of Questions

7.1 What laboratory methods to measure the [Na$^+$] in plasma will provide a lower value if hyperlipidemia is present?

In plasma, Na$^+$ are dissolved only in the water phase (see margin figure). The presence of excessive quantities of nonaqueous volume in the plasma causes a fall in the ratio of Na$^+$ to *total* volume. In hyperlipidemia or hyperproteinemia, there is a marked increase in the nonaqueous phase of plasma. Therefore, although the [Na$^+$] in

[Na$^+$]:
140 mmol/l plasma
154 mmol/kg H$_2$O

1 L

140 mmol of Na$^+$ in 0.93 L of water.

Water phase (the volume in which Na$^+$ is dissolved).

Nonaqueous volume (excludes Na$^+$).

Plasma osmolality
The plasma osmolality may be normal or high even in patients with true hyponatremia plus elevated levels of urea and/or alcohols.

Quantities
—10 g lipid/L
—Density 0.7 g = 1 mL
∴ 10 g occupies 14.3 mL
∴ Na in 1 L is 140 mmol/L × 1000 − 14.3 mL = 138 mmol/L or a decrease of 2 mmol/L/10 g lipid in a liter.

Calculation 1
900 mg/dL rise × 1.4 mmol/L/100 mg/dL glycemia = Fall of 13 mmol/L from 140 to 127 mmol/L

Calculation 2
Convert glucose and urea to mmol/L.
Plasma osmolality = 2 × [Na] + [glucose] + [urea] = (2 × 127) + 55 + 25 = 334 mOsm/kg H_2O

Transuretheral resection of the prostate
See discussion of Question 7.8 for more information.

---

the aqueous phase is normal and the plasma osmolality is normal, the quantity of Na^+ per plasma volume is low. Hence, the term "pseudohyponatremia" applies because the problem is apparent, not real. The diagnosis can be confirmed by inspecting plasma for lipids or by measuring the plasma osmolality.

From the laboratory perspective, a number of different methods are used to detect the $[Na^+]$ in plasma. Some of them require a major dilution of plasma (e.g., the flame photometer, certain types of ion-selective electrodes). Because the plasma is diluted, the original Na^+:plasma volume is reflected, and pseudohyponatremia will be evident. In contrast, if a Na^+-selective electrode or a conductance method is used on undiluted plasma, the $[Na^+]$ (Na^+:H_2O ratio) will approach 152 mmol/kg H_2O. In this case, the machine "back-calculates" the value to 140 mmol/L in order not to confuse the clinician, but this procedure confuses the physiologist.

7.2 A diabetic patient has renal failure. His blood sugar is 1000 mg/dL (55 mmol/L), $[Na^+]$ is 127 mmol/L, and blood urea nitrogen is 70 mg/dL (urea is 25 mmol/L). What is his calculated plasma osmolality? Has hyperglycemia changed his ECF and/or ICF volumes?

Hyperglycemia causes water to shift out of muscle cells (muscle cells contain the bulk of the ICF volume and close to half of body water). Quantitatively, a 900 mg/dL (50 mmol/L) rise in the concentration of glucose causes the $[Na^+]$ to fall by about 13 mmol/L (see margin calculations and Chapter 12, page 499, for the details of this calculation).

The ECF volume is therefore expanded by the water that shifted out of the ICF of muscle. Because renal failure is present, no osmotic diuresis has occurred; hence, the usual clinical finding of ECF volume contraction with severe hyperglycemia is not present.

Summary. The ICF volume of muscle is contracted; the ICF volume is expanded in the liver; and the ICF volume of the brain is probably close to normal (see Figure 12.5).

7.3 In what circumstances will the plasma osmolality help or be misleading with respect to diagnosis in a patient with hyponatremia?

It is common practice to use the plasma osmolality to help in the diagnosis of the basis for hyponatremia (see Figure 7.5). The authors believe that while useful information can be gleaned from a measurement of the plasma osmolality, this will be truly helpful only in a small number of patients.

Plasma Osmolality May be Helpful
There are two circumstances in which measuring the plasma osmolality is helpful. First, consider the patient who has received an infusion of hypo-osmolar organic solute with a volume of distribution equal to the ECF volume (e.g., many of the lavage solutions used in surgery for TURP or endometriosis). In this setting, one cannot tell to what degree the fall in natremia was due to the infusion of the osmole-free water (OFW) as compared with the infusion of isosmolar solution. With administration of OFW, the plasma osmolality will decline, whereas it will not change for

the isosmolar solution. It is only the component of hyponatremia due to a gain of OFW that is important with respect to the brain-cell size (see discussion of Question 7.10).

Second, one can on occasion be surprised that pseudohyponatremia is present if one had no knowledge that a condition like multiple myeloma or hyperlipidemia was present (and one did not know that the plasma was creamy in appearance). In this setting, the plasma osmolality is normal.

Plasma Osmolality Is Not Needed

Hyperglycemia. In almost every case, one has measured the plasma glucose concentration when the plasma Na^+ was measured, so one need not measure the plasma osmolality to reveal that hyperglycemia is present (i.e., a fall in the plasma $[Na^+]$ of 14 mmol/L is accompanied by a rise in glycemia of 900 mg/dL (50 mmol/L)).

7.4 Three patients have hyponatremia (120 mmol/L). In case A, it is due to water gain; in case B, Na^+ loss; in case C, hyperglycemia. Which patient(s) will have swelling of brain cells? Give reasons for your answer.

The plasma $[Na^+]$ indicates the ICF volume if there is no gain of particles in the ECF, like glucose in Case C or a large loss of particles from the ICF (K^+ salts), which would lead to a shift of water out of cells. Of greater importance, if defense of the ICF volume of brain cells has occurred, the ICF volume of brain cells will return toward normal despite the presence of hyponatremia.

Cases A and B. The cells of all organs other than the brain are swollen to the same degree in both patients A and B because the plasma $[Na^+]$ is 120 mmol/L in each case, and there are no other "effective" osmoles to deal with.

With respect to brain cells, if the hyponatremia is chronic, brain-cell size in both of these patients will be close to normal because particles were extruded. If hyponatremia is acute, brain cells will be swollen in both of these patients.

Case C. Hyperglycemia causes a shift of water from muscle cells; this shift results in hyponatremia with a relatively high plasma osmolality. It is important to recognize that water shifts caused by hyperglycemia do not affect all cells equally (see Figure 12.5).

7.5 How can the kidney generate 1 L of EFW if isotonic saline is the only fluid administered?

Two factors are needed: a source of EFW and ADH to prevent its excretion. EFW is generated by desalination (see Figure 7.2). The additional fact that must be known is that the maximum value for the urine $[Na^+ + K^+]$ is close to 300 mmol/L. Hence, to generate 1 L of EFW when isotonic (150 mmol/L for easy arithmetic) saline is the only fluid administered, you must infuse 2 L of that solution and excrete 1 L with a [Na + K] of 300 mmol/L. The remaining 1 L of EFW remains in the body because ADH is acting. The rationale

Clinical pearls
- The plasma osmolality is very helpful in evaluating whether a patient has a high level of alcohol in plasma. The authors use the plasma osmolal gap for this purpose (see Chapter 2 for more discussion).
- By raising the plasma osmolality, a high concentration of urea might lead one to the mistaken belief that pseudohyponatremia or hyperglycemia is present.

Hyponatremia resulting from hyperglycemia
In quantitative terms, expect a 1.4 mmol/L fall in the $[Na^+]$ for every 100 mg/dL (5.5 mmol/L) rise in the glucose concentration; the $[Na^+]$ falls 1 mmol/L with a 4 mmol/L (70 mg/dL) rise in blood glucose concentration. This calculation incorporates the fact that the glucose concentration in the ICF of the liver (and other noninsulin-sensitive cells with respect to glucose transport) is the same as that in the ECF.

for infusing large volumes of saline during surgery is in the margin note.

Rationale for intravenous therapy in patients undergoing surgery
The rationale is to ensure a normal "effective" circulating volume. Because anesthetic agents reduce venoconstriction and vasoconstriction, it is common practice to infuse 2–3 L of isotonic saline during the surgical procedure (the amount given depends on the nature of the operation and the size of the patient). One should not give EFW unless the plasma [Na$^+$] exceeds 140 mmol/L because these patients have a reduced ability to excrete EFW because of the release of ADH. In addition, large volumes of isotonic saline should be avoided (see Figure 7.2).

7.6 If a person on a low-salt diet has surgery, what features might be present in the postoperative period to minimize the degree of hyponatremia in the acute postoperative period?

When ADH acts, the excretion of EFW is low. Notwithstanding, the low-salt diet will cause Na$^+$ to be reabsorbed avidly, so little will be excreted. Therefore, the patient should have edema and will not have a "desalination." This inhibits the generation of EFW and thereby minimizes the potential risk of developing hyponatremia.

7.7 A patient had surgery. Although the plasma [Na$^+$] was in the range of 139–141 mmol/L 1 week before surgery, the preoperative plasma [Na$^+$] was 136 mmol/L. Why? The plasma [Na$^+$] was 128 mmol/L 36 hours after surgery. Why?

The preoperative plasma [Na$^+$] was low because of EFW intake in the presence of ADH actions. The anxiety and anticipation of surgery were sufficient to drive the patient to drink coffee or tea and release ADH. This response probably accounts for the wide normal range of plasma [Na$^+$] in hospitalized patients.

The plasma [Na$^+$] fell in the postoperative period because of a positive balance for EFW and ADH actions. Although the physician avoided routine D$_5$W, a prophylactic antibiotic was given in this solution, and the patient drank postoperatively because his throat was sore and his mouth was dry.

7.8 What volume of an IV solution containing 856 mmol/L Na$^+$ (5% saline) must be infused to raise the plasma [Na$^+$] by 1 mmol/L in a 70-kg patient? (Ignore the water infused, for simplicity.)

Because a 70-kg person has 40 L of water, and water moves rapidly across cell membranes, one must give 1 mmol of Na$^+$ for each liter of total body water even though Na$^+$ remain in the ECF. To give 40 mmol of Na$^+$ from hypertonic saline, one must infuse 48 mL (see margin note).

Calculation
• Volume hypertonic saline:
856 mmol Na$^+$ is in 1000 mL.
1 mmol is in 1000/856 = 1.2 mL.
40 mmol is in 40 × 1.2 = 48 mL.

7.9 Why do surgeons use solutions that are electrolyte-free to lavage the prostatic bed during a transurethral prostatic resection? (Hint: There is considerable bleeding in this procedure.)

During a TURP, the urologist may need to use an electric cautery and lavage the prostatic bed. The lavage solution needs osmoles to avoid hemolysis (a variable quantity of fluid is absorbed systemically), but the fluid cannot contain electrolytes because such a solution conducts electricity. The solute must also be nontoxic. The "solution" for this problem is the use of organic osmolytes such as mannitol, sorbitol, glycerol, or glycine in half-osmolal to isosmolal strength. When these solutions are absorbed systemically, hyponatremia can result, but it is usually transient in nature. Although a severe degree of hyponatremia may develop, its net effect on swelling of brain cells may be mild. Quantitative issues are discussed more fully in the discussion of Question 7.10.

7.10 A 50-kg patient (total body water 30 L) absorbed and retained 3 L of a half–iso-osmotic solution of mannitol during his TURP. What is the quantitative role of mannitol and EFW in causing his hyponatremia (plasma [Na⁺] fell from 140 mmol/L to 113 mmol/L)? What happens to the ICF volume and plasma [Na⁺] once the mannitol is excreted as a 300 mOsm/kg H₂O solution?

When 3 L of EFW is retained, it is distributed into body fluid compartments in proportion to their size—2 L to the ICF and 1 L to the ECF (left side of Figure 7.6).

The patient who gained 3 L of half-isosmolar solution has a much larger gain of Na⁺-free water in the ECF and a more severe degree of hyponatremia; there is also much less swelling of the ICF volume (right side of Figure 7.6).

7.11 Should hyponatremia in patients who undergo a TURP be classified as a form of translocational hyponatremia akin to that of hyperglycemia?

No. This is not translocational hyponatremia because EFW entered cells; EFW did *not* exit from cells.

7.12 What properties of glycine make this compound unique in the pathogenesis of the post-TURP hyponatremia syndrome?

The unique features of glycine are that it is an amino acid and a neurotransmitter. It distributes slowly into muscle cells and almost not at all into the CNS. In the post-TURP syndrome, glycine could cause a delayed hyperammonemia with behavioral or functional changes in the CNS. There is also a urea load.

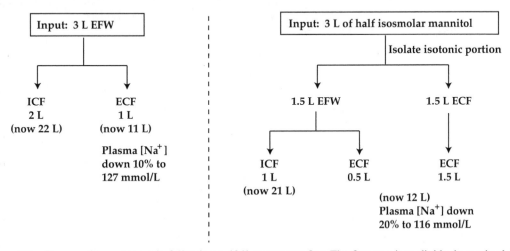

Figure 7.6   Degree of hyponatremia following a 10% water surplus. The first step is to divide the retained fluid into an isotonic component (remains in the ECF only) and the remainder, which is EFW. The left portion of the figure illustrates the changes in ICF volume and plasma [Na⁺] when 3 L of EFW is retained. The right portion of the figure represents events when half-isosmotic lavage fluid is retained. After the mannitol is excreted as 1.5 L of an isosmolal solution (300 mmol/L), the ECF volume declines by 1.5 L to 10.5 L, and the plasma [Na⁺] rises to 133 mmol/L. Note this 20 mmol/L rise in natremia is not accompanied by any change in the ICF volume. (1997. *The Acid Truth and Basic Facts,* 4th ed., ML Halperin, RossMark Medical Publishers, Stirling, Ontario, Canada.)

7.13 How much water must a normal person drink to produce hyponatremia? Would it matter if this person is on a low-salt diet?

A person with normal kidneys can excrete 12 L of EFW per day. Hence, water intake that exceeds this amount can be the sole cause of hyponatremia due to primary psychogenic polydipsia.

Recall that each liter of maximally dilute urine contains some Na^+. To excrete 15 L with a urine $[Na^+]$ of 5 mmol/L, a person will lose 75 mmol of Na^+ (15 L × 5 mmol/L, or 75 mmol). Failure to provide electrolytes in the diet means that endogenous Na^+ must be excreted. As a result, the ECF volume will contract, and ADH will be released. These actions obviously compromise further EFW excretion and can lead to a severe degree of hyponatremia. This pattern can be seen in patients with an excessive beer intake (see margin note).

7.14 Match the four separate causes of hyponatremia with the critical parameter for diagnosis.

Etiology	Critical parameter measured
(1) Chronic diuretic intake	**(a) Normal plasma osmolality**
(2) Hyperlipidemia	**(b) Normal ECF volume and low urine osmolality**
(3) Excess ADH	**(c) ECF volume contraction and hypokalemia**
(4) Compulsive water consumption	**(d) Low plasma and high urine osmolality**

The answers are as follows:

1. Chronic diuretic intake may lead to a degree of ECF volume contraction and hypokalemia consequent to the actions of aldosterone (c).

2. In hyperlipidemia, pseudohyponatremia may occur and will be evident if the plasma osmolality is normal (a).

3. With hyponatremia from excessive ADH action, the plasma osmolality will be low, and the urine osmolality will be high (d).

4. In the compulsive water drinker, the ECF volume will be normal, and the urine osmolality may be very low (b).

7.15 What is the average urine osmolality in a 24-hour urine sample from a normal subject? Is the urine composition in a patient with SIADH different? If so, in what way?

A normal person produces 500 mmol of urea and consumes approximately 200 mmol of NaCl plus KCl (400 mOsm); thus, the urine contains 900 mOsm. If a typical urine volume is 1.5 L, the osmolality of a 24-hour urine is close to 600 mOsm/kg H_2O.

In a chronic condition (SIADH), the subject is in balance so the patient will have the identical urine composition. The problem is it is an inappropriate urine composition for a patient with hyponatremia (the $[Na^+ + K^+]$ in the urine would be much lower if ADH were absent).

7.16 What conclusions can be drawn when the urine osmolality is high?

A high urine osmolality indicates that ADH is acting and that the renal medulla has a high osmolality. The impact on the plasma $[Na^+]$ cannot be deduced from just the urine osmolality; a high urine osmolality may lead to hypernatremia or hyponatremia. Consider the following two examples in which nothing was ingested. First, when urea is the sole osmole excreted in 1 L of hyperosmolar urine (600 mOsm/kg H_2O), a rise in the ECF $[Na^+]$ occurs (the plasma Na^+:H_2O ratio rises) because water without Na^+ was excreted. In contrast, the excretion of a urine with the same osmolality and a $[Na^+]$ of 200 mmol/L (higher than the plasma Na^+:H_2O) favors the development of hyponatremia in the absence of hyperosmolar intake.

7.17 A patient with hyponatremia (127 mmol/L) excretes urine with an osmolality of 176 mOsm/kg H_2O. How would you know if this excretion was due to a reset osmostat type of SIADH?

The presence of hyponatremia and a urine osmolality that is low, but not the expected minimal value of 20–80 mOsm/kg H_2O, suggests that some ADH is present. There are four possible reasons for the low urine osmolality.

1. A Reset Osmostat
If the clinical setting suggests a reset osmostat type of SIADH, the patient, if given a water load, will be able to excrete it promptly. The patient will also have a much higher urine osmolality after water is restricted. The plasma $[Na^+]$ should be similar before and after either treatment. In response to exogenous ADH, the urine osmolality will rise.

Reset Osmostat—Some Speculations. A reset osmostat is a curious condition. On the one hand, cells could defend their normal volume in the face of hyponatremia by having a deficit of intracellular particles. This in turn means a loss of the principal anions in the ICF (organic phosphate such as RNA or phospholipids) and their attendant K^+ ions. This used to be called a "sick cell syndrome" and was thought to reflect a catabolic setting.

A second prototype of a reset osmostat is one in which excessive afferent influences, by the vagus nerve for example, could alter the responsiveness of the "tonicity receptor" such that they require a larger degree of hyponatremia (cell volume increase or stretch) to suppress thirst and inhibit the release of ADH. This type of scenario could explain the relatively high incidence of a reset osmostat (close to 1/3) in patients who have SIADH.

2. Partial Therapy of Central DI
A low urine osmolality might occur if the ADH that was administered for treatment of central DI has almost "worn off" and if the patient drinks a large quantity of water out of habit. There should be an obvious history of central DI and a fall in urine osmolality with time. Rapid (too rapid) correction of hyponatremia should be anticipated and controlled with ADH administration.

3. Psychogenic Polydipsia

The history will usually reveal a psychiatric problem and polydipsia. As discussed in Case 7.7, a recurring cycle develops. With water ingestion, a maximally dilute urine will be excreted. If there is an inadequate osmole load for excretion, Na^+ will be lost. A fall in the ECF volume will ensue, ADH will be released, and there will be an excretion of urine with a somewhat higher osmolality. After the patient ingests water the next day, the cycle will repeat itself. The diagnosis is established by demonstrating that a normal plasma $[Na^+]$ will occur once the ECF volume is restored (NaCl is given, but the rate of correction of hyponatremia must be slow because the hyponatremia is often chronic).

4. Cause for Release of ADH Is Wearing Off

If a patient had taken a drug that caused the release of ADH (see Table 7.4) and the effects of this drug were wearing off, this hyponatremic patient could now excrete a dilute urine. A similar scenario could occur in a patient with a phobia or chronic nausea who had these stimuli for the release of ADH abate.

7.18 The brain has an acute (1–3 h) and a chronic (1–3 days) mechanism to avoid too great a degree of increase in its overall volume when hyponatremia develops. What is the acute mechanism? What is the chronic mechanism?

Acute Mechanism. This is in essence an extracellular defense. When hyponatremia develops, there is a shift of water into cells, and this increases the intracranial pressure. As a result, ECF in the brain is driven into the cerebrospinal fluid (CSF), and from there fluid is pushed into the systemic circulation. This loss of CSF minimizes the rise in intracranial pressure, but it has only a limited capacity to do so. This process is repaired rapidly and does not lead to problems in therapy (see margin note).

Chronic Mechanism. This is an intracellular defense. To minimize the degree of cell swelling, cells of the brain lower their osmotic content by extruding some of their particles. In a qualitative sense it is easy to define some of the particles that are lost: these include organic compounds, such as glutamate, taurine, and sugar derivatives, and ions such as K^+ and intracellular anions. The particles lost are much harder to define in quantitative terms. Although this loss of intracellular particles is essential for survival with a severe degree of hyponatremia, one must recognize that, when designing therapy, it takes a long time (days) to reaccumulate these particles; failure to correct hyponatremia slowly enough is likely to be responsible for the development of the ODS.

Clinical pearl
In a patient who has acute and severe hyponatremia (e.g., plasma $[Na^+]$ 120 mmol/L) and a contracted ECF volume, rapid expansion of the ECF volume with isotonic saline could provoke symptoms due to an acute increase in intracranial pressure. Hence, use hypertonic saline in this setting.

7.19 When a 60-kg patient with hyponatremia (100 mmol/L) and a near-normal ECF volume received 150 mmol of hypertonic NaCl, the plasma $[Na^+]$ rose to 115 mmol/L. Why did it rise: Na^+ gain or water loss?

This question highlights the relative importance of Na^+ gain and water loss in rapid correction of hyponatremia. The concept is that as Na^+ are retained, EFW will shift from the ICF, so total body water must be used as the denominator of the Na^+:H_2O ratio in this case. If the total body water is 30 L, for easy arithmetic, the administered 150 mmol of Na^+ can only raise the plasma $[Na^+]$ by 5 mmol/L. Because there was a much larger rise in the plasma $[Na^+]$, there must be another reason for this change (e.g., a water diuresis caused by a suppressed release of ADH as a result of reexpansion of the ECF volume).

7.20 Could Na^+ loss have occurred via the renal route if the urine is now Na^+-free?

Yes. If a patient took a diuretic "yesterday" and had the natriuresis then (and did not ingest Na^+ today), that patient would have ECF volume contraction and the appropriate renal response of minimal Na^+ and Cl^- in the urine today when the diuretic is no longer acting. This example is presented to emphasize that one must suspect the antecedent intake of diuretics in patients with a contracted ECF volume (intake of diuretics might even be denied by the patient).

Note
To use the urine electrolytes in a more sophisticated way to determine the basis for a contracted ECF volume, see Table 4.5.

7.21 A 50-kg person (30 L total body water) is in a positive balance of 3 L of EFW in steady state; the plasma $[Na^+]$ is 127 mmol/L. Moreover, the ECF volume is normal. What are the total body and ECF balances, and what should be done about this? Consider three parts for your answer: first, the positive balance of EFW only; second, how the ECF volume returns to normal; third, your therapy.

EFW Considerations
Initially, the 3-L positive balance for EFW is distributed as 2 L in the ICF and 1 L in the ECF. The plasma $[Na^+]$ declines by 10% to 127 mmol/L due to the extra 1 L in the ECF.

Return the ECF Volume to Normal
This occurs because of enhanced excretion of Na^+ in response to an expanded ECF volume. With a normal ECF volume (10 L), he has a deficit of 13 mmol/L, which is a total deficit of Na^+ of 130 mmoles. To see how much Na^+ must be excreted to generate 1 L of EFW for the ICF, see Figure 7.7.

Therapy
In balance terms, to restore the ICF volume to normal, there must be a negative balance of 3 L of EFW. To restore the ECF composition to normal, there must be a positive balance of 130 mmol Na^+.

7.22 Why do patients with adrenal insufficiency commonly present with hyponatremia?

There are two major reasons why hyponatremia occurs in the presence of adrenal insufficiency.

1. Aldosterone deficiency leads to renal Na^+ wasting and ECF volume contraction, which causes ADH release (this may be exacerbated by poor cardiac output due to low levels of cortisol).

2. Cortisol deficiency per se leads to enhanced hypothalamic production of ADH (it is no longer believed that glucocorticoids influence water permeability in the collecting duct).

Caution. Treatment with replacement doses of glucocorticoids and mineralocorticoids and replacement of the Na^+ deficit will correct

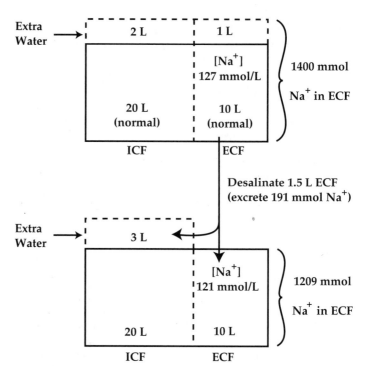

**Figure 7.7   Degree of hyponatremia following a 10% water surplus
while maintaining a normal ECF volume.** The solid rectangle represents
30 L of total body water, 20 L of ICF, and 10 L of ECF. The top portion
of the figure illustrates the changes in ICF volume and ECF volume when
3 L of EFW is retained. The bottom portion of the figure represents events
when enough Na^+ without water are excreted to return the ECF volume to
10 L. The calculation can be thought of as converting 150% of the volume
of ECF that you want to shift into the ICF (1.5×1 L) from isotonic saline
(127 mmol/L in this example) to EFW so that 191 mmol of Na^+ must be
excreted. (1997. *The Acid Truth and Basic Facts,* 4th ed., ML Halperin,
RossMark Medical Publishers, Stirling, Ontario, Canada.)

the hyponatremia. Do not let this correction occur too rapidly;
administration of ADH may be necessary to slow the rate of the
water diuresis.

**7.23 If a 60-kg woman has a plasma $[Na^+]$ of 110 mmol/L, how
quickly will her $[Na^+]$ rise due to water loss with a restriction of water intake to 1 L/day in fluids and food? (Assume
that the urine osmolality is 600 mOsm/kg H_2O and that
she has 600 mOsm to excrete.)**

The key data required are the urine osmolality and the osmole
excretion rate. She excretes 600 mOsm at 600 mOsm/kg H_2O;
hence, her urine volume must be 1 L of water, the quantity she
ingested. The only negative water balance is her loss via the skin
because water production from metabolism equals water loss via
respiration. If she loses a few hundred mL per day, her plasma
$[Na^+]$ will rise close to 1 mmol/L/day.

**7.24 What role might K^+ depletion play in determining the
severity of hyponatremia?**

K^+ depletion is expected when there is hyponatremia and decreased ECF volume. A contracted ECF volume leads to the release of aldosterone, which augments K^+ excretion if delivery of Na^+ and volume to the CCD are sufficient. Where do these urinary K^+ come from? As shown in Figure 9.12, many of these K^+ are derived from muscle ICF and require Na^+ to shift from the ECF to the ICF. This shift depletes Na^+ in the ECF and further accentuates the degree of hyponatremia (this portion of hyponatremia is corrected by KCl therapy, as discussed in Case 7.1). Therefore, in patients with hypokalemia and chronic hyponatremia, there is a risk to aggressive KCl replacement because it may lead to too rapid a rise in plasma $[Na^+]$ and ECF volume as Na^+ exit the ICF.

7.25 If K^+ is lost from the ICF with an accompanying ICF anion, hyponatremia will develop. Will this type of hyponatremia be accompanied by a rise or fall in the ICF volume?

Deductions concerning ECF vs ICF volume loss are not so straightforward with the loss of K^+ (Figure 7.8). A loss of K^+ is not equivalent to a loss of Na^+ with respect to the degree of hyponatremia induced because Na^+ are always associated with monovalent anions (2 particles per Na^+), whereas K^+ are associated with macromolecular intracellular anions and therefore represent a loss of closer to 1 particle per K^+ lost.

Loss of K^+ with Cl^-. In this case, a cation should move from the ECF into cells to maintain electroneutrality (Cl^- is predominantly an ECF anion). There are only 2 cations present in a sufficiently large quantity, H^+ and Na^+. In the former case, HCO_3^- or possibly organic anions would have to accumulate in the ECF in stoichiometric amounts to K^+ lost because the ECF has too few free H^+.

Figure 7.8 Change in the ICF volume when K^+ is lost from the ICF. The solid circle represents the normal ICF volume, and the dashed line represents the ICF volume after the negative K^+ balance. The rectangles represent excretion into the urine. Note the ICF volume should expand with KCl loss and contract when K^+ are excreted with an anion that led to a loss of ICF anions (N° = neutral precursor; A^- = organic anion).

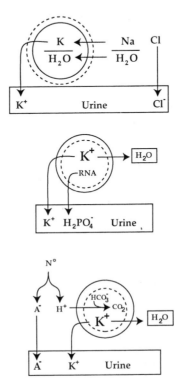

The more likely scenario is a shift of Na^+ into cells when K^+ exited to be excreted with Cl^-. This would result in net loss of NaCl from the ECF without a net change in the number of ICF particles. The ensuing hyponatremia would then lead to an increase in the ICF volume.

Loss of K^+ with Phosphate. If phosphate was derived from cells, its major source is macromolecules such as RNA, DNA, and phospholipids, all of which are esters of monovalent phosphate; accordingly, this loss of monovalent phosphate along with its matching cation, K^+, would result in a net loss of close to 1 particle from the ICF. This will decrease the ICF volume and aggravate the degree of hyponatremia.

Loss of K^+ with Other Anions. The catabolism of neutral substances may lead to the production of a H^+ and the accompanying anion (A^-). If there is no rise in the plasma anion gap, this anion will be excreted with K^+ in the urine. If the plasma HCO_3^- concentration does not change appreciably, virtually all the H^+ produced entered the ICF in an equimolar amount to K^+ that exited. So far there has been no change in the number of particles in the ICF because K^+ were lost and H^+ accumulated in this compartment. Nevertheless, H^+ entering cells must be buffered either by intracellular HCO_3^- or by proteins for the most part. If H^+ were buffered by HCO_3^-, the net result is a loss of 2 particles (H^+ plus HCO_3^-) from cells (see Figure 7.8, bottom panel). Alternatively, if buffering occurs with intracellular proteins, the net loss is 1 particle from the ICF (K^+), and the proteins in the ICF become more positively charged. In either case, the net result is water movement from the ICF to the ECF, causing cell shrinkage and ECF volume expansion; its degree is greater with ICF buffering by HCO_3^-.

8

Hypernatremia

OBJECTIVES

☐ To indicate that hypernatremia, while representing an increase in the amount of Na^+ relative to water in the extracellular fluid (ECF), signals generalized intracellular fluid (ICF) volume depletion in almost every case.

☐ To emphasize that hypernatremia is almost always due to a negative balance for electrolyte-free water (EFW), which most frequently reflects its excretion in the urine. By examining the urine osmolality plus its $[Na^+ + K^+]$ and flow rate, the basis for the large excretion of EFW can be deduced.

☐ To emphasize that a significant degree of hypernatremia will not develop if the thirst mechanism is intact and there is access to EFW.

☐ To stress that one must evaluate the urine $[Na^+ + K^+]$ and not its osmolality to know the impact of the urine losses on the ICF volume.

☐ To provide a diagnostic approach to the causes of hypernatremia based on an evaluation of the ECF volume, weight, and the physiologic responses to a water deficit or Na^+ gain.

☐ To provide a diagnostic approach to patients with polyuria.

☐ To provide the basis for rational decision-making in the treatment of patients with hypernatremia.

Outline of Major Principles

1. Hypernatremia is not a specific disease: look for its cause and treat the underlying disease.

2. In almost all patients with hypernatremia, the ICF volume is contracted. The brain is most susceptible, and a CNS hemorrhage is more likely to ensue if hypernatremia is acute and/or severe.

3. Thirst is such a powerful urge that patients will not permit a significant degree of hypernatremia to develop if their thirst mechanism is intact and they have access to EFW. Hence, most patients who have excessive excretion of EFW simply drink equally large volumes of water. Their clinical problems are management of polyuria and avoidance of settings in which their ability to drink is curtailed.

Clinical pearls
1. If hypernatremia is present, find out why water intake was inadequate.
2. Calculate a tonicity and not an osmole balance.

4. Urine osmolality helps in differentiating the three major causes of water loss: diabetes insipidus (large volume of hypo-osmolar urine), osmotic or pharmacologic diuresis (large volume of slightly hyperosmolar urine), and nonrenal water loss without water intake (minimum volume of maximally hyperosmolar urine).

5. A gain of Na^+ is rarely responsible for hypernatremia. Detect a

Na$^+$ gain by finding an expanded ECF volume, and then estimate the quantity of Na$^+$ retained in the ECF.

6. In terms of salt and water, treatment of a patient with hypernatremia has two components: first, stop EFW loss, if possible; second, administer a hypotonic solution relative to the patient if oliguria is present or relative to the urine if polyuria is present. Hypotonic saline and glucose in water are two intravenous (IV) solutions that contain EFW. Do not give glucose faster than the patient can metabolize it (see discussion of Question 8.10), and do not correct chronic hypernatremia too quickly. The best way to administer EFW is by the oral route.

Importance of the plasma [Na$^+$]

A concentration, which is a ratio (e.g., glucose:water), is generally used to gain insight into the numerator (e.g., how much glucose is present). The plasma [Na$^+$] provides insight into the denominator of the Na$^+$:water ratio.
- **Hyponatremia** reflects an increased ICF water.
- **Hypernatremia** reflects the opposite.
- Nothing is learned about the total body Na$^+$ content from the plasma [Na$^+$].

INTRODUCTORY CASE
Treat the Patient Before He (DI)es
(Case discussed on page 349)

A patient developed acute meningitis, and was confused by the time of admission. The plasma [Na$^+$] was 140 mmol/L, the ECF volume was slightly low, and the urine volume was low. Shortly thereafter, a convulsion occurred; it was treated with a large dose of the anticonvulsant phenytoin (Dilantin). Over the next 8 hours, polyuria developed, but thirst was not present. Physical examination revealed a modest degree of ECF volume contraction and a weight loss of 5 kg. The plasma [Na$^+$] rose to 157 mmol/L and urine osmolality was 100 mOsm/kg H$_2$O.

Of what significance is the modest degree of contraction of the ECF volume?

Why was thirst absent?

Of what significance is the loss of body weight?

What is the significance of the polyuria?

Can any inference be made from the urine osmolality and the acuteness of the onset?

What should the therapy be?

PART A

Etiology of Hypernatremia

Background

[Na$^+$]

The true normal plasma [Na$^+$] is 152 mmol/kg H$_2$O. If measured per liter of plasma, however, the plasma [Na$^+$] is 140 mmol/L because each liter contains 6–7% nonaqueous volume (lipids, proteins), and Na$^+$ are distributed only in the aqueous phase. The

Methods to measure the [Na⁺]

If the plasma [Na⁺] is measured using a Na⁺-selective electrode or a conductance method (i.e., measuring the Na⁺-to-water ratio) on an undiluted sample, the normal value is 152 mmol/L; notwithstanding, the laboratory will back-calculate this value and report it as 140 mmol/L. There is no "correction factor" needed for hyperlipidemia or hyperproteinemia in these cases. If the method used determines the [Na⁺] per volume of plasma (flame photometry), a "factitious" hyponatremia will result from an increased nonaqueous phase (e.g., hyperlipidemia; see Chapter 6).

Osmole excretion rate

Urine volume $\times$ urine osmolality.

or

$$\text{Urine volume} = \frac{\text{osmole excretion rate}}{\text{urine osmolality}}$$

Osmole excretion rate

Refers to the total number of osmoles excreted per day. The major osmoles are urea; Na⁺, K⁺, and their anions; and glucose if glycosuria is present. See Table 8.1.

normal range of plasma [Na⁺] is said to be 136–144 mmol/L. If blood lipids or proteins are excessively high, the laboratory values for the plasma [Na⁺] may be much lower than the actual Na:H_2O ratio if certain methods are used to measure the [Na⁺] (see margin note).

Urine Osmolality (or Specific Gravity)

There is no normal value for urine volume and osmolality. The kidneys respond to a change in tonicity of body fluids by excreting the difference between what the body needs and what is consumed. If no water was taken in, the kidneys should excrete the minimum volume (400–800 mL/day) with the maximum osmolality (1200 mOsm/kg H_2O, specific gravity 1.030); a lower osmolality is observed in the presence of renal disease or if there is a very low intake of protein (urea production). If the osmole excretion rate is low, much lower urine volumes should be expected for any given urine osmolality.

Minimum Urine Volume

Traditional view: The minimum urine volume is determined by the number of osmoles that the patient must excrete and the maximum urine osmolality that the patient can achieve. If the patient has 600 mOsm to excrete in a day and can achieve a urine osmolality of 1200 mOsm/kg H_2O, the minimum urine volume is 500 mL. Urine volumes will be less than 400 mL/day with a low solute excretion rate. They should not be considered as excessively low (oliguric) because they represent the urine volume needed to excrete the current osmole load.

Authors' View

In the traditional view, all urinary solutes have the same physiologic properties. Notwithstanding, the major urinary solute is urea (Table 8.1). When antidiuretic hormone (ADH) acts, urea becomes a permeable solute in the terminal inner medullary collecting duct due to the insertion of the urea transport protein (vasopressin-responsive urea transporter; see Appendix to Chapter 6, page 274, where this subject is considered in detail). Accordingly, the minimum urine

TABLE 8.1 **Major Constituents in the 24-Hour Urine**

Data are from a 70-kg adult eating a typical Western diet. The average urine volume is 1.5 L.

Constituent	Content (mmol)	Concentration (mmol/L)
Urea	400	275
Creatinine	15	10
Na⁺	150	100
K⁺	75	50
Cl⁻	150	100
NH₄⁺	40	26
Phosphate	30	20
Sulfate	15	10
Osmolality	—	600

volume actually depends on the number of tonomoles (impermeable solutes that are electrolytes for the most part) and their concentration in interstitial fluid. Accordingly, the equation describing the minimum urine volume that the kidney can excrete is:

$$\text{Urine volume} = \frac{\text{No. impermeable solutes excreted}}{[\text{Impermeable solutes in the urine}]}$$

QUESTIONS

(Discussions on pages 359–360)

8.1 *Consider the following four examples where the concentration of non–urea solutes is 600 mOsm/kg H$_2$O in the urine (and in the interstitial fluid because ADH is acting).*

Patient	Urea (mOsm/day)	Electrolytes (mOsm/day)
A	400	400
B	50	400
C	400	1600
D	50	100

What is the urine volume and osmolality in each patient?
What is a likely diagnosis in each case?

8.2 *You are asked to see two patients in the intensive care unit because they have a urine output of only 15 mL/h (360 mL/ day). Patient A had cardiac surgery, and edema fluid is present, whereas patient B has a low ECF volume and a normal heart. Both have virtually no Na$^+$ or Cl$^-$ in their urine.*

How could you tell if the glomerular filtration rate (GFR) has fallen?
What would you measure in the urine to determine why the urine rate is so low?

Thirst

Thirst is initiated by a rise in the plasma [Na$^+$] of 2 mmol/L. Look for this response in all hypernatremic patients.

Clinical Approach

- Hypernatremia is almost always due to water loss in the presence of a thirst defect.

In chronic hypernatremia, adaptive mechanisms help restore the volume of brain cells to normal, so therapy should be slow here as it was in chronic hyponatremia (see Chapter 7).

By answering the following four questions, the cause(s) of hypernatremia can usually be deduced (Figure 8.1).

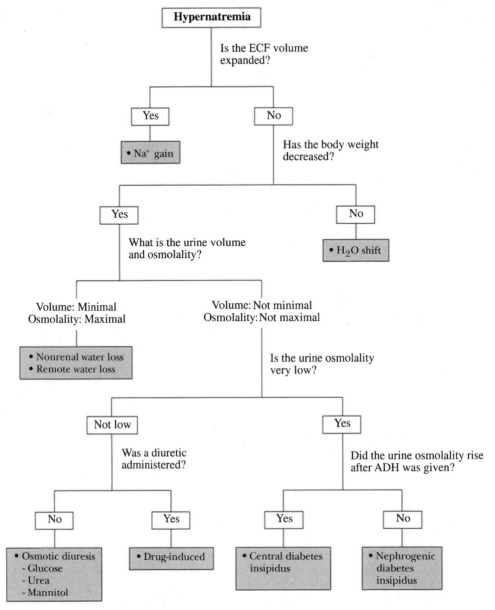

Figure 8.1   Approach to the patient with hypernatremia. The final diagnoses appear in the shaded boxes.

1. What is the ECF volume?
2. Has the body weight changed?
3. Is the thirst response to hypernatremia normal?
4. Is the renal response to hypernatremia normal?

What Is the ECF Volume?

A gain of Na^+ is characterized by ECF volume expansion and is rarely the sole cause of hypernatremia. All other causes of hypernatremia are due primarily to water loss (i.e., there is no ECF volume expansion).

QUESTIONS

(Discussions on pages 360–361)

8.3 *You are confronted with three patients; each has hypernatremia (154 mmol/L). One patient drank sea water, another lost pure water, and the third lost hypotonic saline (from sweating or via a diuretic). What parameter on physical examination would distinguish these three patients? What is (are) the major threat(s) to life in each case?*

8.4 *Two 70-kg patients present with hypernatremia (150 mmol/L). The first patient continues to excrete a very large amount of water; his ECF volume is normal (15 L). The second patient has excreted a large urine volume; the $[Na^+]$ in the urine is close to 50 mmol/L, and the ECF volume is low (13 L). What is the mechanism of hypernatremia in each patient?*

Has the Body Weight Changed?

Very rarely, water shifts from the ECF into the ICF (e.g., with a convulsion or rhabdomyolysis). In this case, hypernatremia is accompanied by a decrease in the ECF volume and no loss of body weight (see margin note).

QUESTION

(Discussion on page 361)

8.5 *Why does water shift into cells with a convulsion or rhabdomyolysis?*

Is the Thirst Response to Hypernatremia Normal?

A 2% rise in plasma tonicity provokes a powerful urge to drink; therefore, hypernatremia should be accompanied by thirst. Failure to drink could occur if the patient was unable to access water (was in a desert, was paralyzed, etc.). The absence of thirst should prompt the clinician to suspect a generalized or localized central nervous system (CNS) lesion.

Is the Renal Response to Hypernatremia Normal?

The appropriate renal response to hypertonicity of body fluids is the excretion of urine with the highest "effective" osmolality that the kidneys can achieve (not just above isotonicity but more than 1000 mOsm/kg H_2O if the blood urea nitrogen is not low) and a urine volume that is the minimum value that can be excreted (about 0.75 L/day on a typical Western diet). Deviations from this response signal an ADH or renal problem (a disorder involving the renal medulla or an osmotic load). Table 8.1 shows the usual osmoles excreted by an adult.

Gain of particles during a convulsion

Excessive muscle contraction causes:

   Creatine phosphate → Creatine + Pi

   ATP → ADP + Pi or AMP + 2 Pi

There are more particles to the right of each arrow, which means that the osmolality of the ICF has increased. In addition, if lactic acid is produced, the [lactate] is higher in the ICF, *and* if its H^+ are buffered by ICF proteins, there is a further increase in ICF osmolality. For these reasons, EFW will shift into cells.

Renal response to hypernatremia
- Urine volume = 20 mL/h (0.5 L/day) unless there is a high rate of excretion of tonomoles ("effective" osmoles or tonomoles).
- Urine osmolality >1000 mOsm/kg H_2O.

QUESTION

(Discussion on page 361)

8.6 *A patient with cirrhosis of the liver and ascites has a urine output of 0.4 L/day (see margin note). Is this patient excreting the lowest possible urine volume?*

Hypernatremia Due To Water Loss

Nonrenal Water Loss

Water loss via the respiratory tract and skin (a hypotonic solution with an even lower [Na$^+$] when its volume is high) is, on average, close to 0.5 L/day. Losses in perspiration can increase dramatically in hot environments and with exercise. Similarly, water losses in patients who are febrile and hyperventilating are higher. If the patient has a generalized or localized CNS lesion involving the thirst mechanism or is unable to obtain water, hypernatremia may develop because water loss is not matched by water intake. Infants may also experience hypernatremia from nonrenal water loss because they cannot specifically complain of thirst. Water loss from the gastrointestinal (GI) tract can be hypotonic if HCl reacts with NaHCO$_3$ or if organic osmoles are produced and the resultant fluid is isosmotic to plasma.

Renal Water Loss

> • In the presence of a thirst defect, renal water loss is the most common cause of hypernatremia. It is usually accompanied by polyuria. The usual causes of polyuria with hypernatremia are diabetes insipidus and an osmotic diuresis.

It is well known that patients with hypernatremia who excrete large volumes of hypo-osmolar urine suffer from diabetes insipidus (DI) (see margin note). If the urine volume can be lowered and the urine osmolality raised appreciably following the administration of ADH, the defect is in the synthesis of ADH or its release from the brain; this disorder is termed *central DI* (Table 8.2). Alternatively,

TABLE 8.2 **Etiology of Central DI**

Trauma (especially basal skull fractures)
Neurosurgery (hypophysectomy, other)
Space-occupying lesions
Neoplasm
Primary (craniopharyngioma, pineal cyst, pituitary tumors)
Secondary (metastatic)
Granuloma
Sarcoid, histiocytosis X
Infection (meningitis, encephalitis)
Vascular (aneurysm)
Posthypoxia
Drugs interfering with ADH release (e.g., phenytoin)
Idiopathic central DI (may be familial)
Presence of a vasopressinase (see margin note)

if the urine remains hypo-osmolar or close to isosmolar and the volume is large after biologically active ADH administration, nephrogenic DI is present.

Central DI

> • Central DI is due to lack of ADH. The major symptoms are polydipsia and polyuria. The plasma [Na$^+$] will be very high only if there is a thirst defect or limited access to water. With ADH administration, the urine volume declines, and osmolality rises.

A rise in the plasma [Na$^+$] (but not hyperosmolality from hyperglycemia or a high urea concentration) stimulates the hypothalamic tonicity receptor and leads to an augmented synthesis of ADH in the paraventricular and supraoptic nuclei. This ADH is then transported by axonal flow to the posterior pituitary. A lesion at any of these sites will produce central DI. The common causes for a lesion are trauma (especially basal skull fractures), infections, space-occupying lesions, and neurosurgical procedures (see Table 8.2). In close to 50% of cases of central DI, no specific cause is identified (called *idiopathic central DI*).

Selective removal of the posterior pituitary usually produces only a transient central DI (it seems that ADH can be released from the hypothalamic neurons that synthesize it). In almost every case, the onset of symptoms of polyuria and polydipsia are abrupt (see margin note).

If central DI is caused by surgery or trauma, there may be an initial polyuria for up to a couple of days (because of inhibition of ADH release). Antidiuresis for up to a few days may ensue (stored ADH is released from the degenerating gland), but permanent central DI often follows.

The diagnosis of central DI is usually easy to confirm. The patient has a CNS problem together with a history of polyuria and polydipsia (cold liquids are usually preferred). Physical examination may help in identifying the underlying disorder. The ECF volume is usually normal or not appreciably reduced. Laboratory examination should show a normal or, more likely, a slightly high plasma [Na$^+$]; a very high plasma [Na$^+$] will only be present if thirst or access to water is compromised. The urine volume will be high (3–20 L/day) unless the GFR is low, and the urine osmolality will be less than 150 mOsm/kg H$_2$O. The diagnosis is confirmed when hypernatremia and polyuria occur with judicious water restriction and when ADH administration results in a prompt rise in the urine osmolality (to above that of plasma but not necessarily to maximum values because time is required for the osmolality in the medullary interstitium to become elevated).

Anything that diminishes the delivery of filtrate to the distal nephron can lower EFW excretion. Hence, polyuria is less dramatic in the presence of ECF volume contraction or anterior pituitary resection, which involves a loss of the hemodynamic benefits of cortisol and thyroid hormone.

An enigma
Why should slowly progressive lesions result in the abrupt onset of polyuria?

Of interest
The volume of water reabsorbed in the medullary collecting duct (MCD) may be higher in DI than in antidiuresis mainly because of the very large volume of delivery to the MCD. This increased reabsorption can contribute to a medullary interstitial "wash-out."

Urine osmolality in DI
For complete DI, the urine osmolality should be less than 70 mOsm/kg H$_2$O. Greater values suggest partial central DI or a low distal delivery of solutes.

Note
- Urine flow rate

$$= \frac{\text{No. osmoles excreted/min}}{\text{Urine osmolality}}$$

- Urine flow rate

$$= \frac{\text{No. "effective" osmoles/min}}{\text{Uosm} - \text{Urea (mmol/L) in the urine}}$$

- Expected values in a patient with hypernatremia on a typical Western diet (400 mOsm of non-urea solutes/day)
1. Flow rate: < 0.7 L/day
2. Uosm: > 900 mOsm/kg H_2O
3. Osmole excretion rate: 0.5 mOsm/min

Abbreviation
Uosm = Urine osmolality

Note
1440 min = 24 h

Bedside Tools for Determining the Basis of Hypernatremia. The use of the urine osmolality, urine flow rate, and the urine "effective" osmolality (see margin note) has been discussed. Expected values for these parameters in a patient with hypernatremia are also provided in the margin note.

Osmole Excretion Rate. For easy arithmetic, if a normal individual excretes 720 mOsm/1440 min, the osmole excretion rate is 0.5 mOsm/min (see margin note). Values greatly exceeding this indicate an osmotic diuresis.

Tonicity Balance. To decide whether the patient's plasma [Na^+] will rise or fall, compare the tonicity of infused fluids with those that are lost. The excretions in the urine are the predominant loss. For water, simply compare the volumes in and out. Do the same for $Na^+ + K^+$ in the input and output. An example of this approach can be found in the discussion of Case 8.4.

QUESTION

(Discussion on pages 361–362)

8.7 *A patient had a stroke that resulted in aphasia. All laboratory test results were normal. She was transferred to a chronic care facility, where tube-feeding was instituted; no drugs were given. She was readmitted to the hospital several weeks later, at which time her ECF volume was contracted. The plasma [Na^+] was 160 mmol/L, the urine osmolality was 450 mOsm/kg H_2O, and the urine volume was 3–4 L per day. The urine glucose was negative.*
What is the diagnosis?

Nephrogenic DI

This disorder can be divided into two major categories:

1. In some instances, ADH fails to increase the water permeability of the collecting duct, and thus osmotic equilibrium does not occur between the interstitial fluid and the hypo-osmolal luminal fluid (see margin note).

2. There is a group of diseases in which a loss of medullary hypertonicity occurs in response to a major medullary interstitial defect or infiltrate (Table 8.3).

A note of caution
If your patient fails to develop an increase in urine osmolality in response to the ADH that was administered, ensure that the preparation of ADH contained biologically active material before making the diagnosis of nephrogenic DI. This precaution provides an ideal opportunity to demonstrate renal physiology to a willing colleague by administering an ADH analogue in the course of water diuresis.

Note
For a summary of molecular advances, see the appendix to this chapter.

In the latter category, the typical urine output is only 3 L/day, and the urine osmolality is generally close to that of plasma. These values differ from the extreme polyuria and maximally dilute urine of central DI and from the values encountered when nephrogenic DI is characterized by a failure to respond to ADH. By definition, patients with nephrogenic DI do not have changes in urine volume or osmolality when ADH is given.

QUESTION

(Discussion on page 362)

8.8 *If a person has nephrogenic DI, drinks an adequate volume of* *water to avoid hypernatremia, has a normal diet, and has a urine osmolality that is consistently close to 300 mOsm/kg H₂O, what will the daily urine volume be?*

TABLE 8.3   **Etiology of Nephrogenic DI**

Failure to insert AQP-2 water channels in the distal nephron
- Lithium
- Demethylchlortetracycline
- Congenital nephrogenic DI
- Hypokalemia
- Marked hypercalciuria

Loss of medullary hypertonicity
- Renal medullary pathology
  —Infiltrations (amyloid, etc.)
  —Infections (pyelonephritis)
  —Drug-induced (analgesics)
  —Hypoxic damage (sickle-cell anemia)
  —Obstructive uropathy
  —Loop diuretics, transient phenomenon
- Generalized kidney disease
  —Polycystic disease
  —Hypokalemia

Idiopathic nephrogenic DI

Hypernatremia Due To Na⁺ Gain

- Hypernatremia is very rarely due to a gain of Na⁺.

A gain of Na⁺ is observed in several clinical situations (Table 8.4): when the patient receives a hypertonic Na⁺ salt intravenously (e.g., NaHCO₃ during treatment for a cardiac arrest), when sea water is ingested, when sugar is replaced with salt in a pediatric formula, and, most commonly, when hypotonic Na⁺ loss is replaced with isotonic saline (e.g., during the treatment of diabetic ketoacidosis). In the latter case, the urine in a patient with an uncomplicated osmotic diuresis should have a [Na⁺] of close to 50 mmol/L; a gain of Na⁺ occurs when isotonic (152 mmol/L) or half-normal (76 mmol/L) saline is infused at the same rate as the urine output.

If hypernatremia is severe, confusion or convulsions may be present. In all cases, the ECF volume is expanded. Treatment in these examples is to increase Na⁺ loss with a diuretic and to give

TABLE 8.4   **Causes of Hypernatremia Resulting From a Gain of NaCl**

---

1. Treatment of polyuria with an infusion that contains a higher [Na⁺] than in the urine
   - Half-normal saline in lithium-induced nephrogenic DI
   - Isotonic saline in a patient with a glucose-induced osmotic diuresis
2. Treatment of cardiac arrest with large volumes of hypertonic NaHCO₃
3. Salt poisoning in infants
4. Ingestion of sea water
5. Dialysis error (use of hypertonic dialysate)
6. Combination of a low capacity to excrete ingested hypertonic NaCl and a thirst center defect

---

Limited rate of glucose metabolism
The maximal rate of glucose oxidation in an ill patient is close to 0.25 g/kg/h, which is equivalent to 0.3 L of D_5W in a 70-kg person. Therefore, administration of more D_5W could result in hyperglycemia and an osmotic diuresis, which could aggravate the degree of hypernatremia.

water by mouth, if possible. Recall that there is a limited amount of glucose in water that can be safely administered intravenously (see margin note).

QUESTION

(Discussion on page 362)

8.9 *What is the cause of hypernatremia in the following case? The plasma $[Na^+]$ rose to 180 mmol/L overnight in a confused patient. He received no medications. His body weight had not changed, but his ECF volume was contracted. His blood sugar was 90 mg/dL (5 mmol/L), the urine volume was extremely low, and the urine osmolality was close to 1200 mOsm/kg H_2O.*

PART B

Symptoms of Hypernatremia

Common Symptoms

The only symptom directly related to a modest degree of hypernatremia is mild confusion (and thirst, if the thirst mechanism is intact); however, during severe hypernatremia, major CNS dysfunction can occur and can ultimately lead to coma and hemorrhages (subarachnoid or intracerebral). The exact $[Na^+]$ that can produce symptoms is lower if the onset of hypernatremia is acute (160 mmol/L seems to be close to the value at which symptoms are common). In contrast, symptoms may be absent if the hypernatremia develops gradually.

The polydipsia of central DI is associated with a strong preference for ice-cold liquids, a preference that is not as common in other polyuric states. Some patients can suppress frequency of voiding and thus urinate very large volumes (close to 1 L) less often; they may develop a dilated bladder, hydroureter, and even hydronephrosis. The onset of polyuria in central DI is often a sudden one.

Polyuria

Definitions of Polyuria

- Polyuria is the excretion of too much urine for a given clinical setting.
- Interpret polyuria by considering each component of the osmole excretion formula:

  Urine volume = osmole excretion/urine osmolality

There are two definitions of polyuria. The first is based on the urine flow rate and is an arbitrary value (greater than 1.5–2 mL/min, or 2.5 L/day, in an adult). The second definition, the one the authors prefer, is based on pathophysiology. In essence, it is a greater rate of excretion of water than one would expect in that clinical setting.

Polyuria as a Function of the Osmole Excretion Rate

Normally, people excrete close to 900 mOsm/day. If we presume, for simplicity, that a patient can achieve a urine osmolality of only 900 mOsm/kg H_2O today, the 24-hour urine volume will be 1 L (900 mOsm at 900 mOsm/kg H_2O). If this patient had an osmotic diuresis with 1800 mOsm to excrete per day at this same urine osmolality, the urine volume would be 2 L in 24 hours, and polyuria would be present.

Two further points need to be emphasized. First, it is extremely difficult to find an extra 900 mOsm to excrete in a day. For example, an extra 900 mmol of urea is equivalent to the catabolism of almost 1 kg of muscle or the digestion of 1 L of blood (see margin note). The only other osmoles of endogenous origin to consider are glucose and salts—neither can be lost at this rate for any sustained period using endogenous supplies. The only way to excrete an extra 900 mOsm is to have an exogenous input, and the solute will almost always be glucose (see the "drinker" subtype of hyperglycemic hyperosmolar syndrome in Chapter 12).

The second point, and a very important one, is that during an osmotic diuresis, the urinary osmolality is unlikely to remain at 900 mOsm/L as in the preceding example (see margin note). Although one can achieve a very high urine osmolality (1200 mOsm/kg H_2O) at low urine flow rates, the renal medullary osmolality falls at very high urine flow rates. It is therefore not surprising to find that the urine osmolality is closer to 450 mOsm/kg H_2O during an osmotic diuresis; the urine volume will be at least 4 L/day when a patient excretes these 1800 mOsm daily (1800 mOsm/450 mOsm/kg H_2O).

Polyuria Based on an Unexpectedly Low Urine Osmolality

There are two major reasons to have an unexpectedly low urine osmolality. First, the renal medulla can be damaged by a number of diseases. If this damage occurs, the urine osmolality will be close to that of plasma when ADH acts (i.e., close to 300 mOsm/kg H_2O, for easy calculating). Accordingly, while one excretes the usual 900 mOsm/day, the daily urine volume will be 3 L (900 mOsm/300 mOsm/kg H_2O). Many clinical nephrologists consider this urine volume to be a form of nephrogenic DI.

A second basis for an unexpectedly low urine osmolality is a lack of ADH (central DI) or a failure of this hormone to insert aquaporin-2 water channels in the late distal convoluted tubule, the cortical collecting duct (CCD), and the MCD (nephrogenic DI). The urine volume now depends on the extent of the lesion. For example, if the urine osmolality is 90 mOsm/kg H_2O, the daily urine volume will be 10 L, but if the urine osmolality is 45 mOsm/kg H_2O, the daily urine volume will be 20 L (900 mOsm ÷ 90 or 45 mOsm/kg H_2O, respectively; see margin note).

Calculation
- One kg of muscle contains 200 g of protein (80% water).
- Protein is 16% nitrogen (N).
- 0.16×200 g = 32 g of N.
- The atomic weight of nitrogen is 14, and urea has two nitrogens. Therefore, 32000 mg/28 = 1143 mmol of urea.
- One liter of blood has 188 g protein:
- 140 g of hemoglobin,
- 48 g of protein (80 g/L but 0.6 L of plasma).

Therefore
For large urine volumes in an osmotic diuresis, the urine osmolality must not be very high.

Note
The same volume of EFW (e.g., 10 L) can be excreted at two different urine osmolalities (e.g., 90 vs 45 mOsm/kg H_2O) by having two different osmole excretion rates (e.g., 900 vs 450 mOsm/day, respectively).

Primary Polydipsia

The excretion of a very large volume of urine in a patient who drinks a large volume of water is called polyuria in the first definition (polyuria based on arbitrary large volumes of urine) but not in our second definition because the appropriate volume of urine is being excreted based on physiologic signals. A "slave to proper definitions" would call this type of excretion a secondary form of polyuria—secondary to polydipsia.

One final point merits emphasis. Using the strict definition of polyuria as a urine volume that is inappropriately high for the clinical setting, a patient with primary polydipsia and hyponatremia can be oliguric while excreting 9 L of urine per day. A look at the numbers makes our point: with an excretion of 900 mOsm/day and a urine volume of 9 L/day, the urine osmolality is 100 mOsm/kg H_2O. But if the expected urine osmolality is 45 mOsm/kg H_2O, the urine volume should be 20 L/day.

Why do we make this seemingly trivial point? An examination of the data in Case 7.6 indicates that ADH is present and acting at some times (urine osmolality greater than 100 mOsm/kg H_2O; see margin note) but possibly not at others (reexpansion of the ECF volume by water ingestion or administration of salt). This view has one major advantage. By recognizing that ADH is acting and suppressing maximal water excretion by close to 50% in Case 7.6 (daily urine volume was 10 instead of the maximum of 20 L), one will not make the mistake of reexpanding the ECF volume (by administering saline) without observing and later limiting the rate of EFW excretion (this rate can be lowered by giving ADH once the desired quantity of water is being excreted). This approach will yield the desired rate of rise in the plasma [Na^+].

Note

It is not possible to deduce the lowest possible urine osmolality in the absence of ADH action without knowing the rate of excretion of osmoles.

- e.g., 10 L of urine/day.
- With an osmole excretion rate of 600 mOsm/day, a Uosm of 60 mOsm/kg H_2O will be required for a 10 L daily urine volume. In contrast, the Uosm will be 90 mOsm/kg H_2O if the osmole excretion rate is 900 mOsm/day and the daily urine volume is still 10 L.

Causes of Polyuria

Because polyuria is very commonly associated with hypernatremia, the authors believe it is appropriate to introduce an approach to polyuria at this point, even though not all causes of polyuria are associated with hypernatremia. Three major causes of polyuria can be identified on the basis of urine osmolality: hyperosmolar, isosmolar, and hypo-osmolar (Figure 8.2). A more detailed approach to polyuria follows.

Hyperosmolar Urine

Clinical pearl

Judging from the level of glucose and urea in plasma plus an estimate of the GFR, deduce whether there were enough filtered osmoles to sustain the osmotic diuresis (see Case 8.5 for an example).

For a large volume of hyperosmolar urine to be excreted, there must be a source of these osmoles. If the urine osmolality is 400 mOsm/kg H_2O, and 5 L of urine are produced per day, 2000 mOsm must be identified (normal is less than half this quantity). If the urine contains much less than 150 mmol/L of Na^+ plus K^+, then look for an osmotic diuretic (close to 300 mmol/L of glucose or urea). A high excretion rate of urea occurs with high-protein feeding, trauma, GI hemorrhage, catabolic state (neoplasm or sepsis), or a high blood urea level (recovery from obstructive uropathy or renal failure; other factors also operate to cause polyuria in these conditions). It is not necessary to administer ADH to establish the diagnosis in this group of patients.

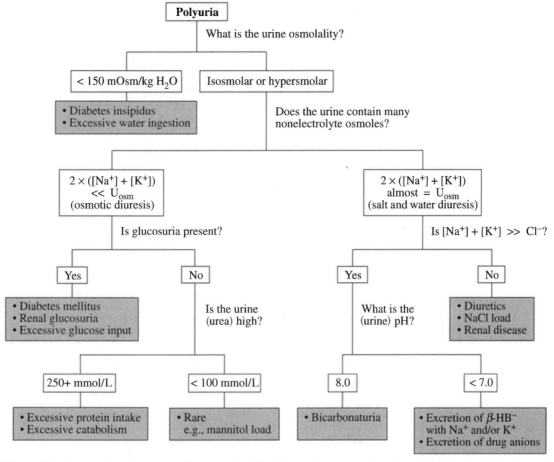

Figure 8.2 Approach to patients with polyuria. The information required to determine the cause of polyuria is shown in the clear boxes, and the final diagnoses are shown in the shaded boxes.

It should be emphasized that each liter of urine excreted during an *osmotic diuresis* is expected to contain close to 50 mmol/L Na^+ and 25–50 mmol/L K^+. If the administration of Na^+ and K^+ is less than 150 mmol/day, deficiency states will ensue and lead to ECF volume contraction and hypokalemia.

Osmotic Diuresis

The challenge is to:
• Identify the osmole.
• Reduce its excretion.
• Replace Na^+, K^+, and water deficits.

Isosmolar Urine

The major differential diagnosis is summarized under "loss of medullary hypertonicity" in Table 8.3. These patients do not show an appreciable increase in urine osmolality following the administration of ADH. It is possible that patients with partial central DI can have isosmolar urine on presentation. In addition, a patient with DI, marked ECF volume contraction, and a low urine flow rate can have urine that is close to isosmolal. In partial central DI, expect at least a significant rise in urine osmolality with ADH administration. The patient undergoing a "saline diuresis" as a result of NaCl administration or loop diuretics may also have isosmolar urine.

Hypo-osmolar Urine

Most hypernatremic patients with very hypo-osmolar urine have central DI; they excrete hyperosmolar urine when ADH is given. Also, certain patients with nephrogenic DI (lithium or demethyltetracycline therapy, congenital nonresponsiveness to ADH) do not have an appreciable increase in urine osmolality after ADH administration.

PART C

Treatment of a Water Deficit

> - Stop the ongoing water loss.
> - Replace the deficit slowly, by the oral route, if possible. If you must give EFW by the IV route, use hypotonic saline plus a limited quantity of glucose in water.

The major objectives of therapy for patients with hypernatremia caused by water loss are to treat the underlying medical problems, to minimize ongoing water losses, and to replace the water deficit.

Stopping the Water Loss

The physician must curtail large ongoing water losses, if possible. The problem of ADH deficiency can easily be rectified with appropriate replacement therapy. If an osmotic diuresis is present, the source of the osmotic agent must be addressed, if possible, and ongoing Na^+ and K^+ losses should be replaced.

Replacing the Water Deficit

Clinical pearls
1. Permit the plasma $[Na^+]$ to decline by close to 10% per day in most patients.
2. A more rapid decline in the plasma $[Na^+]$ is the objective if the hypernatremia is acute or if serious CNS symptoms (coma, seizure) are present.

The water deficit should be calculated, and only a portion (see margin note) should be replaced during the next 12 hours. Total correction should occur over several days. The oral route of water replacement is preferable if the patient is conscious and alert because it avoids the problems of hyperglycemia and glucosuria associated with IV glucose in water administration. The advantages and disadvantages of the IV solutions used for EFW administration are discussed in the following paragraphs.

Glucose in Water (D_5W)

D_5W appears to have ideal properties to deliver EFW intravenously; it is isosmotic initially (thus avoiding hemolysis), and later the osmoles (glucose) disappear as a result of metabolism (see the discussion of Question 8.10 for more information).

QUESTION

(Discussion on page 363)

8.10 *How quickly can the glucose infused in one L of D_5W be metabolized in a patient with hypernatremia?*

Half-Normal Saline

As mentioned earlier, it is important to stop water losses early because it is difficult to administer large volumes of EFW safely. Therapy with just "half-normal" (75 mmol/L) saline is not appropriate if polyuria is present and the $[Na^+]$ in the urine is less than that in the infusion (see margin note).

In patients with a degree of contraction of the ECF volume and no polyuria, the deficit of water should be replaced with half-normal saline and possibly small quantities of D_5W (a maximum of 0.3 L/h). Care should be taken to avoid a serious Na^+ overload. Because each liter of half-normal saline has 500 mL of EFW that distributes throughout total body water, only 333 mL will enter the ICF. In quantitative terms, if the ICF volume is 30 L, then 11 mL of EFW for each liter of half-isotonic saline given will be added to each liter of ICF (the brain contains less than 1 L of ICF). More EFW can be administered if even more hypotonic saline solutions are infused (0.25% or 0.33%), but there is now a risk of hemolysis.

Note
If the $[Na^+]$ in the urine is <100 mmol/L, the "effectiveness" of half-normal saline in the therapy of hypernatremia can be enhanced by increasing the $[Na^+]$ of the urine with a loop diuretic. The difference in $[Na^+]$ between the urine and the IV solution represents the EFW administered.

Distilled Water

Do everything possible to avoid giving distilled water intravenously. If a patient is severely hypertonic, is in congestive heart failure, is severely hyperglycemic, and cannot tolerate dialysis or oral water therapies, it may be necessary to administer sterile water intravenously. This water should be given by central vein, and several liters may be administered per day by this route. Extreme caution and frequent monitoring are required in this setting; the major risk is hemolysis if the water is given too quickly.

Calculation of the Water Deficit in the ICF

When calculating a water deficit, the simplest approach is to obtain quantitative estimates of ECF and ICF volume deficits (see margin note).

Calculation of the water deficit in the ICF
As the hypernatremic patient may have severe ECF volume contraction or expansion, it is best to calculate the water deficit in the ICF and ECF separately.

Data

Imagine that a 70-kg patient lost enough water for the plasma $[Na^+]$ to rise from 140 to 160 mmol/L. The ECF volume, however, is judged to be normal on physical examination. The patient's usual values are an ICF volume of 30 L and an ECF volume of 15 L.

Long Form of the Calculation

The first step is to calculate body water balance by assessing the current vs the expected ICF and ECF volumes.

Usual "effective" osmoles in the ICF
- Assume that a 70-kg adult has 30 L of ICF and a plasma [Na$^+$] of 140 mmol/L.
- 2 (140 mmol/L) $\times$ 30 L = 8400 mOsm.

Change in ICF Volume. One can calculate this change by using the "effective" osmolality and by assuming a constant number of effective osmoles. Normally, the total number of effective osmoles in the ICF is the product of the ICF volume (30 L) and 2 $\times$ plasma [Na$^+$], or 8400 mOsm. After the water loss, assume no change in number of effective osmoles in the ICF. Thus, the new effective osmolality is 320 mOsm/kg H$_2$O (2 $\times$ new plasma [Na$^+$]). Dividing 8400 by 320 yields the new ICF volume of 26.25 L, a fall of 3.75 L.

Short Form of the Calculation of the ICF Water Deficit

Assume total ICF osmoles do not change. Let ["e"] represent the concentration of effective osmoles, which is equal to 2 $\times$ [Na$^+$].

$$\text{ICF volume}_{normal} \times [\text{"e"}]_{normal} = \text{ICF volume}_{abnormal} \times [\text{"e"}]_{abnormal}$$

Sample Calculation

- [Na$^+$] = 160 mmol/L.
- Effective osmolality = 2 $\times$ 160 mmol/L = 320 mOsm/L.
- Normal ICF volume = 30 L.
- Therefore, 30 L $\times$ 280 = new ICF volume $\times$ 320.

New ICF volume = 26.25 L.

Calculation of Deficits in the ECF

Change in ECF Volume. The ECF volume is not revealed by the plasma [Na$^+$]. It is based on a clinical assessment of the vascular volume and, more importantly, the *interstitial volume*. This estimate is imprecise. A 10% decrease in ECF volume will have subtle manifestations; a 20% reduction will be associated with symptoms; and shock will usually accompany a 30% deficit in ECF volume.

[Na$^+$] in interstitial fluid
- With a Donnan factor of 0.95 for cations, the [Na$^+$] in interstitial fluid would be lower than plasma.
- Because there is nonaqueous volume present (6%), the plasma [Na$^+$] is 94% of the actual value (152 mmol/kg H$_2$O).
- Overall, these two factors virtually cancel each other, so the plasma and interstitial [Na$^+$] are almost equal.

Change in Na$^+$ Balance in the ECF. The second step is to calculate the change in content of Na$^+$ in the ECF. The normal content of Na$^+$ is the product of the [Na$^+$] in the ECF (for simplicity, assume 140 mmol/L, the same as that in plasma; see margin note) and the normal ECF volume (15 L). The current content of Na$^+$ in the ECF is the measured [Na$^+$] in plasma multiplied by the clinical estimate of the ECF volume. If the current content of Na$^+$ exceeds the original value, Na$^+$ must have been gained; if the current content of Na$^+$ is less than the original value, Na$^+$ must have been lost.

Contraction of the ECF volume
This 70-kg patient is assessed to have a 20% reduction of the ECF volume (normally 15 L).

Sample Calculation. If the plasma [Na$^+$] was 160 mmol/L and there was a 3 L or a 20% decrease in ECF volume, the content of Na$^+$ in the ECF is 12 L $\times$ 160 mmol/L = 1920 mmoles, whereas the normal ECF content is 2100 mmol (15 L $\times$ 140 mmol/L) (see margin note). Therefore, in addition to the 3-L deficit of water in the ECF, there is a deficit of 180 mmol of Na$^+$. One can view the ECF deficit as 1.2 L of 0.9% saline and 1.8 L of EFW. Therefore, the patient's total deficits are 5.6 L of EFW (3.75 ICF and 1.8 ECF) and 1.2 L of isotonic saline.

Details of Therapy

- Objectives
  1. To calculate mass balance for Na⁺.
  2. To calculate mass balance for water.
  3. To estimate changes present in the ECF and ICF volumes.
  4. To correct the ECF volume quickly if it is contracted and the patient is hypotensive.
  5. To correct the ICF volume slowly unless the patient is seriously symptomatic.

Estimate Mass Balances for Na⁺ and Water

- Replace the ECF volume quickly if the patient is hypotensive.
- Loss of K⁺ without phosphate is matched for the most part by a shift of Na⁺ into cells.

Na⁺

Another consideration for total body Na⁺ is the quantity of Na⁺ that might have shifted into cells in conjunction with a negative balance for K⁺ that is independent of the loss of intracellular anions (monovalent phosphate). Assume that most of this deficit of K⁺ was matched by a shift of Na⁺ into cells (see the discussions of Cases 7.1 and 10.1 for more information).

Ongoing losses of Na⁺ will have to be replaced to achieve the desired change in Na⁺ balance. To create a negative balance for Na⁺, administer a loop diuretic, but reinfuse all losses of water and K⁺.

QUESTION

(Discussion on page 363)

8.11 *If a 70-kg patient has a [Na⁺] of 154 mmol/L and a very marked degree of ECF volume contraction, what is the most likely pathophysiology for this lesion?*

Water

- The asymptomatic patient requires a slow replacement of ICF volume.

There are two ways to give EFW and expand the ICF volume: first, one can administer EFW, two-thirds of which should distribute in the ICF in normal individuals; second, one can cause a loss of isotonic saline and replace all the electrolytes that were lost in a larger volume (see margin note).

One can remove Na⁺ but not water from the ECF; this option

Clinical pearl
During therapy, administration of KCl is similar to administration of NaCl as far as the ECF is concerned (K⁺ leave the ICF mainly in "exchange" for Na⁺); the reverse occurs as K⁺ are lost.

Goal of therapy
- Give 1 L of EFW.

Treatment Part 1
Give a loop diuretic and measure what is excreted (see diagram below).

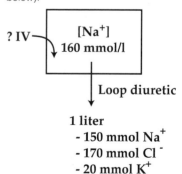

Treatment Part 2
Give: 2 liters of half-isotonic saline (75 mmol NaCl per liter) + 20 mmoles KCl.

Balance
The net result is a positive balance of 1 liter of EFW.

should be considered only if the ECF volume is expanded. To lose Na^+ but not water, administer a loop diuretic to lose Na^+, K^+, Cl^-, plus water; then replace all the K^+ as KCl, and water without replacing $Na^+ + Cl^-$.

It is easiest to calculate the changes in the ECF and ICF volumes independently. The change in ECF volume is assessed clinically, and the change in ICF volume in liters is calculated as described on page 346.

- During therapy, decrease the $[Na^+]$ by close to 0.5 mmol/L/h if the patient is not seriously symptomatic (up to a total of 12 mmol/L/24 h).

Sample calculation

In a 70-kg patient with hypernatremia (160 mmol/L), to lower the $[Na^+]$ by 1 mmol/L/h the positive water balance should be 250 mL/h.

- Percent decline in $[Na^+]$ × total body water = positive water balance.
- $((160 - 159)/160) \times 40$ L = 250 mL.

Note

If the patient is hyperglycemic, do not use D_5W; instead, use hypotonic saline (half the volume of half-normal saline is EFW, or, better still, three-fourths of the volume of quarter-normal saline is EFW).

Note of caution

The $[Na^+]$ in plasma can rise by close to 15 mmol/L during a convulsion.

To achieve a positive water balance and a fall in the plasma $[Na^+]$, the $[Na^+]$ in the IV solution should be compared with that in the patient if the patient is oliguric and with the $[Na^+]$ plus the $[K^+]$ in the urine if the patient is polyuric (see margin note). Examples are provided in the Cases for Review section.

If the patient is experiencing a convulsion, it is possible that the change in brain-cell size has contributed to this emergency (see margin for a note of caution). Aside from the usual means of treating a patient who is convulsing, it is advisable to change the $[Na^+]$ to the value it was before the convulsion. In effect, the $[Na^+]$ should decrease quickly by less than 6 mmol/L. This change can be implemented with the administration of enough EFW (D_5W, $D_{2.5}W$). The volume to infuse should be calculated as follows for a patient with a plasma $[Na^+]$ of 160 mmol/L:

—Assume no change in ICF osmoles.
—Let ["e"] represent the concentration of effective osmoles, which is approximately equal to $2 \times [Na^+]$.
—Initial ["e"] was 2×160 mmol/L = 320 mOsm/L.
—Final ["e"] should be about 2×156 mmol/L (i.e., a decline of 4 mmol/L) = 312 mOsm/L.
—ICF volume at a $[Na^+]$ of 160 was 26.25 L (see page 346).
—Therefore, $320 \times 26.25 = 312 \times$ new ICF volume.
New ICF volume = 27 L, a gain of 0.75 L.

To keep the extra 0.75 L of water in the ICF, one needs to administer 1.125 L, given that approximately two-thirds of the water given remains in the ICF. One need not consider water excretion because it should be small over a very short time span.

QUESTIONS

(Discussions on pages 363–365)

8.12 *Lydia, age 85, was transferred from a nursing home because of a low blood pressure (90/60 mm Hg) and a rapid pulse rate of 110 BPM; her jugular venous pressure is 2 cm below the sternal angle. Her laboratory values reveal the following:*

		Plasma	Urine
Na$^+$	mmol/L	170	40
K$^+$	mmol/L	3.0	60
Cl$^-$	mmol/L	127	—
HCO$_3^-$	mmol/L	30	—
Osmolality	mOsm/kg H$_2$O	360	600

Why is she hypernatremic?
Detail your fluid and electrolyte management.

8.13 *A 70-kg patient has DI, hypernatremia (154 mmol/L), and a normal ECF volume. What is the most likely pathophysiology to explain this set of findings? Provide a quantitative answer. What are the objectives for therapy?*

8.14 *A patient has a clinical syndrome that resembles central DI. One unusual finding is present: the urine osmolality rises when DDAVP is given but not when ADH is given. How does this finding help in defining the etiology?*

PART D

Review

DISCUSSION OF INTRODUCTORY CASE
Treat the Patient Before He (DI)es
(Case presented on page 331)

Of what significance is the modest degree of contraction of the ECF volume?

Hypernatremia is due to Na$^+$ gain or water loss from the ECF. The reduced ECF volume indicates that the hypernatremia in this case is due primarily to loss of water.

Why was thirst absent?

Hypernatremia elicits a thirst response unless a CNS lesion is present (a generalized CNS problem such as confusion, a specific lesion involving the thirst center, or a communication problem). This patient was confused and thus had an inability to translate thirst into access to water.

Of what significance is the loss of body weight?

The loss of weight indicates that the cause of hypernatremia is water loss from the body (not a shift of water into muscles; this could have occurred with a convulsion).

What is the significance of the polyuria?

Polyuria suggests a problem of either diabetes insipidus (DI) or the presence of a diuretic. Because the urine is quite hypo-osmolar in the presence of hypernatremia, the patient has DI.

Can any inference be made from the urine osmolality and the acuteness of the onset?

The low osmolality and the acuteness of onset both suggest a diagnosis of central rather than nephrogenic DI. In this case, the meningitis and/or the phenytoin could have caused a low ADH release. This impression can be confirmed by an appropriate renal response to exogenous ADH (a rise in osmolality and a decrease in the volume of urine).

What should the therapy be?

Leverage for therapy
- Increase water intake. A person who has 900 mOsm to excrete and a urine osmolality of 100 mOsm/kg H_2O needs more than 9 L input per day. You just cannot infuse that volume of water safely.
- Stop water loss. This is where the leverage exists in this patient; give ADH.

Therapy has two major aims. First, stop water loss by giving ADH (see margin note); second, water must be given as half-normal saline (a danger is ECF volume over-expansion) or as glucose in water, provided that hyperglycemia is not present. Do not give more than 0.3 L D_5W/h (dangers are hyperglycemia and a glucose-induced osmotic diuresis, which will cause additional water loss).

Cases for Review

CASE 8.1
The Shrink Shrank the Cells
(Case discussed on pages 352–353)

Manny, a 37-year-old, has been suffering from a bipolar affective disorder for the past 5 years. Lithium has helped him tremendously, but he drinks several liters of water each day. Elective surgery is planned for the near future.

To avoid the complications of lithium-induced nephrogenic DI, what preparations should be made for Manny before and during this operation?

Supplemental Question

Postoperatively, Manny is passing 3 mL urine/min with an osmolality of 150 mOsm/kg H_2O and a [Na^+] of 35 mmol/L; he is now hypernatremic (154 mmol/L). What advice would be appropriate now? Estimate his urine volume over the next 24 hours (assume no change in urine osmolality).

CASE 8.2
Who Put the Na⁺ in Mrs. Murphy's Breast Milk?
(Case discussed on pages 353–354)

Lois, age 2 weeks, has had a rough time. She was normal at birth, weighing 3.5 kg (7.7 lb). She has deteriorated since then and has lost 1 kg (2.2 lb) of weight. She is breast-fed. Diarrhea and vomiting were not present, and she has not taken medications. No other information was provided on history. On presentation, she has a very contracted ECF volume and is virtually anuric. The only laboratory data available are a plasma [Na$^+$] of 180 mmol/L, glucose of 1.1 mmol/L (20 mg/dL), and urea of 75 mmol/L (210 mg/dL). A brilliant intern sent a sample of breast milk for analysis, and the results were unexpected ([Na$^+$] was 107 mmol/L instead of the usual 7 mmol/L).

Is the hypernatremia due to the consumption of "hypernatric" breast milk?
What role might the high [Na$^+$] in breast milk play in this case?
What role might the hypoglycemia play?
What treatment should Lois receive?

CASE 8.3
Steve Is Pee(d) Off
(Case discussed on page 355)

After exams, the class partied. In the competition to see who could drink the most alcohol, Steve won! He went home and slept off his victory. He was very polyuric and was brought to the emergency room the next day. His ECF volume was mildly contracted. His laboratory values follow.

		Plasma	Urine
Na$^+$	mmol/L	152	5
K$^+$	mmol/L	4.0	10
Glucose	mmol/L (mg/dL)	4.0 (72)	0
Urea	mmol/L (mg/dL)	2.0 (5.6)	20
Osmolality	mOsm/kg H$_2$O	420	287

How do your explain Steve's hypernatremia and polyuria?

CASE 8.4
Central DI in an Unbalanced Setting
(Case discussed on page 355)

Adam had neurosurgery for a tumor near his pituitary. The surgery was successful, and the surgeons were expecting central DI in the acute postoperative period. They placed the patient on an IV solution containing EFW (half-isotonic saline, 75 mmol/L for easy calculation) and stated that the rate of infusion should be equal to the urine output.

At the 10-hour postoperative time, the urine flow rate was 12 mL/min (0.7 L/h); the urine osmolality was 100 mOsm/kg H$_2$O, and the plasma [Na$^+$] was 154 mmol/L. Because the patient had received 3 L of isotonic saline and 100 g of mannitol during surgery, the differential diagnosis was central DI and/or an osmotic diuresis.

What data are essential to diagnose central DI in this setting?
Why did hypernatremia develop (Na$^+$ gain or water loss)?
What is your treatment?
What will you use to reflect the actions of ADH?
What is the osmole excretion rate? Is an osmotic diuresis due to mannitol important in this case?

CASE 8.5
Osmotic Diuresis, Not a Solute Decision
(Case discussed on pages 356–358)

A 59-year-old diabetic male had hypercalcemia and a lymphoma. His main symptoms were polydipsia, polyuria, and bone pain. He was on no medication other than an oral hypoglycemic agent for his long-standing non–insulin-dependent diabetes mellitus; there was no history of prior treatment with lithium.

On physical examination, his ECF volume was contracted as evidenced by hypotension (blood pressure 100/60 mm Hg) and low jugular venous column height (1–2 cm below the sternal angle).

Over 24 hours, his urine output was 6 L. A spot urine sample revealed an osmolality of 600 mOsm/kg H_2O; the urine did not contain glucose or ketone bodies.

		Plasma	Random Urine
Na^+	mmol/L	147	49
K^+	mmol/L	3.5	30
Ca^{2+}	mmol/L	3.7	—
Glucose	mmol/L (mg/dL)	3.2 (61)	0
Urea	mmol/L (mg/dL)	10 (28)	—
Creatinine	μmol/L (mg/dL)	197 (2.3)	—
Osmolality	mOsm/kg H_2O	306	600

Can polyuria be due to an osmotic diuresis?

If this is predominantly a water diuresis, why was his urine osmolality so high in a random urine?

What might the role of hypercalcemia be with respect to the urine volume and osmolality?

Discussion of Cases

DISCUSSION OF CASE 8.1
The Shrink Shrank the Cells
(Case presented on page 350)

To avoid lithium-induced nephrogenic DI, what preparations should be made for Manny before and during this operation?

Lithium-induced nephrogenic DI may or may not be reversed when lithium is discontinued. In consultation with Manny's psychiatrist, lithium was discontinued for 3 weeks. His 24-hour urine volume still remained at 5 L/day. He is normonatremic, so a brief period of water restriction will distinguish between habitual polydipsia and nephrogenic DI. With water restriction, his [Na^+] rose, and he was still polyuric; there was no change in urine volume or osmolality following the administration of ADH. Hence, Manny has nephrogenic DI, which seems to be a permanent condition.

Manny should have hypotonic solutions infused in the postoperative period; the [Na^+] in the IV solution should be close to that in the urine. Hyperglycemia should be avoided, and his plasma [Na^+] should be monitored closely.

Supplemental Question

Postoperatively, Manny is passing 3 mL urine/min with an osmolality of 150 mOsm/kg H$_2$O and a [Na$^+$] of 35 mmol/L; he is now hypernatremic (154 mmol/L). What advice would be appropriate now? Estimate his urine volume over the next 24 hours (assume no change in urine osmolality).

Manny was infused with half-normal saline to match his urine output throughout his surgery and postoperative period. This IV solution had a lower [Na$^+$] than his plasma. Hypernatremia developed because 75 mmol of Na$^+$ was infused for every liter of urine excreted (each liter of urine contained only 35 mmol of Na$^+$), and he was therefore in positive balance of 40 mmol of Na$^+$ per liter throughput. This balance should lead to the development of hypernatremia and an expanded ECF volume.

Advice Concerning Balance for Na$^+$. His ECF volume is normal, but each liter contains an extra 14 mmol of Na$^+$. Therefore, he must lose 210 mmol of Na$^+$ (15 L × 14 mmol/L). To achieve this loss, stop the intake, and promote the excretion of Na$^+$; it might be necessary to use a diuretic. This component of the analysis deals with balance for Na$^+$ but not water.

Advice Concerning Balance for Water. His ECF volume is normal, and his ICF volume is down 3 L (10% of an ICF volume of 30 L; see margin note); he therefore needs 3 L of positive EFW balance; ongoing losses must also be replaced. Use the oral route to administer water, if possible.

Practical Considerations. If one gives Manny furosemide, induces a diuresis, and replaces the urine with D$_5$W, after 2 L of urine output Manny will lose 200 mmol of Na$^+$ (the urine [Na$^+$] is most likely to be 100 mmol/L). D$_5$W should not be given at a rate that exceeds 300 mL/h.

If Manny's ECF volume had been contracted, one would have replaced total body water with 3 L of EFW—2 would have gone to the ICF and 1 to the ECF. The ECF volume would have been coincidentally restored with isotonic saline.

TONICITY BALANCE

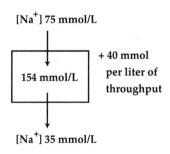

[Na$^+$] 75 mmol/L

154 mmol/L

+ 40 mmol per liter of throughput

[Na$^+$] 35 mmol/L

Note
A [Na$^+$] of 154 is 10% higher than the normal value of 140 mmol/L.

DISCUSSION OF CASE 8.2
Who Put the Na$^+$ in Mrs. Murphy's Breast Milk?
(Case presented on pages 350–351)

Is the hypernatremia due to the consumption of "hypernatric" breast milk?

No. If one ingests NaCl with little water, hypernatremia may develop, but the ECF volume will be expanded, not contracted. With time and an expanded ECF volume, Na$^+$ will be excreted. Therefore, the ECF volume will return to normal or even become mildly contracted because of a natriuresis induced by hypernatremia. Nevertheless, shock is a very unlikely outcome.

Deficit of Na⁺
Normal = 140 mmol (140 mmol/L
    × 1 L)
Admission = 126 mmol (180 mmol/
    L × 0.7 L)
Difference = 14 mmol deficit

Calculation
- Osmolality of breast milk equals the osmolality of the mother.
- Subtract 2 × ([Na⁺] + [K⁺]) for the maximum concentration of lactose.

Calculation
- 100 g of protein = 16 g of nitrogen.
  16 g of nitrogen = 572 mmol of urea (molecular weight of nitrogen = 14, and there are two nitrogen atoms per urea).
- 100 g of protein = 60 g of glucose.
  60 g of glucose = 333 mmol (molecular weight of glucose = 180).
- 572/333 = 1.7

If Lois' ECF volume was initially 1 L (for easy arithmetic) and is now 0.7 L, she will have a total body deficit of Na⁺ (see margin note).

What role might the high [Na⁺] in breast milk play in this case?

To understand the pathogenesis of Lois' problem, one must appreciate that breast milk is isotonic to her mother's plasma (285 mOsm/kg H_2O). Lactose normally constitutes the majority of osmoles (220 mOsm/kg H_2O; electrolytes constitute 45 mOsm/kg H_2O). In this case, with a [Na⁺] of 107 mmol/L in breast milk, there is "room" for, at most, 45 mOsm/kg H_2O lactose (285 − 2 × (107 + 13) mmol/L Na⁺ and K⁺, respectively), which is an insufficient nutritional supply. Therefore, Lois is carbohydrate-starved and must obtain the glucose for her brain from gluconeogenesis and glycogenolysis.

What role might the hypoglycemia play?

Lois' hypoglycemia led to the production of glucose from her body proteins because her stores of glycogen were depleted. For every millimole of glucose formed, 1.7 mmol of urea is formed (see margin note). Excretion of this extra urea will lead to an osmotic diuresis in this setting because the immature kidneys do not reabsorb Na⁺ as well as normal adult kidneys. Hence, Lois excreted large volumes of water with a [Na⁺] that is likely to be in the 50 mmol/L range. This excretion, driven by the urea load, could explain the low ECF volume and the hypernatremia.

What treatment should Lois receive?

Avoid Hypoglycemia. Give enough glucose (5 mmol, 90 mg) to raise the concentration of glucose to normal acutely (ECF volume + 1/4 ICF volume); then give enough glucose to maintain euglycemia, but avoid hyperglycemia because it will lead to shrinking of cells and further osmotic diuresis.

Reexpand the ECF Volume. Give 300 mL of saline with a [Na⁺] close to that of Lois, and replace urine losses when they occur.

Reexpand the ICF Volume Slowly. Give a positive water balance of close to 150 mL to lower the [Na⁺] 12 mmol/L/day.
—Assume no change in ICF osmoles.
—Let ["e"] represent the concentration of effective osmoles, which is close to 2 × [Na⁺].
—Initial ["e"] was 2 × 180 mmol/L = 360 mmol/L.
—Final ["e"] after 24 hours should be 2 × (180 − 12) mmol/L = 336 mmol/L.
—ICF volume at an [Na⁺] of 180 was close to 2 L.
—Therefore, 360 × 2 = 336 × new ICF volume.
New ICF volume = 2.15 L, a positive balance of 0.15 L, or 150 mL, is needed.

Improve Her Nutritional State. Bottle and IV feeding should be sufficient.

DISCUSSION OF CASE 8.3
Steve Is Pee(d) Off
(Case presented on page 351)

How do you explain Steve's hypernatremia and polyuria?

Hypernatremia. Hypernatremia implies Na^+ gain or water loss. There was no Na^+ intake by history, and his ECF volume was mildly contracted, so he had water loss from the ECF.

Water could have shifted into his cells, but there was no evidence of a convulsion or rhabdomyolysis. Subsequent investigations did not support this diagnosis, either.

Water loss was occurring via the kidneys. Although Steve had excessive water intake with alcohol, the water loss was inappropriate because he was hypernatremic. Hypernatremia and excessive renal water loss imply very low actions of ADH. Although nephrogenic DI is possible, it does not develop this quickly.

We speculate that the basis for the low levels of ADH was suppression of its release by ethanol. Note that Steve had a plasma osmolal gap of 110 mOsm/kg H_2O ($420 - (2 \times 152) - 4 - 2$), consistent with astronomic levels of ethanol in plasma (later confirmed by direct assay).

Two other points merit emphasis. First, the urine osmolality was very high considering the large loss of water that induced hypernatremia. The osmolal gap of the urine reveals that most of the osmoles were ethanol, an "ineffective" osmole with regard to water shifts. Hence, Steve's nonethanol osmolality was close to 100 mOsm/kg H_2O, consistent with central DI. Second, his natural history was interesting. As Steve metabolized ethanol in his body, his urine osmolality rose to 456 mOsm/kg H_2O 8 hours later without treatment. The ethanol level was 56 mmol/L in plasma at that time.

Polyuria. Even though Steve's osmole excretion rate was above normal, most of the osmoles were ethanol, and ethanol does not cause an osmotic diuresis. He had ethanol-induced suppression of ADH release, not nephrogenic DI or an osmotic diuresis.

DISCUSSION OF CASE 8.4
Central DI in an Unbalanced Setting
(Case presented on page 351)

What data are essential to diagnose central DI in this setting?

There are three mechanisms to consider in diagnosing central DI. First, one needs to find a stimulus for the release of ADH; that stimulus was hypernatremia. Second, the urine should be far less than maximally concentrated, and the urine flow rate should be inappropriately high. Third, in response to ADH, the urine volume should decline significantly, and the urine osmolality should rise to at least that in plasma.

Why did hypernatremia develop (Na^+ gain or water loss)?

To decide whether the hypernatremia is due to Na^+ gain or water loss, a tonicity balance should be calculated (see Figure in margin).

(i) Water balance: Because the infusion of water was equal to the urinary loss, there was no appreciable negative balance for water.

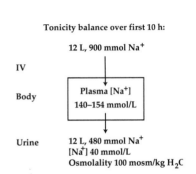

Tonicity balance over first 10 h:

IV   12 L, 900 mmol Na^+

Body   Plasma [Na^+] 140–154 mmol/L

Urine   12 L, 480 mmol Na^+
[Na^+] 40 mmol/L
Osmolality 100 mosm/kg H_2O

(ii) Hypernatremia developed because 900 mmol of Na^+ was infused, and 480 mmol of Na^+ was excreted. The positive balance for Na^+ was 480 mmol and virtually equal to the rise in the plasma $[Na^+]$ (14 mmol/L) $\times$ total body water of 30 L.

What is your treatment?

The first step in the treatment is to stop the excretion of EFW. This is accomplished by giving ADH. The next step is to induce a negative balance of 480 mmol of Na^+. If the urine output is very low, give a loop diuretic to increase Na^+ loss. You can treat this hypernatremia rapidly because it is acute.

What will you use to reflect the actions of ADH?

The urine osmolality should rise, indicating ADH actions. At first, the osmolality should be somewhat greater than that of plasma; it will rise much further once the plasma urea level rises. Another parameter to evaluate is the $[Na + K]$ in the urine. The expected value is 150–300 mmol/L; values approaching 300 mmol/L will be seen with time. The second indicator of ADH actions is a fall in the urine flow rate.

What is the osmole excretion rate?

The osmole excretion rate is 1200 mOsm for 12 hours (100 mOsm/L $\times$ 12 L), more than double the normal rate, so there is excessive excretion of osmoles in this patient with central DI.

Is an osmotic diuresis due to mannitol important in this case?

The next step is to examine the nature of the osmoles excreted—they are almost all Na^+ salts—the nonelectrolyte osmoles $(100 - (2 \times 40)$ mOsm/L) times 12 L is 240 mOsm/12 h, close to the expected value, so this is not a urea- or mannitol-induced osmotic diuresis.

Final Diagnosis: Central DI Due to Surgery

Tonicity Balance. Hypernatremia due to positive balance for Na^+ because the patient could not excrete urine with a high enough $[Na^+]$ (lack of ADH).

Osmole Excretion Rate. This was very high and was due either to the excessive Na^+ load infused or to "cerebral salt wasting" (see discussion of following case).

DISCUSSION OF CASE 8.5
Osmotic Diuresis, Not a Solute Decision
(Case presented on page 352)

Can polyuria be due to an osmotic diuresis?

To explain his urine volume of 6 L/day, either the number of osmoles excreted must be very large and/or the urine osmolality must be very low (see margin note). Because the urine osmolality is 5–10 times greater than that characteristically seen in a water

Note

Volume $\times$ osmolality = No. osmoles

$\therefore$ Volume $= \dfrac{\text{No. osmoles excreted}}{\text{urine osmolality}}$

diuresis (600 vs 50–80 mOsm/kg H_2O), the number of osmoles should be examined first.

Osmole Excretion Rate. This patient appears to have a very high osmole excretion rate (3600 mOsm/day, 600 mOsm/kg H_2O × 6 L/day; persons on a typical diet excrete only 600–900 mOsm/day). The majority of these osmoles are organic because electrolytes are the minor solutes in his random urine. Organic solutes that usually cause an osmotic diuresis are glucose, mannitol, and urea. Because the patient was not given mannitol and did not have glucosuria, the only compound left to evaluate was urea.

A urea-induced osmotic diuresis is not present because his kidneys did not filter 3600 mmol of urea per day (GFR of 100 L/day and plasma [urea] of 10 mmol/L; because his plasma creatinine is twice normal, the authors assume that his GFR was 100 L/day). Therefore, this cannot be a urea-induced osmotic diuresis.

In the absence of a staggeringly high level of ethanol (not present in plasma; plasma osmolality was 303 mOsm/kg H_2O), it follows that the urine sample analyzed cannot be similar in composition to the usual 24-hour urine sample. Hence, the values in the random urine seem to be best explained by the hypothesis that at times the patient was excreting a very dilute urine, whereas at other times he was able to concentrate his urine. A possible resolution to this problem is considered in the discussion of the following question.

If this is predominantly a water diuresis, why was his urine osmolality so high in a random urine?

A water diuresis of 5 L/day can be the result of drinking a similar volume of water; nevertheless, patients with psychogenic polydipsia do not become hypernatremic. Thus, central and/or nephrogenic DI is (are) now the main cause(s) of a water diuresis to consider.

Central DI. The finding of a urine osmolality of 600 mOsm/kg H_2O in a random urine specimen should rule out most causes of nephrogenic DI (hereditary causes, lithium ingestion). Therefore, attention was directed at central DI. The urinary osmolality rose to 600 mOsm/kg H_2O when ADH was administered, so permanent central DI was not a likely cause for his water diuresis. The basis for the central DI, if present, is an "on-again, off-again" action of ADH (see Table 7.3). Support for this theory was found in a review of the fluid balance records. Despite little variation in oral intake, urine volumes in three successive 8-hour shifts differed markedly (1.3, 0.45, and 2.3 L, respectively). Further, values for the osmolality of randomly collected urine samples ranged from 100 to 600 mOsm/kg H_2O. We presumed that his release of ADH was stimulated by afferent input to the ADH center by the low ECF volume, anxiety, nausea, and/or pain.

Nephrogenic DI. Nephrogenic DI might be related to hypercalcemia, as discussed in the next question.

What might the role of hypercalcemia be with respect to the urine volume and osmolality?

Hypercalcemia causes nephrogenic DI; however, why might nephrogenic DI not lead to a consistently hypo-osmolal urine in this setting? Here is where newer insights in physiology may help

Note
Filtered load = GFR × [urea]
1000 mmol = 100 L/day × 10 mmol/L

to understand the clinical findings. When the urine-ionized Ca^{2+} concentration is excessively high, Ca^{2+} binds to a receptor in the lumen of the MCD and, as a result, causes itself *and* aquaporin-2 (AQP-2) water channels to leave the luminal membrane of the MCD despite ADH actions (Figure 8.3). At this time, there is a large water diuresis. At other times (speculation), urinary Ca^{2+} excretion declines, either due to a fall in GFR (low ECF volume) and/or a lower plasma $[Ca^{2+}]$ (the authors noted variations in the plasma $[Ca^{2+}]$ before treatment of 3.7 mmol/L (peak) and 3.2 mmol/L (nadir)). When urinary ionized Ca^{2+} excretion is low enough, AQP-2 remains in the luminal membrane. Note that hypernatremia is present, and this should cause ADH levels in plasma to be high if the pituitary/hypothalamus axis is intact, so control of water excretion depends on whether AQP-2 channels are inserted in the luminal membrane (no polyuria) or remain in vesicles in the cytosol (polyuria) (see margin note).

Note

Although this is an attractive theory, the authors have their doubts because the highest urine $[Ca^{2+}]$ occurs with the smallest urine volumes.

Summary of Main Points

- Hypernatremia is an increase in the Na^+ content relative to that of water. Although hypernatremia provides no insight into the ECF volume status, it does indicate that the ICF volume is contracted.
- Hypernatremia is most commonly due to net water loss and is rarely due to excess retention of exogenous Na^+.
- Hypernatremia indicates either a defect in water acquisition and/or excessive water excretion.
- The hypernatremic patient should be thirsty and should excrete the minimum volume of maximally concentrated urine (>1000 mOsm/kg H_2O).
- Brain cells can regulate their ICF volume in hypernatremia by gaining particles. Therefore, the rate of correction of hypernatremia should be dictated by the clinical symptoms and not by the plasma $[Na^+]$. Generally, unless the CNS symptoms are severe, the $[Na^+]$ should be lowered at a rate of 0.5–1 mmol/L/h, up to a maximum of 12 mmol/L/day.

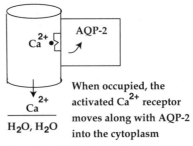

When occupied, the activated Ca^{2+} receptor moves along with AQP-2 into the cytoplasm

Figure 8.3 Putative role of Ca^{2+} in the MCD. The barrel-like structure is the IMCD and the rectangle is a cell. There is a luminal Ca^{2+} receptor on the luminal membrane. If occupied, there is a recycling process that pulls this receptor and the water channel (aquaporin-2) together into the cytosol, where they exist in a vesicle; this could theoretically produce nephrogenic DI if the ionized $[Ca^{2+}]$ in luminal fluid rose to very high levels.

Discussion of Questions

8.1 Consider the following four examples where the concentration of non–urea solutes is 600 mOsm/kg H_2O in the urine (and interstitial fluid because ADH is acting).

Patient	Urea (mOsm/day)	Electrolytes (mOsm/day)
A	400	400
B	50	400
C	400	1600
D	50	100

What is the urine volume and osmolality in each patient?

The urine volume in each patient is the ratio of the number of milliosmoles of electrolytes divided by 600 mOsm/kg H_2O, the non–urea osmolality. Hence, it is 0.67 L/day in patients A and B, 2.67 L in patient C, and 0.167 L in patient D.

The urine osmolality in each of these patients is the sum of the urea plus electrolytes in mOsm/day divided by the daily urine volume. Values in mOsm/kg H_2O are 1200 in patient A, 675 in patient B, 750 in patient C, and 900 in patient D.

What is a likely diagnosis in each case?

Patient A: A normal person who is deprived of water.

Patient B: Given the low urea excretion, this is someone who is eating a very low protein diet.

Patient C: Given the high rate of excretion of electrolytes, this is someone who either has been given a large amount of saline or one who is excreting Na^+ at an excessive rate, e.g., a "cerebral salt waster."

Patient D: Given the low excretion of electrolytes and of urea, this patient is probably being treated for advanced liver disease, with a low-salt and low-protein diet.

Note

An adult who consumes a typical diet excretes close to 800 mOsm/day

8.2 You are asked to see two patients in the intensive care unit because they have a urine output of only 15 mL/h (360 mL/day). Patient A had cardiac surgery, and edema fluid is present, whereas patient B has a low ECF volume and a normal heart. Both have virtually no Na^+ or Cl^- in their urine.
How could you tell if the GFR had fallen?
What would you measure in the urine to determine why the urine flow rate is so low?

How could you tell if the GFR has fallen?

If the low urine flow rate was associated with a fall in the GFR, a progressive rise in the plasma creatinine concentration would be expected.

What would you measure in the urine to determine why the urine flow rate is so low?

Urine

Na$^+$	mmol/L	5
K$^+$	mmol/L	10
Cl$^-$	mmol/L	8
Uosm	mosm/kg H$_2$O	700

Note

See discussion of Question 8.6 for an example of another cause for reduced urine output.

The urine parameters must be considered together with the clinical state to fully analyze the case and determine the therapeutic approach. Consider two patients with identical urine findings (see margin note).

The first patient presents as post–cardiac surgery, with hypotension, an elevated pulmonary capillary wedge pressure, and crackles in the chest. The second presents with severe gastroenteritis and hypotension. Both patients show evidence of ADH action (high urine osmolality) in keeping with this clinical state. Both have a low Na$^+$ + Cl$^-$ excretion rate, implying that there is a message to the kidney to retain Na$^+$ and Cl$^-$. In the first case, there is renal underperfusion due to poor cardiac output ("substandard myocardium"), and the appropriate therapy is to enhance the cardiac output with inotropes and promote the excretion of Na$^+$ with diuretics if the need arises. Do not infuse NaCl.

In the second case, there is poor renal perfusion due to ECF volume contraction; the appropriate therapy is to restore the ECF volume with isotonic NaCl.

8.3 You are confronted with three patients; each has hypernatremia (154 mmol/L). One patient drank sea water, another lost pure water, and the third lost hypotonic saline (from sweating or via a diuretic). What parameter on physical examination would distinguish these three patients?

The high Na$^+$:H$_2$O ratio of 154 mmol/L indicates that the ICF volume is contracted to the same degree in all cases. However, the patient who ingested sea water has ECF volume expansion. In contrast, the patient who lost hypotonic saline has a very reduced ECF volume from loss of Na$^+$. The loss of water per se causes only a small degree of ECF volume contraction.

What is (are) the major threat(s) to life in each case?

In each case, the major organ at risk is the brain (hemorrhage could result). In addition, in the patient who drank sea water, there is the potential danger of congestive heart failure. In the patient who lost hypotonic saline, shock could ensue.

8.4 Two 70-kg patients present with hypernatremia (150 mmol/L). The first patient continues to excrete a very large amount of water; his ECF volume is normal (15 L). The second patient has excreted a large urine volume; the [Na$^+$] in the urine is close to 50 mmol/L, and the ECF volume is low (13 L). What is the mechanism of hypernatremia in each patient?

Basis of Hypernatremia. The basis of hypernatremia is water loss and Na$^+$ gain in the first patient and water loss with some Na$^+$ loss in the second patient. Apart from the renal water loss, both patients should have a powerful urge to drink; water intake should prevent the development of hypernatremia. Hence, each has a problem with thirst appreciation, the ability to communicate thirst, and/or a problem with access to water.

Balance for Na⁺. In the first patient, when a negative balance for water occurs, the ECF and ICF volumes tend to contract. As a result of the lower ECF volume, there is a signal for the reabsorption of Na⁺ by the kidney. Therefore, the ingestion of Na⁺ will result in a positive balance for Na⁺. Looked at in another way, each liter of ECF has retained an extra 10 mmol of Na⁺. With a normal ECF volume (15 L), the patient has a positive balance of 150 mmol of Na⁺ (15 L × 10 mmol/L) and will need to lose this quantity of Na⁺ during therapy.

The second patient has lost Na⁺ and water. This loss is a major cause of the marked degree of contraction of the ECF volume (see margin note). Because the ECF volume is 13 vs the normal 15 L, as suggested, the content of Na⁺ is 1950 mmol (13 L × 150 mmol/L); the normal content of Na⁺ is 2100 mmol (15 L × 140 mmol/L). Hence, this patient will need a positive balance for Na⁺ of 150 mmol during therapy.

Note
When the ECF volume is contracted from water (+ Na⁺) loss, the majority of this loss is from the interstitial fluid because the rise in the colloid osmotic pressure plus a fall in capillary hydrostatic pressure tends to defend the intravascular volume.

8.5 Why does water shift into cells with a convulsion or rhabdomyolysis?

Water shifts into cells when cells gain particles or when the ECF gains water or loses particles (Na⁺, Cl⁻). In the examples cited, muscle cells gain particles because macromolecules break down to smaller molecules (inorganic phosphate for the most part).

8.6 A patient with cirrhosis of the liver and ascites has a urine output of 0.4 L/day. Is this patient excreting the lowest possible urine volume?

To determine if the urine volume is a minimum one, assess the maximum urine osmolality and the osmole excretion rate. For simplicity, assume the maximum urine osmolality that this patient can achieve is 600 mOsm/kg H_2O. If the patient is on a low-protein diet and the urine is electrolyte-free, this patient could be excreting 100 mOsm per day. If the minimum urine volume is being excreted, the urine volume would be 0.167 L/day, less than half the current urine output (see margin note). Hence, this patient is not really conserving water maximally because the osmole excretion rate is so low.

Calculation
Urine osmolality = 600 mOsm/kg H_2O.

Excretion = 100 mOsm.

Urine volume =
$$\frac{osmoles}{Uosm} \times \frac{100}{600} = 0.167 \text{ L}$$

With a stimulus for release of ADH (the low "effective" arterial volume), any urine volume >0.167 L/day is in fact a form of polyuria in this setting.

8.7 A patient had a stroke that resulted in aphasia. All laboratory test results were normal. She was transferred to a chronic care facility, where tube-feeding was instituted; no drugs were given. She was readmitted to the hospital several weeks later, at which time her ECF volume was contracted. The plasma [Na⁺] was 160 mmol/L, the urine osmolality was 450 mOsm/kg H_2O, and the urine volume was 3–4 L/day. The urine glucose was negative. What is the diagnosis?

Because hypernatremia was associated with ECF volume contraction, it was due to water loss (and Na⁺ loss). The water loss was renal because the patient was polyuric; the urine osmolality of 450 mOsm/kg H_2O indicates that that the water loss was not a simple water diuresis. Therefore, an osmotic diuresis is the most likely cause (no drugs were given). In the absence of glucosuria, a urea-induced diuresis should be suspected (to confirm, measure the urea in urine; it should be at least 300 mmol/L). The urea load was probably due to the high-protein feeding.

Note the absence of (or failure to communicate) thirst, a consequence of the previous stroke with resulting aphasia.

In addition, an osmotic diuresis can lead to Na^+ loss when there is a renal abnormality—hence, the prominent degree of ECF volume contraction.

Osmole-free water
This is an antiquated term because clinicians are interested in the quantity of water excreted that influenced body tonicity.

Electrolyte-free water
Divide the urine into two parts (ignore urea):
1. Electrolyte excretion that is isotonic to the patient ((urine $[Na^+] + [K^+])/[Na^+]$ in plasma);
2. Pure water loss.

8.8 If a person has nephrogenic DI, drinks an adequate volume of water to avoid hypernatremia, has a normal diet, and has a urine osmolality that is consistently close to 300 mOsm/kg H_2O, what will the daily urine volume be?

On a normal diet, one can expect an osmole excretion rate that is close to 900 mOsm/day. If these osmoles are excreted at 300 mOsm/kg H_2O, the urine volume will be 3 L.

8.9 What is the cause of hypernatremia in the following case? The plasma $[Na^+]$ rose to 180 mmol/L overnight in a confused patient. He received no medications. His body weight had not changed, but his ECF volume was contracted. His blood sugar was 90 mg/dL (5 mmol/L), the urine volume was extremely low, and the urine osmolality was close to 1200 mOsm/kg H_2O.

The patient did not receive Na^+ salts, and the ECF volume was contracted; therefore, hypernatremia was not due to Na^+ gain. Although GI secretions may have a $[Na^+]$ that is less than 140 mmol/L, there was no clinical evidence to support the accumulation of very large volumes of these fluids (marked contraction of the ECF volume and an acid-base disorder). Because there was no change in body weight, hypernatremia was not the result of water loss from the body (water loss should have caused a weight loss of more than 5 kg), and the renal response to hypernatremia was normal (low volume of maximally concentrated urine). Hence, the rise in $[Na^+]$ was due to a shift of water from the ECF to another compartment.

Because the plasma $[Na^+]$ increased by 40 mmol/L (140 to 180 mmol/L), the osmolality rose by almost 30%; this increase could occur if close to 3.3 L of water shifted from the ECF (plus an additional water shift from the ICF of other organs that were not involved in the pathologic condition) to the ICF of the diseased organ. Judging by the relative masses of individual organs, water must have accumulated in muscle.

For water to shift into cells, the number of particles in these cells must have increased (and Na^+ did not accumulate in these cells). Rhabdomyolysis, which involves a breakdown of intracellular muscle macromolecules into a larger number of smaller particles that are retained in the ICF of muscle, could have resulted in an increased tonicity of these cells.

From a clinical viewpoint, it is essential to realize that although water shifted into muscle cells, it shifted out of other normal cells (e.g., brain cells). Shrinkage of these cells could be life-threatening. Therefore, therapy should defend both the ECF volume and the ICF volume of nonmuscle tissues (e.g., brain cells); half-normal saline is the best solution for these purposes. A further expansion of the ICF of muscle should be anticipated with therapy, and specific steps may be necessary to cope with this expansion (i.e., decompression).

8.10 How quickly can the glucose infused in one L of D₅W be metabolized in a patient with hypernatremia?

One liter of D_5W contains 278 mmol (50 g) of glucose. The total glucose content of the body when the blood glucose concentration is 5 mmol/L (90 mg/dL) (5 mmol/L $\times$ 15 L ECF + 4 L ICF) is only 95 mmol (17.1 g). Without metabolism, 1 L of D_5W can increase the blood glucose concentration threefold, and, because several liters of D_5W are required for water replacement during severe hypernatremia, this addition could cause a severe degree of hyperglycemia in a hyperosmolar state.

Approximately 0.5 g of glucose can be metabolized per kilogram of body weight per hour, providing that a fat-derived fuel is not available for oxidation. However, during fasting, when ketoacids are oxidized, less than 0.1 g of glucose/kg of body weight is metabolized to CO_2. Therefore, in a stressful setting, oxidative metabolism of glucose in major organs is close to 7 g/h in a 70-kg person. Because the liver does not oxidize large quantities of circulating glucose to CO_2, and because the conversion of glucose to glycogen in the liver and muscle is rather limited in acutely ill patients, the maximum rate of glucose metabolism is close to 7 g/h. Taken together, these factors should alert the clinician to the life-threatening danger of profound hyperglycemia consequent to large D_5W infusions. The authors advise that the rate of administration of D_5W not exceed 0.3 L/h (17 g glucose) in a 70-kg adult. Monitor the blood sugar and slow the rate of glucose infusion when this value approaches 10 mmol/L (180 mg/dL).

8.11 If a 70-kg patient has a [Na⁺] of 154 mmol/L and a very marked degree of ECF volume contraction, what is the most likely pathophysiology for this lesion?

Hypernatremia implies the presence of a thirst defect. If the hypernatremia were due to water loss, the ECF volume would be contracted by only 10%. Hence, the pathophysiology must reflect a thirst defect, a loss of water, and a loss of Na^+. These three aspects could occur together in a patient with a stroke who is fed a high-protein diet (urea-induced osmotic diuresis).

8.12 Lydia, age 85, was transferred from a nursing home because of a low blood pressure (90/60 mm Hg) and a rapid pulse rate 110 BPM; her jugular venous pressure (JVP) is 2 cm below the sternal angle. Her laboratory values reveal the following:

		Plasma	Urine
Na⁺	mmol/L	170	40
K⁺	mmol/L	3.0	60
Cl⁻	mmol/L	127	—
HCO₃⁻	mmol/L	30	—
Osmolality	mOsm/kg H₂O	360	600

Why is she hypernatremic?

Given the contracted ECF volume, hypernatremia is not due solely to Na^+ gain but to water loss for the most part. The urine osmolality is 600 mOsm/kg H_2O, so ADH is present. Because only 200 mOsm/

kg H_2O is due to Na^+ and K^+ and their anions, one would want to know the nature of the remaining urine osmoles and their excretion rate. The urine did not contain glucose, and the concentration of urea was 370 mOsm/kg H_2O. Therefore the major urine osmole is currently urea. If a protein supplement was given and the urea excretion rate was high, the most likely basis for hypernatremia would be a urea-induced osmotic diuresis. In the elderly, urea may augment the excretion of Na^+; the balance data are calculated as follows.

Detail your fluid and electrolyte management.

Begin by calculating the deficits.

Water in the ICF. The patient weighs 60 kg, and 50% of the body weight is water (elderly have a reduced muscle mass). Therefore, her ICF volume was 20 L and ECF volume 10 L. Her ICF "effective" osmoles were (and remain) $20 \times 140 \times 2 = 5600$ mOsm. At a plasma $[Na^+]$ of 170 mmol/L, the current ICF volume is 5600/(170×2) = 16.5 L. Therefore, there is an ICF deficit of 3.5 L of water.

Na^+ in the ECF. The patient is hypotensive, so it is reasonable to assume that the ECF volume is decreased by 20%, or 2 L. The current Na^+ content in the ECF is 8 L $\times$ 170 mmol/L = 1360 mmol. Because the normal ECF Na^+ content is 1400 mmol Na^+ (10 L $\times$ 140 mmol/L), there is no major change in the ECF Na^+ content. You can appreciate that if one were to administer several liters of normal saline, she would have a significant surplus of Na^+ if this Na^+ were not excreted.

Total Body Water Deficit. The total deficit is 5.5 L: 3.5 L from the ICF and 2 L estimated from the ECF.

Intracellular Composition. A deficit of K^+ is likely to be present but difficult to quantitate; it may well be several hundred millimoles. A substantial component of the ICF K^+ deficit may have been replaced with Na^+ as K^+ exited the ICF. Therefore, there is likely to be a surplus of Na^+ in the body, which will become evident when KCl is given (Na^+ will exit from the ICF and enter the ECF).

Therapy. You want to stop renal EFW loss, which involves addressing the source of the urea. If the patient is receiving high-protein feedings, they should be stopped. If the patient is catabolic from sepsis, appropriate antibiotics should be given, and if there was blood loss into the GI tract, this problem must be addressed.

As the patient is hypotensive, the ECF volume should be reexpanded promptly, accepting that the patient may not have a Na^+ deficit (initially, it is more appropriate to restore the ECF volume aggressively). A reasonable solution would be half-isotonic saline (75 mmol/L) containing 40 mmoles KCl/L. Two liters of this solution should be given over 2–3 hours while the clinician watches her JVP and cardiac status. With this therapy, the patient received 2 L of water containing 230 mOsm of electrolytes (2 (75 + 40 mmol/L)). This is equivalent to 1.35 L of fluid isotonic to the patient (170 mmol/L) saline and 0.65 L of EFW. The former should improve the blood pressure by reexpanding the ECF volume. The impact of the EFW on the plasma $[Na^+]$ is calculated as follows:

With the administration of the 1.35 L of isotonic fluid, her total body water volume was 26.85 L (25.5 L at presentation plus 1.35 L administered). Therefore total osmoles were $170 \times 2 \times 25.5$ L $= 8670$ mOsm. After the administration of 0.6 L of EFW, the plasma [Na$^+$] will be 0.5 (8670/26.85 L, or 167.7 mmol/L). Thus, her plasma [Na$^+$] has fallen by 2.3 mmol/L over 3 hours, an acceptable initial rate of fall.

To maintain a fall in the plasma [Na$^+$] of 0.5 mmol/L/h will require: $(0.5/167) \times 26.85 =$ close to 80 mL EFW per hour, plus replacement of urine losses. The urine cations (Na$^+$ + K$^+$) should be replaced with K$^+$ to accommodate the Na$^+$ exit from the ICF as K$^+$ enter the ICF.

8.13 A 70-kg patient has DI, hypernatremia (154 mmol/L), and a normal ECF volume. What is the most likely pathophysiology to explain this set of findings? Provide a quantitative answer.

The pathophysiology includes a thirst defect, a loss of water (3 L), and a gain of close to 210 mmol of Na$^+$ (14 mmol extra Na$^+$ in each of the 15 L of ECF). One example of such a defect can be seen in Case 8.1.

What are the objectives for therapy?

The objectives for therapy are to lose 210 mmol of Na$^+$ while gaining 3 L of water. These objectives can be achieved by giving 3 L of water orally and by replacing renal and nonrenal losses of water and electrolytes (except for the 210 mmol of Na$^+$).

The reason for the thirst problem must be explored.

8.14 A patient has a clinical syndrome that resembles central DI. One unusual finding is present: the urine osmolality rises when DDAVP is given but not when ADH is given. How does this finding help in defining the etiology?

The response to DDAVP and the lack of response to ADH suggest that something is present that destroys ADH when this is given or produced, but not DDAVP. The differences chemically are the absence of an amino terminal (desamino) and the presence of D-instead of L-arginine in DDAVP. The answer to the problem is the presence of an enzyme (a "vasopressinase" produced by the placenta of the patient) that destroys only ADH because it has an amino terminal.

Appendix

Molecular Advances

Diseases where AQP-2 is not inserted properly in the luminal membrane of the MCD:

There are a number of disorders characterized by too few AQP-2 channels in the terminal distal nephron membranes (see Figure 6.7).

1. **Lack of ADH:** Obviously, if ADH is needed to insert AQP-2 in the luminal membrane, a lack of ADH (central DI) will cause too few of them to reside in the luminal membrane of the late distal nephron. The disorder is reversed by giving

Note

If ADH was present and acted in the cortex, the urine osmolality would equal that of plasma. Therefore, a Uosm < Posm implies a cortical defect as well.

Note

The low luminal K^+ availability also limits NaCl reabsorption and the ability to generate a hyperosmolar medullary interstitial fluid. This may help explain NaCl wasting in patients with hypercalcemia.

Note

Ca^{2+} ion reabsorption occurs between cells, is large, and is driven by a lumen-positive potential difference generated by K^+ ion entry.

ADH or a compound that mimics the V_2 receptor activity of ADH (e.g., DDAVP).

2. **Nephrogenic DI due to lithium:** Lithium enhances the excretion of osmole-free water because it leads to a striking lack of AQP-2 in the distal nephron. One mechanism involved is that lithium diminishes signal transduction elicited by ADH.

   This defect involves both the renal cortex and medulla because the urine osmolality is much less than that of plasma (often in the range of 100–150 mOsm/kg H_2O; see margin note). Interestingly, these effects of lithium may last for a very long time, long after the drug was discontinued; the basis for this is not clear.

3. **Nephrogenic DI due to hypokalemia:** With hypokalemia, there is a decreased density of AQP-2 water channels in the luminal membrane of the distal nephron.

   Hypokalemia also diminishes signal transduction and cAMP formation in response to ADH.

4. **Nephrogenic DI due to hypercalcemia:** Studies have provided a molecular basis for the nephrogenic DI that occurs with hypercalcemia (Figure 8.4). Ultimately, AQP-2 water channels are removed from the luminal membrane of the distal nephron. To understand this story, one must appreciate how the $[Ca^{2+}]$ becomes elevated in the luminal fluid of the distal nephron.

   First, there is an ionized Ca^{2+} receptor on the basolateral membrane (blood side) of the thick ascending limb of the loop of Henle cells (see Figure 8.4). When occupied (high–plasma-ionized Ca^{2+}), a signal results, blocking the luminal K^+ ion channel. Hence, there is less luminal positive voltage generated in the lumen and less Ca^{2+} (Mg^{2+} and Na^+) ion reabsorption here (see margin note) with more Ca^{2+} delivery to the MCD.

   Second, there is a receptor for ionized calcium in the luminal membrane of the IMCD. When the luminal $[Ca^{2+}]$

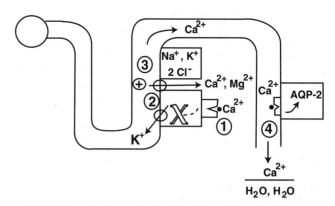

Figure 8.4   Sites of action of ionized calcium. When the plasma ionized Ca^{2+} rises and binds to its receptor on the basolateral side of the thick ascending limb cells (site 1), the luminal K^+ ion channels in these cells are inhibited (site 2). The lumen becomes less positively charged, and this retards the absorption of Na^+, Ca^{2+} and Mg^{2+} ions. In addition, with less K^+ in the lumen, there is less reabsorption of Na^+ and Cl^- by the Na^+, K^+ 2 Cl^- cotransporter (site 3). In the IMCD, if the luminal $[Ca^{2+}]$ rises sufficiently, water reabsorption is impaired due to internalization of the Ca^{2+} receptor paired with AQP-2 (site 4).

exceeds 8 mmol/L, the Ca^{2+}-bound luminal receptor internalizes into a vesicle in the cytosol. Of great interest, the AQP-2 water channels co-localize with this Ca^{2+}-receptor, and they are internalized together (see Figure 8.4). The net effect is to prevent water reabsorption in the inner MCD and thereby also prevent a further rise in luminal $[Ca^{2+}]$, minimizing the risk of stone formation; the "price to pay" is ADH-insensitive water excretion (nephrogenic DI) so long as luminal Ca^{2+} remain high (see Case 8.5).

Potassium

CHAPTER

9

Potassium Physiology

Concepts in Potassium Physiology

1. Potassium ions (K^+) play a key role in the generation of the resting membrane potential (RMP), which in turn influences many important biologic events.
2. The clinical importance of K^+ is that a surplus or deficit of K^+ in the extracellular fluid (ECF) may predispose the patient to cardiac arrhythmias.
3. The kidneys adjust overall K^+ homeostasis by increasing or decreasing the rate of excretion of K^+.

OBJECTIVES

☐ To emphasize that K^+ are the primary intracellular cations and to explain the mechanisms responsible for the distribution of K^+.

☐ To demonstrate that there are two components of K^+ excretion, the $[K^+]$ in the urine and the rate of urine flow, and to explain the regulation of each.

Outline of Major Principles

1. The major clinical concern in a patient with hyperkalemia or hypokalemia is a cardiac arrhythmia.

2. Almost all (98%) K^+ are in cells, held there by an electrical force (inside negative). This charge separation across cell membranes is called the resting membrane potential (RMP).

3. There are two important factors leading to the RMP: first, the electrogenic $Na^+K^+ATPase$ creates a high intracellular $[K^+]$ (3 Na^+ are pumped out and 2 K^+ enter); second, and more importantly, K^+ diffuse out of cells, down their concentration difference. The entry of Na^+ into cells is limited because the permeability of these membranes to Na^+ is so much lower than the permeability to K^+. Most anions do not diffuse out of cells down their electrical gradient because the quantitatively important ones are impermeable macromolecular compounds.

4. Excretion of K^+ is the product of the $[K^+]$ in the urine times the urine flow rate. The $[K^+]$ in the lumen of the cortical collecting duct (CCD) is determined by the lumen-negative trans-epithelial potential difference (TEPD). This TEPD is generated by the reabsorption of Na^+ at a faster rate than the reabsorption of Cl^- (called *electrogenic reabsorption of Na^+*). The major factors that adjust this TEPD are aldosterone and possibly the $[HCO_3^-]$ in the luminal fluid; the delivery of Na^+ is rarely a limiting factor. The other major influence on K^+ excretion is the

Electrogenic reabsorption of Na^+
When Na^+ are reabsorbed without Cl^-, a lumen-negative voltage drives the countermovement of K^+ and/or H^+.

volume of fluid delivered to the terminal CCD (this volume determines the number of K^+ that enter the lumen to reach electrochemical equilibrium).

Electroneutral reabsorption of Na$^+$
When Na$^+$ are reabsorbed equimolarly with Cl$^-$, a lumen-negative voltage to drive the countermovement of K$^+$ and/or H$^+$ is not created.

INTRODUCTORY CASE
Lee's [K$^+$] (K)rashed
(Case discussed on page 393)

Lee, discussed in Chapters 1, 2, 3, and 6, has been unwell for 2 weeks with an upper respiratory tract infection. She presented to the emergency room and was diagnosed as having diabetic ketoacidosis. She was treated with isotonic saline and insulin.

		Admission	4 Hours Later
Na$^+$	mmol/L	130	134
K$^+$	mmol/L	5.6	3.2
Cl$^-$	mmol/L	93	98
HCO$_3{}^-$	mmol/L	10	12
Glucose	mmol/L (mg/dL)	25 (450)	20 (360)

What was the total body K^+ content at the time of presentation and why?

What factors led to her hyperkalemia?

Why did hypokalemia develop 4 hours later?

PART A

Distribution of K$^+$ in the ICF

Overview of K$^+$ Distribution

- The ICF contains 98% of K^+ in the body.
- When faced with a load of K^+, entry of K^+ into cells is rapid. This shift is the body's initial defense mechanism.

Concepts
1. Potassium ions (K$^+$) play a key role in the generation of the resting membrane potential (RMP), which in turn influences many important biologic events.
2. The clinical importance of K$^+$ is that a surplus or deficit of K$^+$ in the ECF may predispose the patient to cardiac arrhythmias.

Most (98%) of the K^+ in the body are in cells (40–50 mmol/kg body weight). In contrast, the total content of K^+ in the extracellular fluid (ECF) is quite low, less than 1 mmol/kg body weight, a quantity similar to the dietary intake of an adult on a typical Western diet. A steady state is maintained with a [K^+] in the intracellular fluid (ICF) that is close to 35-fold greater than that in the ECF. To avoid important changes in this [K^+] gradient, regulatory mechanisms must be rapid and extremely sensitive to small variations in the input and output of K^+ (see the discussion of Question 9.1).

Factors influencing the [K+] in the ICF

- There are several ways to change the [K+] in the ICF. One can change the RMP by changing the activity of the Na+K+ATPase and/or by increasing the permeability of the cell membrane to Na+. One can also lower the permeability of this membrane to K+.
- K+ movement across cell membranes requires either the countermovement of a cation (Na+ or H+) or a parallel movement of an anion (phosphate in most cells).
- The number of K+ that must move to generate the RMP is very small.

Quantities in a 70-kg adult

- **K+ in ICF:** Close to 4000 mmol
- **K+ in ECF:** Close to 60 mmol

Key facts

1. Na+ can enter cells in an electroneutral fashion (exchange for H+). When these Na+ are pumped out of cells by the Na+K+ATPase, there is a more negative RMP, and this leads to a fall in the [K+] in the ECF. Conversely, when 1 Na+ enters cells via its Na+ channel, more positive charges enter than leave, so the RMP becomes less negative, and this leads to a rise in the [K+] in the ECF.
2. The architecture around muscle cells is important. Most K+ are released locally into T-tubules on depolarization so that they can be taken back into cells on repolarization, preventing large and sudden changes in the plasma [K+]. This physiology can be disturbed with muscle wasting.

Ultimately, all K+ ingested in excess of nonrenal losses must be excreted to maintain balance for K+.

QUESTION

(Discussion on page 394)

9.1 *What quantity of K+ of dietary origin (70 mmol) will be distributed in cells if there is no excretion of K+ and no change in the RMP? What will the plasma [K+] be?*

The Resting Membrane Potential

There are two major factors that generate the RMP, an active one—the Na+K+ATPase—and a passive one—the diffusion of K+ from the ICF, where the [K+] is high (150 mmol/L), to the ECF, where the [K+] is low (4.1 mmol/L). Further diffusion of K+ is retarded by an electrical force (negative charge inside cells, the RMP). Quantitatively, the Na+K+ATPase creates a minor component of the RMP by pumping 3 Na+ out of cells in exchange for 2 K+ entering cells. The passive diffusion of K+ out of cells is responsible for generating the majority of the RMP.

In addition to the two factors, low permeability of the cell membrane to Na+ and the fact that the intracellular anions are mostly macromolecular help maintain the RMP (Figure 9.1).

In the paragraphs to follow, the factors influencing the distribution of K+ between the ECF and ICF will be considered in more detail (Table 9.1).

Na+K+ATPase

- Hydrolysis of 1 molecule of adenosine triphosphate (ATP) pumps 3 Na+ out of cells for every 2 K+ that enter; therefore, this pump is electrogenic.

TABLE 9.1 **Factors Influencing a K+ Shift from the ICF to the ECF**

Hormones
  Lack of insulin, β_2-adrenergic antagonists, lack of aldosterone
Acid-Base Disturbances
  Acute HCl gain or NaHCO$_3$ loss (other acid-base disturbances have little direct effect on K+ distribution)
ICF Anion Change
  Catabolism, loss of organic phosphates
Cell Necrosis
Rare Factors
  Cellular depolarization (e.g., succinylcholine)
  Decrease in K+ permeability (barium poisoning)
  Unusual cation accumulations in the ICF (lysine/arginine toxicity)
  Hypertonicity, which decreases the ICF volume (an overrated factor; see the discussion of Question 9.5).
  Hyperkalemic periodic paralysis, hypokalemic periodic paralysis

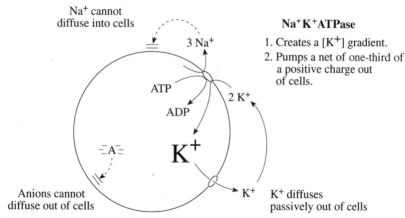

Na$^+$ cannot
diffuse into cells

Na$^+$K$^+$ATPase

3 Na$^+$

1. Creates a [K$^+$] gradient.
2. Pumps a net of one-third of
   a positive charge out
   of cells.

ATP

2 K$^+$

ADP

$_\equiv$A$_\equiv$

K$^+$

Anions cannot
diffuse out of cells

K$^+$ K$^+$ diffuses
passively out of cells

Figure 9.1   Generation of the RMP. The RMP is due largely to the activity of the Na$^+$K$^+$ATPase and the passive diffusion of K$^+$, but not Na$^+$ or anions, across cell membranes.

Almost every cell contains Na$^+$K$^+$ATPase, an ion translocating pump that pumps 3 Na$^+$ out of cells for every 2 K$^+$ that enter these cells (see margin note). The net result of having a normal activity of the Na$^+$K$^+$ATPase is a large transmembrane cation gradient with a very low intracellular [Na$^+$] of close to 10 mmol/L (vs 150 mmol/L in interstitial fluid); the converse applies to K$^+$ (150 mmol/L inside most cells and 4.3 mmol/L in interstitial fluid). These [Na$^+$] and [K$^+$] gradients have implications for many vital functions of the cell (Figure 9.2).

Note
Some cells do not have the Na$^+$K$^+$ATPase as their principal ion translocating pump. For example, the H$^+$ATPase is the principal ion pump in α- and β-intercalated cells in the CCD and medullary collecting ducts (MCD).

GENERATIONS	**EFFECTS**
1. K$^+$ diffuses from the ICF to the ECF.	1. Na$^+$/H$^+$ antiport
2. Na$^+$K$^+$ATPase pumps one-third of a charge from the ICF to the ECF.	2. Na$^+$/Ca^{2+} exchange
	3. Na$^+$/nutrient cotransport
	4. K$^+$ secretion
	5. Lower RMP

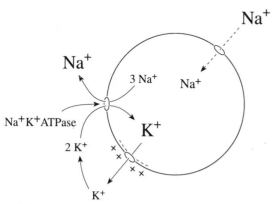

Na$^+$

Na$^+$

3 Na$^+$ Na$^+$

Na$^+$K$^+$ATPase

K$^+$

2 K$^+$

K$^+$

Figure 9.2   The role of the [Na$^+$] gradient across cell membranes. The generators of the [Na$^+$] gradient are shown on the left side of the figure, and the effects of this gradient are shown on the right side of the figure.

QUESTIONS

(Discussions on page 395)

9.2 *What is the intracellular cation composition in the red blood cells of a dog? These cells lack Na$^+$K$^+$ATPase pumps.*

9.3 *Why does the entry of Na^+ into cells increase the RMP when augmented by insulin but decrease the magnitude of the RMP in hyperkalemic periodic paralysis?*

Factors Influencing the Activity of the $Na^+K^+ATPase$ Pump

The major factors influencing the activity of the $Na^+K^+ATPase$ pump are the $[Na^+]$ in the ICF and the number and/or activity of individual pump units.

Intracellular $[Na^+]$. In general, the activity of the $Na^+K^+ATPase$ is enormous relative to the quantity of Na^+ that need to be pumped because cell membranes have an extremely low permeability to Na^+. The $Na^+K^+ATPase$ extrudes Na^+ rapidly when the $[Na^+]$ rises transiently in the ICF. Hence, it follows that the principal regulator of pump activity is the $[Na^+]$ in the cytosol in immediate proximity to this pump (see margin note). Given this pump-leak system, if the activity of the $Na^+K^+ATPase$ changes, the $[Na^+]$ in the ICF will have to change in a reciprocal way because this pump does not seem to be involved in an equilibrium system (see margin note).

Activity of the $Na^+K^+ATPase$. The $Na^+K^+ATPase$ has α and β subunits. The assembly of these inactive precursors permits rapid changes in activity to occur. Phosphorylation and dephosphorylation also modulate the activity of the $Na^+K^+ATPase$. Longer-term control is exerted by synthesis of new α and β subunits. A commonly used inhibitor of this pump is ouabain, a compound in the digitalis family of drugs. There is evidence of the existence of endogenous compounds with ouabain-like actions.

Factors Influencing a Shift of K^+ Across Cell Membranes

Hormones

Hormones can influence the quantity of Na^+ pumped by the $Na^+K^+ATPase$ in three general ways (Table 9.2). First, they can increase the electroneutral entry of Na^+ into cells (activate the Na^+/H^+ antiporter), which will lead to more pumping of Na^+ out of cells via this electrogenic pump. Second, hormones may activate existing $Na^+K^+ATPase$ enzymes in cell membranes via phosphorylation.

TABLE 9.2 **Effects of Some Hormones on Distribution of K^+ Between ICF and ECF**

Hormone	Possible Mechanisms	Quantitative Role
Insulin	• Increased entry of Na^+ via activation of NHE-1	• A lack of insulin leads to an acute rise in the $[K^+]$ in the ECF of close to 0.5 mmol/L
$β_2$-Adrenergics	• Activation of $Na^+K^+ATPase$	• Pharmacologic doses can bring the $[K^+]$ in the ECF below 3.0 mmol/L
Aldosterone	? (see margin note)	• If aldosterone is given to a patient who lacks this hormone, the $[K^+]$ in the ECF can fall by about 0.5 mmol/L

Third, hormones may induce the net synthesis of more Na$^+$K$^+$ ATPase enzyme molecules.

> • The most important hormones are insulin and the β-adrenergics.

Insulin. Insulin causes K$^+$ to shift into cells. The most important mechanism seems to be the activation of the electroneutral Na$^+$/H$^+$ antiporter. For full expression of this effect, supraphysiologic doses of insulin may be required. Once Na$^+$ have entered cells, the [Na$^+$] in the ICF will rise transiently. When these Na$^+$ are pumped out of cells, there will be an increased flux through the electrogenic Na$^+$K$^+$ATPase (Figure 9.3). Quantitatively, if the basal insulin concentration halves, the [K$^+$] in the ECF rises by about 0.5 mmol/L within 30 minutes.

On a clinical note, administration of insulin causes a significant fall in the [K$^+$] in the ECF; this fall is especially important during treatment for diabetic ketoacidosis and for hyperkalemia with ECG changes.

Catecholamines. The effects of catecholamines on the [K$^+$] in the ECF are complex. β$_2$-Adrenergics stimulate the movement of K$^+$ into cells, possibly via effects on the Na$^+$K$^+$ATPase. The mechanism may involve a rise in cyclic adenosine monophosphate (AMP) and, as a result, phosphorylation and activation of the Na$^+$K$^+$ ATPase.

Catecholamines can also act in an indirect fashion. For example, they stimulate glycogenolysis, which leads to hyperglycemia and the release of insulin from β cells of the pancreas. Insulin causes K$^+$ to move into the ICF as just described.

α-Adrenergic actions lead to a direct shift of K$^+$ out of cells.

Other actions of insulin
Insulin causes the synthesis of phosphate esters in the ICF (hexose phosphates, RNA, etc.). An increase in intracellular anions could "attract" K$^+$ into cells. This effect is usually slow and small.

Other actions of catecholamines
β$_1$-Adrenergics, which stimulate renin release from the kidneys, increase aldosterone production and, as a result, promote the excretion of K$^+$.

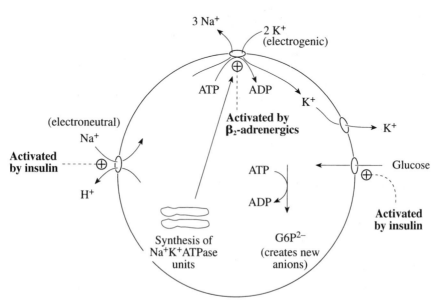

Figure 9.3 Hormones that cause K$^+$ to shift into cells. The major hormones involved are insulin and β$_2$-adrenergics. Both permit the Na$^+$ to be pumped out of cells, leaving the ICF with a more negative net charge, thereby causing K$^+$ to enter cells. Insulin uses NHE-1. β$_2$-adrenergics use existing intracellular Na$^+$.

Hormones with this action may also influence the $[K^+]$ in plasma indirectly. In addition, because they inhibit release of insulin from pancreatic β cells, their actions may also lead to development of hyperkalemia.

Aldosterone. If a patient lacking aldosterone is hyperkalemic and is given aldosterone, the plasma $[K^+]$ falls promptly before excretion of K^+ rises appreciably. Therefore, aldosterone seems to permit the entry of K^+ into cells in this setting. In contrast, when aldosterone is given to normal individuals, there is no acute fall in the plasma $[K^+]$. Hence, aldosterone does not promote K^+ entry if its level was not extremely low initially.

QUESTION

(Discussion on page 395)

Note
Question 9.4 needs independent exploration.

9.4 *What property of the $Na^+K^+ATPase$ might allow it to bind K^+ at a $[K^+]$ of 4 mmol/L in the ECF yet also permit K^+ to dissociate from this pump at a $[K^+]$ of 150 mmol/L in the ICF?*

Acid-Base Changes

> • Only metabolic acidosis caused by loss of $NaHCO_3$ (or gain of HCl) leads to a shift of K^+ across cell membranes and hyperkalemia. With time, normal kidneys and aldosterone response return the plasma $[K^+]$ to normal.
> • A gain of an organic acid does not cause hyperkalemia.
> • Lack of insulin or hypoxia may lead to hyperkalemia.
> • There is little K^+ shift across cell membranes during acute respiratory acid-base disorders.

Data in Animals. When HCl was infused into nephrectomized dogs, there was a rise in the $[H^+]$ in the ECF and a shift of H^+ into the ICF; some K^+ moved out of cells for charge balance. In contrast to HCl, infusion of organic acids, L-lactic acid, and keto-acids did not cause a net shift of K^+ out of cells as a result of ICF buffering because L-lactate and ketoacid anions entered the ICF to almost the same degree as protons (Figure 9.4). Therefore, when metabolic acidosis is due to the accumulation of these organic acids, factors other than the acidemia per se cause hyperkalemia (if it is present).

Respiratory acid-base disorders cause only small changes in the plasma $[K^+]$. Therefore, if the $[K^+]$ changes with a $Paco_2$ change, look for a cause other than the simple acid-base disturbance (see margin note).

Shift of K^+ in acute respiratory acid-base disorders
During acute respiratory acidosis or alkalosis, there is little change in the $[HCO_3^-]$ in the ECF and only a very small movement of K^+ across the cell membrane. In acute experiments, no appreciable change in the $[K^+]$ in the ECF was detected when the change in $Paco_2$ was in the range of 20–80 mm Hg.

Intracellular Anions

> • The $[K^+]$ in the ICF is "electrically balanced" mainly by intracellular macromolecular anions, largely organic phosphates; these anions are restricted to the ICF compartment.

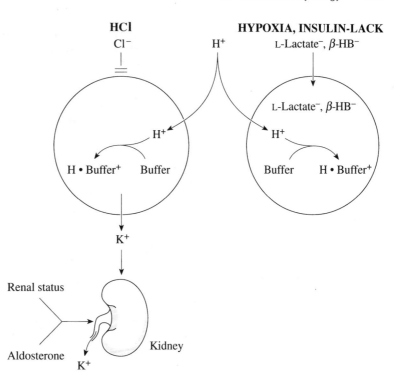

Figure 9.4 Buffering of H⁺ and the consequent K⁺ shift. The circles represent the cell membrane. Although Cl⁻ remain largely in the ECF (left circle), organic anions enter the ICF (right circle). Hence, hyperkalemia is due to a shift of K⁺ with HCl only. Hyperkalemia should stimulate aldosterone release and result in excretion of the extra K⁺. Therefore, a steady-state hyperkalemia in hyperchloremic metabolic acidosis should be seen only if there is low excretion of K⁺. A decrease in excretion of K⁺ may occur during renal insufficiency or low aldosterone bioactivity.

The positive and negative charges in a compartment are virtually equal in number. In the ICF, many of the negatively charged molecules do not cross cell membranes (mainly the organic phosphates, DNA, RNA, adenosine triphosphate creatine phosphate; intracellular proteins do not make a major net contribution to this anionic charge). The intracellular anionic composition is normally relatively constant (although the specific phosphate compounds differ from organ to organ). However, loss of organic phosphates (largely RNA), as can occur in specific disease states (e.g., diabetic ketoacidosis (DKA)), leads to the parallel loss of K⁺. The reason for the fall in RNA is the lack of the actions of insulin (i.e., degradation of ribosomal RNA needed for protein synthesis—the catabolic state of a relative lack of insulin); this topic is explored further in the discussion of Question 9.7. The converse will occur during states with anabolism (i.e., recovery from DKA).

Ion Channels

Periodic Paralysis. Molecular studies have led to many new discoveries concerning the function of various ion transport proteins and the uncovering of important associations between changes in their structure and function. Certain inherited disorders result in abnormal shifts of K⁺ across cell membranes and are the result of ion channels that do not function in a normal fashion.

In the resting state, the Na⁺ channel is inactive because the voltage in resting skeletal muscle cells is sufficiently negative. With the arrival of a nerve impulse, there is a sudden activation, or opening, of these voltage-gated Na⁺ channels and thereby a rapid increase in the permeability to Na⁺, allowing Na⁺ (positive voltage) to enter the ICF. This depolarization is transient for three reasons. First, depolarization diminishes the magnitude of the negative volt-

Net charge on intracellular proteins

At the ICF pH, the anionic charges on proteins are on the C-terminal carboxyl group and on the anionic amino acids glutamate and aspartate. The positive charges on ICF proteins are on the N-terminal amino group and on the cationic amino acids lysine, arginine, and close to half of the histidines. Simple arithmetic shows that the anionic groups do not exceed the cationic residues in most proteins. Hence, proteins are not likely to be major ICF anions unless very marked changes in the pK of amino acids occur in specific ICF environments.

age inside these cells, which in turn leads to inactivation of this Na^+ channel. Second, the negative intracellular voltage activates (opens) voltage-gated K^+ channels—i.e., now when K^+ exit down their electrochemical gradient, the interior of the cell again becomes more negatively charged. Third, the Na^+ are extruded by the electrogenic Na^+, K^+, ATPase.

When there is a defect in sarcolemmal excitability, one can expect to see either myotonia or periodic paralysis. The latter is characterized by episodic weakness or paralysis of voluntary muscles in the absence of motor neuron disease or in abnormality of the neuromuscular junction. Attacks are most frequently associated with changes in the plasma $[K^+]$. These disorders are often familial and have a higher incidence in certain races. Electrophysiologic studies have revealed abnormalities in skeletal muscle ion conductances.

Molecular Basis for Hyperkalemic Periodic Paralysis (HYPP). This disorder is the result of a mutation in the skeletal muscle Na^+ channel gene. HYPP is closely associated with paramyotonia congenita and K^+-activated myotonia. The paralysis in HYPP is often brought on by the hyperkalemia associated with heavy physical exercise. The basis for the lesion is a failure to completely inactivate a small subpopulation of these voltage-gated Na^+ channels in skeletal muscle cells when the $[K^+]$ in the ECF is raised. This leads to electrical inexcitability of the skeletal muscle. This spontaneous depolarization is blocked by tetrodotoxin, which blocks voltage-gated Na^+ channels, and this returns the RMP to its normal value.

Molecular Basis for Hypokalemic Periodic Paralysis (HOPP). HOPP is an autosomal-dominant skeletal muscle disorder in which episodes of weakness occur. The first symptoms typically occur in teenage years. The characteristic clinical association is weakness and hypokalemia, which might be very severe at times (<2.0 mmol/L). In HOPP, the RMP is 10–15 mV less negative than in normal muscle fibers, even if the $[K^+]$ in the ECF is normal. Its basis is not a specific problem with the voltage-gated Na^+ channel as in HYPP, so tetrodotoxin has no effect on spontaneous depolarization in a low K^+ environment.

Genetic analysis links HOPP to the dihydropyridine-sensitive receptor, which in turn is linked to a Ca^{2+} channel. It is not completely clear how the effects on the RMP and plasma $[K^+]$ are produced in HOPP. Voltage-gated Ca^{2+} channels in skeletal muscle act as voltage sensors in excitation-contraction coupling, and it might be that the rapid inactivation in these mutant channels interferes with this process.

QUESTIONS

(Discussions on pages 395–396)

9.5 *How much will the plasma $[K^+]$ change when 1 L of pure water is shifted from the ICF to the ECF? Assume a constant RMP.*

9.6 *Will a drug that depolarizes cell membranes cause a change in the plasma $[K^+]$?*

9.7 *Why does the loss of intracellular phosphate anions cause hyperkalemia in DKA but not in poliomyelitis?*

9.8 *During K^+ depletion, Na^+ replace K^+ in cells. How does this exchange affect the $Na^+K^+ATPase$?*

PART B

Renal Regulation of K^+ Excretion

Physiology of K^+ Excretion

- Events controlling K^+ excretion have their greatest impact in the CCD.
- To analyze K^+ excretion, assess both the $[K^+]$ in urine and the urine volume.
  K^+ excretion
  $$\text{Urine } [K^+] \times \text{Urine volume}$$
  - Aldosterone
  - HCO_3^- in the lumen
  - Na^+ and H_2O intake
  - Diuretics
  - Urea

Concept
3. The kidneys adjust overall K^+ homeostasis by increasing or decreasing the rate of excretion of K^+.

Each day, the kidneys must excrete virtually all the K^+ that were absorbed from the gastrointestinal (GI) tract; in adults ingesting a typical Western diet, this amounts to about 1 mmol/kg body weight. Excretion of K^+ requires two major events: the $[K^+]$ in each liter of fluid traversing the CCD must be increased, and there must be a sufficient number of liters traversing this portion of the nephron.

Other nephron segments also influence the excretion of K^+ (Figure 9.5). A very important point to emphasize is that the amount of K^+ delivered out of the loop of Henle is similar to that ingested and excreted per 24 hours (see margin note).

K^+ delivery to the CCD
A reasonable estimate of the volume of fluid delivered to the early distal convoluted tubule in humans is 20–30 L. With a $[K^+]$ of 3 mmol/L, 60–90 mmol of K^+ could be delivered here. This amount is equivalent to the quantity of K^+ consumed and excreted daily by most adults on a typical Western diet.

Events in the CCD

- Virtually all regulation of urinary K^+ occurs in the CCD.

In the CCD, the cell involved in K^+ secretion is the principal cell. For secretion of K^+, Na^+ are reabsorbed through an ion-specific channel, the epithelial Na^+ channel (ENaC) (induced or activated by aldosterone and inhibited by K^+-sparing diuretics such as amiloride).

In this nephron segment, reabsorption of Na^+ is either electrogenic or electroneutral (Figure 9.6). If more Na^+ than Cl^- are reabsorbed, there is electrogenic reabsorption, which creates the electrical driving force that augments the net secretion of K^+. In contrast, if equal quantities of Na^+ and Cl^- are reabsorbed in the

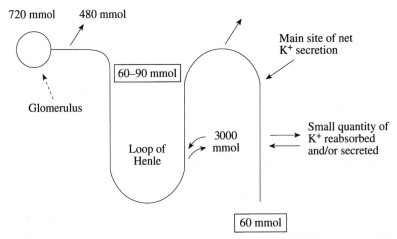

Figure 9.5   Handling of K⁺ in segments of the nephron. Most of the filtered K⁺ (720 mmol/day in an adult) is reabsorbed in the proximal convoluted tubule (480 mmol); the [K⁺] in the luminal fluid is not very different from that in the ECF. In the loop of Henle (LOH), close to 3000 mmol of K⁺ is secreted and then reabsorbed in the thick ascending limb via the Na⁺, K⁺, 2 Cl⁻ cotransporter. This cycle permits Na⁺ and Cl⁻ to be reabsorbed. The [K⁺] in the luminal fluid that exits the LOH is close to 3 mmol/L. The CCD is the main site of K⁺ secretion; the 60-90 mmol in the rectangle represents the number of mmol of K⁺ delivered out of the loop of Henle.

CCD, the reabsorption is electroneutral and does not "drive" the net secretion of K⁺. In the following section, the components responsible for the net secretion of K⁺ are considered.

Delivery of Na⁺ to the CCD

The delivery of Na⁺ to the CCD rarely influences net secretion of K⁺. This delivery falls to limiting values if the ECF volume is markedly contracted (see margin note).

Reabsorption of Na⁺ in the CCD

More detailed information on the molecular physiology of the renal handling of K⁺ is provided in the appendix to this chapter. In the CCD, Na⁺ are reabsorbed through the ENaC, which is regulated in part by the availability of aldosterone (aldosterone opens the ENaC). The ENaC is inhibited by the diuretic amiloride. Entry of Na⁺ into cells of the CCD has two effects:

1. It makes the membrane potential across the luminal membrane more electronegative; this action favors the secretion of K⁺ into the lumen.

2. The transient small elevation in the [Na⁺] in the cell increases flux through the basolateral Na⁺K⁺ATPase and thereby brings K⁺ from the fluid adjacent to the basolateral membrane into principal cells. The net effect is movement of K⁺ from the ECF to the lumen. Said another way, the actions of aldosterone lead to an elevated luminal [K⁺] that is approximately 10-fold higher than that in the ECF (Figures 9.7 and 9.8).

Cl⁻ Reabsorption in the CCD

The mechanisms that regulate the reabsorption of Cl⁻ in the CCD are relatively unclear. The bulk of Cl⁻ movement is believed to

[Na⁺] in the lumen of the CCD
The luminal [Na⁺] required for half-maximal rates of K⁺ secretion in the CCD is 10–15 mmol/L in the rat. No comparable data are available in humans, so the authors assume a similar value for the human CCD. Because the osmolality of fluid in the terminal CCD is equal to that in plasma when ADH acts, and because the maximum concentration of urea in the lumen of the CCD is close to 100 mmol/L in normal individuals, electrolytes represent close to 200 mOsm/L. Half of these milliosmoles are cations, the bulk of which are Na⁺. Thus, the [Na⁺] can be less than 15 mmol/L only when the concentration of urea exceeds 200 mmol/L in this fluid (i.e., with a marked degree of contraction of the ECF volume).

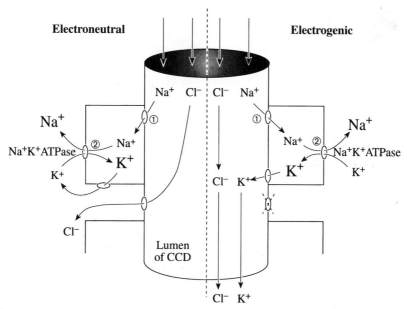

Figure 9.6   Electrogenic and electroneutral reabsorption of Na⁺. The barrel-shaped structure is the CCD. When Na⁺ and Cl⁻ are reabsorbed in equimolar amounts, there is no voltage created to favor net secretion of K⁺; this reabsorption, termed electroneutral, is shown on the left side of the figure. In contrast, reabsorption of Na⁺ without Cl⁻ is electrogenic and generates a transepithelial potential difference (lumen negative), which drives the net secretion of K⁺ (right side of the figure). There are two components to Na⁺ reabsorption: (1) the ENaC in the luminal membrane, and (2) the Na⁺K⁺ATPase on the basolateral membrane.

occur via a paracellular rather than transcellular route, driven in part by the lumen-negative transepithelial potential difference (TEPD) and limited by the permeability of the luminal membrane to Cl⁻ (see Figure 9.6). Intracellular and luminal events may also regulate this permeability to Cl⁻. The influence of HCO_3^- is considered next.

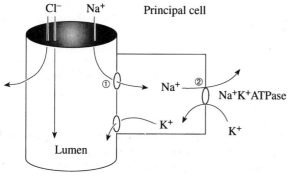

Figure 9.7   Physiology of aldosterone-induced K⁺ secretion. The barrel-shaped structure represents the lumen of the CCD, and the square represents a principal cell. The actions of aldosterone open the ENaC (1) and cause more Na⁺K⁺ATPase units to be inserted in the basolateral membrane (2). Reabsorption of Na⁺ in the CCD can be electroneutral or electrogenic, depending on whether Cl⁻ are more or less permeable in the CCD luminal membrane. If the flux of Cl⁻ is less than that of Na⁺, a TEPD is generated, and K⁺ secretion increases.

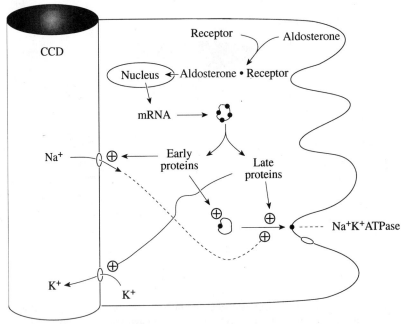

Figure 9.8 Summary of actions of aldosterone on principal cells of the CCD. Aldosterone enters the principal cell via the basolateral membrane and binds to a specific receptor. This hormone receptor complex enters the nucleus and causes the synthesis of new proteins. The early action of aldosterone is the opening of luminal Na^+ channels and, possibly, the synthesis of the precursor of the $Na^+K^+ATPase$. The later actions of aldosterone include the insertion of more $Na^+K^+ATPase$ units into the basolateral membrane and K^+ channels into the luminal membrane.

Role of Anions Other Than Cl^- in the Lumen of the CCD

Among anions that influence the excretion of K^+, HCO_3^- seem to be unique; they lead to a very high rate of excretion of K^+ (provided that aldosterone is also present) by permitting a very high $[K^+]$ in the luminal fluid of the CCD. There are two possible mechanisms of action:

1. **HCO_3^- may act simply as poorly reabsorbed anions in the CCD (like SO_4^{2-}):** A high TEPD will be generated if Na^+ reabsorption is electrogenic (without Cl^-). For this electrogenic reabsorption, Cl^- should be absent from the luminal fluid. Because HCO_3^- cause a high transtubular $[K^+]$ gradient (TTKG) even if Cl^- are present in the urine, the mechanism of action cannot simply be as a poorly reabsorbed anion (see margin note).

2. **HCO_3^- inhibit the reabsorption of Cl^- in the CCD:** The mechanism is not known, but some data are consistent with it. Clinically, conditions associated with enhanced delivery of HCO_3^- to the CCD (e.g., vomiting, treatment of proximal renal tubular acidosis (RTA) with $NaHCO_3$, the use of carbonic-anhydrase-inhibitor type of diuretics such as acetazolamide, and the subgroup of distal RTA that results from a defect in distal nephron H^+ secretion) have in common hypokalemia with an inappropriately high $[K^+]$ in the urine. The authors' speculation on the ways in which HCO_3^- might enhance net secretion of K^+ is considered in the discussion of Question 9.12.

Note
SO_4^{2-} causes a high TTKG when given with aldosterone *only* if the $[Cl^-]$ in the urine is very low.

Associations Between Excretions of K⁺ and HCO₃⁻

1. **Diurnal excretion of K⁺:** The excretion of K^+ is highest around noon and lowest overnight (Figure 9.9). Peak excretion is associated with the alkaline tide urine and plasma pH. Several facts cast doubt on the role of aldosterone as an important mediator of this diurnal variation of K^+ excretion. First, there is no consistent rise in aldosterone in the several hours before noon. Second, a diurnal pattern seems to persist in adrenalectomized rats infused with aldosterone at a constant rate. In addition, there is little rise in the rate of excretion of K^+ when aldosterone is given in the evening.

    One final point merits mention. If bicarbonaturia is induced by administering either $NaHCO_3$ or a drug inhibiting proximal reabsorption of HCO_3^-, aldosterone will cause a rise in K^+ excretion in all portions of its diurnal excretion cycle. Hence, correlative evidence is present linking K^+ excretion and distal delivery of HCO_3^-.

2. **Influence of the plasma [K⁺] on the [K⁺] in the lumen of the CCD:** Hyperkalemia is associated with high values, and hypokalemia (or a K^+ deficit) is associated with low values for the $[K^+]$ in the lumen of the CCD. Of interest, hyperkalemia depresses and hypokalemia enhances proximal reabsorption of HCO_3. Perhaps this could represent a physiologic way for aldosterone to be a K^+-secreting (K^+ surfeit) or not a K^+-secreting hormone (K^+ deficit) in pathophysiologic states. This will be considered in more detail in a subsequent section.

K⁺ Transport in the CCD

> • There are three major pathways for K^+ movement: specific K^+ channels, antiporters, and cotransporters.

Specific K⁺ Channels. The major transport system involved in net K^+ secretion seems to be K^+ channels. There are two major types of K^+ channels in the luminal membrane of the CCD: one that is activated by Ca^{2+} or depolarization, and another that is almost permanently open and apparently makes up the bulk of the luminal K^+ conductance. These latter channels can be inhibited by intracellular acidification and ATP. They are also inactivated by protein kinase C and arachidonic acid; nevertheless, they are usually active enough so that conductance of K^+ does not generally impose a major limit to net secretion of K^+.

Figure 9.9 Diurnal variation in K⁺ excretion. Most of the excretion of K^+ occurs close to noon and is the result of a higher $[K^+]$ in luminal fluid in the CCD.

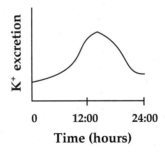

Antiporters. K^+ may be reabsorbed in the CCD and MCD. Reabsorption is, in general, smaller in magnitude and mediated by the major antiport system, the K^+/H^+ antiporter. This antiporter leads to the reabsorption of K^+ and the secretion of H^+ (providing that there is a suitable H^+ acceptor such as HCO_3^-, NH_3, or divalent phosphate in the lumen). The quantity of these H^+ acceptors in the lumen is not large.

Cotransporters. There is also a K^+, Cl^- cotransporter for secretion of K^+, but it seems to operate only when the luminal $[Cl^-]$ is exceedingly low (less than 10–15 mmol/L, a rare event); this transporter may therefore be important only on rare occasions.

The Adrenal Gland and Aldosterone Release

> • Hyperkalemia and ECF volume contraction (via angiotensin II) are the two major stimuli for aldosterone release.

Lesson from molecular advances
Rare patients have hypertension that is associated with high levels of mineralocorticoids. The cause is an abnormality in the adrenal cortex where ACTH drives the synthesis of a compound with aldosterone-like actions. Suppression of ACTH with dexamethasone eliminates the hypertension (called glucocorticoid remedial aldosteronism; see Chapter 10).

The release of aldosterone is stimulated primarily by hyperkalemia and angiotensin II; these two stimuli act in a fashion that is more than additive. The level of angiotensin II rises when renin is released from the juxtaglomerular apparatus of the kidneys. Renin release is stimulated by ECF volume contraction, renal artery stenosis, and β_1-adrenergic stimulation; in contrast, it is inhibited by ECF volume expansion and adrenergic β_1-blockers. Destruction of the juxtaglomerular apparatus by interstitial renal disease also results in lower levels of renin release. In some cases, angiotensin II levels may not be elevated despite high renin levels. Such cases can occur when drugs inhibit the conversion of angiotensin I to its active form, angiotensin II (Figure 9.10).

The release of aldosterone from zona glomerulosa cells is diminished by atrial natriuretic factor.

Integrative Physiology

At times, the principal function of aldosterone will be to promote the reabsorption of NaCl but not the excretion of K^+. In contrast, there will be times when the actions of aldosterone should be to excrete K^+ but not reabsorb excessive amounts of NaCl.

Settings

Reabsorb NaCl But Not Excrete K^+. Consider a person who is without food for 2 weeks. Typically, deficits for NaCl and K^+ are close to 350 mmol. In this setting, the signal for the release of aldosterone is the release of angiotensin II. Because this agent stimulates the reabsorption of $NaHCO_3$ in the proximal and distal tubules, the combination of an open ENaC (aldosterone action to reabsorb Na^+) and little delivery of HCO_3 distally (angiotensin II) plus acidemia (ketoacids), which augments distal H^+ secretion, acts in concert to ensure faster Cl^- reabsorption (little effect of HCO_3^- in the CCD) and make aldosterone a NaCl-retaining but not a K^+-excreting hormone (Figure 9.11).

Eat Fruit Plus a Large Amount of NaCl. In this setting, one must excrete K^+ but not retain NaCl. The signal that releases aldosterone

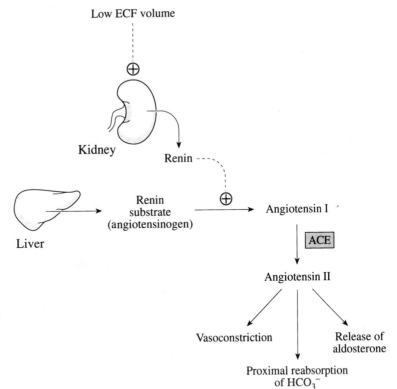

Figure 9.10 Renin-angiotensin system and the site of action of angiotensin-converting enzyme (ACE) inhibitors. An important class of antihypertensive drugs that influence angiotensin II levels is the ACE inhibitors.

is K$^+$, not angiotensin II because the latter is suppressed by the salt load. Because the K$^+$ load suppresses the reabsorption of HCO$_3$$^-$ in the proximal convoluted tubule, there should be an abundant distal delivery of HCO$_3$$^-$. The combined effects of aldosterone

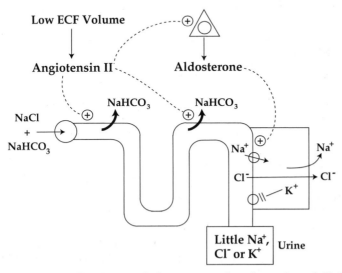

Figure 9.11 Aldosterone and the augmented reabsorption of NaCl. Aldosterone opens the ENaC in the CCD. The secretagogue for the release of aldosterone when the ECF volume is contracted is angiotensin II. Angiotensin II, by stimulating the reabsorption of NaHCO$_3$ in the PCT and DCT, diminishes distal delivery of HCO$_3$ and thereby does not promote a kaliuresis.

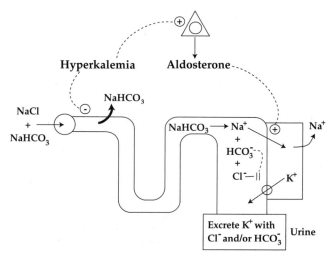

Figure 9.12   Aldosterone and the augmented secretion of K^+. The critical point when the primary role of aldosterone is to promote the excretion of K^+ is that distal delivery of HCO_3^- should be high to augment K^+ excretion. Aldosterone leads to an ("open") ENaC in the CCD. Having hyperkalemia depress proximal reabsorption of HCO_3^-, the aldosterone released in response to hyperkalemia leads to electrogenic reabsorption of Na^+ in the CCD by retarding the reabsorption of Cl^- due to luminal HCO_3^-.

(faster Na^+) and HCO_3^- (slower Cl^-) on reabsorptive rates in the CCD could permit aldosterone to be a K^+-excreting and not a NaCl-retaining hormone in this setting (Figure 9.12).

Overall. The secretagogue for aldosterone permits this hormone, which simply opens the ENaC in the CCD, to be an NaCl-retaining hormone (angiotensin II) or a K^+-excreting hormone (plasma K^+); distal delivery of HCO_3^- could play a central role in the overall picture (see Figure 9.12). This is only an hypothesis at present.

QUESTIONS

(Discussions on pages 396–398)

9.9 *What is the maximum rate of K^+ excretion in 24 hours? (Given: plasma $[K^+]$ is 4 mmol/L, TTKG is 10, 5 L of filtrate reaches the CCD, and there is no medullary K^+ secretion or reabsorption.)*

9.10 *Can you determine whether a high urine $[K^+]$ is due to K^+ addition to the CCD or to water reabsorption in the MCD?*

9.11 *Does the excretion of K^+ conserve Na^+ and thereby defend the ECF volume? This question requires you to consider the origin of the K^+ that is excreted.*

9.12 *A very high $[K^+]$ in the lumen of the CCD occurs in a patient who vomits. A similarly high $[K^+]$ occurs when acetazolamide (a carbonic anhydrase inhibitor) acts. Common to both situations is bicarbonaturia. What might the mechanism be?*

9.13 *Does a normal person excrete more K^+ than a patient with adrenal insufficiency (assuming they eat the same diet)?*

9.14 *Is the volume delivered to the terminal CCD lower in a patient with a normal or reduced GFR (lower by 50%)?*

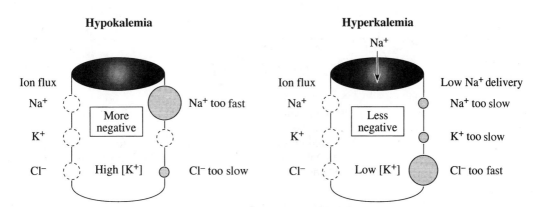

Figure 9.13   Changes in ion channel flux that may be the renal basis of hypokalemia or hyperkalemia. The barrel-shaped structures represent the CCD and the dashed circles represent pathways for ion movement. The potential lesions causing hypokalemia are shown in the left figure, and those causing hyperkalemia are shown in the right figure; possible lesions are depicted in the right side of each figure by the shaded circles. More detailed information is provided in Table 9.3.

Pathophysiologic Approach to Disturbances in the Plasma [K⁺]

Analysis of the rate of excretion of K⁺ in patients with hypokalemia or hyperkalemia can indicate why the renal response is not adequate. This rate should be compared with the expected values for an otherwise normal person with a deficit of K⁺ (excretion less than 10–15 mmol/day) or a surplus of K⁺ (excretion close to 400 mmol/day). If the rate of excretion of K⁺ is abnormal, the next step is to determine whether the fault is with the [K⁺] in the luminal fluid in the CCD or with the flow rate in the CCD. The levels of aldosterone and renin often help in clarifying the basis of the problem. In these analyses, the components leading to a high or low net secretion of K⁺ should be deduced (Figure 9.13, Table 9.3, and the review flow charts on pages 404 and 449).

Note

A decreased conductance or permeability to K⁺ in the luminal membrane of the CCD could theoretically lead to hyperkalemia. In this setting, there would be little augmentation of K⁺ excretion when a diuretic increases the flow rate.

TABLE 9.3   **Potential Lesions in the CCD that May Cause Hypokalemia or Hyperkalemia**

The lesions described are speculative and cause a change in K⁺ homeostasis by changing the [K⁺] in the lumen of the CCD (see Figure 9.13 as well). The other way to change the rate of K⁺ excretion is to change the flow rate in the CCD.

Lesion in CCD	ECF Volume	Renin	Urine [Na⁺] and [Cl⁻] with Low ECF Volume	TTKG + 9αF
Hypokalemia caused by:				
• Faster Na⁺	High	Low	Absent	>6
• Slower Cl⁻	Low	High*	Not <20 mmol/L	>15
Hyperkalemia caused by:				
• Low Na⁺ delivery	Low	High*	Absent	Low or high
• Slower Na⁺	Low	High*	Not <20 mmol/L	Low
• Faster Cl⁻	High	Low	Absent	Low

*The high level of renin can be suppressed by expansion of the ECF volume.

Notes
- 9αF = fludrocortisone, a drug with mineralocorticoid action.
- We switched terminology from "greater open probability" to "faster" for economy of space.
- With a very low flow rate, one can achieve a high [K⁺] in the lumen of the CCD, but only a small quantity of K⁺ will be excreted.

P A R T C

Diagnostic Tests

The clinician may employ any or all of the following tests to evaluate the K^+ secretory process: the rate of excretion of K^+, $[K^+]$ in a random urine sample, the ratio of K^+ to Na^+ in the urine, the fractional excretion of K^+, and the TTKG. Each test has its advantages and shortcomings (Table 9.4).

24-Hour K^+ Excretion Rate

This test is the most important to perform because it indicates whether a renal disorder is present. Expected values are less than 15 mmoL/day during hypokalemia and greater than 200 mmoL/day if hyperkalemia is present. Because there is a diurnal pattern for K^+ excretion, a 24-hour specimen is ideal, but it is not necessary given the wide ranges of expected values.

$[K^+]$ in a Random Urine Sample

One major advantage of this test is its simplicity. Nevertheless, on its own, the urine $[K^+]$ may be frankly misleading because reabsorp-

Rise in $[K^+]$ in the MCD
Three-fourths of the water content can be reabsorbed from MCD fluid (rise of urine osmolality from 300 to 1200 mOsm/kg H_2O) in the MCD.
- This reabsorption will elevate the $[K^+]$ fourfold, from a maximum of 40 to 160 mmol/L.
- Therefore, a 120 mmol/L rise in the $[K^+]$ can be due to water reabsorption.

TABLE 9.4 **Tests Used to Monitor the K^+ Excretion Process**

For a description, see the text.

Test	Strengths	Weaknesses	Expected Value HypoK	HyperK
Measure of K^+ excretion				
• 24-hour K^+ excretion (mmol/day)	• Valuable	• Does not indicate pathophysiology	<15	>200
• K^+ per creatinine (mmol/mmol)	• Can use random urine	• Must know expected rate of creatinine excretion	<1	>20
TTKG	• Physiologic basis • "Translates" urine to CCD • Separates $[K^+]$ from urine flow rate	• Many unverified assumptions	<2	>10
Less useful tests				
• Random urine $[K^+]$	• Simple	• Does not consider MCD water reabsorption	None	None
• K^+/Na^+	• None	• Depends on dietary Na^+	?	?
• Fractional excretion of K^+	• None	• Expected values depend on GFR • Is not based on the physiology of K^+	Need nomogram	

tion of water in the MCD has a great influence on the $[K^+]$ in the urine (see margin note). The other major disadvantage of a simple random urine sample is that the sample might be nonrepresentative (not usually a major concern).

With either of two manipulations, the $[K^+]$ in a random urine sample can be very useful. First, the daily rate of excretion of K^+ can be deduced by dividing the $[K^+]$ in the random urine sample by the concentration of creatinine in that sample multiplied by an estimate of the 24-hour creatinine excretion (the daily rate of excretion of creatinine is both constant and predictable; see margin note). This calculation will provide results that are satisfactory at the bedside. Second, the TTKG can be calculated (see three sections following). It will permit a separate analysis of the $[K^+]$ and the volume components of the K^+ excretion formula as well as provide a way to "translate" data from the urine to the CCD.

Ratio of K$^+$ to Na$^+$ in the Urine

This ratio has been suggested to give some insights into aldosterone action. In our opinion, it is not useful because the denominator, the $[Na^+]$ in urine, depends primarily on dietary intake of NaCl and/or diuretics. Therefore, unless the patient is on a fixed diet, the test is useless; even with a fixed diet, the test has little merit.

Fractional Excretion of K$^+$

This frequently performed calculation relates the quantity of K^+ excreted to that filtered. It does not provide any insights as to the mechanisms in the CCD, and it depends heavily on the rate of filtration of K^+. One needs to carry a nomogram to interpret the fractional excretion. For these reasons, we do not recommend it (see the discussion of Question 9.15 for more detail).

QUESTION

(Discussion on page 398)

9.15 *In what way does the calculation of the fractional excretion of K^+ differ from that of the TTKG?*

Transtubular [K$^+$] Gradient

The TTKG is a test designed to reflect the driving force for K^+ secretion. Before describing the calculation, the authors present the premise and then consider the weaknesses and assumptions required for this calculation. Remember that the excretion of K^+ is a function of the $[K^+]$ in the lumen of the CCD and the distal flow rate.

Premise

To calculate the $[K^+]$ in the lumen of the CCD, adjust the $[K^+]$ in the urine to "correct" for changes in the $[K^+]$ caused by the reabsorption of water in the MCD.

Use of creatinine excretion
In any individual, the rate of excretion of creatinine is relatively constant throughout the day. It depends on muscle mass, and the daily rate is close to 20 mg (0.2 mmol)/kg body weight. If a person excretes 10 mmol of creatinine per day and the urine has a $[K^+]$ of 40 mmol/L and a creatinine concentration of 5 mmol/L, the 24-hour K^+ excretion rate should be close to 80 mmol (40 mmol/L K^+/5 mmol/L creatinine × 10 mmol creatinine per day = 80 mmol of K^+/10 mmol of creatinine).

Assumptions

1. **Reabsorption of water in the MCD can be estimated:** The quantity of water reabsorbed in the MCD is calculated by comparing the rise in the osmolality of the fluid from the terminal CCD (same as that of plasma when ADH is acting) with that in the final urine. A twofold rise in urine osmolality implies that half the water was reabsorbed in the MCD, provided that no particles were reabsorbed in the MCD. This assumption is true for urea, NH_4^+, and K^+ for the most part, but it is not true for Na^+ (see Figure 9.14 and the discussion of Question 9.16).

2. **K^+ are not reabsorbed or secreted in the MCD:** In the rat, K^+ are not usually secreted or reabsorbed. Nevertheless, with profound K^+ depletion, there is net K^+ reabsorption, and when "subindustrial" doses of K^+ are given, there is net secretion of K^+ in the MCD. The authors assume that humans do have this capacity, but perhaps only in these extremes. Because this assumption is impossible to verify, one must have "faith" and a sense of caution when using the TTKG.

3. **The osmolality is known in the terminal CCD:** Knowing the osmolality of the tubular fluid in the CCD is a critical component of the calculation of the TTKG. If the urine osmolality is not greater than the plasma osmolality, the TTKG cannot be used because one does not know how much water was reabsorbed in the MCD. In contrast, with a higher urine osmolality, it is safe to assume that the fluid in the CCD has the same osmolality as that in the plasma.

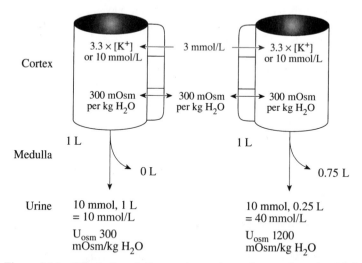

Figure 9.14   Effect of medullary water reabsorption on the urine [K^+]. The barrel-shaped structures represent the CCD, and the arrows below them the MCD. In both examples, there is a TTKG of 3.3. Consider what happens when 1 L of fluid traverses the MCD. In the left-hand example, there is no medullary water reabsorption but, in the right-hand example, 75% of the water is reabsorbed. In both cases, no K^+ are reabsorbed or secreted in the medulla. Therefore, although the excretions of K^+ are equal in both cases, the [K^+] in urine is fourfold higher (40 mmol/L) when water is reabsorbed in the medulla (right side). This increase must be considered when assessing the urine [K^+].

4. **The [K^+] in plasma reflects that in the peritubular fluid around the CCD:** This assumption cannot be verified, but the [K^+] in plasma should be representative unless K^+ excretion rates are enormous (see the discussion of Question 9.17).

Calculation of the TTKG

$$TTKG = [K^+]_{urine}/(urine/plasma)_{osm}/[K^+]_{plasma}$$

If the [K^+] in urine is divided by the urine-to-plasma osmolality ratio ([K^+]$_{urine}$/(urine:plasma)$_{osm}$), a reasonable approximation of the [K^+] at the end of the CCD can be deduced. This value will be high (7 or more times the plasma [K^+]) if mineralocorticoids are acting and low (less than 2 times the plasma [K^+]) if they are not. It is critical to ensure that the urine is not hypo-osmolal to plasma before doing this calculation.

QUESTIONS

(Discussions on page 399)

9.16 *If NaCl is reabsorbed in the MCD, in what direction will the TTKG change?*

9.17 *If all the filtered K^+ were excreted (100% fractional excretion), how would the calculated value for the TTKG change?*

PART D

Review

DISCUSSION OF INTRODUCTORY CASE
Lee's [K^+] (K)rashed
(Case presented on page 373)

What was the total body K^+ content at the time of presentation and why?

At the time of presentation, most patients with DKA have a reduced total body K^+ content primarily because of renal loss of K^+ subsequent to the glucose-induced osmotic diuresis. The degree of K^+ depletion depends on the antecedent intake of K^+ and, more importantly, on prior loss of K^+. In this regard, a history of vomiting or diuretic use might suggest excessive K^+ loss. On the other hand, an underlying kidney problem might limit the degree of K^+ depletion.

What factors led to her hyperkalemia?

The primary factor is insulin deficiency. A contributing factor may be that hyperglycemia caused a shift of water from K$^+$-rich ICF; this shift raised the [K$^+$] in the ICF (not a very important factor; see the discussion of Question 9.5).

Several other factors could influence the degree of hyperkalemia.

1. Acidemia is not an important factor.
2. Although the rate of excretion of K$^+$ is not high now, it might have been higher when her GFR was not so low (before the development of a markedly contracted ECF volume caused by the glucose-induced osmotic diuresis).
3. Intrinsic renal disease caused by long-standing diabetes mellitus could have compromised her renal excretion of K$^+$.
4. Certain drugs often given to diabetics may impair the excretion of K$^+$ (e.g., angiotensin-converting enzyme inhibitors).

Why did hypokalemia develop 4 hours later?

Patients with DKA have a large deficit of K$^+$ but are hyperkalemic because of a lack of insulin. Hypokalemia can develop after 2 hours when insulin promotes the entry of K$^+$ into cells. To a very minor extent, dilution will occur when the ECF is reexpanded with saline that contains no K$^+$.

In DKA there is little renal excretion of K$^+$ on admission despite hyperkalemia (the mechanism is unclear, but it prevents further K$^+$ depletion; for the authors' speculation, see margin note).

Summary of Main Points

- Potassium, principally an intracellular cation, is electrically balanced primarily by large macromolecular anions that are not free to leave the ICF.
- The ratio of the [K$^+$] in the ICF to that in the ECF (35–40:1) is due to the electrogenic Na$^+$K$^+$ATPase and diffusion of K$^+$ from the ICF to the ECF. This distribution, which is primarily influenced by hormones (insulin and β-adrenergics), generates the RMP across cell membranes, an important determinant of cell function.
- Renal excretion of K$^+$ is a function of the [K$^+$] in the urine and the urine flow rate. The major determinant of the [K$^+$] in the urine is the electrogenic reabsorption of Na$^+$ in the CCD; the major determinant of the flow rate in the CCD is the rate of excretion of osmoles when ADH acts.

Discussion of Questions

9.1 What quantity of K$^+$ of dietary origin (70 mmol) will be distributed in cells if there is no excretion of K$^+$ and no change in the RMP?

The calculation is based on the following facts: the distribution of K$^+$ between the ICF and the ECF is 35–40:1 at the usual RMP.

Because the RMP did not change, the ingested K^+ will distribute at a 35–40:1 concentration ratio, and the ICF volume is twice that of the ECF. Because 70 mmol of K^+ was ingested, approximately 1 mmol will remain in the ECF and 69 mmol will enter the ICF.

What will the plasma [K⁺] be?

The ECF volume is 15 L, so the rise in $[K^+]$ is 1/15, or 0.067 mmol/L.

9.2 What is the intracellular cation composition in the red blood cells of a dog? These cells lack Na⁺K⁺ATPase pumps.

If there is no $Na^+K^+ATPase$, the $[Na^+]$ will be very high (close to 140 mmol/L), and the $[K^+]$ will be very low (close to 9 mmol/L) in these cells. Perhaps this is why we refer to dogs as canines.

9.3 Why does the entry of Na⁺ into cells increase the RMP when augmented by insulin but decrease the magnitude of the RMP in hyperkalemic periodic paralysis?

The answer becomes obvious when the number of positive charges that move is counted.

Insulin. The entry of Na^+ into cells is electroneutral because it occurs in conjunction with the export of H^+ from cells; flux is via the NHE-1. When Na^+ are pumped out of cells via the electrogenic $Na^+K^+ATPase$, a net of one-third of a positive charge exits the cell per Na^+ that entered via the NHE-1; this movement increases the electronegativity of the RMP (see margin note).

Periodic Paralysis. The entry of Na^+ is electrogenic; Na^+ enter via their ion-specific channels, so 1 positive charge enters the cell per Na^+. As discussed, only a net of one-third of a charge exits the cell per Na^+ pumped via the $Na^+K^+ATPase$. Hence, the net effect is net positive charge entry and a diminished magnitude of the RMP.

Na⁺K⁺ATPase
One-third of a positive charge is exported per Na^+ pumped (3 Na^+ are pumped out and 2 K^+ enter).

9.4 What property of the Na⁺K⁺ATPase might allow it to bind K⁺ at a [K⁺] of 4 mmol/L in the ECF yet also permit K⁺ to dissociate from this pump at a [K⁺] of 150 mmol/L in the ICF?

This question is challenging and the answer is unknown. The affinity for K^+ has to be considerably less in cells than in the ECF (smaller by orders of magnitude). The authors offer the following suggestions: a conformational change in the K^+-binding subunit of the $Na^+K^+ATPase$ that occurs once it is in the intracellular domain and/or the presence of a nearby positive charge in the cell that helps "repel" K^+ from this ion pump.

Note
Question 9.4 is for the more curious and needs further exploration.

9.5 How much will the plasma [K⁺] change when 1 L of pure water is shifted from the ICF to the ECF? Assume a constant RMP.

The assumption requires that the ratio of the $[K^+]$ in the ICF to the $[K^+]$ in the ECF remain constant. If 1 L leaves the ICF, its volume declines by 1/30, or 3.33%. This decline raises the $[K^+]$ in the ICF (and ECF) by 3.33% because the ratio of the $[K^+]$ in the ICF to the $[K^+]$ in the ECF remains constant. Therefore, the $[K^+]$ in plasma will rise from 4 to 4.13 mmol/L at steady state, a trivial rise. If hyperosmolal states cause hyperkalemia, a simple shift of water is not the primary mechanism involved. Rather, hyperosmolality leads to a lowering of the RMP, or it is associated with decreased excretion of K^+.

9.6 Will a drug that depolarizes cell membranes cause a change in the plasma [K⁺]?

Yes. With depolarization, the RMP falls; thus, the ratio of the $[K^+]$ in the ICF to the $[K^+]$ in the ECF falls, and hyperkalemia will be present.

9.7 Why does the loss of intracellular phosphate anions cause hyperkalemia in DKA but not in poliomyelitis?

The answer derives from three facts: first, the major anions in the ICF are organic phosphates; second, the major cation is K^+; third, electroneutrality must be preserved.

Poliomyelitis. In this disorder, there is a wasting of muscles and the loss of phosphate, water, and K^+ in the same proportion as they exist in cells. There is no change in the RMP. Thus, there is just a smaller (but otherwise normal) ICF compartment in this disorder. There is ample time to excrete the K^+ and phosphate.

DKA. In this acute catabolic setting, there is a loss of organic phosphates (RNA, etc.), K^+, and water from the ICF. The key to hyperkalemia is the fall in the RMP associated with a lack of insulin; this fall means that more K^+ will be distributed into the ECF. The degree of hyperkalemia will also depend on the rate of excretion of K^+ (osmotic diuresis) in DKA. Usually in DKA there is a large total body deficit of K^+ and a redistribution of K^+ from the ICF to the ECF.

Clinical pearl
Close to half of the deficit of K^+ in DKA is due to the parallel loss of K^+ and phosphate. Await the anabolic effects of insulin and a supply of phosphate to replace this deficit of K^+ (takes several days).

9.8 During K⁺ depletion, Na⁺ replace K⁺ in cells. How does this exchange affect the Na⁺K⁺ATPase?

A rise in the intracellular $[Na^+]$ should make the $Na^+K^+ATPase$ pump more quickly. Faster pumping should, in turn, lower the $[Na^+]$ in cells back to normal. If the elevated $[Na^+]$ persists, something else must have happened. Perhaps there was also a fall in the number of $Na^+K^+ATPase$ units or their activity. There may also have been a lower affinity of the $Na^+K^+ATPase$ pump for Na^+. At least one of these events must have occurred for a higher intracellular $[Na^+]$ to be present in steady state.

9.9 What is the maximum rate of K⁺ excretion in 24 hours? (Given: plasma [K⁺] is 4 mmol/L, TTKG is 10, 5 L of filtrate reaches the CCD, and there is no medullary K⁺ secretion or reabsorption.)

Note
K^+ excretion = Urine $[K^+]$ × Urine volume.

The luminal $[K^+]$ increases to almost 10-fold above the plasma $[K^+]$ when stimulated by aldosterone. If the plasma $[K^+]$ is 4 mmol/L, then the luminal $[K^+]$ is 40 mmol/L (i.e., 10×4 mmol/L). If distal delivery is 5 L, then 200 mmol of K^+ could be excreted; alternatively, a 10 L delivery could result in the excretion of 400 mmol at the same TTKG. Hence, the importance of the volume of filtrate delivered to this nephron site can be appreciated. In addition, it has been reported that the $[K^+]$ in luminal fluid can be 20 times the plasma $[K^+]$ if bicarbonaturia is present. Therefore, there is the potential to augment the excretion of K^+ considerably; the highest excretion rates reported are close to 400 mmol/day.

9.10 Can you determine whether a high urine [K⁺] is due to K⁺ addition to the CCD or to water reabsorption in the MCD?

The $[K^+]$ is the $K^+:H_2O$ ratio. If the $[K^+]$ were to rise from the reabsorption of water in the MCD, the particle:H_2O ratio (osmolality) would also rise in fluid traversing the MCD if the particles themselves were not reabsorbed (half of the particles are normally urea, and urea is not reabsorbed in the MCD to an appreciable extent). Hence, if the urine osmolality has not risen above that of plasma, the rise in $[K^+]$ is due to the net secretion of K^+, a cortical action. In contrast, a rise in urine osmolality implies a role for water reabsorption in the MCD. This issue is examined quantitatively in the section addressing the TTKG, pages 391–393.

9.11 Does the excretion of K⁺ conserve Na⁺ and thereby defend the ECF volume? This question requires you to consider the origin of the K⁺ that is excreted.

To answer this question, consider the actions of aldosterone in terms of Na^+ and K^+ physiology, as depicted in Figure 9.15. The first step in aldosterone action is the reabsorption of Na^+ in the CCD. This reabsorption does not necessarily conserve Na^+ for the ECF. Consider pathway (1a), for example: to reabsorb Na^+, K^+ are transported from the ECF to the urine. Because the ECF has a small quantity of K^+, the source of the K^+ is really the ICF. To transport most of the K^+ out of the ICF, Na^+ enter this compartment. Therefore, the net effect is the excretion of intracellular K^+ in the urine and the placement of Na^+ from the ECF into the ICF. These actions do not appear to defend either the ECF volume (Na^+ content) or the ICF composition (K^+); however, in a different context, the reabsorption of Na^+ may indeed defend the ECF volume.

If the source of the urinary K^+ was dietary K^+ (1b), if Na^+ reabsorption was linked to the excretion of NH_4^+ (hypokalemia stimulates ammoniagenesis), or if a Na^+ and Cl^- were reabsorbed, the ECF volume would be defended. Hence, it is necessary to obtain a broad overview to integrate Na^+, K^+, and acid-base physiology.

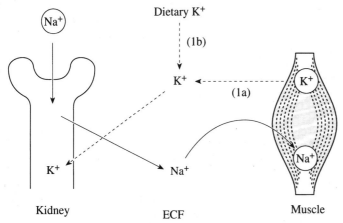

Figure 9.15 The source of excreted K⁺ and the defense of the ECF volume. The reabsorption of filtered Na^+ with K^+ excretion will result in the preservation of the ECF volume only when the source of the K^+ is dietary.

9.12 A very high [K⁺] in the lumen of the CCD occurs in a patient who vomits. A similarly high [K⁺] occurs when acetazolamide (a carbonic anhydrase inhibitor) acts. Common to both situations is bicarbonaturia. What might the mechanism be?

The mechanism has not yet been defined, but the authors offer the following speculation. For HCO_3^- to cause such a high TTKG, it seems that HCO_3^- inhibit the reabsorption of Cl^- in the CCD. Assume that the mouth of the Cl^- channel contains a positively charged group, such as the epsilon amino group in lysine (pK close to 9). These positive charges "attract" Cl^- to the mouth of the channel, where they are permitted or encouraged to enter. In contrast, if HCO_3^- enter this environment, alkalization occurs. The epsilon $R\text{-}NH_3^+$ group dissociates (the equation following is driven to the right by the fall in the $[H^+]$).

$$R\text{-}NH_3^+ \leftrightarrow RNH_2 + H^+$$

The uncharged RNH_2 group is very reactive and will combine with CO_2 to form a carbamino compound that bears a negative charge (the equation in the margin is drawn with HCO_3^- for convenience).

This anionic carbamino compound may face the lumen, repel Cl^- from the mouth of the Cl^- channel, and diminish the reabsorption of Cl^-. The authors emphasize that this explanation is highly speculative.

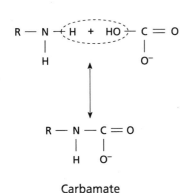

Carbamate

9.13 Does a normal person excrete more K⁺ than a patient with adrenal insufficiency (assuming they eat the same diet)?

Adrenal insufficiency is a chronic condition, so the patient is in balance; all the K^+ ingested and absorbed are excreted. Thus, both people eat and excrete the same quantity of K^+. The difference is that the normal person uses aldosterone to "drive" K^+ excretion, but the patient who lacks aldosterone requires hyperkalemia to achieve excretion of K^+ and K^+ balance. Nevertheless, K^+ excretion would be much higher in a normal individual with a large intake of K^+ (i.e., has aldosterone).

9.14 Is the volume delivered to the terminal CCD lower in a patient with a normal or reduced GFR (lower by 50%)?

The volume delivered to the terminal CCD depends on the osmole excretion rate if ADH is acting. When ADH acts, the osmolality in this fluid is the same as in plasma (e.g., 300 mOsm/kg H_2O). If 900 mOsm is excreted per day with a normal or 50% reduction in GFR, the volume delivered to the terminal CCD is the same in both examples: 3 L/day (see margin illustration).

Delivery to CCD: 3 L

300 mOsm/L

900 mosmoles

9.15 In what way does the calculation of the fractional excretion of K⁺ differ from that of the TTKG?

The TTKG "adjusts" for water reabsorption in the MCD, and the fractional excretion adjusts for water reabsorption throughout the nephron. They differ in the methods used to monitor water reabsorption—osmolality vs creatinine.

The formulas for these two calculations are as follows (U = urine and P = plasma):

$$\text{Fractional excretion} = (U/P)_{[K^+]} \div (U/P)_{\text{creatinine}}$$
$$\text{TTKG} = (U/P)_{[K^+]} \div (U/P)_{\text{osmolality}}$$

9.16 If NaCl is reabsorbed in the MCD, in what direction will the TTKG change?

If more particles are reabsorbed in the MCD, for the same urine osmolality, one will underestimate the volume of water reabsorbed in the MCD. With more water reabsorption, the [K$^+$] or the K$^+$:urine volume will be higher. Hence, the value back-calculated for the [K$^+$] in the CCD will be higher than it should be, and thereby the TTKG will overestimate the ratio of tubular fluid to plasma [K$^+$].

Note
See discussion of Bartter's and Gitelman's syndromes in Chapter 10.

9.17 If all the filtered K$^+$ were excreted (100% fractional excretion), how would the calculated value for the TTKG change?

Because close to one-fourth of renal plasma flow is filtered, one-fourth of the K$^+$ is removed and excreted when the fractional excretion is 100%. Therefore, the [K$^+$] in the peritubular fluid (and renal vein plasma) is 3 vs 4 mmol/L. Hence, the TTKG using systemic venous blood will underestimate the TTKG, and the result will be 75% of the real value.

Appendix to Chapter 9

New Information in the Molecular Physiology of Renal Handling of Potassium

The major nephron segment involved is the cortical distal nephron, and the main cell type is the principal cell.

Overall Process

1. Basolateral Membrane
Use the Na$^+$, K$^+$, ATPase located on the basolateral membrane to lower the intracellular [Na$^+$]. The molecular anatomy (α, β, γ subunits) is unchanged (see Chapter 6).

2. Luminal Membrane
a) ENaC
Function
ENaC permits Na$^+$ ions to move from the lumen, where their concentration is high, to the ICF, where their concentration is low. Moreover, the interior of the cell has a net negative charge, facilitating this entry of Na$^+$ ions.

Molecular Anatomy
There are three subunits. The α subunit is the most important one for Na$^+$ conductance. The β and γ subunits are sites for regulation.

Disease Correlations
Inhibition by Drugs. Cationic drugs such as amiloride, triamterene, trimethoprim, and pentamidine inhibit the ENaC.

Inherited Diseases. Mutations in the β or γ subunits lead to a more open configuration of this ENaC (Liddle's syndrome, Chapter 10). Conversely, a less open configuration is called pseudohypoaldosteronism type 2b (Chapter 11).

(b) K$^+$ Ion Channels.
There is a family of K$^+$ ion channels; because they do not seem to regulate K$^+$ secretion, they are not further discussed here.

Note
Cortisol also binds avidly to the aldosterone receptor, activating a response.

(c) Important Hormone Receptors

The receptor for ADH resides in the basolateral membrane (Chapter 6), whereas the receptor for aldosterone resides in the cytoplasm.

Aldosterone or Type I Mineralocorticoid Receptor

This receptor has a high affinity for aldosterone and for cortisol.

11 β-Hydroxysteroid Dehydrogenase. To make the aldosterone receptor a specific one for aldosterone, it must be linked to a specific enzyme system, 11-β hydroxysteroid dehydrogenase (11 β-HSDH). Actually, there is a pair of enzymes in the basolateral membrane that catalyzes the complete destruction of cortisol before it can enter the cytosol. The first of these enzymes destroys most of the cortisol quickly (high capacity, lower affinity), and the second destroys the remaining cortisol (low capacity, high affinity).

Disease Correlations

In some patients, 11 β-HSDH is absent (apparent mineralocorticoid excess syndrome), whereas in others 11 β-HSDH is inhibited (licorice), overwhelmed by super-high cortisol levels (ACTH-producing tumors), or its catalytic activity is avoided (fludrocortisone).

10

Hypokalemia

Hypokalemia
• Plasma [K$^+$] <3.5 mmol/L.
• Threats are cardiac arrhythmias, respiratory failure, and hepatic encephalopathy.

Summary
After being consumed, K$^+$ are stored in cells temporarily and are then excreted several hours later (close to the noon hour).

Note
For the cell to lose 400 mmol of K$^+$, there must be a loss of 400 mEq of intracellular anions or a gain of 400 mmol of Na$^+$ and/or H$^+$ in the ICF. Hence, major changes in the ICF environment should be expected.

OBJECTIVES

☐ To provide a clinical approach to the patient with *hypokalemia* based on an assessment of K$^+$ intake, shift of K$^+$ into cells, and increased loss of K$^+$, with an appreciation that most clinical problems are in the renal loss category.

☐ To describe how to evaluate both components of renal K$^+$ loss—the [K$^+$] in the luminal fluid of the cortical collecting duct (CCD) and the volume of fluid delivered to the terminal CCD.

☐ To illustrate how an assessment of the urine electrolytes (Na$^+$, Cl$^-$, and K$^+$) helps to elucidate the basis of excessive renal excretion of K$^+$.

☐ To provide a plan of treatment based on physiologic principles.

Outline of Major Principles

1. **General considerations:** Because the extracellular fluid (ECF) contains only 2% of K$^+$ (60 mmol), physicians monitor total body K$^+$ through a tiny and inadequate window. The ratio of the [K$^+$] across the cell membrane is 150 mmol/L/4.3 mmol/L, or close to 35:1. If the plasma [K$^+$] falls from 4 to 3 mmol/L, and this ratio of [K$^+$] remains constant, the fall in the content of K$^+$ in the intracellular fluid (ICF) would be 25% of the total, or close to 1125 mmol (0.25 × 4500 mmol). Because the deficit of K$^+$ is much less than half of this value in clinical studies (100–400 mmol), the transcellular ratio of [K$^+$] must rise (i.e., the ratio of [K$^+$] in the ICF to that in the ECF is higher; see margin note). A rise in this ratio implies that the resting membrane potential (RMP) has hyperpolarized (i.e., more positive charges (K$^+$) diffused out of cells down their higher concentration difference).

2. **Etiology of hypokalemia:** Loss of K$^+$ occurs most often in patients who vomit, have nasogastric suction or diarrhea, or who use (abuse) diuretics, but in each case the major route of K$^+$ loss is renal. The clues are found in the history (vomiting, laxative abuse, diuretics—all of which the patient may deny) and the physical finding of ECF volume contraction. If there is no ECF volume contraction, look for a primary reason for high levels of aldosterone. The presence of hypertension is a useful clue when deducing the cause of hyperaldosteronism. A shift of K$^+$ into cells can occur under the influence of hormones, metabolic alkalosis, or recent anabolism; however, these causes are uncommon for chronic and severe hypokalemia.

3. **Diagnosis of hypokalemia:** Clinical suspicion is essential because weakness is a late symptom and is not present until K$^+$ depletion is quite severe; hypokalemia is most often found on "routine" analysis of electrolytes, as a result of electrocardiogram (ECG) changes, or in patients with a history of disorders associated with renal K$^+$ loss. Urine electrolyte levels are most helpful in establishing the cause, and a useful approach is to interpret the urine [K$^+$] by adjusting it for water reabsorption in the renal medulla to reflect the [K$^+$] in the lumen of the CCD (i.e., the transtubular potassium gradient [TTKG]; see Chapter 9, pages 391–393).

4. **Dangers of hypokalemia:** The major danger of hypokalemia is a cardiac arrhythmia (see margin note), especially in the presence of *digitalis*. A second danger is hypoventilation in the patient with a severe degree of metabolic acidosis because high values for alveolar ventilation are required to maintain a very low Pa_{CO_2}; hypoventilation is often due to muscle weakness when associated with hypokalemia. A third setting in which hypokalemia may be detrimental is hepatic encephalopathy. The hypokalemia may aggravate toxicity by permitting more NH_4^+ to accumulate in cells (hypotheses mentioned include enhanced production of NH_4^+ in the kidney and their distribution in cells because of acidosis of the ICF).

5. **Treatment:** Large quantities of K^+ must be given when the total body deficit is great. In most cases, KCl is needed; $KHCO_3$ should be given to patients with hypokalemia and a severe degree of metabolic acidosis. In the patient receiving digitalis and in the patient with diabetic ketoacidosis in whom K^+ will shift into cells 1–2 hours following insulin administration, K^+ must be replaced more aggressively. When a large quantity of KCl is given, there may be a significant expansion of the ECF volume because Na^+ will move from the ICF to the ECF when K^+ enter cells (Figure 10.1).

Note

The major danger of hypokalemia and hyperkalemia is cardiac arrhythmias.

Digitalis

A glycoside that is given to improve myocardial contractility or to slow atrioventricular conduction.

DEVELOPMENT

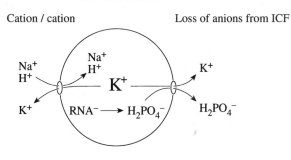

THERAPY

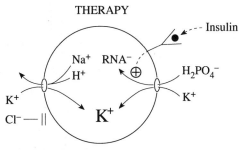

Figure 10.1   The effect of KCl administration in a patient with K^+ deficiency. As shown on the top portion, K^+ can be lost from the ICF by two mechanisms: a cation-cation pathway on the left and a loss of K^+ plus an ICF anion (phosphate) on the right. During therapy (bottom portion), if the entire K^+ deficit was not produced by the cation-cation exchange, KCl alone will not correct the ICF deficit of K^+ because Cl^- is predominantly an ECF anion. To replace the entire deficit of K^+ in the ICF, some K^+ must be given along with phosphate once anabolism occurs. This is most relevant in the repair of the K^+ deficit of diabetic ketoacidosis because anabolism is stimulated by insulin.

INTRODUCTORY CASE
Toby Is Losing More Than Weight
(Case discussed on page 429)

Toby, the ballerina (see Chapter 4, Introductory Case) is on the verge of landing a job with a prestigious ballet company. She believes that a possible impediment is a gain of weight. She tries measures that worked in the past during her adolescence. Although she loses weight, her stamina is not the same as it used to be. She sees a physician for advice. She denies taking medications and vomiting. On physical examination, a degree of contraction of the ECF volume is detected. Laboratory results follow.

		Plasma	Urine (Random Sample)
Na^+	mmol/L	136	7
K^+	mmol/L	3.1	22
Cl^-	mmol/L	108	84
HCO_3^-	mmol/L	19	0
pH		7.35	5.6
Osmolality	mOsm/kg H_2O	278	589
Glucose	mmol/L (mg/dL)	5 (90)	0

Review flow chart
Causes of hypokalemia with excessive excretion of K^+
The causes of excessive excretion of K^+ are too high a flow rate in the CCD (left limb) and too high a $[K^+]$ in the lumen of the CCD (right limb). Both flow rate and $[K^+]$ in the CCD should be evaluated in each patient. Final considerations are shown in the shaded boxes. (ECFV = extracellular fluid volume.)

What is her total body K^+ deficit?
Was a shift of K^+ into cells a major cause of hypokalemia?
What factors could have contributed to a renal loss of K^+?
What tests might be helpful in this regard?

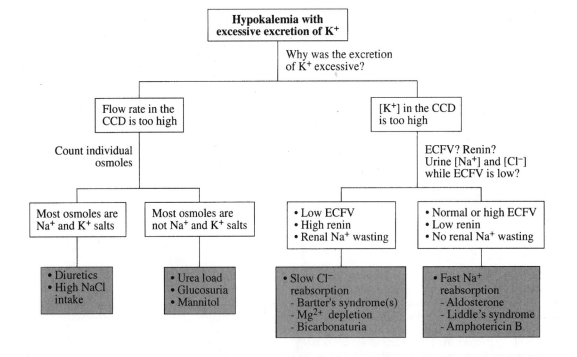

Diagnosis

Approach to the Patient with Hypokalemia

Because hypokalemia can lead to a life-threatening event, one might have to embark on therapy before the investigation can be completed (Figure 10.2). If there is an important change in the ECG, if digitalis is being used in a patient with a cardiac problem, or if respiratory failure or hepatic encephalopathy is imminent, proceed directly with treatment (see pages 425–429); otherwise, use the steps outlined in Figure 10.2 to make a diagnosis. The questions to ask are as follows:

1. **Is the rate of excretion of K⁺ excessive?** A rate of excretion of K⁺ that is less than 15 mmol/day in an adult with hypokalemia indicates two possibilities: first, the hypokalemia may not be due to excessive excretion of K⁺; second, renal K⁺ loss may have occurred at an earlier time, but the provocative agent or event is not present now (e.g., remote vomiting or diuretic use). Nevertheless, in most patients with hypokalemia, there is excessive renal excretion of K⁺ (greater than 15 mmol/day).

2. **Why is the rate of excretion of K⁺ high?** The first step to take to understand why the rate of excretion of K⁺ is too high

Dangers
1. Cardiac arrhythmias
2. Respiratory weakness
3. Hepatic encephalopathy

Excretion of K⁺
K⁺ excretion =
   Urine [K⁺] × Urine volume

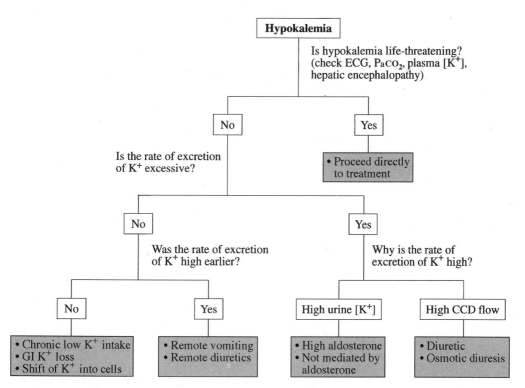

Figure 10.2 Investigation of hypokalemia. The final diagnostic groups are shown in the shaded boxes (for a more detailed discussion, see the text).

TABLE 10.1 **Urine Electrolyte Levels During Chronic Severe Hypokalemia of Renal Origin**

Electrolyte	Vomiting	Diuretics
Na^+	• High if vomiting was recent despite ECF volume contraction; otherwise <10 mmol/L.	• <10 mmol/L unless use of diuretics was recent.
K^+	• High relative to plasma value; absolute value depends on medullary water abstraction.	• Can be >20 mmol/L even if no diuretics were used recently.
Cl^-	• Always <10–15 mmol/L.	• <10 mmol/L if ECF volume is low and there was no recent use of diuretics.
HCO_3^-	• Abundant with recent vomiting.	• Zero unless carbonic anhydrase inhibitor–type of diuretics.

is to determine whether a high $[K^+]$ or a high flow rate in the CCD is responsible. First, consider the $[K^+]$ in the urine: if the TTKG is greater than 4, one cause of the high rate of excretion of K^+ is a high $[K^+]$ in the terminal CCD. The question at this point is to determine whether the high $[K^+]$ is due to actions of aldosterone. This aspect will be considered in detail later.

The other major contributor to a high rate of excretion of K^+ is a large flow rate in the CCD, driven by an osmole excretion load. The osmoles can be electrolytes (usually caused by a diuretic; Table 10.1) or nonelectrolytes (usually from an osmotic diuresis caused by glucose or urea).

QUESTIONS

(Discussions on pages 441–442)

10.1 *What is the most likely cause of K^+ loss in patients A, B, C, and D? They all have hypokalemia, ECF volume contraction, and metabolic alkalosis.*

Urine electrolyte		Patient			
		A	B	C	D
Na^+	mmol/L	25	25	25	0
K^+	mmol/L	60	60	60	10
Cl^-	mmol/L	0	85	0	0
HCO_3^-	mmol/L	85	0	0	0

10.2 *Will a patient consuming a very high NaCl load become hypokalemic as a result of enhanced renal K^+ excretion? With respect to K^+ homeostasis, how does such a patient differ from one who receives a loop diuretic? Assume equal Na^+ excretion rates.*

Etiology of Hypokalemia

Three factors must be examined to determine the most likely basis for hypokalemia: intake of K^+, distribution of K^+ in the ICF, and the excretion of K^+. The most important of these factors is excessive renal excretion of K^+ in a patient with chronic hypokalemia.

Decreased Intake of K^+

- Hypokalemia is almost never due solely to low intake of K^+.

A deficiency of K^+ develops slowly if its basis is low intake of K^+ because renal excretion of K^+ falls to very low levels (10–15 mmol/day) in K^+-depleted subjects. Two major populations are at risk for low dietary K^+ intake: first, the urban poor, because they do not consume the meat and vegetables that contain abundant K^+ (Table 10.2); second, populations that live in rural, near-equatorial regions, such as the northeast area of Thailand, because their diet consists mostly of polished rice (high in carbohydrates, low in K^+), and they do not ingest other foods rich in K^+.

Given the ability of the kidneys to diminish the excretion of K^+ so efficiently and so promptly, it should take weeks to months to lower the overall K^+ content by 100 mmol. Notwithstanding, a less severe restriction in K^+ intake can contribute to hypokalemia if there is a greater loss of K^+. This tendency becomes important when people lose K^+ by sweating excessively and when diuretics are given to people who eat a low quantity of foods that contain K^+ (e.g., the elderly who are hypertensive; see the discussion of Case 10.1).

Usual K^+ intake
1. In an adult on a Western diet the intake of K^+ is 1 mmol/kg body wt.
2. Most of the K^+ ingested is absorbed. Certain materials, such as resins, bind K^+ so that K^+ cannot be absorbed. This binding can be considered a decrease in the "net intake" of K^+. In therapy of hyperkalemia, gastrointestinal loss of K^+ can be promoted with K^+-binding resins.

QUESTION

(Discussion on page 442)

10.3 *A patient takes a diuretic, which causes the excretion of an extra 60 mmol of K^+ per day. The doctor recommended that this patient consume bananas to replace the K^+ lost each day. If all the kcal were retained as stored fat (9 kcal/g), what would be the weight gain at the end of 1 year?*

TABLE 10.2 **Examples of Foods that Supply 60 mmol of K^+**

Foods	Weight (g)
Vegetables	
Potatoes and beans	500
Peas	5000
Fruits	
Bananas and cantaloupe	800
Oranges	1200
Meats	
Beef and chicken	600

TABLE 10.3 **Causes of a Shift of K⁺ into Cells**

Acid-base disorder
Metabolic alkalosis
Acting via hormones
Insulin, β_2-adrenergic agonists, possibly aldosterone, α-adrenergic antagonists
Anabolism
Growth, recovery from diabetic ketoacidosis, total parenteral nutrition, red blood cell synthesis (e.g., recovery from pernicious anemia)
Rare disorders
Hypokalemic periodic paralysis
Other
Anesthesia? (see margin note)

Anesthesia

In animals, the induction of anesthesia leads to a significant fall in the plasma [K⁺] that is independent of the acid-base status. It may be due to catecholamine release and/or a direct membrane effect of anesthetics. No comparable data are available in humans.

Increased Shift of K⁺ into Cells

The factors promoting a shift of K⁺ into cells are listed in Table 10.3. In general, these factors, when acting individually, lead to a fall in serum [K⁺] of less than 1 mmol/L, but when acting in combination, with very high doses of drugs, or in the right clinical setting (e.g., recovery from diabetic ketoacidosis (DKA)), a much larger fall in the plasma [K⁺] can occur.

In the paragraphs to follow, the factors discussed are the influence of the acid-base state, the actions of hormones, the role of anions in the intracellular fluid (ICF), and the loss of K⁺ by nonrenal and renal routes.

Influence of the Acid-Base States

- In metabolic alkalosis, K⁺ shift into cells; no shift of K⁺ occurs in respiratory alkalosis.

A shift of K⁺ from the ECF into cells should occur as a result of the movement of H⁺ in the opposite direction (Figure 10.3). Because the magnitude of this H⁺ shift is much smaller with respiratory acid-

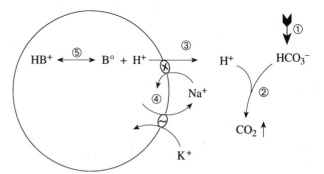

Figure 10.3   The shift of K⁺ from the ECF to the ICF. The addition of HCO_3^- (1) causes the [H⁺] in the ECF to fall (2). This fall causes Na⁺ to enter the ICF in conjunction with H⁺ export on the Na⁺/H⁺ exchanger (3). The Na⁺K⁺ATPase (4) pumps the Na⁺ out of cells while pumping K⁺ into cells. Continued flux requires back-titration of buffers in the ICF (5). There is no way to predict whether Na⁺ or K⁺ will remain in the ICF when H⁺ exit; the "decision" is made by the K_m for Na⁺ of the Na⁺K⁺ATPase (i.e., does this K_m change?).

base disorders, hypokalemia in a patient with respiratory alkalosis is probably due to causes other than this acid-base disorder. In contrast, K$^+$ do shift into cells during metabolic alkalosis.

Actions of Hormones

> • Hormone-induced K$^+$ shifts are due mainly to insulin and β$_2$-adrenergics.

Insulin. Insulin promotes the entry of K$^+$ into the ICF by making the RMP more electronegative. A more negative voltage in cells is the result of the electroneutral entry of Na$^+$ and the electrogenic export of Na$^+$ via the Na$^+$K$^+$ATPase (see Figure 9.2 and margin note); actions of insulin also lead to an increase in the content of anions in the ICF (phosphate esters such as RNA). The major clinical setting in which this action is observed is following the administration of insulin for treating patients with diabetes mellitus in poor control. The fall in plasma [K$^+$] can be quite large (approximately 90 minutes after insulin administration).

Note
Very large doses of insulin can activate NHE-1 and cause a greater electroneutral entry of Na$^+$ and its efflux through the electrogenic Na$^+$K$^+$ATPase.

β$_2$-Adrenergic Activity. β$_2$-Adrenergics lead to the entry of K$^+$ into cells. Elevated levels of these hormones are seen during the response to hypotension, stress, exercise, hypoglycemia, and in the clinical setting of delirium tremens, among others. Drugs with these actions are commonly given to alleviate bronchospasm. With the usual dose of β$_2$-agonist, the plasma [K$^+$] can fall by 0.2–0.3 mmol/L, whereas massive overdoses cause a fall of almost 1.5–2.0 mmol/L. In contrast, β$_2$-antagonists cause a much smaller rise in the plasma [K$^+$] (0.3 mmol/L).

Aldosterone. Hypokalemia in patients with high aldosterone activity is due primarily to renal K$^+$ loss rather than a shift of K$^+$ into cells. Nevertheless, in patients with a deficiency of aldosterone, there may also be a diminished capacity to retain K$^+$ in the ICF (mechanism unknown), and administration of aldosterone to these patients may be associated with a significant fall in plasma [K$^+$].

Gain in ICF Anions. During acute anabolic states, such as recovery from diabetic ketoacidosis or when malnourished subjects are given a nutritional supplement, organic phosphate anions accumulate in cells (e.g., RNA, DNA, phospholipids); for electrical balance, K$^+$ will also return to cells, and hypokalemia will develop if the intake of K$^+$ is not increased appropriately.

QUESTIONS

(Discussions on pages 442–443)

10.4 *Elite athletes often have a [K$^+$] in plasma that is close to 3.0 mmol/L at rest. What mechanisms might be involved?*

10.5 *If an individual is K$^+$-depleted and has lost 300 mmol of K$^+$, what is the most likely change in ionic composition of the ICF, and what adjustments were needed to permit this change?*

10.6 *The result of the lesion in hypokalemic periodic paralysis may be a higher open probability of Na$^+$ channels in the plasma*

Note
These questions require further exploration.

membrane. How might this lesion cause hypokalemia? In what way is this lesion different from that in hyperkalemic periodic paralysis in which Na+ channels also have a more open probability?

CASE 10.1
Kay Has His Ups and Downs
(Case discussed on page 433)

Kay, age 52 years, works as an elevator repairman. He fell five stories and sustained severe head and soft-tissue injuries. On arrival in the hospital, he was comatose and required vigorous life-support efforts, including an infusion of an adrenaline-like compound to maintain his blood pressure. Laboratory results follow.

Time (Hours)		0	3.0	3.5	15	16
Plasma						
Na$^+$	mmol/L	140	140	138	140	136
K$^+$	mmol/L	3.6	3.2	1.6	3.2	9.2
HCO$_3^-$	mmol/L	22	22	20	20	19
Glucose	mmol/L (mg/dL)	5 (90)	5 (90)	6 (108)	5 (90)	5 (90)
Urine						
Volume				← 0.5 L →		

The striking abnormality is a sudden and severe degree of hypokalemia that developed over 30 minutes at the end of 3.5 hours. This was accompanied by ventricular tachycardia (severe cardiac rhythm disorder). He survived.

If there was no excretion of K+ between 3.0 and 3.5 hours, how many millimoles of K+ entered Kay's cells?

What was the most likely reason for his acute fall in plasma [K+] between 3.0 and 3.5 hours?

What is the largest amount of K+ a clinician might have to infuse into Kay?

By what route and how much K+ should the clinician infuse into Kay in the first minute of therapy?

Enhanced Loss of K+

- Renal excretion of K+ is the major method of K+ loss.
- Certain types of diarrhea cause hypokalemia via actual gastrointestinal (GI) K+ loss.

Gastrointestinal Tract

The [K+] of upper gastrointestinal secretions is usually 15 mmol/L or less (Table 10.4). Because gastric secretions have such a low [K+], hypokalemia due to vomiting or nasogastric suction actually results from K+ loss in the urine (see the discussion of Question 10.7). In contrast, loss of colonic contents can lead directly to hypokalemia (see margin note). When diarrhea is due to more distal colon involvement (villous adenoma of the rectum), the K+ content

Obligate loss of K+
- Nonrenal
  1. Sweat (close to 10 mmol/L, but volume can vary from 0.2 to 12 L/day); losses of K+ in sweat are higher in cystic fibrosis
  2. Stool loss (100 mmol/L × 0.1 L/day)
  3. Diarrhea ([K+] close to 40–50 mmol/L)
- Renal
  1. Minimum of 10 mmol of K+ per day

TABLE 10.4 **Representative Electrolyte Contents and Volumes of Upper Gastrointestinal Secretions**

Values are representative for a typical 70-kg adult.

Site	Volume L/day	$[Na^+]$ mmol/L	$[K^+]$ mmol/L	$[Cl^-]$ mmol/L	$[HCO_3^-]$ mmol/L
Gastric	1.5	20	10	130	0
Duodenal	3–8	110	15	115	10
Pancreas	0.5	140	5	30	115
Bile duct	0.5	140	5	100	25
Jejunal	3.0	140	5	100	20
Ileal	0.5	80	10	60	75

Note

In cholera, for example, 6 L of water containing 750 mmol of Na^+ and 100 mmol of K^+ can be lost in 24 hours.

Laxative abuse

The loss of K^+ is much larger when a phenolphthalein type of laxative is used instead of an osmotic or bulk type of laxative.

might be two or three times higher. Suspect that diarrhea is the cause of hypokalemia when metabolic acidosis with a normal plasma anion gap is present and the rate of excretion of NH_4^+ is not low (greater than 100 mmol/day, see Discussion of Introductory Case).

QUESTIONS

(Discussions on pages 443–444)

10.7 *What is the cause of hypokalemia in patients who vomit and have metabolic alkalosis?*

10.8 *When a person starves for 3 weeks, there is a negative balance for K^+ of close to 300 mmol, but the subject is normokalemic. What changes may have occurred in cells to cause this intracellular K^+ deficit?*

10.9 *Should the deficit of K^+ in a starved person be replaced during the fast?*

Urinary K^+ Loss

- Excretion of K^+ is high when there is either a higher $[K^+]$ in the CCD or higher volume of fluid traversing the terminal CCD.
- Although hypokalemia can result from decreased intake of K^+, shift of K^+ into cells, or K^+ loss, virtually all cases with chronic hypokalemia have increased renal K^+ loss.

Note

This mechanism requires release of aldosterone or a setting that leads to mineralocorticoid-like effects.

From a clinical perspective, patients with hypokalemia on a chronic basis usually have hypokalemia caused by excessive renal excretion of K^+. This form of hypokalemia should be suspected if patients were treated with diuretics (usually for hypertension or edema states) or if vomiting or nasogastric suction was prominent in the clinical picture (see margin note). As stated, the two components of the K^+ excretion formula—$[K^+]$ and the flow rate in the CCD—should be examined independently.

A high $[K^+]$ in the CCD is seen with
- Mineralocorticoid-like actions
- Bicarbonaturia
- Low urine $[Cl^-]$

High $[K^+]$ in the Urine. A TTKG that is greater than 4 in a patient with hypokalemia indicates that certain factors have raised the $[K^+]$ in the terminal CCD. These factors form part (or all) of the basis

Secretagogues for mineralocorticoids
- Normal adrenal gland
  Angiotensin II
  Hyperkalemia
- Abnormal adrenal gland
  Adrenocorticotropic hormone
  Tumor
  Genetic defect

for the hypokalemia. In this setting, look for stimulators of this process: first, aldosterone or compounds with aldosterone-like actions (Table 10.5 and page 423); second, bicarbonaturia; and third, a very low [Cl^-] in the luminal fluid in the CCD.

1. **Plasma aldosterone:** In the patient with excessive renal loss of K^+, hypertension, and a normal ECF volume, the plasma renin and aldosterone levels help one to differentiate adrenal from nonadrenal causes of hyperaldosteronism (see Table 10.5). The diagnostic efficacy of these hormone assays is improved by expanding the ECF volume with saline to suppress endogenous renin release; one should make these measurements while the patient is recumbent (when the patient is in the upright position, the ECF volume redistributes and thereby stimulates the release of renin).

2. **Bicarbonaturia:** Bicarbonate in the lumen of the CCD causes the [K^+] to rise markedly at this location if aldosterone is also present (e.g., vomiting). The mechanism is not clear but could involve inhibition of reabsorption of Cl^- at this nephron site (see Chapter 9, page 385).

3. **A low [Cl^-] in the luminal fluid of the CCD:** When Na^+ are delivered to the CCD with an anion other than Cl^-, reabsorption of Na^+ will be electrogenic if aldosterone acts. This electrogenic reabsorption makes the lumen more negative and thereby increases the [K^+] in the lumen of the CCD (provided that Cl^- are not present in appreciable amounts).

There are seven causes for high mineralocorticoid action identified in Figure 10.4 with the following numbers.

Those with High Levels of Aldosterone in Plasma

1. High renin (e.g., renal artery stenosis, renin-producing tumors).

2. Cells (e.g., adenoma) in the adrenal cortex producing aldosterone or a compound with mineralocorticoid bioactivity.

3. ACTH stimulating aldosterone production because there is a genetic lesion in the adrenal gland in which the ACTH promoter

TABLE 10.5 **Causes of a Hypermineralocorticoid Action**

See Figure 10.4 for a visual representation of these states of high mineralocorticoid-like actions.

Endogenous release of aldosterone
Associated with increased renin levels
- Low effective circulating volume usually caused by diuretics or vomiting, less commonly the result of intrinsic renal disorders such as Bartter's syndromes
- Renal artery stenosis
- Juxtaglomerular apparatus hypertrophy or tumor
Associated with low renin levels
- Primary adrenal cortical hyperplasia or adenoma
- Defects in enzymes of the adrenal gland
Nonaldosterone-mediated (associated with low renin levels)
Endogenous compounds with mineralocorticoid effects
- Cushing's syndrome or tumors that secrete excessive ACTH
- Dexamethasone-suppressible release of aldosterone (GRA)
- Defects in enzymes of the adrenal gland
- Apparent mineralocorticoid excess syndrome (defect 11 β-HSDH)
Exogenous compounds
- Excessively high levels of hydrocortisone (ACTH-producing tumor)
- Licorice, swallowed chewing tobacco, carbenoxolone, which block 11 β-HSDH

HIGH MINERALOCORTICOIDS

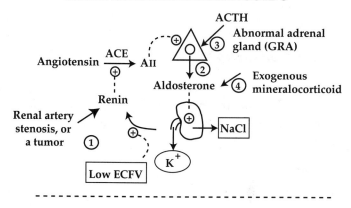

- -

LOW MINERALOCORTICOIDS

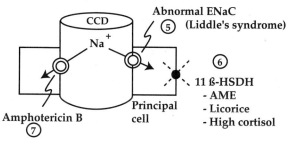

Figure 10.4　Causes of hypokalemia. The figure is divided into two sections. The top portion deals with hypokalemia associated with high levels of aldosterone or an aldosterone-like compound in plasma. The bottom portion represents high aldosterone bioactivity when aldosterone levels in plasma are low. The triangular figure is the adrenal gland. The outer layer (zona glomerulosa) produces and releases aldosterone.

drives the synthesis of a compound with mineralocorticoid bioactivity. Suppressing ACTH with glucocorticoids decreases their production (glucocorticoid remedial aldosteronism (GRA), a genetic chimera).

Those with Low or Absent Levels of Aldosterone in Plasma

4. Exogenous compounds mimicking the actions of aldosterone, such as fludrocortisone.

5. An epithelial Na^+ ion channel (ENaC) in the luminal membrane, which is permanently in an open conformation due to a mutation (Liddle's syndrome).

6. Blocking the destruction of cortisol in principal cells by creating a relatively low activity of 11 β-hydroxysteroid dehydrogenase (11 β-HSDH) (e.g., licorice).

7. Insertion of an artificial Na ion channel in the luminal membrane of the CCD (e.g., amphotericin B).

QUESTIONS

(Discussions on pages 444–445)

10.10 *Can excessive delivery of Na^+ to the CCD augment the rate of excretion of K^+?*

10.11 *How do poorly reabsorbed anions lead to an augmented excretion of K⁺?*

Clinical Features

> • Unless the plasma [K⁺] is less than 3 mmol/L, few symptoms should be attributed to the hypokalemia.

Symptoms

Symptoms have a high degree of variability from patient to patient. A classification of these symptoms with respect to the organ affected is in Table 10.6.

Cardiac Muscle

Severely hypokalemic patients are likely to develop a number of cardiac arrhythmias. This tendency is important if the patient is on digitalis or has underlying myocardial disease.

Skeletal Muscle

The most common complaint related to hypokalemia is weakness or easy fatigability. Symptoms become prominent at a plasma [K⁺] below 3.0 mmol/L. Low levels can ultimately lead to paralysis (see margin note). This consequence is especially important during metabolic acidosis because respiratory muscle weakness can compromise ventilation and result in a life-threatening fall in pH in cells. The pattern of muscle weakness caused by K⁺ deficiency seems to be most evident in the lower extremities. With time and/or continuing K⁺ loss, the trunk and upper extremities become involved. Rarely, patients may also complain of cramps, muscle tenderness, and tetany.

With a severe degree of hypokalemia, the patient is at greater risk of developing *rhabdomyolysis*. If hypokalemia remains untreated for a prolonged time, muscle atrophy could occur.

Note
Some individuals with marked degrees of hypokalemia do not have weakness; the authors do not know how to explain this difference.

Rhabdomyolysis
A disorder in which macromolecules in skeletal muscle are hydrolyzed and retained; they may also be released. This disorder occurs more frequently in patients with hypokalemia and hypophosphatemia. Interestingly, it is not a common cause of severe hyperkalemia.

TABLE 10.6 **Symptoms of Hypokalemia**

Muscular
  Cardiac muscle
    Arrhythmias (especially if digitalis or heart disease is present)
  Skeletal muscle
    Weakness, cramps, myalgias, rhabdomyolysis with extreme K⁺ depletion
  Smooth muscle
    Intestinal disturbances (constipation, ileus)
Renal
  Concentrating defect (polyuria, nocturia)
  Medullary interstitial disease (a direct consequence of K⁺ deficiency and a result of enhanced NH₃ availability)
Neurologic
  Thirst, decreased deep tendon reflexes, paresthesias

Smooth Muscle

With hypokalemia, GI motility might decline and lead to constipation and, in the extreme, an ileus (see margin note).

Renal Problems

Polydipsia is a common complaint during severe hypokalemia and may be due to a more direct effect on the thirst center. Because of a reduction in renal-concentrating ability during severe hypokalemia, polyuria and nocturia may develop (see margin note). These symptoms occur when the K^+ deficiency is chronic and severe (greater than 200 mmol). The renal lesion may ultimately become irreversible because of interstitial fibrosis and tubular damage. In contrast, the ability to excrete a dilute urine is relatively preserved during hypokalemia.

Other Factors

The central nervous system seems to be spared in hypokalemia. The $[K^+]$ in the cerebrospinal fluid is constant despite wide swings in the plasma $[K^+]$.

ECG Changes During Hypokalemia

Hypokalemia is associated with a more negative RMP. Nevertheless, although ECG changes occur, they correlate poorly with the plasma $[K^+]$. In general, the earlier changes include T-wave flattening or even inversion. The ST segment becomes depressed and may have a "trough-like" appearance. A U wave may also appear (see margin note). In addition, severe hypokalemia tends to promote arrhythmias and conduction disturbances. The Q–T interval is normal, or it may be prolonged during hypokalemia, and this difference may help distinguish the ECG effects of hypokalemia from those seen with digitalis toxicity. The ECG abnormalities of hypokalemia are exaggerated if hypercalcemia is also present.

Importance of ECF Volume Status and/or Hypertension

From a clinical perspective, it is helpful to subdivide groups of patients presenting with hypokalemia based on their ECF volume and blood pressure (Figure 10.5).

Contracted ECF Volume and Lower Blood Pressure

Patients with a contracted ECF volume commonly have vomiting or diuretic use (abuse) as the most likely basis (see discussion of Question 10.1). Less often, Bartter's syndromes may be present.

Normal or Expanded ECF Volume and Hypertension

In those patients who do not have a contracted ECF volume, the presence of hypertension suggests that hyperaldosteronism is present; its basis should be sought (see Figure 10.4).

Patients with Mg^{2+} depletion may have high aldosterone levels despite hypokalemia. The mechanism for aldosterone release is not

Clinical pearl
If patients with hypokalemia and low GI motility are given K^+ supplements orally, K^+ may accumulate in the GI tract. Later, these K^+ may be absorbed and provide a sudden K^+ load, with a resulting hyperkalemia. Chronic hypokalemia retards subsequent excretion of K^+ for 24 hours or so.

Note
Hypokalemia causes polyuria by having less aquaporin-2 in the luminal membrane of the MCD.

ECG changes in hypokalemia
This ECG is from a patient with a severe degree of hypokalemia. The most prominent findings are the "lazy" ascent of the ST segment and the prominent U wave. Hypokalemia is often associated with hypomagnesemia. This combination of abnormalities may lead to polymorphic ventricular tachycardia (torsades de pointes).

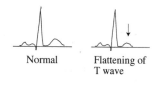

Normal   Flattening of
                T wave

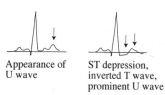

Appearance of   ST depression,
U wave   inverted T wave,
                 prominent U wave

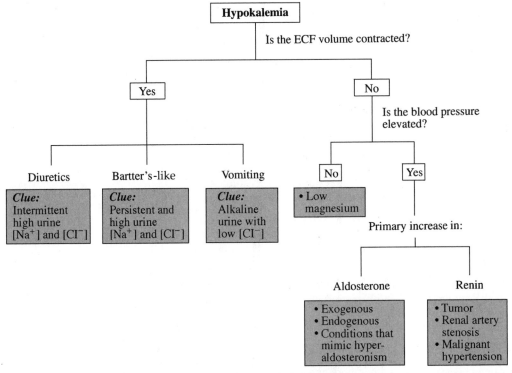

Figure 10.5   Clinical evaluation of the patient with hypokalemia. The major factors to evaluate are the ECF volume and the blood pressure. Refer to Figure 10.4 for more information concerning states with high aldosterone-like activity.

clear. Suspect Mg^{2+} depletion if there is hypocalcemia, alcoholism, and/or a GI problem, or if the patient was treated with drugs that cause Mg^{2+} wasting (large doses of loop diuretics, cisplatin, or aminoglycosides). Mg^{2+} depletion also occurs frequently in Gitelman's syndrome and less commonly in Bartter's syndrome (discussed below).

Application of Basic Physiology at the Bedside

[K⁺] in the CCD
This concentration is the [K⁺] in urine divided by the urine/plasma osmolality, provided that the urine osmolality equals or exceeds that of plasma.

Note
To deliver a small quantity of Cl⁻ to the CCD, the stimulus of a low effective circulating volume must be present, together with the presence of a large delivery of Na⁺ with anions other than Cl⁻ (e.g., carbenicillin, hippurate, or sulfate). Another way to reduce the reabsorption of Cl⁻ is if permeability to Cl⁻ in the CCD is diminished.

- This section is speculative and requires "faith" in possible physiologic mechanisms.

A High [K⁺] in the Lumen of the CCD

For there to be an unduly high [K⁺] in the lumen of the CCD (see margin note), the electrogenic reabsorption of Na⁺ must be augmented creating a higher transepithelial potential difference (TEPD). This augmentation, from an ion movement point of view, means that there was either faster reabsorption of Na⁺ or slower reabsorption of Cl⁻ in the CCD (see margin note, Figure 10.6, and the flow chart on page 404).

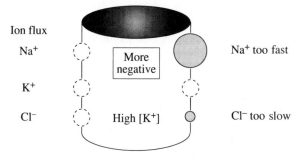

Figure 10.6   Causes of increased [K⁺] in the lumen of the CCD. The "normal size" of the ion channels or conductive pathways responsible for the net secretion of K⁺ is represented on the left side of the figure. The major factors that lead to a high [K⁺] in the CCD are relatively faster Na⁺ reabsorption and relatively slower Cl⁻ reabsorption (shaded circles shown on the right side). Both lead to an increase in the lumen-negative TEPD. Plasma renin levels and urine electrolytes help to confirm clinical suspicions.

Faster Reabsorption of Na⁺ in the CCD

High mineralocorticoid activity causes the ENaC in the CCD to have an open probability that is greater than normal (see Table 10.5). Liddle's syndrome is a rare disorder that results from a greater open probability of ENaC in the CCD. Another form of excessive Na⁺ permeability is the insertion of a nonspecific cation channel, as occurs in *amphotericin B*–induced nephrotoxicity; this channel enables Na⁺ reabsorption independent of factors that regulate the normal Na⁺ channel; it is thus insensitive to amiloride.

As a result of the increased reabsorption of Na⁺, there should be a tendency for ECF volume expansion, low levels of renin, and perhaps even hypertension to go along with the hypokalemia and the high TTKG. The other finding is the ability to excrete a Na⁺-poor and Cl⁻-poor urine when the ECF volume is contracted. With ECF volume contraction, renin levels should be higher.

Slower Reabsorption of Cl⁻ in the CCD

An increase in the electrochemical driving force for K⁺ excretion can occur if there is reabsorption of Na⁺ without enough Cl⁻; this slower reabsorption of Cl⁻ may be due to a reduced delivery of Cl⁻ or a reduced permeability of the luminal membrane of the CCD to Cl⁻. Reduced delivery of Cl⁻ occurs in rare circumstances (marked ECF volume contraction and a high rate of excretion of urea). With normal Na⁺, but a relatively slow reabsorption of Cl⁻ in the CCD, there should be hypokalemia and an excessively high [K⁺] in the urine (a very high TTKG) along with Na⁺ and Cl⁻ in the urine even if the patient has ECF volume contraction. There is a tendency to ECF volume contraction and hyperreninemia and, because of the hypokalemia and ECF volume contraction, metabolic alkalosis (see Chapter 4). Because of their hypovolemia, these patients should not be hypertensive despite high levels of angiotensin II. In many ways, these features resemble Bartter's-like syndromes (see the following section).

Amphotericin B
A drug used to treat certain fungal infections.

Criteria for faster Na⁺ reabsorption in the CCD
1. Hypokalemia, high TTKG.
2. Increased ECF volume and low renin.
3. Urine can be Na⁺-poor if the ECF volume is decreased.

Criteria for slower Cl⁻ reabsorption in the CCD
1. Hypokalemia, high TTKG.
2. Low ECF volume and high renin.
3. Urine [Na⁺] and [Cl⁻] not low when the ECF volume is decreased.

Note
A water diuresis does not cause a high rate of excretion of K^+ even if aldosterone levels are high; perhaps this feature reflects the requirement of ADH for normal K^+ conductance in the luminal membrane of the CCD.

High Flow Rate in the CCD

The two major reasons for a high flow rate in the CCD are a water diuresis and an osmotic diuresis (see margin note). The main factor controlling flow rate in the CCD in the presence of ADH is the rate of delivery of osmoles (Figure 10.7). The two major groups of osmoles are nonelectrolytes (usually urea) and electrolytes. The former reflects primarily the load of protein ingested, and the latter reflects largely the ingestion of salt or the use of diuretics. It is possible that both a high flow rate and a high $[K^+]$ in the CCD may be present in a given patient.

Increased Delivery of Na^+ and Cl^- to the CCD

If a patient has a defect in the reabsorption of Na^+ and Cl^- in nephron segments upstream (more proximal) to the CCD, a larger quantity of Na^+ and Cl^- will be delivered to the CCD. Now the relative rate of Na^+ as compared with Cl^- reabsorption rates could come into play with respect to the excretion of K^+. The authors propose that two circumstances may lead to excessive excretion of K^+ from this enhanced delivery of Na^+ and Cl^-.

Enhanced Excretion of K^+ Due to a Higher Flow Rate Traversing the CCD

When ADH acts, the flow rate in the CCD is a function of the number of osmoles delivered. With a plasma osmolality of 300 mOsm/kg H_2O, the flow rate in the CCD is 1 L/300 mOsm that exits the CCD (i.e., the osmolality of the fluid entering the CCD is 300 mOsm/kg H_2O; see Figure 10.7). Hence, if a loop diuretic resulted in the delivery of 1800 mOsm to the CCD instead of the usual 900 mOsm per day, the flow rate in the CCD would be 6 L instead of the usual 3 L. If the $[K^+]$ in each liter were to remain unchanged, K^+ excretion would double with a loop diuretic—this is the typical effect of an acute administration of a diuretic.

Delivery of More Na^+ and Cl^- than the CCD Can Reabsorb

- The explanation here is speculative, but it could explain the data.

We must imagine that the capacity to reabsorb Na^+ in the CCD is greater than the capacity to reabsorb Cl^- once this nephron segment has responded to chronic ECF volume contraction (enhanced reabsorption capacity for Na^+ and Cl^-). As shown in Figure 10.8, the CCD has a delivery of close to 1000 mmoles of Na^+ and Cl^- each

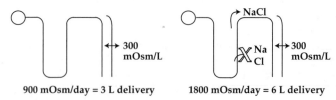

900 mOsm/day = 3 L delivery   1800 mOsm/day = 6 L delivery

Figure 10.7 Flow rate in the CCD. For every 300 mOsm that exits the CCD, 1 L was delivered to the MCD when ADH acts (osmolality equal to plasma). The figure on the right represents events when a loop diuretic acts.

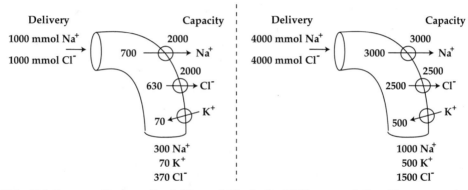

Figure 10.8   Relative capacity to reabsorb Na⁺ and Cl⁻ in the CCD: a speculation. The structure is the CCD. The setting on the right represents chronic exposure to increased delivery of Na⁺ and Cl⁻ to the CCD that exceeds their enhanced reabsorptive capacities. The numbers inside the nephron represent quantities reabsorbed, whereas the transport capacity is depicted to the right of the nephron.

day (3% of the filtered load). Two other points could be valid. First, this nephron segment has a large capacity to reabsorb Na⁺ and Cl⁻, but this capacity is not expressed because one has a smaller rate of delivery of Na⁺ and Cl⁻ under normal circumstances. The second point is that with chronic ECF volume contraction, there is stimulation of the capacity to reabsorb Na⁺ and Cl⁻. If, in this setting, Na⁺ were reabsorbed at a relatively faster rate than Cl⁻, the net result would be enhanced excretion of K⁺ (see right portion of Figure 10.8).

Specific Disorders in Which Hypokalemia Is a Prominent Feature

Bartter's Syndrome

The cardinal features of Bartter's syndrome are hypokalemia, a variable degree of renal Na⁺ and Cl⁻ wasting, a contracted ECF volume, metabolic alkalosis, hyperreninemia, and, in many cases, a deficiency of Mg^{2+} caused by excessive excretion of this cation. Secondary features include hypertrophy of the juxtaglomerular apparatus, a resistance to the vasoconstrictor actions of angiotensin II, and a high rate of excretion of Ca^{2+}.

The pathophysiology of Bartter's syndrome has recently been clarified. The following lesions have been proposed:

- The pathophysiology can be considered as having a loop diuretic acting 24 hours a day.

Common Lesions. Molecular studies have shown that the most common variant of Bartter's syndrome is a defect in the Na⁺, K⁺, 2 Cl⁻ electroneutral cotransporter (NKCC) in the luminal membrane of the thick ascending limb of the loop of Henle; this is the transporter inhibited by the loop diuretic furosemide. The net effect of this defect is to cause the delivery of Na⁺ and Cl⁻ to the CCD to be much higher on a chronic basis than normal. As a result, there could be enhanced excretion of K⁺, NaCl wasting, and a low ECF volume with a resulting high level of renin (Figures 10.8 and 10.9).

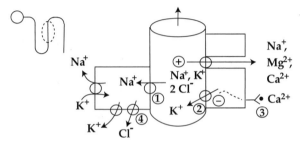

Figure 10.9 Possible lesions for Bartter's syndrome. The barrel-shaped structure represents the lumen and the rectangle represents a cell in the thick ascending limb of the loop of Henle. The possible lesions are the NKCC (1), the luminal K^+ channel (2), occupation of the basolateral Ca^{2+} receptor (3), or the Cl ion channel (4).

Other Lesions. There are other molecular lesions that can cause Bartter's-like syndrome. One variant is a mutation in the K^+ ion channel in the luminal membrane of the thick ascending limb of the loop of Henle. Other putative lesions are a defect in the Cl^- ion channel in the basolateral membrane or the delivery of a signal to close this luminal K^+ ion channel. Examples of the latter are seen when the calcium ion receptor is activated in the basolateral membrane in these cells. A ligand known to do this is hypercalcemia; as well, cationic drugs such as gentamicin and tobramycin and possibly cationic proteins could make Ca^{2+} a more effective ligand to express its effect.

Associated Findings. The net effect of the lesions is that the lumen does not have its usual positive voltage. As a result, there is less reabsorption of Ca^{2+} (hypercalciuria), magnesium (tendency for hypomagnesemia), and Na^+ (ECF volume contraction) and a defect in the ability to achieve a high maximum value for the urine osmolality when ADH acts. In the CCD, there is a tendency for faster reabsorption of Na^+ than Cl^-, leading to renal K^+ wasting. There is now some evidence that this renal K^+ wasting is more prominent with hypomagnesemia. While all mechanisms remain speculative, requiring Mg^{2+} for "faster" reabsorption of Cl^- could explain the diminished renal K^+ wasting when Mg^{2+} is infused and the plasma Mg^{2+} level is restored.

Gitelman's Syndrome

- The pathophysiology can be considered as having a thiazide diuretic acting 24 hours a day.

Molecular Lesions. The majority of patients have a mutation that involves the Na^+:Cl^- cotransporter in the early distal convoluted tubule. Nevertheless, there are some patients who have all the clinical features of Gitelman's syndrome without a recognized mutation in this transporter. Possible lesions would be a defect in a protein needed for "docking" this transporter in the luminal membrane or a defect in one of its activators.

Clinical Manifestations. Patients have many features in common with those with Bartter's syndrome (NaCl wasting, low ECF volume, high renin levels, renal K⁺ wasting, hypomagnesemia), but there are two notable differences. First, there is no defect in the ability to have a maximum urine osmolality when ADH acts (unless there is a second lesion that damaged the medulla, such as caused by chronic hypokalemia or long-term treatment with drugs such as nonsteroidal antiinflammatory agents, for example). Second, there is a very low rate of excretion of Ca^{2+}. Clinicians use the Ca^{2+}:creatinine ratio in the urine to reflect this enhanced reabsorption of Ca^{2+}. The mechanism, which is likely due to a lower intracellular Ca^{2+} concentration, is the result of a lower intracellular $[Na^+]$ (less Na^+ reabsorbed due to low activity of NaCl cotransporter)—this lower $[Na^+]$ means less Na^+ exit via the $(Na^+)_2:Ca^{2+}$ antiporter on the basolateral membrane and thereby less entry of Ca^{2+} (figure in margin).

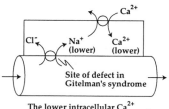

The lower intracellular Ca^{2+} promote the reabsorption of Ca^{2+}

A comparison of the clinical features of Bartter's and Gitelman's syndromes are in Table 10.7, and a diagnostic flow chart is provided as Figure 10.10.

Therapy for patients with Bartter's syndrome or Gitelman's syndrome is not satisfactory. Usually, high intake of KCl provides only partial benefit. A high-salt diet is beneficial for the low ECF volume but may be detrimental for K⁺ balance (see the discussion of Question 10.12). Other measures advised, such as *nonsteroidal antiinflammatory drugs* (NSAIDs), may lead to long-term problems (interstitial nephritis), so the minor, short-term benefit must be weighed against this theoretical detrimental effect. Although dietary supplements of Mg^{2+} make sense, absorption may not be sufficient to achieve a therapeutic benefit; high doses cause diarrhea. The other therapeutic option to consider is the use of the drug amiloride, but this K⁺-sparing diuretic may be of only modest benefit. One

NSAIDs
The rationale for NSAIDs is that they depress the synthesis of prostaglandins of the E_2 family, and PGE_2 levels are raised in states with marked deficiency of K⁺.

TABLE 10.7 **Hereditary Diseases and Hypokalemia**

All the disease categories present with hypokalemia and excessive excretion of K⁺ with a higher than expected urine $[K^+]$. Abbreviations: GRA = glucocorticoid remediable aldosteronism; AME = apparent mineralocorticoid excess; 11 β-HSDH = 11 β-hydroxysteroid dehydrogenase; TAL = thick ascending limb of the loop of Henle; DEX = dexamethasone; NKCC = Na^+, K^+, 2 Cl^- cotransporter in TAL of LOH; DCT = distal convoluted tubule; Uosm = urine osmolality

	Gitelman's	Bartter's	Liddle's	GRA*	AME
Molecular Lesion	Inhibited NaCl cotransporter in DCT	Inhibited NKCC or ROM-K⁺ channel	Activated ENaC in the CCD	Chimeric gene: ACTH-driven mineralocorticoid synthesis	Defect in 11 β-HSDH in principal cells
Presenting Feature	Tetany; unexpected laboratory finding	Failure to thrive; laboratory finding	Hypertension; hypokalemia; family history	Severe hypertension	Hypertension
Age of First Symptoms	Teenage	Children	Young, if severe	Young adult	Children
Mimicked by Drugs	Thiazides	Loop diuretics	Amphotericin B	Mineralocorticoids	Licorice; carbenoxolone
Plasma Mg²⁺	Low	Low	Normal	Normal	Normal
ECF Volume	Contracted	Contracted	Expanded	Expanded	Expanded
Hypertension	No	No	Yes	Yes	Yes
Key Diagnostic Feature	Hypocalciuria	Lower than expected maximum Uosm; hypercalciuria	Hypertension	Suppression of aldosterone by dexamethasone; excess cortisol C-18, oxidation metabolites	Urine cortisone-to-cortisol ratio

*Some members of families with this disorder do not have hypokalemia.

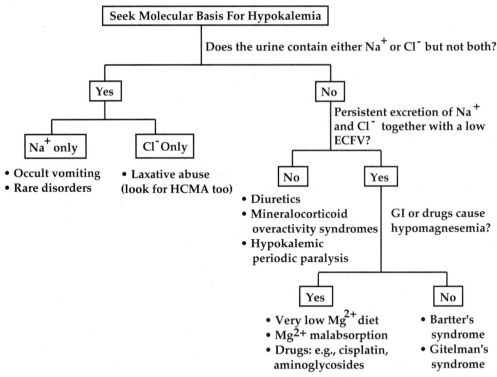

Figure 10.10   Differential diagnosis of hereditary causes of hypokalemia. The initial step is to rule out common causes of hypokalemia that may be denied by the patient. Here, the urine electrolytes become very important (see Table 10.1). A finding of persistent excretion of Na^+ and Cl^- despite a contracted ECF volume narrows the differential diagnosis to causes where there is obvious basis for hypomagnesemia or not. Finding Mg^{2+}-poor urine will suggest a low intake or poor GI absorption of Mg^{2+}. Failure to find an obvious cause for renal Mg^{2+} wasting suggests that Bartter's or Gitelman's syndrome may be present.

could consider using angiotensin-converting enzyme inhibitors (ACE-I) in patients who are significantly symptomatic from hypokalemia and resistant to other therapies. ACE-I lead to a lower plasma aldosterone level by decreasing angiotensin II levels (Figure 9.11). ACE-I could be poorly tolerated because of hypotension and other recognized side effects (e.g., cough). On a theoretical basis, the patients who respond would be those whose excessive K^+ excretion was driven by aldosterone but in whom distal delivery of HCO_3^- was not an important factor (stimulated by a lack of angiotensin II). It is not clear how large a population this represents.

QUESTIONS

(Discussions on pages 445–446)

10.12 *In a patient with Bartter's syndrome, in what ways will a greater salt intake increase the rate of excretion of K^+? What are the dangers of giving a small load of NaCl to this patient?*

10.13 *When a patient presents with all the features characteristic of Bartter's syndrome, a clinician must rule out surreptitious use (abuse) of diuretics, vomiting, and laxative abuse. What features should a clinician rely on in each of these settings?*

Hypokalemia Following Vomiting and Diuretics

Hypokalemia as a result of vomiting and the use of diuretics was considered in detail in Chapter 4. During vomiting, the excessive loss of K^+ is due to a very high $[K^+]$ in the CCD that results from both the high level of aldosterone and, of special importance, the presence of bicarbonaturia.

With diuretic abuse, the high levels of aldosterone are secondary to ECF volume contraction; the abuse is associated with a high delivery of osmoles and therefore volume to the CCD. These factors lead to an augmented rate of excretion of K^+. Nevertheless, the degree of hypokalemia is generally quite mild (3.0–3.5 mmol/L). Greater degrees of hypokalemia can occur if the dietary intake of K^+ is very low (e.g., in the aged; see the discussion of Case 10.2) or if hyperaldosteronism is present for other reasons (e.g., primary hyperaldosteronism).

Primary Hyperaldosteronism

A tumor of the adrenal cortex leads to high levels of aldosterone, ECF volume expansion, hyporeninemia, and hypertension. The characteristic electrolyte finding is hypokalemia in the range of 3.0 mmol/L. All these findings suggest that the lesion in the CCD is of a Na^+ channel with a greater open probability. The patients are in K^+ balance because they excrete the usual K^+ content of the diet. Typical values for the TTKG are close to 6 and perhaps reflect the influence of hypokalemia and K^+ depletion. Treatment is surgical removal, if feasible. Medical therapy includes aldosterone antagonists such as spironolactone.

11β-Hydroxysteroid Dehydrogenase and Hypokalemia

11β-HSDH exists in cells that respond to mineralocorticoids; there are actually two enzymes acting in sequence. The first has a high

Note
Diuretics are a commonly used therapy for hypertension. Therefore, as primary hyperaldosteronism is a cause of hypertension, it is possible to have a patient with hypokalemia who, when receiving diuretics, has an excessive degree of K^+ depletion.

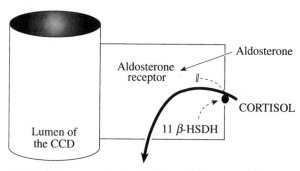

Figure 10.11   Influence of 11β-HSDH on "aldosterone-like" actions in the CCD. Cortisol has a very high affinity to the aldosterone receptor. As cortisol enters principal cells of the CCD, the enzymes 11β-HSDH inactivate it before it can bind to the aldosterone receptor. There are three circumstances in which cortisol will successfully bind to the aldosterone receptor: when there is a deficiency of 11β-HSDH (apparent mineralocorticoid excess syndrome), when an inhibitor of 11β-HSDH is present (e.g., licorice), and possibly when there is an excess supply of cortisol relative to the normal activity of 11β-HSDH (perhaps ectopic production of ACTH by a tumor).

capacity but lower affinity for cortisol so it removes most, but not all, of this potential activator of the mineralocorticoid receptor. A second high-affinity, low-capacity enzyme completes the removal of cortisol from the cytosol of principal cells. Hence, this pair of enzymes converts cortisol to an inactive product so that cortisol will not occupy the aldosterone receptor illicitly and mimic the actions of aldosterone in these cells. Cortisol, if permitted to enter and accumulate in principal cells of the CCD, would bind to the aldosterone receptor and lead to activation of the K^+ secretory process.

Cortisol is present in much higher levels than is aldosterone. Therefore, the enzyme 11β-HSDH exists in principal cells to inactivate cortisol before it can "contaminate" the aldosterone message (see margin note). There are three circumstances in which cortisol might have aldosterone-like actions. First, if the enzyme 11β-HSDH has a low activity or is absent on a congenital basis, principal cells will behave as if they were continuously exposed to aldosterone because of the high intracellular levels of cortisol (Figure 10.11). This condition is called the "apparent mineralocorticoid excess syndrome." Second, at excessively high levels of cortisol (as may occur with ACTH-producing tumors), this hormone may "overwhelm" the activity of 11β-HSDH and activate the aldosterone receptor because not all of the intracellular cortisol has been destroyed. Third, 11β-HSDH may be inhibited, as occurs when licorice is consumed, when chewing tobacco is swallowed, or when the drug carbenoxolone is ingested.

Note
A receptor has a much higher affinity for a ligand than does an enzyme. Therefore, 11β-HSDH must act before cortisol enters the cytoplasm.

Dexamethasone-Responsive Aldosteronism

A chromosomal crossover has been documented: ACTH promotes the synthesis of aldosterone and other steroids in addition to the usual glucocorticoids. Surprisingly, hypokalemia is often absent. Suppressing ACTH with dexamethasone ameliorates the hypertension and the hypokalemia, if present. It has been suggested that steroids other than aldosterone may contribute to the hypertension, which may be unduly severe.

Liddle's Syndrome

Note
See page 404 for a review flow chart on the causes of hypokalemia with excessive excretion of K^+.

In 1963, Liddle described a patient with chronic hypokalemia, excessive excretion of K^+, metabolic alkalosis, and a severe degree of hypertension associated with hyporeninemia and near-absent levels of aldosterone. There were no abnormal levels of steroid hormones. The TTKG was in the range of 10, and the flow rate in the CCD was normal, as judged by the osmole excretion rate. The urine contained a small quantity of Na^+ and Cl^- when the ECF volume was contracted. Taken together with the hyporeninemia, the lesion behaved as if there were a more open probability of the ENaC in the CCD. Moreover, these abnormalities responded to blockers of the ENaC in the CCD but not to aldosterone antagonists. Of extreme interest, renal transplantation relieved all of these abnormalities. Recently, the molecular basis for this lesion has been confirmed on the ENaC (see margin note).

Molecular lesion in Liddle's syndrome
The mutations compromise the ENaC. The net result is an ENaC with a greater open probability.

Hypokalemic Periodic Paralysis

Hypokalemic periodic paralysis is a rare disorder that results in a net shift of K^+ from the ECF to the ICF. It occurs more frequently in people of Asian descent and, in many of these cases, it occurs in conjunction with hyperthyroidism. Affected individuals suffer abrupt attacks of mild to severe degrees of hypokalemia; these attacks often last 6–24 hours. The major symptoms relate to weakness, which might be severe enough in degree to cause paralysis. Some patients may develop a cardiac arrhythmia during an attack (see Chapter 9). Factors that might precipitate an acute attack are a high carbohydrate load and conditions associated with high levels of adrenergic activity.

Therapy for this disorder is largely symptomatic or empiric. Patients are advised to avoid carbohydrate-rich meals and take β-blockers if symptoms are related to sympathetic activity. Hyperthyroidism is treated in the usual fashion. If this treatment fails, patients should take 250–750 mg of acetazolamide daily. Acetazolamide acts via unknown mechanisms; its benefits are based on empiric observations.

PART B

Treatment

Because hypokalemia may have many causes, there is no universal therapy. In this section, only the replacement of the deficit of K^+ is considered. The urgency for this replacement is dictated by a number of factors (Table 10.8):

1. the presence of drugs (e.g., digitalis) or heart disease, which may increase the likelihood of a cardiac arrhythmia;

2. the possibility that K^+ will shift into cells (e.g., during recovery from diabetic ketoacidosis or with β_2-adrenergic administration);

3. the development of severe weakness in the patient, who must have maximum hyperventilation because of metabolic acidosis;

4. the severity of the deficit and the continuing K^+ losses;

5. the patient with advanced liver disease and hepatic encephalopathy.

TABLE 10.8 **Indications for Initiating K^+ Therapy During Hypokalemia**

Absolute Indications
  Digitalis therapy
  Therapy for diabetic ketoacidosis because insulin will act
  Presence of symptoms (e.g., respiratory muscle weakness causing
    hypoventilation)
  Severe hypokalemia (<2.0 mmol/L)
Strong Indications
  Myocardial disease
  Anticipated hepatic encephalopathy
  Anticipated increase in another factor that causes a shift of K^+ into the ICF
    (e.g., β_2-adrenergics)
Modest Indications
  Development of glucose intolerance
  Mild hypokalemia ([K^+] closer to 3.5 mmol/L)
  Need for better antihypertensive control

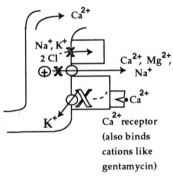

Figure 10.12   Events in the Loop of Henle. Ca^{2+} reabsorption occurs between cells in the thick ascending limb of the loop of Henle and is driven by a lumen-positive potential difference. This lumen-positive charge is generated by K^+ ion entry through the K^+ channel (ROM K^+-1). If there is no K^+ entry by this pathway, there cannot be a lumen-positive charge to drive the reabsorption of Ca^{2+}, Mg^{2+} and some Na^+. The absence of K^+ entry stops NaCl reabsorption by the Na^+, K^+ 2 Cl^- cotransporter as well.

At the bedside, it is helpful to monitor the ECG and assess the possibility of hypoventilation and the degree of weakness.

Quantity of K⁺ to Administer

Rise in [K⁺] with therapy
During chronic hypokalemia, renal mechanisms are called into play to minimize the aldosterone-induced rise in the TTKG; this effect may persist for 24–36 hours. Hence, aggressive therapy with K⁺ can lead to retention of K⁺ and an undue but transient degree of hyperkalemia.

When considering the quantity of K^+ to administer, the aim should be to get the patient out of danger quickly but to replace the entire K^+ deficit more slowly (see margin note). How quickly can K^+ be administered? The consideration here is to deliver enough K^+ to the cell membrane of the heart before a life-threatening arrhythmia occurs. This approach requires an assessment of the dose required and proper mixing of K^+ in the venous blood (administration should be through a large central vein because K^+ are very irritating to smaller veins where the concentration must be raised considerably). Therefore, the emergency replacement of K^+ is by a central vein, with the patient on a cardiac monitor.

Calculation of the Bolus of KCl to Administer

If a 70-kg adult has a very severe degree of hypokalemia (1.5 mmol/L) and an abnormal ECG, the aim will be to raise the plasma $[K^+]$ from 1.5 to 3.0 mmol/L in 1 minute. To do so, one should infuse 4.5 mmol of KCl over 1 minute into a central vein, a minimum estimate. The basis for this decision is as follows: the total blood volume (5 L) circulates each minute (cardiac output is 5 L/min). Because 60% of this blood volume is plasma (3 L), and the target for the plasma $[K^+]$ might be 3.0 mmol/L, then 1.5 mmol/L $\times$ 3 L must be given over 1 minute. The infused K^+ will mix with interstitial fluid (4 $\times$ the plasma volume) before reaching the cell membrane, so there will be a much smaller rise in $[K^+]$ next to cell membranes. Following this bolus, the rate of infusion of K^+ should be reduced to 1 mmol/min, and measurement of the plasma $[K^+]$ should be repeated in 5 minutes. If the plasma $[K^+]$ is still much less than 3.0, the above procedure can be repeated. The rate of infusion of K^+ should be much slower once the plasma $[K^+]$ approaches 3.0 mmol/L.

Replacement of the Deficit of K⁺

> • To correct severe hypokalemia, several hundred mmol of K⁺ are usually required.

It is difficult to relate accurately the degree of hypokalemia to the extent of total body K⁺ deficit. A fall in the plasma [K⁺] from 4 to 3 mmol/L is usually associated with a total body K⁺ deficit of 100–400 mmol; a much larger deficit is required to lower the plasma [K⁺] from 3 to 2 mmol/L. Nevertheless, if the patient also has a shift of K⁺ into or out of cells, the magnitude of this deficiency is not accurately reflected by these numbers (see margin note).

Clinical pearl
Although there are rough guidelines for relating the deficit of K⁺ to the degree of hypokalemia, these are very unreliable in an individual patient. The "clinical trial" in a patient is critical and requires frequent reassessment.

Methods of K⁺ Administration

Route of K⁺ Administration

The safest route to give K⁺ is by mouth. The conditions demanding intravenous therapy are GI problems that limit intake or absorption of K⁺, a severe degree of hypokalemia with either respiratory muscle weakness or cardiac arrhythmias (especially if digitalis is present), and an anticipated shift of K⁺ into the ICF (recovery from diabetic ketoacidosis).

Clinical pearl
Check for bowel sounds before giving a large amount of K⁺ by the oral route.

Rate of Administration

The rate of K⁺ infusion should not exceed 40–60 mmol/h in most circumstances. The [K⁺] in intravenous solution should be less than 60 mmol/L for use in peripheral veins because a higher [K⁺] leads to local discomfort, venous spasm, or sclerosis. In general, do not administer K⁺ in glucose-containing solutions because the glucose (via insulin) can lead to an initial lowering of the plasma [K⁺]. As discussed, when there is an acute medical emergency (cardiac arrhythmia; extreme weakness, especially if it involves respiratory muscles), K⁺ will have to be given more rapidly intravenously via a central vein. This situation requires extreme caution, cardiac monitoring, and frequent determination of the [K⁺] in plasma.

Preparation of K⁺

The anions accompanying K⁺ are in three major classes. The choice depends on the clinical situation.

KCl

> • The most common K⁺ preparation used is KCl.

In virtually all cases in which hypokalemia is associated with ECF volume contraction, Cl⁻ are essential to correct the K⁺ deficit. Diuretics and vomiting (the two most common clinical causes of K⁺ deficiency) are associated with a Cl⁻ deficit and ECF volume deficit. Because Cl⁻ permit Na⁺ to be reabsorbed, the ECF volume can be restored.

KCl can be obtained as a liquid or in solid form. Enteric-coated KCl can lead to the development of small intestinal ulcerations that are due to local irritation by hypertonic KCl. Because the liquid form of KCl is relatively unpalatable, KCl in a wax matrix or coated microspheres may be preferable.

KHCO$_3$

> • Give KHCO$_3$ only if the patient needs the HCO$_3^-$ load.

Ingesting K$^+$ salts of organic acids (acetate, citrate, gluconate, etc.) is equivalent to ingesting KHCO$_3$ because HCO$_3^-$ are produced when these organic anions are metabolized. Administer these salts when the patient has lost KHCO$_3$ (e.g., in diarrhea). Obviously, administration of KHCO$_3$ is a poor choice for K$^+$ replacement if the patient has a high plasma [HCO$_3^-$] (metabolic alkalosis) or if the patient is unlikely to metabolize the accompanying anion (hypoxia, etc.). Moreover, bicarbonaturia may promote the renal excretion of K$^+$.

K$^+$ Phosphate

> • Give phosphate (<6 mmol/h) to ensure that K$^+$ will stay in the ICF during anabolism.

Note
Close to half of the deficit of K$^+$ in patients with DKA is the loss of K$^+$ with phosphate. Do not try to replace this rapidly.

If the K$^+$ deficit is due to or associated with a loss of intracellular anions (phosphate), the K$^+$ deficit will be corrected only when phosphate is administered. Clinically, the need for K$^+$ phosphate is most evident in anabolism during total parenteral nutrition (TPN) or in the recovery from diabetic ketoacidosis. Nevertheless, clinicians may satisfy this need indirectly by giving KCl while relying on the patient to eat the phosphate (plus Mg^{2+}, etc.) required for ICF replacement. Recall that a large phosphate load has the danger of inducing hypocalcemia and metastatic calcification.

Dietary K$^+$

The best way to replace K$^+$ deficits or to keep up with ongoing losses is to use the oral route. The diet should contain the phosphate, Cl$^-$, Mg^{2+}, and HCO$_3^-$ needed. Foods rich in K$^+$ are fresh fruits, juices, and meats (see Table 10.2). However, a disadvantage may be that these foods contain a significant number of calories—a problem for obese patients.

Controversy Concerning Hypokalemia and K$^+$ Therapy

The clinician must decide whether a hypokalemic patient needs to receive K$^+$ supplements. Apart from the replacement of existing deficits (to avoid more serious degrees of K$^+$ depletion), the basis of K$^+$ therapy is to prevent serious cardiac arrhythmias. On the opposite side of the argument, there is a significant cost: the real danger of hyperkalemia when patients are taking certain drugs (K^+-sparing diuretics, β-blockers, ACE inhibitors), when an ileus is intermittent, or when renal function is poor. There is lack of proof that treating modest hypokalemia (3.0–3.5 mmol/L) really does diminish the cardiac arrhythmias and improve the patient's well-being. If the patient is taking a digitalis preparation, however, KCl treatment should be given. Furthermore, in other acute clinical situations in which there are factors that will cause a shift of K^+ into cells (treatment of severe metabolic acidosis), K^+ therapy for hypokalemia is mandatory. Therefore, at present, prudent patient selection should avoid most of the dangers of KCl therapy.

QUESTION

(Discussion on page 446)

10.14 *What is the time course and the expected degree of hypoka-lemia with diuretic therapy? At the usual doses, is the hypo-kalemia particularly severe with one class of diuretics?*

PART C

Review

DISCUSSION OF INTRODUCTORY CASE
Toby Is Losing More Than Weight
(Case presented on page 404)

What is her total body K^+ deficit?

Without a major shift of K^+ into the ICF, a 1 mmol/L fall in the $[K^+]$ would imply that the deficit of K^+ is 100–400 mmol. In patients with high levels of catecholamines, a shift of K^+ into cells can occur without a deficit of K^+. Therefore, it is not possible to be sure of her actual deficit of K^+ at present; it may be as large as 400 mmol, but its magnitude will become clear during therapy.

Was a shift of K^+ into cells a major cause of hypokalemia?

A shift of K^+ into cells rarely causes a large change in the plasma $[K^+]$. Metabolic acidosis will not cause a fall in the $[K^+]$ in the ECF. Of the hormones, insulin is not likely to be important because the blood sugar is normal; $β_2$-adrenergic activity secondary to hypoten-sion could have caused some K^+ to shift into cells, but it is difficult to be quantitative here.

What factors could have contributed to a renal loss of K^+?

Aldosterone, bicarbonaturia, and a high rate of urine flow cause high rates of K^+ loss in the urine. ECF volume contraction should lead to aldosterone release and contribute to the high [K$^+$] in the random urine sample. Bicarbonaturia is not present, but it might have been present earlier in her history if she had induced vomiting to lose weight.

What tests might be helpful in this regard?

To establish the basis for renal K$^+$ loss, measure the urine flow rate, osmole excretion rate, and [K$^+$]. Because the TTKG is high, it seems that aldosterone is acting. The low plasma [HCO$_3^-$] in conjunction with a high urine [Cl$^-$] and a negative urine net charge (metabolic acidosis with increased renal NH$_4^+$ excretion) makes laxative abuse more likely. Alternatively, vomiting of fluid rich in intestinal secretion with or without the presence of achlorhydria could produce these results (see margin note). At this point, it will be necessary to have a chat with Toby to see if she needs more serious counseling regarding a self-induced metabolic disorder (long-term K$^+$ depletion can lead to progressive renal interstitial disease).

Note

The blood pH may be different in young children who vomit if pyloric stenosis is present. If present, metabolic alkalosis is found (loss of HCl); metabolic acidosis is common (loss of NaHCO$_3$) with a patent pylorus.

Cases for Review

CASE 10.2
Diuretics in the Elderly
(Case discussed on page 434)

Emily is 73 years old; her usual lifestyle involves entertaining visitors in her home. She enjoys toast with jam along with her traditional cup of tea (a large cup). Visitors come because she is such a great conversationalist.

On her annual checkup, her physician noted that her blood pressure was high (170/95 mm Hg), so the physician prescribed a thiazide diuretic. Emily has not felt as well since she began taking this medication. She becomes lightheaded when she stands up, she feels weak, and she is less able to perform at her high intellectual level.

On physical examination, her blood pressure is now 150/90 mm Hg, and she now has a postural fall in blood pressure of 15 mm Hg. No other abnormalities are observed.

The results of blood and urine tests follow. Her urine volume is 0.5 L/day.

		Plasma	**Urine**
Na$^+$	mmol/L	107	3
K$^+$	mmol/L	1.9	12
Cl$^-$	mmol/L	67	7
HCO$_3^-$	mmol/L	30	0
pH		7.47	5.1
Urea	mmol/L (mg/dL)	1.5 (4.2)	-
Glucose	mmol/L (mg/dL)	6.0 (108)	0
Osmolality	mOsm/kg H$_2$O	220	405

Compare her results with those of her son, Jerry, Case 7.5.

What is the basis of the hyponatremia?

What is her anticipated K^+ deficit (her weight is 50 kg)?

What is her Na^+ balance?

What is her total body water balance?

What dangers should be anticipated during acute therapy?

What therapy should be recommended initially?

CASE 10.3
I Told You I Do Not Vomit
(Case discussed on page 436)

Alicia has always been concerned about her body image but claims that she is more realistic now. She has vomited in the past but vigorously denies vomiting recently. She says food intake is now normal. She has no specific complaints.

When Alicia appeared for her routine physical examination, she was hypokalemic (2.7 mmol/L). On more detailed investigation, she denied vomiting and the use of diuretics or laxatives. Her blood pressure was on the low side (90/55 mm Hg), and she had clinical signs suggesting that her ECF volume was indeed contracted (low jugular venous pressure (JVP), low blood pressure).

Laboratory values follow.

		Plasma	**Urine**
Na^+	mmol/L	138	36
K^+	mmol/L	2.7	61
Cl^-	mmol/L	99	57
HCO_3^-	mmol/L	28	0
Mg^{2+}	mmol/L (mg/dL)	0.5 (1.2)	4
Creatinine	μmol/L (mg/dL)	88 (1.0)	-
Osmolality	mOsm/kg H_2O	287	563

Do these urine values suggest that Alicia is a surreptitious vomiter or diuretic abuser?

In what way might the hypomagnesemia help with the diagnosis?

Why is her excretion of K^+ not low?

What is the final diagnosis?

CASE 10.4
Hypokalemia in a Patient with Malignancy
(Case discussed on page 437)

Alfie, age 57 years, has cancer of the lung with hepatic metastases. He has not been doing well and was admitted to the hospital. He is not taking any medications. The physical examination was not very helpful. The only new recent finding was an expanded ECF volume.

Laboratory investigation on admission revealed the following results.

		Plasma	Urine
Na$^+$	mmol/L	141	38
K$^+$	mmol/L	1.9	22
Cl$^-$	mmol/L	96	27
HCO$_3^-$	mmol/L	31	0
pH		7.43	6.0
Creatinine	μmol/L (mg/dL)	89 (1.0)	Not done
Urea	mmol/L (mg/dL)	5.9 (16)	Not done
Magnesium	mmol/L	0.7	Not done
Osmolality		288	306

Was the rate of excretion of K$^+$ high and, if so, what is the most likely reason for excessive excretion of K$^+$?

What could be responsible for the lesion?

What should be done for therapy? Focus on the hypokalemia.

CASE 10.5
Amy Developed Hypokalemia in the Hospital
(Case discussed on page 438)

Amy has a long medical history. When she was young, she was very concerned about her body image and was desperate to lose weight. She admitted to alternating bouts of starvation and binge eating, self-induced vomiting, and the use of a thiazide diuretic. On many of her past admissions, she was hypokalemic ([K$^+$] 2.5–3.0 mmol/L) and had a contracted ECF volume and metabolic alkalosis (HCO$_3^-$ 35–38 mmol/L). She denies these practices now.

Her current admission was for a urinary tract infection. This was treated with the antibiotics ampicillin and gentamicin. This infection is responding well to therapy. In routine blood work, hypokalemia and metabolic alkalosis are present, similar to past admissions, although her plasma [K$^+$] was normal on this admission. Physical examination now reveals a modest degree of ECF volume contraction.

		Plasma			Urine
		Past	Admission	Now	
Na$^+$	mmol/L	136	140	136	52
K$^+$	mmol/L	2.9	3.8	2.9	45
Cl$^-$	mmol/L	89	103	89	63
HCO$_3^-$	mmol/L	36	25	36	<5
pH		7.48	7.40	7.48	6.1
Mg^{2+}	mmol/L	0.7	0.7	0.4	3.1
Mg^{2+}	mg/dL	1.7	1.7	1.0	(high)
Ca^{2+}	mmol/L	2.4	2.4	2.4	(high)
Creatinine	μmol/L	70	60	108	5.0
Creatinine	mg/dL	0.8	0.7	1.2	—
Urea	mmol/L	3.1	3.0	7	200
BUN	mg/dL	9	8	20	—
Osmolality	mOsm/kg H$_2$O	—	—	—	402

Is the excretion of K$^+$ excessive in Amy?

How likely is vomiting to be the best explanation of her results?

How would you rule out diuretics as a major cause of her hypokalemia?

Which nephron segment is not functioning properly, and could this malfunction lead to her hypokalemia?

What role might drugs have played in her hypokalemia?

CASE 10.6
Is This Bartter's Syndrome?
(Case discussed on page 439)

A 50-year-old paraplegic male has a neurogenic bladder, the result of a motor-vehicle accident. He developed a urinary tract infection and was treated with intravenous saline and an aminoglycoside antibiotic, gentamicin (80 mg three times a day), for the past 2 weeks. There were no special findings on physical examination other than the obvious; his ECF volume was not low (plasma renin level was low).

Laboratory results were striking (see the following table); his plasma [K$^+$] decreased from 3.8 mmol to 1.6 mmol during the course of 2 weeks; moreover, hypokalemia did not improve much despite treatment with 200 mmol KCl/day; the highest plasma [K$^+$] with K$^+$ supplements was 2.1 mmol. Urine output ranged 2–5 L/day.

With long-term follow-up, the urinary tract infection resolved, and all the electrolyte abnormalities disappeared with 6 weeks of discontinuing the aminoglycoside.

		Plasma (Admission)	Plasma (Day 14)	Urine (Random) (Day 14)
Na$^+$	mmol/L	140	140	49
K$^+$	mmol/L	3.8	1.6	36
Cl$^-$	mmol/L	105	91	82
HCO$_3^-$	mmol/L	26	38	0
pH		7.40	7.48	5.5
Creatinine	μmol/L (mg/dL)	60 (0.7)	52 (0.6)	—
Urea (BUN)	mmol/L (mg/dL)	4.0 (11)	3.6 (10)	—
Mg^{2+}	mmol/L (mg/dL)	0.9 (2.2)	0.9 (2.2)	—
Volume	L/day	—	—	3

What is the major basis for his hypokalemia?

What role might the aminoglycoside have in causing his hypokalemia?

Discussion of Cases

DISCUSSION OF CASE 10.1
Kay Has His Ups and Downs
(Case presented on page 410)

If there was no excretion of K$^+$ between 3.0 and 3.5 hours, how many millimoles of K$^+$ entered Kay's cells?

The fall in plasma [K$^+$] was 1.6 mmol/L. If his ECF volume was 15 L, then only 24 mmol of K$^+$ entered cells. Notice how small this amount is relative to the ICF K$^+$ content of greater than 4000 mmol. Nevertheless, this tiny fall in K$^+$ content in his ECF could cause the

Calculation

1.6 mmol/L $\times$ 15 L = 24 mmol

cardiac arrhythmia because it was associated with a large change in the RMP.

What was the most likely reason for his acute fall in plasma [K⁺] between 3.0 and 3.5 hours?

Because there was a small urine volume, there was little K⁺ excreted so K⁺ shifted into his cells. To shift K⁺ into cells, a larger intracellular negative voltage is needed. In essence, this means pumping intracellular Na⁺, or Na⁺ that entered cells electroneutrally, out of cells by the Na⁺K⁺ATPase. In this case, because there was no reason for insulin release, but there was a very high adrenergic response to his head injury plus the adrenergic agents administered to defend his hemodynamics, the β₂-adrenergic stimuli are the most likely causes for the shift of K⁺ into his cells.

What is the largest amount of K⁺ a clinician might have to infuse into Kay?

The largest amount of K⁺ that could shift into his cells independent of a change in plasma [HCO₃⁻] is equal to the ICF Na⁺ content. With 30 L of ICF and a [Na⁺] of 15 mmol/L, 450 mmol of K⁺ is the maximum amount to bring the plasma [K⁺] back to normal. In fact, this patient required just over 600 mmol of K⁺ to raise his plasma [K⁺] to 2.5 mmol/L.

There is a future danger, however. This K⁺ will come out of cells, and the clinician must be prepared to deal with the hyperkalemia that will ensue. Notice that this indeed occurred abruptly 15–16 hours after arrival in the hospital.

> **Note**
>
> If the plasma [HCO₃⁻] has not changed, it is reasonable to assume that few H⁺ exited the ICF in association with K⁺ entry.
>
> **Calculation**
>
> 15 mmol/L × 30 L = 450 mmol

By what route and how much K⁺ should the clinician infuse into Kay in the first minute of therapy?

The first step is to select a desired plasma [K⁺] to minimize the risk of an arrhythmia; 3–4 mmol/L will do. For easy arithmetic, raise the plasma [K⁺] by 2 mmol/L, but do this only in plasma for a margin of safety. With a blood volume of 5 L, the [K⁺] in each of the 3 L of plasma should be raised by 2 mmol/L. Therefore, give 6 mmol of K⁺ over 1 minute (cardiac output 5 L/min).

The options of giving 6 mmol of K⁺ are by 100 mL of a 60 mmol/L solution or 40 mL of a 150 mmol/L K⁺ solution, or by 10 mL of a 600 mmol/L solution in 1 minute. Notice the advantage of giving hypertonic K⁺ solution (even a smaller volume to infuse).

DISCUSSION OF CASE 10.2
Diuretics in the Elderly
(Case presented on page 430)

What is the basis of the hyponatremia?

Emily has three components contributing to her hyponatremia.
1. **Water intake:** Emily always drank a relatively large volume by habit (her cup of tea). Now she may drink even more because of thirst secondary to her ECF volume contraction.
2. **Less water excretion:** There are two factors to consider in this regard. First, she has a higher urine osmolality than

expected because of ADH actions. ADH was released as a result of low ECF volume. Second, she has a low osmole excretion rate, largely because of her low-protein diet. Her urine osmolality is 405 mOsm/kg H_2O, and she is excreting only 200 mOsm, so she can excrete only 0.5 L of water in urine. In contrast, if she excreted the usual 800 mOsm, she could excrete close to 2 L of water per day. Her diet, which is low in protein ("tea and toast"), provides little urea for excretion (note the low concentration of urea in plasma). This low urea excretion limits her ability to excrete water by limiting the delivery of fluid to the terminal CCD when ADH acts.

3. **Loss of Na^+:** As a result of the actions of the diuretic, she lost Na^+ from her ECF; this loss decreased the Na^+:H_2O ratio in plasma. She then shifted Na^+ from her ECF to her ICF as K^+ exited the ICF. The loss of Na^+ could result in ADH release if the ECF volume were appreciably low.

What is her anticipated K^+ deficit (her weight is 50 kg)?

This deficit is difficult to assess. Without a major reason for a sudden shift of K^+ into cells, the K^+ deficit could easily be 200–400 mmol, perhaps even more. She is unlikely to lose a vast quantity of intracellular anions (largely phosphate esters such as DNA, RNA, phospholipids, adenosine triphosphate, creatine phosphate) in the absence of a major catabolic disease. For K^+ to leave the ICF and electroneutrality to be maintained, a large number of cations must enter cells. Because the degree of metabolic alkalosis is mild, she probably has a very large gain of Na^+ in her ICF (see margin note).

What is her Na^+ balance?

If her ECF volume is nearly normal (on physical examination) and is normally 10 L, she should have lost close to 330 mmol of Na^+ from her ECF (see margin note). Now, if her ICF gained 200–400 mmol of Na^+ during the K^+ deficit, she could be virtually in Na^+ balance but have a large maldistribution of Na^+—more in the ICF and less in the ECF.

What is her total body water balance?

Her ECF volume is near normal, but the plasma $[Na^+]$ indicates an expanded ICF volume. If the formula in the margin note is used to calculate her ICF volume, you find that her ICF volume should be expanded by close to 6 L.

What dangers should be anticipated during acute therapy?

The major dangers to anticipate are cardiac arrhythmias (from the hypokalemia) and excessively rapid water diuresis once ADH levels are suppressed (via reexpansion of her ECF volume); the latter could lead to a rapid loss of water in the urine and subsequently to osmotic demyelination with a rapid rise in the $[Na^+]$. Reexpansion of the ECF volume will come about equally well if NaCl is given or if KCl is given (K^+ enter cells and Na^+ exit; see Figure 10.1). Emily is elderly, and her heart may not tolerate rapid expansion of her ECF volume. Therefore, a final risk is the development of

Note
To have a higher $[Na^+]$ in the ICF, the $Na^+K^+ATPase$ activity must be low or, more likely, this enzyme must have a higher K_m for Na^+ in the ICF.

Calculation of Na^+ in the ECF
- Fall in $[Na^+]$ is 33 mmol/L (140 − 107 mmol/L).
- Original and current volume of ECF is 10 L.
- Fall in content of Na^+ = 33 mmol/L × 10 L = 330 mmol.

Calculation
- Assume the content of osmoles in the ICF does not change.
- 2 $[Na^+]$ × normal ICF volume of 20 L = number of milliosmoles normally in the ICF.
- 2 [140] × 20 L = 2 [107] × new ICF volume.
- New ICF volume = 26 L.

congestive heart failure (CHF) subsequent to KCl therapy, which will probably be equivalent to NaCl administration as far as the ECF is concerned. To prevent this, a loop diuretic may be needed.

What therapy should be recommended initially?

If you keep in mind the preceding balance data, the dangers to anticipate, and the fact that Emily is not symptomatic from her hyponatremia, you may decide that she is not likely to need Na^+ now. Therefore, the initial recommendation should be the slow, oral replacement of her K^+ deficit with KCl. The dose of KCl to choose depends on the desired rate of correction of her hyponatremia. Because the initial aims are to replace the K^+ deficit and to raise the $[Na^+]$ in plasma by only 0.3 mmol/L/h, 0.3 mmol of KCl should be given per liter of total body water for each of the first several hours. Emily has close to 35 L of total body water, so 10–12 mmol of KCl should be given per hour as a starting therapy. Look for a positive balance of K^+; urine losses should be monitored. In total, her plasma $[Na^+]$ should rise by 8 mmol/L in a 24-hour period, and her plasma $[K^+]$ should not be permitted to rise above 3.5 mmol/L on the first day. Her ECG should be monitored closely (for arrhythmias), as should her plasma $[K^+]$ (for hyperkalemia), her urine volume (for rapid water diuresis), and her plasma $[Na^+]$ (to see the expected rise in her $[Na^+]$). ADH should be given if her urine volume increases suddenly; such an increase could lead to too rapid a loss in water and ultimately to too rapid a rise in her plasma $[Na^+]$.

Watch for the early signs of CHF (increasing JVP, crackles in the chest), and be prepared to use a diuretic. If the urine $[Na^+]$ is lower than her plasma $[Na^+]$, and she has a substantial diuresis, be careful of the rate at which the plasma $[Na^+]$ rises.

DISCUSSION OF CASE 10.3
I Told You I Do Not Vomit
(Case presented on page 431)

Do these urine values suggest that Alicia is a surreptitious vomiter or diuretic abuser?

Vomiting. These values do not suggest vomiting. The hallmark for a diagnosis of vomiting is near-absent excretions of Cl^- in the urine.

Diuretics. With a recent intake of diuretics, the urine $[Na^+]$ and $[Cl^-]$ may be high. Because the concentrations of Na^+ and Cl^- were both high in a patient with a low ECF volume, these values in the urine are typical for diuretic abuse. Diuretic abuse was the initial clinical diagnosis, but two facts made this diagnosis unlikely. First, every random urine sample contained a high $[Na^+]$ and $[Cl^-]$. Second, urine assays for diuretics were consistently negative. Therefore, a renal salt-wasting syndrome is present, and the nephron site responsible for the salt-wasting is not the CCD because of the very high TTKG (>10).

In what way might the hypomagnesemia help with the diagnosis?

The principal nephron site that regulates the renal excretion of Mg^{2+} is the thick ascending limb of the loop of Henle. Because this patient has hypomagnesemia, renal excretion of Mg^{2+}, a low ECF volume, and renal excretion of Na^+ plus Cl^-, the thick ascending limb of the loop of Henle seems to be involved. The high TTKG is also consistent with this interpretation. Hypomagnesemia is associated with use of loop diuretics, GI disease, chemotherapy, and Bartter's syndrome.

Why is her excretion of K^+ not low?

During hypokalemia, the excretion of K^+ should be low. Alicia has a high rate of excretion of K^+ because the $[K^+]$ in the urine is too high (TTKG is close to 11); it does not appear that her osmole excretion rate is excessive, but more data will be needed (urine flow rate and osmolality) to confirm this suspicion.

The cause of the high TTKG should be sought. Perhaps it is due to the presence of a high level of aldosterone. This hormone could be released as a result of ECF volume contraction. She has a high delivery of Na^+ with Cl^- to the CCD, and perhaps this increased delivery contributes to her unexpectedly high rate of excretion of K^+ and the high $[K^+]$ in the urine. She behaves as if the luminal membrane of the CCD has a relatively slower reabsorption of Cl^-.

Note
See page 404, which has a flow chart on the causes of hypokalemia with excessive excretion of K^+.

What is the final diagnosis?

The authors believe that she has Bartter's syndrome.

DISCUSSION OF CASE 10.4
Hypokalemia in a Patient with Malignancy
(Case presented on page 431)

Was the rate of excretion of K^+ high and, if so, what is the most likely reason for excessive excretion of K^+?

Rate of Excretion of K^+. The helpful data provided are the urine $[K^+]$ (22 mmol/L) and the urine osmolality (306 mOsm/kg H_2O). Because normal adults excrete 600–900 mOsm/day at a relatively consistent rate (see margin note), and the random urine osmolality is 306 mOsm/kg H_2O, one could extrapolate (at some risk) that his 24-hour K^+ excretion is two to three times 22 mmol, or close to 50 mmol/day. Hence, the rate of excretion of K^+ is much greater than 15 mmol/day, so it is excessive for a patient with hypokalemia.

Note
Patients who eat little protein and salt will have a much lower rate of excretion of osmoles.

Reasons for a High Excretion of K^+. A high excretion of K^+ is due to a high volume and/or a high $[K^+]$ in the CCD. The former cannot be assessed (the authors do not know the osmole excretion rate), so we can only comment on the latter. The TTKG is very high, close to 10. A high TTKG implies electrogenic reabsorption of Na^+ in the CCD. Two possibilities are an increased conductance for Na^+ or a decreased Cl^- reabsorptive rate (see Figure 10.6 and the flow chart on page 404). Given the expanded ECF volume and

TTKG in subjects with a deficit of K⁺ and hyperaldosteronism
The TTKG falls to close to 6 in these subjects and does not rise with exogenous mineralocorticoids unless the K⁺ deficit is repaired or bicarbonaturia is induced.

the high TTKG, the results favor a higher conductance for Na^+. This view would be reinforced if the patient could elaborate a Na^+-poor and Cl^--poor urine with a contracted ECF volume (he was able to do so).

What could be responsible for the lesion?

High levels of aldosterone could be a possibility, but the $[K^+]$ in plasma is too low for the diagnosis of primary hyperaldosteronism alone. Nevertheless, aldosterone levels in plasma should be measured. When measured, the level of this hormone was not elevated; hence, another explanation should be sought. The authors' hypothesis is illustrated in Figure 10.4. We speculate that high levels of cortisol have resulted from ACTH production by the tumor. This cortisol could be "acting like aldosterone" in the principal cells of the patient's CCD because the 11β-HSDH activity is not high enough to deal with such a high load of cortisol. Both ACTH and cortisol were measured and found to be extremely high on several occasions during the day. An ACTH-producing tumor (along with little intake of K^+) is our best guess for the principal cause of hypokalemia.

What should be done for therapy? Focus on the hypokalemia.

The patient's dietary NaCl should be restricted, and he needs KCl supplements. Perhaps amiloride will be needed if these measures do not cause his plasma $[K^+]$ to rise to 3.0 mmol/L.

Monitor the plasma $[K^+]$ carefully when using the combination of amiloride and KCl therapy because of the patient's risk of developing hyperkalemia later when the GI tract absorbs the K^+.

DISCUSSION OF CASE 10.5
Amy Developed Hypokalemia in the Hospital
(Case presented on page 432)

Is the excretion of K⁺ excessive in Amy?

Yes. Do not compare urine values with those in normal patients (same as in Amy). Rather, compare these values with the ones expected for a person with a deficit of K^+ (<10–15 mmol/day). Because she has urine creatinine of 5 mmol/L, her 24-hour urine volume exceeds 1 L, and her K^+ excretion rate likely exceeds 45 mmol/day.

How likely is vomiting to be the best explanation of her results?

Key to this decision is the urine $[Cl^-]$; it should be virtually 0 in vomiting; the authors would not like this diagnosis as the sole one. She could have vomited and taken a thiazide diuretic; given the past history, the authors cannot absolutely rule out vomiting at present.

How would you rule out diuretics as a major cause of her hypokalemia?

There are two steps—frequent and unannounced random urines

analyzed for Na^+ and Cl^-. A sample devoid of both of these electrolytes would make the authors very suspicious of diuretic abuse. If you are still not sure, measure diuretic levels in urines containing $Na^+ + Cl^-$. The test result for diuretics was negative.

Which nephron segment is not functioning properly, and could this malfunction lead to her hypokalemia?

The key findings we have to explain are hypokalemia, renal wasting of Na^+ and Cl^-, renal Mg^{2+}-wasting, a high normal urine Ca^{2+}, and a urine osmolality lower than expected (check this again after ADH was given—it remained close to 400 mOsm/kg H_2O). All this adds up to a lesion in the thick ascending limb of the loop of Henle (see Figure 10.12, page 426).

What role might drugs have played in her hypokalemia?

We are looking for a drug that has a loop diuretic–like action, but not a loop diuretic (assay negative). The authors strongly suspect gentamicin.

DISCUSSION OF CASE 10.6
Is This Bartter's Syndrome?
(Case presented on page 433)

What is the major basis for hypokalemia?

Our approach to the patient with chronic hypokalemia is that there is a very low K^+ intake and/or excessive loss of K^+ from the ECF (almost always a renal problem). Given the high intake of KCl and persistent hypokalemia, low K^+ intake is not the problem. The presence of metabolic alkalosis could contribute to a shift of K^+ from the ECF to the ICF, but the degree of hypokalemia is too large for this as a sole diagnosis in view of the especially high rate of excretion of K^+.

Whereas a normal person who has a low K^+ input excretes as little as 10–15 mmol of K^+ per day, this patient has excessive K^+ excretion (K^+ excretion close to 100 mmol/day).

The next step is to decide to what extent K^+ excretion is driven by a high flow rate and/or a high urine $[K^+]$ (see margin note). Given that the osmole excretion rate is not excessive, the flow rate in the CCD is not large and the major reason for the excessive renal K^+ excretion is a high urine $[K^+]$. A possible reason for the high urine $[K^+]$ is considered in the discussion of the next question.

Note
K^+ excretion
$= $ Flow rate $\times$ Urine $[K^+]$
$= 3$ L $\times$ 36 mmol/L

What role might the aminoglycoside have in causing his hypokalemia?

The subtype of hypokalemia with excessive K^+ excretion accompanied by hypercalciuria, hypomagnesemia, and a renal concentrating defect is called Bartter's syndrome. There are three genetic defects identified in these patients, and two are in the luminal membrane of the thick ascending limb of the loop of Henle—one is a defect in the Na^+, K^+, 2 Cl^- cotransporter and the other is in the ROM-K^+ channel (see Figure 10.9). A third genetic defect is in the Cl^- channel in the basolateral membrane. In effect, all look like a loop

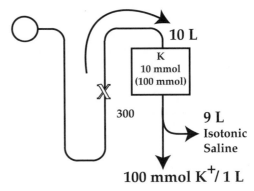

Figure 10.13   High urine [K⁺] due to the reabsorption of NaCl in the MCD. The white "X" represents a lesion in the thick ascending limb of the loop of Henle; the net result is a large (10 L/day) delivery of isotonic saline to the CCD (the rectangle in the nephron). Each liter contains 10 mmol K⁺, so the total delivery of K⁺ is 100 mmoles. When 9 L of isotonic saline is reabsorbed in the MCD, the 100 mmol of K⁺ is excreted in 1 L. This is not recognized by the TTKG.

diuretic acting 24 hours a day. Gentamicin, a cation in plasma, binds to the basolateral membrane of the thick ascending limb to its ionized Ca^{2+} receptor. Acting via a G-protein signal system, the net effect is to block the entry of K^+ and positive charges into the lumen (see Figure 10.12). The small supply of K^+ in the lumen of the thick ascending limb of the loop of Henle limits NaCl reabsorption by the Na^+, K^+, 2 Cl^- cotransporter. The lack of positive charge in the lumen retards the reabsorption of Na^+, Ca^{2+}, and Mg^{2+} ions through the intercellular space.

Overall. So much NaCl is delivered to the CCD that volume delivery is exceedingly high. Even if the luminal $[K^+]$ is only 10 mmol/L here, the reabsorption of the bulk of NaCl but not K^+ in the MCD leads to the excretion of urine with both a high K^+ content and concentration (Figure 10.13). There are also negative balances for Na^+, Cl^-, Ca^{2+}, and Mg^{2+}.

Summary of Main Points

- Potassium is primarily an intracellular cation, and its concentration in the ICF relative to the ECF is the major reflector of the RMP. As hypokalemia develops, the RMP becomes more electronegative (hyperpolarized) (i.e., the ratio of K^+ in the ICF to K^+ in the ECF increases). The magnitude of a K^+ deficit is difficult to determine from the plasma $[K^+]$.
- Renal K^+ excretion has two components: the $[K^+]$ in CCD fluid and the flow rate through the CCD. The former is determined primarily by the open probability of the ENaC (mineralocorticoid action or Liddle's syndrome) and bicarbonaturia, the latter by osmole delivery to the CCD.
- The most prevalent cause of hypokalemia is renal K^+ loss, the most likely basis being diuretic use and vomiting.

• In some circumstances, replacement of large K^+ deficits constitutes an emergency. Cardiac arrhythmias may occur (more likely in patients receiving a digitalis preparation); hypoventilation may result from hypokalemic muscle weakness; and some patients may have a shift of K^+ into the ICF (e.g., recovery from diabetic ketoacidosis).

Discussion of Questions

10.1 What is the most likely cause of K^+ loss in patients A, B, C, and D? They all have hypokalemia, ECF volume contraction, and metabolic alkalosis.

		Patient			
		A	**B**	**C**	**D**
Urine electrolyte					
Na^+	mmol/L	25	25	25	0
K^+	mmol/L	60	60	60	10
Cl^-	mmol/L	0	85	0	0
HCO_3^-	mmol/L	85	0	0	0

   A. The major clue is the anion present in the urine. In this case, it is HCO_3^-. Because the patient has a high content of HCO_3^- (metabolic alkalosis) and is losing HCO_3^- in the urine, there must be an additional source of HCO_3^-. In the absence of HCO_3^- intake, loss of HCl (vomiting) is the most likely cause. The low $[Cl^-]$, which indicates a normal renal response to ECF volume contraction in the presence of Na^+ and HCO_3^- excretion, is further supportive evidence of vomiting as the basis of the findings.
   B. The major clue is the high $[Cl^-]$ in urine. Loop diuretics cause the excretion of NaCl, which leads to ECF volume contraction, and thereby aldosterone release; aldosterone leads to a high $[K^+]$ in the urine. A high urine $[Na^+]$ (and $[Cl^-]$) in view of ECF volume contraction suggests that the diuretic was acting on the kidney at the time the urine was collected. Alternatively, if no diuretics were taken, the patient could have Bartter's syndromes.
   C. The major clue is that the sum of measured cations (Na^+ and K^+) greatly exceeds that of the usual anions (Cl^- and HCO_3^-). Therefore, another anion (e.g., β-HB^-, hippurate, or a drug) is excreted initially as its Na^+ salt. This excretion leads to ECF volume contraction, aldosterone release, and loss of K^+ in the urine.
   D. There is little renal K^+ loss at present; the kidney is behaving normally by conserving Na^+ and Cl^-. If the delivery of Na^+ and volume to the lumen of the distal nephron is low, there is a small quantity of Na^+ for aldosterone to act on. Thus, the diagnostic features of urine electrolytes disappear when the provocative stimulus (vomiting/diuretics) is not a recent event. One can suspect their presence in the past if treatment with NaCl plus KCl readily returns the plasma electrolyte values to normal. Furthermore, frequent random urine electrolyte studies should be done to see if a sudden rise in the concentration of Na^+, K^+, Cl^-, and/or HCO_3^-

Note

In glue-sniffers, toluene is metabolized to hippuric acid, and the hippurate anion is excreted in the urine.

ensues. If it does, either the patient vomited ($[HCO_3^-]$ high in urine) or took diuretics ($[Cl^-]$ high in urine). In the latter case, appropriate urine studies to measure the diuretic at this time may confirm a suspicion of occult diuretic abuse.

10.2 Will a patient consuming a very high NaCl load become hypokalemic as a result of enhanced renal K⁺ excretion? With respect to K⁺ homeostasis, how does such a patient differ from one who receives a loop diuretic? Assume equal Na⁺ excretion rates.

There must be a stimulus for aldosterone release plus a high distal flow rate to get very high rates of K⁺ excretion. The patient who has a high intake of NaCl that increases distal flow rate but does not have ECF volume contraction to stimulate aldosterone release will not become hypokalemic. Thus, this patient differs from the patient who takes a diuretic that causes ECF volume contraction, aldosterone release, and an increase in the distal tubular flow rate.

10.3 A patient takes a diuretic, which causes the excretion of an extra 60 mmol of K⁺ per day. The doctor recommended that this patient consume bananas to replace the K⁺ lost each day. If all the kcal were retained as stored fat (9 kcal/ g), what would be the weight gain at the end of 1 year?

A banana (120 g) contains close to 10 mmol of K⁺; therefore, the patient will have to consume 720 g (1.6 lb) of bananas daily to supply the needed 60 mmol of K⁺. The caloric content of bananas depends on their dry weight and whether the major constituent is carbohydrate (4 kcal/g) or fat (9 kcal/g). Assuming that bananas contain 67% water and that the remaining dry weight has 4 kcal/g, the number of extra kcal ingested per day is close to 1000, the equivalent of 1/4 lb of stored fat (see margin note). Thus, the overall weight gain would be approximately 90 lb/y. This weight gain will be even greater due to the fat content of bananas, which was ignored in the calculation in the margin.

10.4 Elite athletes often have a [K⁺] in plasma that is close to 3.0 mmol/L at rest. What mechanisms might be involved?

The authors are not sure. Either there is a total body deficit of K⁺ or there is a hyperpolarized RMP that maintains more K⁺ in the ICF.

Deficit of K⁺. K⁺ can be lost in sweat or the urine.

1. **Sweat:** Although the [K⁺] in each liter of sweat is low (close to 10 mmol/L), the number of liters lost can be large (>10/ day). Hence, nonrenal loss of K⁺ can be significant. If this loss were the only effect, the urinary excretion of K⁺ would be less than 15 mmol/day, but it is higher and therefore suggests renal mechanisms as well.
2. **Renal excretion of K⁺:** A higher rate of excretion of K⁺ suggests hyperaldosteronism. Perhaps the high levels of aldosterone reflect the state induced by chronic exercise. In response to the threats to the ECF volume during exercise (sweating and shift of water into cells induced by the higher osmolality in muscle cells when muscles contract), the body retains extra Na⁺ to expand the ECF volume. This expansion

Quantities
- Daily surplus of kcal: If the wet weight is 720 g, then the dry weight (33%) = 240 g. 240 g × 4 kcal/g = close to 1000 kcal.
- Stored fat has 9 kcal/g. If 111 g of fat is stored each day (1000 kcal/9 kcal/kg), there will be a weight gain of 1/4 lb/day (1 lb = 454 g and close to 4000 kcal/lb).
- Overall: 365 days × 1/4 lb/day = 91 lb/y.

provides the "reserve" that the athlete needs to fill his or her blood volume (high stroke volume, dilated capillary beds in exercising muscle and skin).

Hence, loss of K^+ may occur by both renal and nonrenal routes.

Shift of K^+ Into Cells. Perhaps higher catecholamine levels or increased sensitivity to β_2-adrenergics can lead to a higher RMP.

10.5 If an individual is K^+-depleted and has lost 300 mmol of K^+, what is the most likely change in ionic composition of the ICF, and what adjustments were needed to permit this change?

To lose 300 mmol of K^+ from the ICF, either 300 mEq of anions must be lost (organic phosphates) or 300 mEq of cations (H^+ or Na^+) must enter cells (see Figure 10.1). Thus, in the former case, cells would have to lose RNA, DNA, ATP, creatine phosphate, or phospholipids; in the latter case, cells would have to become more acidic and/or have a higher $[Na^+]$. To maintain this higher $[Na^+]$, the $Na^+K^+ATPase$ would have to be less active (fewer pumps, inhibited pumps, and/or pumps with a higher K_m for Na^+).

10.6 The result of the lesion in hypokalemic periodic paralysis may be a higher open probability of Na^+ channels in the plasma membrane. How might this lesion cause hypokalemia? In what way is this lesion different from that in hyperkalemic periodic paralysis in which the Na^+ channels also have a more open probability?

In hypokalemic periodic paralysis, some Na^+ channels appear to be more open (mechanism unknown). Thus, there is a large flux of Na^+ into cells. Because a higher $[Na^+]$ in cells could drive the $Na^+K^+ATPase$, some of the positive charges that enter are exported. In quantitative terms, one positive charge enters per Na^+ entry but only one-third of a charge exits per Na^+ pumped via the $Na^+K^+ATPase$; this net entry of positive charges depolarizes the RMP. The fall in RMP should cause K^+ to exit and result in hyperkalemia. Given the fact that hypokalemia is present in hypokalemic periodic paralysis, a possible explanation is that the K^+ channels have a reduced open probability and, as a result, more of the K^+ that enter cells could remain in the ICF. This explanation is the authors' guess as to what might happen.

In the hyperkalemic variety, different mutant Na^+ channels have a consistent higher open probability. Thus, the RMP is also depolarized. If, in this setting, the K^+ channels maintained their high open probability, K^+ would exit from cells because of the fall in RMP and hyperkalemia would be the result.

10.7 What is the cause of hypokalemia in patients who vomit and have metabolic alkalosis?

Vomiting is an example of K^+ loss by more than one route. As outlined in Figure 4.1, the plasma $[HCO_3^-]$ rises and $[Cl^-]$ falls with each loss of gastric HCl. The consequent increase in the filtered load of HCO_3^- exceeds its renal reabsorption and leads to a small loss of Na^+ from the body. The resultant decrease in ECF volume stimulates aldosterone release. Aldosterone action, together with a large distal nephron delivery of Na^+-rich fluid that contains HCO_3^-, produces a large renal loss of K^+.

To a lesser extent, there is a shift of K^+ into the ICF (see Figure 10.3).

The loss of K^+ by the GI tract is quite small; the $[K^+]$ of gastric fluid is usually less than 15 mmol/L.

10.8 When a person starves for 3 weeks, there is a negative balance for K^+ of close to 300 mmol, but the subject is normokalemic. What changes may have occurred in cells to cause this intracellular K^+ deficit?

The loss of K^+ from the ICF could be the result of one of three major reasons.

1. There might be a shift of cations such as H^+ into cells for buffering, but this loss is trivial in ketoacidosis of starvation.

2. There might be a lower quantity of Na^+ pumped by the $Na^+K^+ATPase$ as a result of the low level of insulin.

3. A loss of intracellular anions (phosphate esters such as RNA) occurs during fasting and requires a similar loss of K^+ for electroneutrality. The $[K^+]$ in the ICF need not change because water will be lost as well. This type of K^+ loss is important during chronic fasting. An example is provided in the margin.

10.9 Should the deficit of K^+ in a starved person be replaced during the fast?

Although there is a large negative balance for K^+, much of the intracellular stores of K^+ cannot be replaced before the net synthesis of RNA and phospholipids occurs (insulin acts to stimulate anabolism) and phosphate is ingested. Accordingly, only small supplements of K^+ are advisable during a fast, and larger supplements are needed on refeeding. One can imagine that the renal response that led to the negative K^+ balance was appropriate during fasting because it prevented the development of hyperkalemia (see margin note).

10.10 Can excessive delivery of Na^+ to the CCD augment the rate of excretion of K^+?

To determine whether the delivery of Na^+ to the CCD actually limits net secretion of K^+, one needs to know the $[Na^+]$ in the luminal fluid and the $[Na^+]$ needed for the net secretion of K^+ (a $[Na^+]$ of 15 mmol/L can support half the maximal rate of K^+ transport in the CCD in rats).

$[Na^+]$ in the Luminal Fluid in the CCD. To calculate this $[Na^+]$, one first needs to know the osmolality of luminal fluid. For easy arithmetic, when ADH acts (i.e., most of the day), the osmolality of the luminal fluid is the same as that of plasma, say 300 mOsm/kg H_2O. The next step is to decide how many of these osmoles are urea, because the rest will be largely due to electrolytes. The likely concentration of urea is 100 mOsm/L (see margin note). Therefore, the concentration of electrolytes is close to 200 mOsm/L, half of which are Na^+ plus K^+. Because the $[Na^+]$ exceeds the K_m for the Na^+ needed to augment K^+ secretion by 5- to 10-fold, delivering

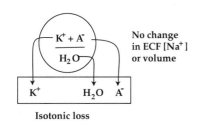

Isotonic loss

Note
A slight degree of hypokalemia helps limit further K^+ loss by decreasing distal delivery of HCO (see Figure 9.11).

more Na$^+$ per se will not drive more K$^+$ secretion unless volume delivery is increased.

10.11 How do poorly reabsorbed anions lead to an augmented excretion of K$^+$?

A poorly reabsorbed anion can augment K$^+$ secretion by two mechanisms. First, it can augment the delivery of volume to the CCD by increasing the osmolar load. This contribution is usually minor. The second way is to deliver more Na$^+$ without Cl$^-$ to the CCD (i.e., during ECF volume contraction). In experiments in humans, a load of poorly reabsorbed anions did not cause a significant kaliuresis in normovolemic subjects because the [Cl$^-$] in their urine was not less than 10–15 mmol/L.

10.12 In a patient with Bartter's syndrome, in what ways will a greater salt intake increase the rate of excretion of K$^+$?

The excretion of K$^+$ can increase if the [K$^+$] in the CCD or the flow rate in this nephron segment rises. A higher delivery of Na$^+$ and Cl$^-$ to the CCD can increase the flow rate in the CCD by raising the rate of excretion of osmoles. Moreover, the [K$^+$] in the CCD can be higher in Bartter's-like syndrome if even more Na$^+$ than Cl$^-$ were reabsorbed here (see Fig. 10.8). Hence, two factors could lead to much higher rates of excretion of K$^+$.

What are the dangers of giving a small load of NaCl to this patient?

If too small a load of NaCl is given, a smaller quantity of K$^+$ will be excreted; nevertheless, if Na$^+$ excretion continues and exceeds its input, the patient might develop a larger deficit of Na$^+$, and the ECF volume will be contracted to a greater extent.

10.13 When a patient presents with all the features characteristic of Bartter's syndrome, a clinician must rule out surreptitious use (abuse) of diuretics, vomiting, and laxative abuse. What features should a clinician rely on in each of these settings?

Diuretic Abuse. The patient probably will not admit to the abuse of diuretics. Therefore, the findings of hypokalemia, low ECF volume (high renin), and a urine with abundant quantities of Na$^+$ and Cl$^-$ provide the common database. At this point the authors would, without prior notice, ask for many random urine samples. If at least one is Cl$^-$-poor or Na$^+$-poor, we would suspect diuretic abuse; assays should be carried out in multiple urine samples. Assays for diuretics would be diagnostic in urine that contains Na$^+$ and Cl$^-$. Finally, hypomagnesemia often is very significant in the patient with Bartter's-like syndrome.

Vomiting. Again, the urine is very helpful. A urine that contains very little Cl$^-$ makes loss of HCl a very likely diagnosis. A urine that contains Na$^+$ and is alkaline should confirm the diagnosis.

Laxative Abuse. If the patient's ECF volume is contracted, the urine should have a small quantity of Na$^+$. If metabolic acidosis is

Calculation
Because 400 mmol of urea is excreted per day, and close to 4 L of GFR will reach the terminal CCD, the concentration of urea in the lumen of the CCD is 100 mmol/L. A higher value for urea occurs during antidiuresis because of urea recycling.

present, more NH_4^+ will be excreted (along with Cl^-). Therefore, in this setting, the quantity of Na^+ (not Cl^-) in urine reflects the ECF volume status. Urine with a low $[Na^+]$ and a high $[Cl^-]$ suggests that NH_4^+ are being excreted in response to acidosis (or hypokalemia). On the other hand, a urine that contains Na^+ but not Cl^- or HCO_3^- suggests that organic anions are being excreted.

As a final caution, patients with a "doctorate in deception" may utilize multiple abusive techniques simultaneously and increase the diagnostic challenge. A high degree of suspicion, an enjoyment of subterfuge, careful observation, and a combination of the preceding analyses can help one unravel these problems.

10.14 What is the time course and the expected degree of hypo-kalemia with diuretic therapy?

The plasma $[K^+]$ falls to its steady-state value within 1 week of diuretic therapy. The degree of hypokalemia is modest—only 5% of patients have values less than 3.0 mmol/L (if lower than 3.0 mmol/L, look for another cause for K^+ loss, including reasons for high aldosterone and/or urine flow rate). Elderly Caucasian women seem to be the most susceptible to developing hypokalemia, perhaps because their diets have a much lower quantity of K^+.

At the usual doses, is the hypokalemia particularly severe with one class of diuretics?

The degree of hypokalemia is not really different with the various classes of diuretics, with the possible exception of acetazolamide, which can cause a greater loss of K^+ due to the associated bicarbona-turia. This difference is, at best, however, very modest.

11

Hyperkalemia

OBJECTIVES

☐ To provide the physiologic background so that a classification of *hyperkalemia* can be developed. Although intake and shift of

K$^+$ from ICF may contribute to hyperkalemia, reduced excretion of K$^+$ in the urine is virtually always present in chronic hyperkalemia.

☐ To emphasize that the components of renal K$^+$ excretion are the [K$^+$] in the urine and the urine volume.

☐ To elucidate the factors that lead to a rise or fall in the urine [K$^+$] and the urine volume and to recognize their impact on maintaining hyperkalemia.

☐ To provide an approach to the therapy of hyperkalemia.

Outline of Major Principles

1. **General considerations**: Hyperkalemia may produce serious side effects when the plasma [K$^+$] is greater than 6 mmol/L. The correlation between the plasma [K$^+$] and untoward effects (arrhythmias) is not reliable. In general, the rate at which hyperkalemia develops is as important as its degree in determining its overall threat to the body.

2. **Etiology of hyperkalemia**: Chronic hyperkalemia implies that the rate of excretion of K$^+$ is lower than expected in almost every case. In the absence of renal failure, suspect low aldosterone bioactivity or diminished distal nephron flow. A shift of K$^+$ out of cells is a less common cause for severe hyperkalemia; it occurs with hormone deficiency, certain types of metabolic acidosis, catabolism, or a metabolic abnormality such as hyperkalemic periodic paralysis.

3. **Diagnosis of hyperkalemia**: Hyperkalemia may be suspected clinically and confirmed by measuring the plasma [K$^+$]. Urine electrolytes help in establishing the cause of chronic hyperkalemia.

4. **Treatment**: Eliminate K$^+$ intake. Antagonize the cardiac effects of K$^+$ with calcium (a very rapid effect). Shift K$^+$ into cells with insulin and possibly NaHCO$_3$ (requires 0.5–2 hours). If hypoaldosteronism or a low urine flow rate is present, promote K$^+$ loss in the urine. Induce K$^+$ loss in the GI tract with resins (a slow process). Be prepared to promote loss of K$^+$ by dialysis if hyperkalemia is severe or rapidly progressive (i.e., if there is an ongoing K$^+$ load).

Hyperkalemia
- Definition: plasma [K$^+$] > 5.0 mmol/L.
- Expected renal responses: >200 mmol of K$^+$ excreted/day, TTKG > 10.
- The main danger is a cardiac arrhythmia.
- The diagnosis is usually made by the routine determination of plasma electrolytes supported by clinical suspicions.

INTRODUCTORY CASE
Lee's [K$^+$] Is on a High
(Case discussed on page 468)

Lee is our noninsulin-dependent diabetic. Now, glycemic control is relatively poor (blood glucose is 360 mg/dL, or 20 mmol/L), and she is hyperkalemic (5.4 mmol/L). On physical examination, there is evidence of a mild degree of ECF volume contraction.

Pertinent laboratory values follow.

		Plasma	Urine (Random Sample)
Na$^+$	mmol/L	130	53
K$^+$	mmol/L	5.4	20
Cl$^-$	mmol/L	99	51
HCO$_3^-$	mmol/L	19	0
pH		7.35	5.4
Glucose	mmol/L (mg/dL)	20 (360)	302
Osmolality	mOsm/kg H$_2$O	285	600
Creatinine	mmol/L (mg/dL)	180 (2.0)	—
Urea	mmol/L (mg/dL)	10 (28)	135

What factors contributed to hyperkalemia?

What additional information is needed to understand the relative importance of each factor?

What initial therapy would be most appropriate?

Flow chart: Causes of hyperkalemia with low excretion of K$^+$

The causes of a low rate of excretion of K$^+$ are too low a flow rate in the CCD (left limb) and too low a [K$^+$] in the lumen of the CCD (right limb). Both flow rate and [K$^+$] in the CCD should be evaluated in each patient. Final considerations are shown in the shaded boxes. In renal failure, the excessive flow rate per nephron limits electrogenic reabsorption of Na$^+$ and thereby causes the kidneys to behave as if there is slow reabsorption of Na$^+$. (ECFV = extracellular fluid volume.)

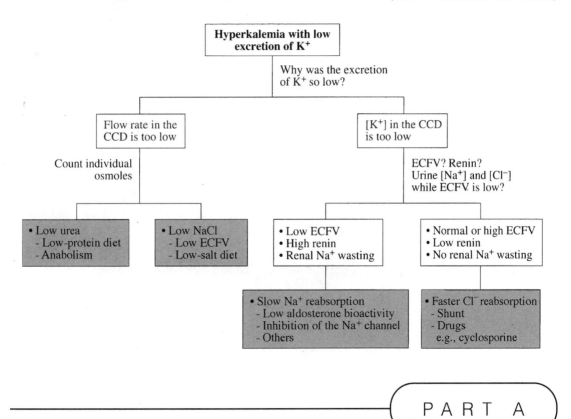

$\Big)$ PART A

Patients with Hyperkalemia

Clinical Approach

The clinical approach the authors recommend is illustrated in Figures 11.1*A* and 11.1*B* and outlined in Table 11.1. It requires answers to the following questions:

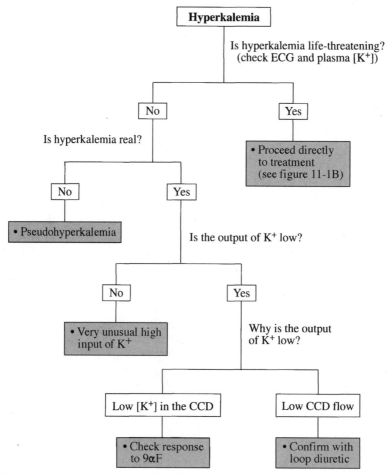

Figure 11.1A Diagnostic approach to hyperkalemia. The final diagnostic groups are shown in the shaded boxes. For details, see the text.

1. Is hyperkalemia life-threatening?

Hyperkalemia endangers patients by provoking cardiac arrhythmias. There is no specific plasma [K$^+$] at which an arrhythmia occurs. In general, hyperkalemia is better tolerated in the very young and if the hyperkalemia is chronic. The factors that suggest the possibility of an arrhythmia are changes in the ECG (see page 462), a sudden rise in the degree of hyperkalemia, the likelihood that K$^+$ will be released into the ECF (cell lysis and recovery from an ileus, especially if oral K$^+$ were given), and the presence of medications that may permit hyperkalemia to worsen (e.g., β-blockers). The absence of these factors does not mean that an arrhythmia will not occur.

If a patient is in danger from hyperkalemia, address therapy first (see Figure 11.1*B*). The steps here are to antagonize the effects of hyperkalemia, a benefit that occurs in minutes (with Ca^{2+}); to promote progressive entry of K$^+$ into cells (with insulin and possibly NaHCO$_3$), and, as more remote therapy, to promote the excretion of K$^+$. Details are provided later in this chapter.

On the other hand, if the danger of an arrhythmia is judged to be small, the authors recommend limiting K$^+$ intake and proceeding toward a diagnosis, as shown on the left side of Figure 11.1*A*.

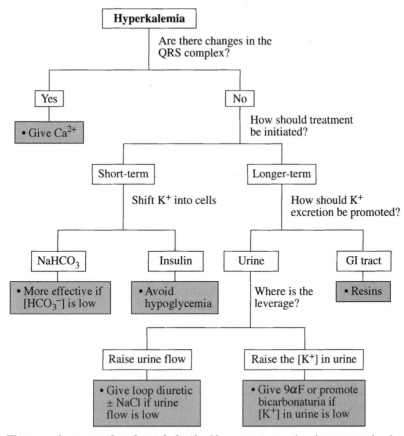

Figure 11.1B   Therapeutic approach to hyperkalemia. If treatment must be given promptly, the steps to take are as shown. In a patient with hyperkalemia, multiple treatment interventions are usually required.

2. Is the hyperkalemia real?

At times (see Figure 11.1A), hyperkalemia may be reported by the laboratory but not represent values in the patient (called *pseudohyperkalemia*). The common causes for this error are improper techniques in drawing blood and lysis of blood cells. A relatively common way to achieve an artificial elevation in the $[K^+]$ in plasma is to draw blood from a patient who clenches his fist excessively; the muscular contraction leads to depolarization of cell membranes and, as a result, release of K^+ from cells. This release of K^+, however, does not usually go into the general pool of interstitial fluid but, rather, enters *T tubules*. Certain patients, especially those with *cachexia* and/or those whose veins are difficult to puncture (more fist clenching), are more prone to release K^+ into their venous blood.

Alternatively, K^+ may be released from red blood cells that have lysed. In this case, the plasma is red. Platelets can rupture during clotting or if they contact glass; nevertheless, significant hyperkalemia is only evident if the platelets are abnormally large in diameter. Given the very small size of platelets, an abundant number (thrombocytosis) does not correlate well with pseudohyperkalemia (see the discussion of Question 11.1). In rare instances, circulating tumor cells (leukemias) can be unduly fragile. To minimize these errors, blood should be drawn slowly into a silicone-coated tube

Pseudohyperkalemia
An elevated $[K^+]$ in plasma that does not represent events in vivo. It is usually due to cell rupture or depolarization of cell membranes during withdrawal of blood. A useful clue is that there are no electrocardiogram (ECG) changes.

T tubules
Invaginations in the plasma membrane of skeletal muscle where most of the K^+ are released during depolarization of muscle cells. The K^+ released are taken up rapidly before they can mix with the general interstitial fluid.

Cachexia
A marked degree of muscle wasting. Disturbed local architecture (T tubules) may permit K^+ to enter interstitial fluid during depolarization.

TABLE 11.1   **Approach to a Patient with Hyperkalemia**

Rule out a life-threatening condition in which therapy for hyperkalemia is the first consideration.
- Antagonize effects of hyperkalemia with Ca^{2+} if there are important ECG changes.
- Allow no K^+ intake.
- Shift K^+ into cells with insulin and possibly $NaHCO_3$.
- Promote K^+ loss in the urine, GI tract, or via dialysis.

Rule out pseudohyperkalemia.
- Determine if the technique for drawing blood was improper.
    Excessive muscular contraction
- Did blood cell lysis occur?
    Red blood cells, fragile tumor cells in blood, enhanced platelet volume

Assess the cause for reduced excretion of K^+ in the urine (see margin note).
- Is the $[K^+]$ in the urine low?
- Is the distal flow rate low?

Assess K^+ intake.
- A high intake will aggravate hyperkalemia if there is compromised renal K^+ loss.

Assess a shift of K^+ from the ICF to the ECF.
- What was the cause of the shift?
    Metabolic acidosis (nonorganic)
    Hormonal causes
      Insulin deficiency
      β_2-Adrenergic blockade
      Aldosterone deficiency
      More than one hormone deficiency can lead to a severe degree of hyperkalemia, aggravated by hyperglycemia.
    Necrosis or depolarization
    Rare disorders (e.g., hyperkalemic periodic paralysis)

Note

Expected rate of excretion of K^+ should be greater than 200 mmol/day.

Note

If the rate of excretion of K^+ exceeds 200 mmol/day or 140 μmol/min, look for a very high intake of K^+; a high K^+ intake is an extremely unlikely sole cause of hyperkalemia.

that contains heparin to avoid the lysis that is caused by a glass surface or that occurs during clotting. To rule out pseudohyperkalemia, one could draw two blood samples simultaneously—one from the arm using the usual technique and another from the femoral vein or an artery using a heparinized, silicone-treated tube.

Once pseudohyperkalemia has been ruled out or proved not to be the sole cause of hyperkalemia, the next stage in the approach is to address the renal response. Chronic hyperkalemia implies a defect in the excretion of K^+ in almost every case.

3. Is the rate of excretion of K^+ low? If so, why?

In almost every case, the excretion of K^+ will be low in a patient with chronic hyperkalemia (see margin note). Because the excretion of K^+ is the product of the $[K^+]$ in the urine and the urine flow rate, each component should be examined independently.

$[K^+]$ in Urine. Two factors lead to a high $[K^+]$ in the urine. First, there must be electrogenic reabsorption of Na^+ in the cortical collecting duct (CCD) to generate the driving force for the net secretion of K^+. Second, the luminal membrane must be permeable to K^+ for this secretion to occur. Both components of the K^+ secretory process can be evaluated by examining concentrations of electrolytes and the osmolality of the urine (see pages 391–393). In practice, calculating the transtubular $[K^+]$ gradient (TTKG) is very helpful.

If the TTKG is lower than expected (less than 10 in a patient with hyperkalemia), one can question whether the level of aldosterone is low or whether there is a lesion in the CCD so that it fails to respond to aldosterone. To answer these questions, blood should be drawn for renin and aldosterone levels (there is a long delay before results are available), and an acute challenge with 100 μg of *9αfludrocortisone* (9αF) should be attempted. If the TTKG rises to greater than 10, suspect a problem with aldosterone synthesis; a problem in the CCD is present if the TTKG does not rise to greater than 10 two hours after 9αF is given.

Volume Delivery to the CCD. Low-volume delivery to the CCD is uncommon as the sole cause of hyperkalemia. In essence, volume delivery is assessed by measuring the osmole excretion rate; details are provided later in this chapter (Figure 11.3). To confirm that a low volume is the reason for the low rate of excretion of K^+, a loop diuretic should be given. Expect the rate of excretion of K^+ to rise to greater than 140 μmol/min at peak diuresis (flow 10 mL/min). If the patient has ECF volume contraction, be sure to replace the Na^+ and water losses.

4. Has either a high intake of K^+ or a shift of K^+ from the ICF to the ECF contributed to the hyperkalemia?

The intake of K^+ has been discussed. The only point to add is that resolution of an ileus might provide an "occult" load of K^+ (see margin note).

A shift of K^+ from cells occurs if there is necrosis, depolarization, hyperchloremic metabolic acidosis, and/or a deficiency of insulin and/or β_2-adrenergic agonists. If present, these disturbances should be addressed.

QUESTION

(Discussion on page 479)

11.1 *What is the total K^+ content in the platelets of 1 L of blood? (Assume 400,000 cells/mm³, a 150 mmol/L [K^+] in the ICF, and a platelet volume of 1 μ³.)*

Etiology of Hyperkalemia

Role of Excessive K^+ Intake

> • Chronic severe hyperkalemia occurs with increased K^+ intake only if the excretion of K^+ is compromised.

After appropriate redistribution, the retention of 70 mmol of K^+ produces only a 0.1 mmol/L rise in the plasma [K^+] in normal individuals (see the discussion of Question 9.1). Notwithstanding, should a defect in K^+ movement into cells be present, severe hyperkalemia could ensue. Extremely high K^+ intake leads to chronic hyperkalemia only in patients with compromised K^+ excretion. In certain cultures, K^+ intake can be 10 or 400 mmol/day.

In special conditions, an unusually large load of K^+ can be administered intravenously (e.g., when large volumes of whole blood are transfused); the degree of this danger depends on the

9αfludrocortisone (9αF)
A drug with mineralocorticoid actions. It is active when given orally. Because this derivative of cortisol is not totally inactivated by 11 β-HSDH, it occupies the mineralocorticoid receptor in principal cells and has an aldosterone-like action.

Occult load of K^+
If a patient with hypokalemia and an ileus receives an oral K^+ load, the K^+ may remain in the gastrointestinal (GI) tract. Once GI motility recovers, there will be a sudden load of K^+ that the kidneys cannot excrete promptly. It may take 24 hours of normokalemia to restore K^+ excretion to normal.

Very high K^+ intake
1. A very high K^+ intake is rare; examples include the use of large quantities of salt substitutes that contain 10–13 mmol of K^+ per gram and the intake of K^+ salts of organic acids (citrate) given to alkalinize the urine.
2. In patients undergoing aortic surgery, rapid reperfusion after clamp removal can result in a sudden bolus of K^+ from the previously ischemic limbs to the heart. An analogous situation may occur following renal transplantation if the transplanted kidney was perfused with a K^+-rich solution during preservation.

preservative, the temperature of the blood, cell lysis, the duration of blood storage, and whether the blood has sedimented (plasma may deliver a large K^+ load because it has a high $[K^+]$ and will be infused faster as a result of a lower viscosity). If the citrate that is used as an anticoagulant acutely lowers the plasma-ionized calcium concentration, the biologic response to hyperkalemia might be more severe. The cardioplegic solution used in cardiac surgery also may provide a substantial K^+ load to the patient.

Excessive Shift of K^+ from Cells

- K^+ will shift from cells with hormone deficiencies, acidosis, or cell damage.

Hormones

Insulin and β_2-adrenergic agonists are the major hormones that cause movement of K^+ into cells. Hyperkalemia is seen if these hormones are relatively inactive.

Insulin. Insulin promotes the entry of K^+ into cells by hyperpolarizing the cell membrane (more flux through the NHE-1 leads to more pumping of Na^+ via the $Na^+K^+ATPase$ and, as a result, a more negative resting membrane potential). Insulin also increases the net anionic charge (organic phosphates) in cells.

The shift of K^+ out of cells during diabetic ketoacidosis is not due to a pH change but is due to the lack of insulin. This cause can be deduced from direct experiments and the amount of time of events (i.e., the plasma $[K^+]$ falls 1–2 hours after insulin is given; at this time there is little change in the acid-base status; see margin note).

β_2-Adrenergic Agonists. β_2-Adrenergic agonists lead to a shift of K^+ into cells; hence, β-blockers may cause hyperkalemia. β_1-Blockers diminish renin release, and this action can reduce aldosterone levels and thereby K^+ excretion. In contrast, α-adrenergic agonists have the opposite effect; they tend to increase the severity of hyperkalemia if there is already a stimulus to move K^+ out of cells.

Aldosterone. Low levels of aldosterone contribute to the serious hyperkalemia that is due primarily to a reduced renal excretion of K^+.

Combined Hormone Deficiency. If a patient has both hypoaldosteronism and low insulin levels, a much greater degree of hyperkalemia can occur. If hyperglycemia develops in this hormonal setting, it can markedly exacerbate the degree of hyperkalemia by mechanisms that are not entirely clear.

Quantities
In acute experiments in which the basal insulin level was halved, the plasma $[K^+]$ rose 0.5 mmol/L.

Note
The plasma $[K^+]$ rises by only a few tenths of a millimole per liter in normal subjects on β-blockers.

QUESTIONS

(Discussions on pages 479–480)

11.2 *What sets the limit on K^+ uptake into cells?*

11.3 *How might β-blockers cause a severe degree of hyperkalemia?*

11.4 *What happens to the plasma $[K^+]$ during exercise?*

11.5 *Why do patients with a problem regenerating ATP in muscle cells suffer from weakness but not hyperkalemia?*

11.6 *How much of a K^+ load might a patient receive if 1 L of blood is digested in the GI tract in the course of a GI bleed?*

Acid-Base Factors

> • Hyperkalemia is not caused directly by respiratory acidosis, ketoacidosis, and L-lactic acidosis.
> • If hyperkalemia accompanies chronic acidosis, look for a problem with K^+ excretion or insulin deficiency.

Acute respiratory acidosis per se does not cause an appreciable rise in the plasma $[K^+]$. Similarly, metabolic acidosis caused by the accumulation of lactic acid or ketoacids does not cause an appreciable exit of K^+ from cells, because H^+ enter the intracellular fluid (ICF) with their conjugate base. In contrast, if a patient has metabolic acidosis from $NaHCO_3$ loss, hyperkalemia may ensue (see margin note). Notwithstanding, if the kidneys and adrenal glands are normal with respect to K^+ handling, hyperkalemia will not persist (see Figure 9.4).

Note
When H^+ enter cells without an anion, a cation must exit. This is usually Na^+ on NHE-1; the fall in the ICF $[Na^+]$ leads to the decreased exit of positive charges on the Na^+, K^+, ATPase, lowering the net negative valence in cells. As a result, K^+ exit from cells.

Cell Damage

Because the $[K^+]$ in the ICF is close to 35-fold higher than that in the ECF, if an appreciable number of cells are damaged, hyperkalemia may result. This type of hyperkalemia is seen in patients suffering from acute organ necrosis or trauma or those given cytotoxic treatment for neoplasms. The degree of hyperkalemia will be more severe if the patient also has a reduced rate of excretion of K^+ or deficiencies of insulin or β_2-adrenergic agonists.

Although not technically an example of cell damage, hyperkalemia can be caused in special circumstances by a cellular K^+ shift in response to "destruction" of the resting membrane potential. In large doses, succinylcholine may depolarize the entire muscle and lead to a severe degree of hyperkalemia (instead of the less than 1 mmol/L transient rise in the plasma $[K^+]$ when the usual dose of succinylcholine is used during anesthesia).

A Rise in "Effective" Osmolality

A rise in plasma effective osmolality is associated with hyperkalemia in a number of settings. Nevertheless, for a shift of K^+ from the ICF to the extracellular fluid (ECF) to cause chronic hyperkalemia, either the resting membrane potential across cell membranes must become less negative (depolarization), or permeability of cell membranes to K^+ must have decreased so that K^+ cannot reenter cells. There are no compelling data to support such a role for hyperosmolality. For example, in the clinical setting of diabetic ketoacidosis, there are other factors, such as deficiency of insulin, that cause the hyperkalemia. Similarly, in experiments in animals in which a rise in the plasma $[K^+]$ was associated with a rise in osmolality, enormous infusions were given, and hyperkalemia was not an isolated finding.

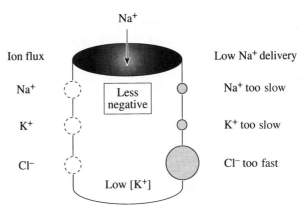

Figure 11.2 Factors that may cause a low [K⁺] in the CCD. The barrel-like structure is the lumen of the CCD. For details, see the text. The potential lesions are a low delivery of Na⁺ to the CCD, fewer open Na⁺ channels, fewer open K⁺ channels, and/or more Cl⁻ permeability in the CCD.

Reduced Excretion of K⁺ in the Urine

Clinical pearls
- Assess the rate of K⁺ excretion first.
- If this rate is low, assess the [K⁺] and volume of urine separately.
- The TTKG reflects the [K⁺] in the CCD relative to that in plasma.
- The osmole excretion rate reflects the volume delivered to the terminal CCD (osmole excretion rate/P_{osm} (plasma osmolality) provides a minimum estimate of the number of liters delivered to the CCD if ADH is acting).

To excrete K⁺, there must be electrogenic reabsorption of Na⁺ in the CCD. It is difficult to establish just what constitutes a reduced rate of excretion of K⁺ in a hyperkalemic patient. Because a normal person can excrete as much as 450 mmol of K⁺ per day when K⁺-loaded, anything less than this amount should constitute a low rate of excretion of K⁺. If the 24-hour K⁺ excretion rate is less than 200 mmol, the rate of excretion of K⁺ is clearly lower than expected in the presence of hyperkalemia. The causes of reduced excretion of K⁺ can be an unexpectedly low [K⁺] in the luminal fluid in the CCD and/or a low delivery of volume to the CCD. In the latter circumstance, the pathophysiology will include a low rate of excretion of osmoles (see margin note).

A low [K⁺] in the fluid in the lumen of the CCD usually reflects a reduced aldosterone bioactivity (Table 11.2) and/or an intrinsic renal lesion. The role of the adrenal gland can be assessed by hormone measurements and by the kaliuretic response to exogenously administered mineralocorticoid (100 μg 9αF).

In the following paragraphs, the authors present a speculative way to assess why the [K⁺] in the lumen of the CCD may not be high enough in a patient with hyperkalemia. We apply newer discoveries in physiology to the bedside (Figure 11.2 and the review flow chart on page 449).

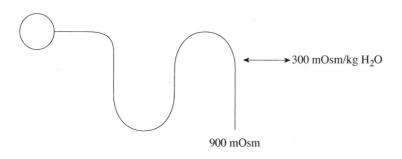

900 mOsm

Figure 11.3 Causes of a low flow rate in the CCD. When ADH acts, the osmolality in the lumen of the CCD is the same as that in plasma, say 300 mOsm/kg H_2O. If 900 mOsm is excreted in a period of time, 3 L of urine traversed the terminal CCD.

TABLE 11.2 **Factors to Evaluate in Patients with Hyperkalemia and Low Aldosterone Bioactivity**

Plasma renin concentration (while ECF volume is low)
   Low
• Problem with juxtaglomerular apparatus
   High
• Converting enzyme inhibitor, angiotensin II receptor blocker
• Adrenal gland problem
• Impaired renal response to aldosterone
Plasma aldosterone concentration
   Low
• Low renin
• Converting enzyme inhibitor, angiotensin II receptor blocker
• Adrenal gland problem
   High
• Renal problem (interstitial nephritis, Cl^- shunt, etc.)
• Aldosterone antagonists
• K^+-sparing diuretics or drugs such as trimethoprim that mimic K^+-sparing diuretics
Renal response to mineralocorticoids (physiologic dose)
   Urine [K^+] not high enough
• Interstitial nephritis or tubular damage
• Very low distal Na^+ delivery
• K^+-sparing diuretics
• Cl^- shunt in the CCD
• Low Na^+ conductance in the CCD
   High urine [K^+]
• Low aldosterone levels because of an adrenal problem

Causes of an Unexpectedly Low [K^+] in the CCD

• This approach is speculative but based on physiologic principles, and the authors find it useful.

Potentially, six lesions may cause hyperkalemia via a low [K^+] in the CCD (see Figure 11.2 and Tables 11.3 and 11.4).

1. Low delivery of Na^+ to the terminal CCD

There are many instances that suggest a low delivery of Na^+, but it is not clear whether the delivery is low enough to limit the net

TABLE 11.3 **Pathophysiologic Classification of Low Excretion of K^+**

For a description, see the text.

Low [K^+] in the lumen of the CCD
• Low delivery of Na^+ (rare)
• Low Na^+ channel open probability
     Low aldosterone bioactivity, amiloride, trimethoprim, congenital disorders
• High Cl^- permeability
     Possibly in some patients taking cyclosporine, in those with diabetes mellitus, in those with Gordon's syndrome
• Increased H^+/K^+ antiporter activity
     In patients with a low TTKG that fails to rise with bicarbonaturia
• Low K^+ conductance
Low volume delivery to the CCD
• Low urea excretion rate plus ECF volume contraction (Figure 11.3)

Note
A high H^+/K^+ antiporter activity and a low K^+ ion conductance are only theoretical possibilities at present.

Quantitative analysis

1. Close to 1000 mmol of Na^+ is delivered to the CCD, and the majority of Na^+ (700 mmol or so) are reabsorbed in an electroneutral fashion with Cl^-. Hence, only 50–70 mmol of Na^+ is reabsorbed daily in an electrogenic manner, and this reabsorption is responsible for ensuring the net secretion of 50–70 mmol of K^+.

2. Close to 90 mmol of K^+ exits the loop of Henle because the volume of fluid that exits from the loop is close to 30 L/day in an adult, and the $[K^+]$ in this fluid is close to 3 mmol/l. A smaller quantity is actually delivered to the CCD because some K^+ are reabsorbed in the distal convoluted tubule.

Criteria

1. Hyperkalemia and low TTKG ± 9αF
2. Somewhat low ECF volume and high renin
3. Na^+ and Cl^- wasting while the ECF volume is contracted

Note

The term *hyporeninemic hypoaldosteronism* does not represent a single entity; it includes a group of conditions that have the features of a Cl^- shunt in most cases.

secretion of K^+. The authors recommend the following approach. When Na^+ are excreted in the urine, one can assume that Na^+ were present in the CCD because Na^+ are not secreted into the lumen of the MCD (see margin note).

How can one deduce what the $[Na^+]$ was in the CCD when Na^+ were not present in the urine? The following data permit an analysis:

(a) The $[Na^+]$ in the CCD required for half-maximal net secretion of K^+ is 10–15 mmol/L in rats.

(b) When ADH acts, the osmolality in the luminal fluid in the CCD is the same as that in plasma (e.g., 300 mOsm/kg H_2O, for easy arithmetic).

(c) If the volume delivered to the terminal CCD is 5 L/day in a 70-kg adult, and if the quantity of urea excreted is 400 mmol/day, the concentration of urea is 80 mmol/L.

(d) Hence, the concentration of electrolytes is close to 200 mmol/L, half of which is Na^+, so delivery of Na^+ will only limit the net secretion of K^+ in very rare circumstances (e.g., marked degree of contraction of the ECF volume with high urea excretion rates).

(e) If one suspects that a low TTKG is due to a low delivery of Na^+ to the CCD, one should administer a loop diuretic and expect to see an increase in the TTKG and K^+ excretion.

2. Low open probability of the Na^+ channel in the luminal membrane of the CCD

The Na^+ channel in the luminal membrane of the CCD (ENaC) is normally regulated by aldosterone (which leads to a greater open probability) and is inhibited by K^+-sparing diuretics, such as amiloride, and by drugs bearing a positive charge, such as the antimicrobial trimethoprim (see margin note).

There are inborn or possibly acquired errors in Na^+ reabsorption in the CCD; a possible example is discussed in Case 11.3. The cardinal features of ENaC with a reduced open probability are tendencies for hyperkalemia and ECF volume contraction. The latter leads to high renin levels and the inability to achieve a Na^+-free and Cl^--free urine when the ECF volume is contracted. Finally, the

TABLE 11.4 **Causes of an Unexpectedly Low $[K^+]$ in the CCD**

The major findings are hyperkalemia and a low rate of excretion of K^+. The lesions are listed below and described in the text.

Suspected Lesion	Major Features	Other Comments
Low delivery of Na^+	• Na^+-free urine • Very low effective arterial volume	• Rare cause of hyperkalemia
Low open probability of the Na^+ channel	• Low ECF volume and a high $[Na^+]$ and $[Cl^-]$ in the urine • High renin	• Adrenal gland may be the problem • Also suspect K^+-sparing diuretics or trimethoprim
High permeability to Cl^-	• ECF volume tends to be expanded • Low renin • Can achieve Na^+-free and Cl^--free urine with ECF volume contraction	• Hypertension may be present • May be called "hyporeninemic hypoaldosteronism" • Can achieve high TTKG with bicarbonaturia

TTKG should be on the low side when a physiologic supplement of a mineralocorticoid is given (100 μg 9αF). A tendency to hypotension could be present in some patients, especially when they consume a low-salt diet.

3. An increased permeability to Cl⁻ in the luminal membrane of the CCD

If the luminal membrane of the CCD had an increased permeability to Cl⁻, there would be an enhanced electroneutral rather than electrogenic absorption of Na^+ because there would be little restriction to the movement of Cl⁻ across the luminal membrane (see margin note). Hence, the cardinal features would be hyperkalemia, a tendency to an expanded ECF volume with low levels of renin, and possibly hypertension in those individuals who are particularly sensitive to an expanded ECF volume despite the low level of vasoconstrictors (i.e., low angiotensin II). Possible clinical examples of this variety of hyperkalemia are found in patients who receive cyclosporine, those with Gordon's syndrome (also called a Cl⁻ shunt or pseudohypoaldosteronism type II), or even those with diabetes mellitus, given the label of *hyporeninemic hypoaldosteronism*. In these patients, bicarbonaturia may lead to a marked rise in the TTKG if aldosterone is present; the authors use this observation to support the speculation that there is a "Cl⁻ shunt" in the CCD.

4. Nonspecific anion permeability in the CCD

Nonspecific anion permeability in the CCD is a theoretical lesion. It would be characterized by a low TTKG, but if the urine volume were to rise (after a loop diuretic is given), one might expect to see a rise in the rate of excretion of K^+. These individuals should be able to have an Na^+-poor and Cl⁻-poor urine when salt-restricted. Bicarbonaturia would not augment kaliuresis or the TTKG with this type of lesion. There would be a tendency to ECF volume expansion and low renin levels.

5. A low open probability of the luminal K⁺ channel

As far as we know, there are no reports that specifically characterize a low open probability of the luminal K^+ channel. We would suspect it if there were hyperkalemia and low excretion of K^+ (low TTKG) and if the TTKG would not rise in the presence of aldosterone and bicarbonaturia. Perhaps the most distinguishing feature would be a lack of an appreciable rise in the rate of excretion of K^+ when the flow rate in the CCD is increased following the administration of a loop diuretic; in this setting the TTKG would fall.

Plasma Aldosterone and Renin

In the hyperkalemic patient, failure to find a high aldosterone concentration suggests an adrenal or a renin problem because hyperkalemia should stimulate the release of aldosterone. If the renin level is high, there are two possibilities: either the problem is in the adrenal gland or there is inhibition of the angiotensin-converting enzyme (see margin note). In contrast, if the patient's ECF volume is low or on the low side of normal and the renin level is not

Criteria
1. Hyperkalemia and low TTKG ± 9αF
2. Somewhat high ECF volume and low renin
3. Can excrete Na^+-poor and Cl⁻-poor urine when the ECF volume is contracted

Hyporeninemic hypoaldosteronism
We do not like to use this descriptive term because it represents a heterogeneous pathophysiology. In the Cl⁻ shunt, the hyporeninemia is due to ECF volume expansion; with primary destruction of the juxtaglomerular apparatus (JGA), however, there is low renin and secondary ECF volume contraction. Treatments in these two categories differ: diuretics and a low-salt diet for the Cl⁻ shunt, and 9αF plus NaCl for the JGA defect.

Note
Some patients who are severely ill behave as if they cannot generate high angiotensin II levels.

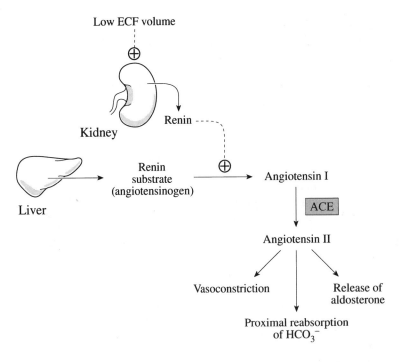

Figure 11.4 The adrenal-renal axis. Renin, which is produced in the kidney, acts on renin substrate from the liver to yield angiotensin I; this latter compound is converted into the biologically active angiotensin II by the angiotensin-converting enzyme (ACE). Angiotensin II is also a stimulator of thirst.

elevated, then the problem is renal in origin (Tables 11.2 and 11.5 and Figure 11.4). In some patients, there may be two renal problems: low renin release and low renal response to aldosterone.

CASE 11.1
Severe Degree of Hyperkalemia with a GI Upset
(Discussion on page 472)

A 69-year-old woman has two chronic medical problems, hypertension (160/100 mm Hg) and hyperkalemia (plasma $[K^+]$ 5.5 mmol/L).

For the past several days, she has had diarrhea, which continued up to the time of admission. She passed three to four liquid bowel movements per day. There was no drug intake before or during this episode. She appears to be very ill.

On physical examination, the striking feature was a profound degree of ECF volume contraction. No other specific findings were evident.

On laboratory examination, she had a life-threatening degree of hyperkalemia (9.2 mmol/L) with ECG changes that were alarming.

Unknown causes
Hyporeninemia may be caused by excessive Na^+ retention and ECF volume expansion (e.g., a Cl^--shunt disorder).

TABLE 11.5 **Causes of Hyporeninemia in Patients with Hyperkalemia**

Destruction of juxtaglomerular apparatus
- Interstitial nephritis or infiltration
  Infection
  Drugs, such as nonsteroidal anti-inflammatory drugs (NSAIDs), and certain antibiotics, including methicillin
  Depositions such as urate or amyloid
- Diabetes mellitus

Pharmacologic blockade with β_1-adrenergic blockers
Unknown causes (see margin note)

		Plasma	**Urine**
Na^+	mmol/L	132	75
K^+	mmol/L	9.5	30
Cl^-	mmol/L	110	82
HCO_3^-	mmol/L	18	0
Urea	mmol/L (mg/dL)	11 (31)	—
Creatinine	μmol/L (mg/dL)	176 (2.0)	10 mM (1.3 g/L)
Glucose	mmol/L (mg/dL)	6.0 (108)	0
Hemoglobin	g/L	155	—
Osmolality	mOsm/kg H_2O	278	600

What emergencies need immediate management, and what should you administer?

Why did such a severe degree of hyperkalemia develop?

Why did her ECF volume become so contracted following this acute GI episode?

At the level of the luminal membrane of her CCD, what is the most likely explanation for her electrolyte disorder at the time of admission?

Clinical Assessment

Symptoms and Signs

The major symptom of hyperkalemia is weakness; ultimately, paralysis may occur. These symptoms appear only with a very severe degree of hyperkalemia. This weakness is first evident in the lower extremities. Often, the patient is asymptomatic, and the diagnosis is "stumbled upon" when the electrolytes are "routinely" determined.

Note
When hyperkalemia is present, the resting membrane potential is less negative than normal (partial depolarization).

Drugs That May Cause or Aggravate the Degree of Hyperkalemia

Table 11.6 contains a list of drugs that can cause hyperkalemia; these drugs are classified according to mechanism of action.

TABLE 11.6 **Drugs That May Cause Hyperkalemia**

Preparations such as KCl and other K^+ salts that contain K^+ (only if renal function is compromised)
Drugs that cause a shift of K^+ from ICF to ECF
- β_2Adrenergic blockers, α-adrenergic agonists
- Drugs that impair insulin release from β cells of the pancreas
- Drugs that depolarize cell membranes (e.g., succinylcholine, massive digitalis overdose)
- Drugs that cause cell necrosis (e.g., in cancer chemothrapy)

Drugs that interfere with excretion of K^+ in the urine
- Drugs that cause acute renal failure
- Drugs that cause interstitial nephritis (e.g., NSAIDs)
- Drugs that interfere with aldosterone bioactivity
    Disrupted release from the adrenal gland
        β_1-Adrenergic blockers, which diminish renin release
        Converting enzyme inhibitors, angiotensin II receptor blockers
        Heparin
    Blocked binding of aldosterone to its renal receptor
        Spironolactone
    Presence of postreceptor blockers
    Na^+ channel blockers in the CCD (e.g., amiloride, trimethoprim)
        Increased Cl^- permeability in the CCD (possibly cyclosporine)

Electrocardiogram

ECG changes during hyperkalemia

1. Increased T-wave amplitude
2. Decreased R-wave amplitude
3. S–T segment depression
4. Decreased P-wave amplitude
5. Prolonged P-R, QRS, and Q-T intervals
6. Absent P waves
7. Bradycardia
8. Sine-wave pattern of QRST
9. Ventricular arrhythmias

The margin note contains a list of the changes that occur in the ECG during hyperkalemia. The plasma [K$^+$] at which the ECG changes is variable. These changes may be seen at a lower [K$^+$] if hypocalcemia, hyponatremia, or acidosis is present; they are more dramatic if the changes in plasma [K$^+$] are acute. Early changes include an increase in T-wave amplitude that leads to tall, narrow, peaked, symmetrical T waves. With a greater degree of hyperkalemia, the R-wave amplitude decreases, the S wave increases, and the S-T segment becomes depressed. The P-R, QRS, and Q-T intervals all become prolonged. The P-wave duration increases, but its amplitude decreases. With extreme hyperkalemia, there is progressive QRS and T-wave widening. Terminally, ventricular tachyarrhythmias may be observed.

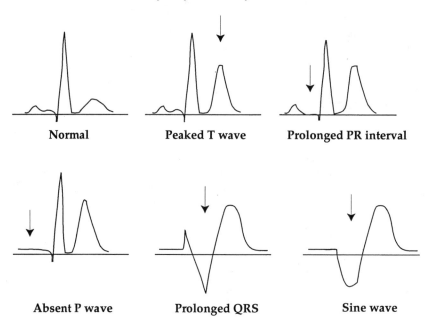

| Normal | Peaked T wave | Prolonged PR interval |
| Absent P wave | Prolonged QRS | Sine wave |

Specific Clinical Examples

Addison's Disease

Clinical pearl
The cardinal feature of Addison's disease is a low rate of excretion of K$^+$ relative to the degree of hyperkalemia.

- K$^+$ excretion = [K$^+$] in urine × Urine volume
             (aldosterone)   (osmole excretion)
             (bicarbonaturia)   (diuretics)

A simple examination of the natural history of patients with aldosterone deficiency illustrates the problems associated with the clinical assessment of reduced excretion of K$^+$. If the patient has chronic hyperkalemia and is in a steady state, the 24-hour urine K$^+$ excretion equals the amount absorbed from the diet. Therefore, to be diagnostic, the 24-hour urine K$^+$ excretion must be interpreted in conjunction with the plasma [K$^+$]. As a generalization, hyperkalemia and aldosterone produce many of the same results in the CCD, but hyperkalemia is less effective. Hence, the K$^+$ excretion rate matches the diet (60–80 mmol/day) but does not reach the expected rate of several hundred mmol/day, which a normal person would excrete if rendered hyperkalemic by K$^+$-loading. The TTKG is close to 5–6 vs the expected value of 10. Given these constraints, patients with Addison's disease have a plasma [K$^+$] in the mid-5 range, day in and day out. A higher plasma [K$^+$] occurs in two circumstances: first, if there is a very low GFR (low urine volume); second, if there is a very high intake of K$^+$ or a shift of K$^+$ from the ICF.

Treatment of hyperkalemia will have two features: saline to restore the ECF volume and the volume of fluid delivered to the CCD; and a mineralocorticoid to augment Na$^+$ reabsorption and K$^+$ secretion in the CCD.

Hyperkalemic Periodic Paralysis

Hyperkalemic periodic paralysis is a rare inborn error of metabolism that has undergone remarkable clarification in the past several years. The clinical picture is dominated by weakness or even paralysis. Symptoms are precipitated by an event that leads to hyperkalemia (e.g., after exercise). At times, patients may suffer from a chronic increase in motor activity (clonus).

From a biochemical perspective, the lesion seems to be in the regulation of specific Na$^+$ channels in the cell membrane (3–15% of Na$^+$ channels, those sensitive to tetrodotoxin, a toxin from uncooked spiny fish from seas near Japan; see margin note). Normally, when a stimulus arrives for muscular contraction, Na$^+$ channels open; as flux of Na$^+$ increases, these cells depolarize. When the RMP approaches -50 mV, normal Na$^+$ channels close. In hyperkalemic periodic paralysis, the mutant channels remain open because of hyperkalemia. Hence, cells have a persistently less negative resting membrane potential (RMP). Depending on the absolute voltage, lesser changes result in myotonia, and larger changes lead to paralysis. Hyperkalemia develops because of the less negative RMP together with relatively open K$^+$ channels.

Treatment, which is directed at measures that avoid hyperkalemia, involves the use of certain drugs, such as acetazolamide, whose mechanisms of action are unclear but empirically effective.

Molecular biology in hyperkalemic periodic paralysis Studies have suggested a similar gene location for growth hormone and the Na$^+$ channel. See Chapter 9 as well.

Chronic Renal Insufficiency

Patients with renal failure develop hyperkalemia when their glomerular filtration rate (GFR) falls toward 20% of normal. This decline results in a lower rate of excretion of K$^+$. Examining the components of this excretion individually (volume, [K$^+$]) suggests that the basis for the low rate of excretion of K$^+$ is not a fall in the volume delivered to the terminal CCD but rather the very rapid rate of flow in the remaining CCDs. In more detail, if a patient with renal failure is excreting the usual 900 mOsm each day, the volume delivered to the terminal CCD is close to the same as in normal individuals, but this volume is traversing many fewer CCDs (see Figure 11.3).

The second component of the analysis is the [K$^+$] in the CCD. Because of an extremely rapid flow rate per CCD, the [K$^+$] in each

CCD cannot be raised to 10 times that in the plasma. Therefore, the TTKG is always less than maximal, even if aldosterone is acting.

In a normal individual, 30 L of dilute urine exits from the loop of Henle, and each liter contains 3 mmol of K^+ per liter. When 80% of this volume is reabsorbed, the $[K^+]$ can rise to 15 mmol/L without additional secretion of K^+. In contrast, in renal insufficiency, many fewer liters of fluid leave the loop, so to have a $[K^+]$ of 15 mmol/L in fluid entering the CCD, more K^+ must be secreted.

PART B

Treatment of Patients with Hyperkalemia

> • Urgency of treatment depends on ECG changes and the anticipated future rise in plasma $[K^+]$.

Because hyperkalemia can arise from many causes, there is no universal therapy for this electrolyte abnormality. The authors assume, for simplicity, that the cause of hyperkalemia is known, all diagnostic tests have been performed, and specific therapy, where applicable, has been initiated. Treatment is now dictated by the degree of ECF volume expansion or contraction and the degree of elevation of the plasma $[K^+]$ together with the anticipated rate of K^+ release from the ICF. The degree of abnormality in the ECG can help the clinician decide on the urgency of therapy because the major aim initially is to prevent cardiac arrhythmia. A normal ECG, however, does not imply that a casual approach should be taken because the ECG can change quickly. A list of the treatment modes and their period for effect is presented in Table 11.7 and Figure 11.5. Table 11.8 summarizes therapy for hyperkalemia.

Note
Rectally administered resins that bind K^+ have a faster onset of action because the rate of secretion of K^+ in the colon exceeds that of the more proximal GI tract.

TABLE 11.7 **Time for the Effect of Therapeutic Agents for Hyperkalemia**

Seconds to minutes
• Antagonist to cardiac effects of hyperkalemia (intravenous Ca^{2+} salts)
30 minutes–1 hour
• Insulin
• $NaHCO_3$ (isotonic), but the effect is small unless acidemic
1–4 hours
• Aldosterone agonists
• Rectally administered K^+-binding resins
More than 6 hours
• Orally administered K^+-binding resins
Immediate once instituted
• Dialysis

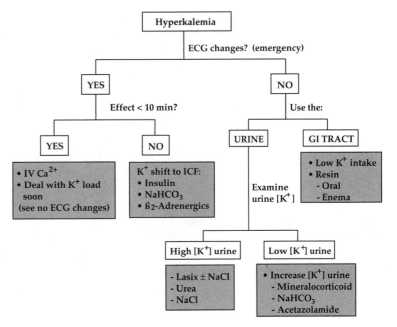

Figure 11.5 Treatment of the patient with hyperkalemia. If an emergency is present (usually cardiac), intravenous Ca^{2+} must be given. This treatment should act promptly. Once the emergency is dealt with, or if there is just a severe degree of hyperkalemia, efforts are now to shift K^+ into cells with insulin $\pm$ $NaHCO_3$. Longer-term strategies are to limit intake of K^+, prevent its absorption in the GI tract, and promote its excretion. In this latter context, examine the urine $[K^+]$ and flow rate to decide leverage for therapy.

Preventing a Further Rise in Plasma $[K^+]$

Intake of K^+

Intake of K^+ should be as low as possible. Do not overlook the fact that certain medications are K^+ salts (certain penicillin preparations, alkalinizing salts).

Preventing a Shift of K^+ from the ICF

In certain cases, preventing a shift of K^+ from the ICF is an important form of therapy. If a patient is in a catabolic state, this catabolism should be arrested. Among the drugs to consider

TABLE 11.8 **Summary of Therapy for Hyperkalemia**

Stop K^+ intake.
Shift K^+ into cells.
• Hormones
    Insulin
• Acid-base factors
    Bicarbonate
• Gain of ICF anions
    Replace phosphate deficits.
Increase K^+ loss from the ECF.
• Bind K^+ in the GI tract.
    K^+ exchange resins
        Oral resins have a slower onset of action.
        Resins given by enema have a faster onset of action.
• Promote urinary K^+ loss.
    Ensure adequate distal Na^+ and volume delivery to the CCD (e.g., give
        diuretics, restore the ECF volume if it is contracted).
    Remove mineralocorticoid antagonists, K^+-sparing diuretics, or other
        Na^+ channel blockers (e.g., trimethoprim).
    Administer mineralocorticoids and acetazolamide, if appropriate.

discontinuing are those that cause cell lysis and those that promote catabolism (anticancer medications, drugs causing hemolysis, etc.). Another potential for cell lysis that should be considered is bleeding into the gastrointestinal tract. Nevertheless, because 1 L of blood has only 0.4 L of red blood cells (the $[K^+]$ in the ICF = 150 mmol/L), the quantity of K^+ released is only 60 mmol/L of blood digested.

Although it may be difficult to stop all of the causes of cell lysis, their presence should dictate a more active role in promoting K^+ loss on a longer-term basis. Without a rapid reversal in causation, a patient who cannot excrete the K^+ released should be considered for dialysis before life-threatening hyperkalemia ensues.

Preventing the Absorption of Dietary K^+

Certain resins bind K^+ avidly enough to diminish the net absorption of K^+. In the process, the cations Na^+, Ca^{2+}, or H^+ (depending on the nature of the resin) are displaced and possibly absorbed. The major resin used is Na^+ polystyrene sulphonate; each gram of resin may bind 1 mmol of K^+. Usually 30 g of resin is given every 2–4 hours with 70% sorbitol to hasten transit to the colon because the colon is the major site of K^+ binding (where K^+ are secreted). Oral resins are therapeutically effective only after many hours; in contrast, if the resins are administered by enema, they are effective much sooner. For administration by enema, give 100 g of resin in as little water as needed to dissolve it (200 mL); keep it in the colon for as long as possible.

Promoting K^+ Loss in the Urine

Two events are required for K^+ loss in the urine: an increase in the $[K^+]$ in the lumen of the CCD (aldosterone) and an increased flow through the CCD. If the patient has a low aldosterone level, administer a physiologic dose of $9\alpha F$ (100 μg). If the urine $[K^+]$ (adjusted for medullary water reabsorption) does not rise in 4 hours to at least $6 \times$ plasma $[K^+]$, the dose may be quadrupled, and the same parameters may be followed (see margin note). Aldosterone action requires a lag period of up to 2 hours, and the maximum biologic effect may take days to develop. If the patient is taking drugs that interfere with aldosterone action (K^+-sparing diuretics, trimethoprim, competitive inhibitors), they should be discontinued if the hyperkalemia cannot be controlled by other measures. In some patients, a large kaliuresis can be achieved if distal delivery of HCO_3^- is enhanced when aldosterone is present (see margin note and the following section).

Reduced K^+ excretion may occur if the volume of fluid reaching the CCD is small. Suspect this occurrence in patients with ECF volume contraction or a low cardiac output. In the former case, saline administration is appropriate. Digitalis and/or a loop diuretic may help patients in the second category. Even if the $[K^+]$ in the CCD is lower than one might hope for, raising the flow rate in the CCD with a loop diuretic can increase the rate of excretion of K^+.

Release of K^+ from tumors
If 1 lb (454 g) of tumor is lysed, there would be a release of close to 60 mmol of K^+ (150 mmol/L in the ICF, 80% of the weight is water, and 1 lb of tumor contains 400 mL of water). The value would be lower if one corrected for water of ECF origin.

Note
If diarrhea is provoked by phenolphthalein rather than by sorbitol, the K^+ loss from the GI tract will be greatly enhanced.

Bicarbonaturia
The most effective agent to increase the $[K^+]$ in the CCD is HCO_3^-; the excretion of HCO_3^- can be enhanced by acetazolamide.

NaHCO₃ Therapy

If the patient had metabolic acidosis caused by loss of $NaHCO_3$, the acidemia could have led to a shift of K^+ into the ECF. This shift can be minimized by administering sufficient $NaHCO_3$ to bring the blood pH toward normal. Even in patients who have a normal blood pH, therapy with $NaHCO_3$ (50 mmol for 5–10 minutes, repeat 30 minutes later if necessary) can be effective in lowering the plasma $[K^+]$. Some, but not all, studies show a synergism with insulin and $NaHCO_3$ in this context. Nevertheless, in clinical trials, $NaHCO_3$ is relatively ineffective unless it augments renal excretion of K^+. The dangers of this therapy are related to the Na^+ load given (ECF volume expansion) and to potential problems of alkalemia (tetany, etc.).

Hormonal Therapy

Two major hormones need to be considered—insulin and β_2-adrenergic agonists. If the patient is severely hyperglycemic, insulin can have a dramatic effect in lowering the plasma $[K^+]$. Insulin therapy can also be dramatic in diabetic patients with aldosterone deficiency.

To lower the plasma $[K^+]$, large doses of insulin may be necessary, but do not rely on this administration as a long-term therapy. As an example, giving 500 mL of 10% glucose in water stimulates endogenous insulin release; if diabetes mellitus is present, give a bolus of 10 units of insulin. A much higher dose of insulin may be required to activate the Na^+/H^+ antiporter.

β_2-Adrenergics shift K^+ into cells. Therefore, β-blockers should be discontinued. Because of the possibility of cardiac arrhythmias, the authors prefer not to administer β_2-adrenergics to lower the plasma $[K^+]$.

Although a lack of an essential ICF constituent such as phosphate or magnesium is not directly related to hormonal or acid-base effects, any deficits should be replaced to promote anabolism and a subsequent shift of K^+ into cells.

Antagonizing the Effects of K⁺ on the Heart

The administration of calcium salts can decrease membrane excitability and thereby protect against the effects of hyperkalemia. This benefit begins within minutes but is relatively short-lived; it "buys 60 minutes" for other forms of therapy (insulin, $NaHCO_3$) to lower the plasma $[K^+]$. The usual dose is 10 mL of 10% Ca^{2+} salt infused for 2–3 minutes. This dose can be repeated in 5–10 minutes if ECG changes persist (note the danger of hypercalcemia-induced digitalis toxicity if cardiac glycosides are being given).

Removing K⁺ by Dialysis

When renal function cannot eliminate sufficient K^+, dialysis therapy should be considered. The major indications for dialysis are ECG changes or a plasma $[K^+]$ that is very high and the anticipation of an ongoing shift of K^+ from cells. Hemodialysis is preferred to peritoneal dialysis because it is more efficient at removing K^+. Although there will be some variation because of characteristics of dialyzer membranes, differences in the $[K^+]$, and blood flow rates,

Emergency treatment of hyperkalemia

- If the QRS abnormality is significant, give 10 mL of 10% Ca^{2+} gluconate.
- Begin an infusion of 500 mL $D_{10}W$ that contains 10 units of regular insulin. If there is no heart failure, add 50 mmol of $NaHCO_3$, and run the infusion at 150–200 mL/h.
- If acidemia is present ($[HCO_3^-] <$ 15 mmol/L and no heart failure), give 50 mmol of $NaHCO_3$ intravenously over 5 minutes.
- Give 100 g of K^+-binding resin by enema.
- If there is renal failure, make plans for dialysis.
- If the patient has heart failure and is acidemic, consider phlebotomy to allow $NaHCO_3$ administration. HCl loss from the stomach can also be promoted (see page 160).

close to 30–50 mmol of K^+ per hour may be removed by hemodialysis and 15–25 mmol of K^+ per hour by peritoneal dialysis.

Apart from the dialysis membrane and the flow rate past this membrane, the major factor influencing the dialysis of K^+ is the $[K^+]$ gradient: the higher the plasma $[K^+]$ and the lower the bath $[K^+]$, the greater the rate of K^+ removal. Therefore, once dialysis is started, one should stop the glucose and insulin drip and reduce the bath glucose to minimize those forces moving K^+ into the ICF.

QUESTIONS

(Discussions on pages 480–481)

11.7 *Does aldosterone act only on the kidney and the ICF-ECF interface to lower the plasma $[K^+]$?*

11.8 *An otherwise healthy patient presents with hyperkalemia associated with mild ECF volume expansion and hypertension, metabolic acidosis with a normal plasma anion gap, and an unexpectedly low urine $[K^+]$. No drugs were taken. What is the lesion in this patient?*

11.9 *A patient has a severe degree of hyperkalemia and ECF volume contraction. A random urine sample has the following values: $[Na^+] = 3$ mmol/L, $[K^+] = 80$ mmol/L, $[Cl^-] = 23$ mmol/L. What should be done to increase the rate of excretion of K^+ promptly?*

PART C

Review

DISCUSSION OF INTRODUCTORY CASE
Lee's [K$^+$] Is on a High
(Case presented on page 448)

What factors contributed to hyperkalemia?

First, pseudohyperkalemia caused by a hemolyzed sample, thrombocytosis, or leukemia and excessive fist-clenching were ruled out. Second, because there is no indication that K^+ intake was excessive, hyperkalemia is probably due to a K^+ shift from the ICF and/or reduced K^+ excretion.

K^+ Shift from the ICF. There is no evidence of excessive destruction of cells, so a single or multiple hormone deficiency should be suspected if there is a major shift of K^+ from cells. Insulin deficiency is present; aldosterone deficiency is discussed later. In the setting of insulin plus aldosterone deficiencies, hyperglycemia exacerbates hyperkalemia. Because the metabolic acidosis was not ketoacidosis, as judged from the normal value for the plasma anion gap, the acidemia may have caused some K^+ to shift out of cells.

Reduced K$^+$ Excretion in the Urine. The GFR is not markedly reduced, and the urine volume is large, so aldosterone deficiency is possibly the cause of a low rate of K$^+$ excretion. All of the following could point to this diagnosis: Lee has ECF volume contraction but is losing Na$^+$ in the urine; the urine [K$^+$] is low (especially when correction is made for water abstraction in the medullary collecting duct); and the TTKG is in the range that suggests a low aldosterone bioactivity (see margin note). To determine if this low TTKG is due to low levels of aldosterone, a physiologic replacement dose of aldosterone (100 μg 9αF) should be given, and the TTKG should be measured. If the TTKG rises toward 10, an adrenal problem is likely; if it remains low, there is a prereceptor or postreceptor problem with the K$^+$ secretory process in Lee's CCD. Additional studies would then be needed.

TTKG
Assume that her plasma osmolality is 300 mOsm/kg H$_2$O for easy arithmetic. Her TTKG is 20/(600/300)/5.4 = close to 2; the expected value would be close to 10 with "perfect" kidneys and adrenals.

What additional information is needed to understand the relative importance of each factor?

When Lee received insulin, her blood glucose concentration fell to less than 180 mg/dL (10 mmol/L), but her plasma [K$^+$] fell to only 4.8 mmol/L.

When Lee received sufficient NaHCO$_3$ to bring the plasma [HCO$_3^-$] to normal, the plasma [K$^+$] fell to 4.3 mmol/L; nonetheless, the Na$^+$ load could have led to an increased renal K$^+$ excretion.

Osmotic diuresis
The glucose-induced osmotic diuresis could help to explain the natriuresis and the low TTKG.

Blood samples were drawn to measure aldosterone and renin. Because the results require several days, a physiologic dose of mineralocorticoids was administered. There was little change in the plasma and urine [K$^+$]. Thus, the major problem seems to be reduced K$^+$ excretion in the presence of normal concentrations of mineralocorticoids. The problem therefore lies in the kidney (the plasma renin and aldosterone levels were found to be high), and the final diagnosis is end-organ (kidney) hyporesponsiveness to aldosterone. One would then further characterize this defect by individually assessing the Na$^+$ and K$^+$ channels and the Cl$^-$ permeability in the CCD (see pages 381–386).

What initial therapy would be most appropriate?

Initial therapy should consist of a low K$^+$ intake, insulin for better glycemic control (and to shift K$^+$ into the ICF), NaHCO$_3$ to correct the metabolic acidosis (and to shift K$^+$ into the ICF), and saline to maintain a normal ECF volume. Because end-organ hyporesponsiveness to aldosterone may be transient, Lee needs to be observed closely.

Cases for Review

CASE 11.2
Ewe Too Can Avoid Hyperkalemia
(Case discussed on page 474)

Ewe, a female sheep, weighs 70 kg. She eats 800 mmol of K$^+$ daily but does not become hyperkalemic because she excretes 800 mmol of K$^+$ in her urine each day.

What quantity of K$^+$ can Ewe store in her cells if she does not change her acid-base status?

What renal mechanisms permit such a large excretion of K^+?

How might a gastric H^+/K^+ ATPase offer Ewe an advantage in excreting her dietary K^+ load?

What factors lead to the delivery of HCO_3^- to her CCD?

CASE 11.3
Channel Your Thoughts
(Case discussed on page 475)

Shirley, age 30 years, was referred by her family physician because the basis of her hypertension (150/110 mm Hg) could not be detected after an extensive work-up, including renal arteriography. The only value that was considered abnormal was a very mild degree of ECF volume contraction on physical examination and hyperkalemia (5.2 mmol/L). Laboratory data from the investigations are provided in the following table. Samples were obtained when Shirley was off all medications. The excretions of Na^+ and K^+ in a 24-hour urine sample (volume 1 L) were 150 and 53 mmol, respectively.

		Plasma	Random Urine Sample
Na^+	mmol/L	138	160
K^+	mmol/L	5.2	46
Cl^-	mmol/L	106	161
HCO_3^-	mmol/L	18	0
Urea	mmol/L (mg/dL)	4.3 (12)	—
Creatinine	μmol/L (mg/dL)	84 (0.9)	—
Albumin	g/L (g/dL)	40 (4.0)	—
Osmolality	mOsm/kg H_2O	285	606

Special Studies

1. The TTKG did not rise after the administration of $9\alpha F$.

2. Plasma renin was very elevated; it fell to normal with salt-loading. Plasma aldosterone levels moved in parallel.

3. In response to ECF volume contraction, the $[Na^+]$ and $[Cl^-]$ in the urine were 46 and 76 mmol/L, respectively.

What might be the pathophysiology of her hyperkalemia?

How might it be related to the hypertension?

What specific therapy might help ameliorate her hypertension and hyperkalemia?

CASE 11.4
Hyperkalemia After Renal Transplantation
(Case discussed on page 476)

Andrea, age 24 years, had a successful renal transplant. Postoperative medications included cyclosporine. On routine examination 6 months later, several abnormalities were detected. First, a mild degree of hypertension developed (a new finding). On laboratory investigation, there was a mild degree of hyperkalemia and metabolic acidosis with a normal plasma anion gap. The only other findings were a very low renin level and a normal value for aldosterone in plasma. There were no changes in K^+ excretion (or the TTKG) when aldosterone was given.

		Plasma	Random Urine Sample
Na^+	mmol/L	137	103
K^+	mmol/L	5.2	46
Cl^-	mmol/L	108	111
HCO_3^-	mmol/L	19	0
pH		7.35	5.1
Creatinine	μmol/L (mg/dL)	123 (1.4)	—
Osmolality	mOsm/kg H_2O	285	606

What is the most likely basis for the hyperkalemia?
What additional studies might help clarify this pathophysiology?
Why was metabolic acidosis present?

CASE 11.5
Treatment Threatens More Than the Protozoa
(Case discussed on page 477)

Pat has had AIDS for several years. He recently developed a nonproductive cough. Because the cough persisted and he developed chills and shortness of breath, he went to the emergency room. His blood pressure was 110/70, and his pulse was 86. The physical examination had normal results, except that he had crackles at both lung bases. His laboratory results were all normal (K^+ = 4.3 mmol/L and creatinine = 86 μmol/L). The chest x-ray showed bilateral interstitial infiltrates. The presumptive diagnosis was pneumocystis pneumonia, so he was started on trimethoprim (240 mg) and sulfamethoxazole (1200 mg) every 8 hours. Three days later, although his pneumonia was stable, his blood pressure fell to 90/70 when he was standing. His jugular venous pulse was not visible. His laboratory results on day 3 are listed in the following table. Because his 24-hour urine volume was 0.8 L, his osmole excretion rate was somewhat low, 480 mOsm/day.

		Plasma	Random Urine Sample
Na^+	mmol/L	131	82
K^+	mmol/L	5.6	18
Cl^-	mmol/L	99	77
HCO_3^-	mmol/L	21	0
pH		7.35	5.1
Creatinine	μmol/L (mg/dL)	111 (1.3)	—
Osmolality	mOsm/kg H_2O	268	577

Why has hyperkalemia developed?
What is the most likely intrarenal defect?
How could one deduce that a nonrenal factor contributed to the degree of his hyperkalemia?
In what ways will an infusion of saline help correct his hyperkalemia?

Discussion of Cases

DISCUSSION OF CASE 11.1
Severe Degree of Hyperkalemia with a GI Upset
(Case presented on page 460)

What emergencies need immediate management, and what should you administer?

1. **Hyperkalemia**: Because of the ECG changes and the very high plasma [K^+], this is an emergency. For its therapy, the authors would infuse calcium gluconate, administer insulin with enough glucose to avoid hypoglycemia, and give 50 mmol $NaHCO_3$ because of the severity of the hyperkalemia.
2. **The very low ECF volume**: For therapy, we would infuse 1 L of isotonic saline over 30 minutes and another liter over 60 minutes if she still had evidence of ECF volume (and "effective" vascular volume) contraction. Further therapy will depend on the response to this initial treatment. Other measures were needed and are discussed below.

Why did such a severe degree of hyperkalemia develop?

As the patient did not ingest a large amount of K^+, the major reason for her hyperkalemia is a shift of K^+ out of cells. Factors that could be responsible are a lack of insulin (due to an α-adrenergic response to her low ECF volume), the α-adrenergic response itself, a mild degree of metabolic acidosis, cell necrosis if present, and the catabolic response to her GI illness.

All of these together are not sufficient to explain her severe degree of hyperkalemia. Part of the rise could have been due to pseudohyperkalemia (ruled out with additional blood tests and remember the ECG abnormalities). There are two other factors to explain her severe degree of hyperkalemia: first, because she was hyperkalemic to begin with, she probably had more K^+ than normal in her cells, which permitted these reasons for a K^+ shift to cause a more severe degree of hyperkalemia; second, she may not have been able to excrete as much of the K^+ that shifted out of her cells as would occur with a normal kidney.

Why did her ECF volume become so contracted following this acute GI episode?

Although there was a loss of Na^+ by the GI tract (diarrhea), given her history and the very small decline in her plasma [HCO_3^-], there seems to be another factor operating. That factor is renal Na^+ wasting, because her urine had a very high [Na^+] and [Cl^-] despite a contracted ECF volume. Hence, the authors would look for a lack of aldosterone or an agent that blocks its actions or inhibits the ENaC, like amiloride or trimethoprim. No exogenous agent was present, so adrenal insufficiency was suspected.

Follow-up studies:

Cortisol levels in plasma were low and failed to rise with ACTH, so adrenal insufficiency was the presumptive diagnosis. The acute exacerbation was presumed to be due to her acute gastroenteritis. Data on aldosterone levels were sent, but results have not been provided. Nevertheless, think about her hypertension and hyperkalemia. She was given replacement therapy for adrenal insufficiency and was asked to return in 2 weeks (after being off her medication for 24 hours) for diagnostic studies.

At the level of the luminal membrane of her CCD, what is the most likely explanation for her electrolyte disorder at the time of admission?

1. **Rate of excretion of K^+**: This is very low as judged by the K^+/creatinine ratio in her urine (expected values would be 40 mmol K/mmol creatinine or 400 mmol/g creatinine with a normal renal response to a K^+ load).

2. **Components of K^+ excretion**:
   Flow rate in the CCD: This is modestly low because her rate of excretion of osmoles is somewhat less than 600 mOsm/day as judged from her osmole/creatinine ratio. This contributes to, but does not totally account for, her low rate of excretion of K^+.
   [K^+] in the CCD: The expected value for her TTKG is 10, but the observed value is very low, less than 2 (urine [K^+] 30 mmol/L/plasma [K^+] of 9.2 mmol/L, and the urine osmolality is more than double that of plasma).

3. **Channel analysis**: The combination of a very low TTKG and evidence for renal Na^+ wasting makes the likely diagnosis "slower" Na^+ rather than "faster" Cl^- reabsorption in the CCD as the basis for the less negative transepithelial voltage in the CCD.

4. **Causes for "slower" Na^+ reabsorption in the CCD**: In the absence of drugs that inhibit ENaC and the very unlikely presence of an inborn error in the ENaC, the authors strongly suspected a deficiency of aldosterone.

Diagnostic studies:

Two weeks after her acute episode, she returned for additional testing off her medications. Her plasma aldosterone results on the original admission were available and they were below the lower limit of normal. Now her physical examination results were normal.

She was given a physiologic replacement dose of a mineralocorticoid (100 µg of an α-fludrocortisone), and the following values were obtained in her urine.

			Urine	
		Plasma	**Before 9αF**	**After 9αF**
Na^+	mmol/L	136	130	181
K^+	mmol/L	6.2	25	42
Cl^-	mmol/L	106	128	156
HCO_3^-	mmol/L	18	0	0
Osmolality	mOsm/kg H_2O	285	521	629
TTKG		—	2	3
Renin		Very low	—	—

Does she have an adrenal and/or a renal problem responsible for her hyperkalemia? What other tests are essential?

Discussion of diagnostic studies:

The fact that her TTKG was so low after $9\alpha F$ suggests that her tubules do not respond to a mineralocorticoid with respect to its kaliuretic actions. At the channel level, the absence of a low ECF volume and the very low renin suggest that her hyperkalemia now is a "faster" Cl^- reabsorption in the CCD. The basis for this is not known, but it could help explain why she has hypertension. She has a normal plasma Mg^{2+} level. Future studies will be performed.

DISCUSSION OF CASE 11.2
Ewe Too Can Avoid Hyperkalemia
(Case presented on page 469)

What quantity of K^+ can Ewe store in her cells if she does not change her acid-base status?

If Ewe wanted to shift K^+ into cells and could neither generate new organic phosphate esters (RNA, DNA, etc.) nor change the $[H^+]$, the only way for K^+ to enter her cells is if Na^+ exit. Because the ICF of a 70-kg adult contains close to 300 mmol of Na^+ (10 mmol/$l \times 30$ L), this amount sets the maximum for net entry of K^+ into cells (one meal's worth). This limit underscores the need for Ewe to have a rapid rate of excretion of K^+.

What renal mechanisms permit such a large excretion of K^+?

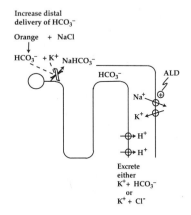

Increase distal
delivery of HCO_3^-

Orange + NaCl

$HCO_3^- + K^+$ $NaHCO_3^-$

HCO_3^- ALD

Na^+

K^+

H^+

H^+

Excrete
either
$K^+ + HCO_3^-$
or
$K^+ + Cl^-$

To have a rapid rate of excretion of K^+, there must be a large volume delivered to the terminal CCD (many osmoles) and a very high $[K^+]$ in the lumen of the CCD. With regard to the former, sheep excrete threefold to fourfold more osmoles than do humans (half are urea). With regard to the latter, the $[K^+]$ in the CCD is higher because aldosterone is present from the K^+ load, and bicarbonaturia is always present (the major anions accompanying K^+ in the diet are organic anions, which are ultimately metabolized and yield HCO_3^- as a product; see the following as well).

How might a gastric $H^+/K^+ATPase$ offer Ewe an advantage in excreting her dietary K^+ load?

To excrete K^+ rapidly, one must ensure that HCO_3^- are delivered to the lumen of the terminal CCD and that aldosterone is present. If H^+ are secreted in conjunction with gastric reabsorption of luminal K^+, the net effect will be the addition of K^+ and HCO_3^- to the venous blood leaving the stomach (see Figure 4.1). Thus, the sheep need not depend on very rapid metabolism of the dietary organic anions to yield HCO_3^-. An advantage of bicarbonaturia is the initiation of a high rate of kaliuresis.

What factors lead to the delivery of HCO_3^- to her CCD?

For a high $[K^+]$ in the lumen of the CCD, one needs a high

[HCO$_3^-$] in the luminal fluid and a high level of aldosterone in plasma. To have a high [HCO$_3^-$] in the CCD, more HCO$_3^-$ must be filtered and/or less must be reabsorbed. Reabsorption of HCO$_3^-$ in the proximal tubule is inhibited mainly by ECF volume expansion (low angiotensin II) and hyperkalemia (possibly via ICF alkalemia). The overall effect of providing K$^+$ and HCO$_3^-$ to the body is that together they augment the delivery of HCO$_3^-$ to the CCD by the following mechanisms: the alkalemia should depress the indirect reabsorption of filtered HCO$_3^-$ in the PCT; a higher plasma [K$^+$] also depresses this reabsorption and ensures delivery of Na$^+$ and HCO$_3^-$ to the CCD. In the presence of aldosterone actions, there will be a very high TTKG (close to 20). HCO$_3^-$ can still be reabsorbed in the MCD if stimulated by a fall in the plasma [HCO$_3^-$] because there are many H$^+$ATPase pumps in this nephron segment.

DISCUSSION OF CASE 11.3
Channel Your Thoughts
(Case presented on page 470)

What might be the pathophysiology of her hyperkalemia?

Because long-term homeostasis for K$^+$ is maintained by regulation of renal excretion, the first step is to assess the renal response to hyperkalemia. The expected value for the rate of excretion of K$^+$ with hyperkalemia and normal kidneys is the excretion of several hundred mmol/day; 24-hour K$^+$ excretion in Shirley was only 53 mmol/day. Because K$^+$ excretion is the product of the [K$^+$] and the volume of urine, there are two major components that could be responsible for her low rate of excretion of K$^+$: a low volume of urine or a decreased ability to raise the [K$^+$] (reduced K$^+$ secretion in the CCD).

Volume in the CCD. The volume of urine and osmole excretion rate were not particularly low; therefore, the problem must be a low [K$^+$] in the CCD.

TTKG. The measured value of the TTKG was 4.2 (see margin note), much lower than the expected value of 10. This low TTKG may indicate the lack of a stimulator, the presence of an inhibitor, or an intrinsic defect in the K$^+$ secretory process. The latter seems to be the case because the TTKG failed to rise in response to 9αF. Moreover, the levels of renin and aldosterone in her plasma were elevated. Therefore, lack of mineralocorticoids was not the cause of hyperkalemia with a low TTKG.

Authors' Approach. The subnormal kaliuretic response to hyperkalemia and the tubular insensitivity to aldosterone may result from low delivery of Na$^+$ to the CCD, low open probability of the Na$^+$ or K$^+$ conductive pathways, or high permeability to Cl$^-$ in the CCD (see Figure 11.2).

Less Availability of Na$^+$. In the rat, the [Na$^+$] required for half-maximal rates of K$^+$ secretion in the CCD is 10–15 mmol/L. Because Shirley had a much higher [Na$^+$] in her urine and because some Na$^+$ are normally reabsorbed in the MCD, reduced delivery of Na$^+$ to the CCD was very unlikely to limit her K$^+$ secretory system.

Note
See page 449 for a flow chart on causes of hyperkalemia with low excretion of K$^+$.

Note
TTKG =
    46/(606/285)/5.2
    = 4.2

High Permeability to Cl⁻ in the CCD. Failure to generate a favorable transepithelial potential difference (TEPD) in the CCD because of increased "permeability" to Cl⁻ in the CCD, the so-called "Cl⁻-shunt disorder" has been postulated as one lesion that could cause hypertension, hyperkalemia, low levels of renin, and a low rate of excretion of K⁺ in a patient with a normal GFR. The shunting of Cl⁻ when Na⁺ are reabsorbed (electroneutral reabsorption of NaCl) leads to ECF volume expansion and suppression of the renin-angiotensin-aldosterone system. These features were not present in Shirley.

Low Na⁺ Channel Activity in the CCD. The mild degree of contraction of the ECF volume on clinical examination, the presence of high renin and aldosterone, and the high concentrations of Na⁺ and Cl⁻ in urine suggest this pathophysiology for the hyperkalemia and the tubular insensitivity to mineralocorticoids in Shirley. Failure to reabsorb Na⁺ in the CCD could diminish the TEPD in the CCD and thereby reduce the driving force to secrete K⁺. Moreover, this wasting of Na⁺ could lead to a degree of contraction of the ECF volume, which would in turn stimulate the release of renin and aldosterone; all are consistent with Shirley's case.

How might it be related to the hypertension?

A second lesion is necessary to explain the presence of hypertension. Not only does Shirley need high levels of vasoconstrictors, but there must also be an increase in sensitivity to these agents to produce hypertension because the ECF volume is contracted.

If her hypertension is due to the ECF volume contraction, salt-loading would decrease the levels of vasoconstrictors and benefit her blood pressure.

What specific therapy might help ameliorate her hypertension and hyperkalemia?

There are two therapeutic options with respect to the hyperkalemia. One is to increase the urine flow rate; if the TTKG does not change, excretion of K⁺ will rise. A diet high in NaCl will not only increase the flow rate, but will also reexpand the ECF volume. The other strategy is to try to increase the TTKG by causing bicarbonaturia (Na⁺ load with NaHCO₃) to reduce Cl⁻ reabsorption.

One also can maintain her on a low-K⁺ diet.

DISCUSSION OF CASE 11.4
Hyperkalemia After Renal Transplantation
(Case presented on page 470)

What is the most likely basis for the hyperkalemia?

Chronic hyperkalemia is due, at least in part, to a low excretion of K⁺. The basis for the low excretion was an unexpectedly low TTKG (close to 4; see margin note). The components of K⁺ excretion indicate that there was a reasonable urine volume and osmole excretion rate (see margin note), and Na⁺ delivery was not rate-limiting for K⁺ excretion, as judged by the urine [Na⁺]. One

Note
An infusion of 1 L of isotonic saline caused a prompt fall in her blood pressure to normal levels.

TTKG
[K⁺] in urine (46)
÷ (U/P)ₒₛₘ (606/285)
÷ [K⁺] in plasma (5.2)
= 4

Volume to the CCD
= Uₒₛₘ (606) × urine volume (1 L)
÷ Pₒₛₘ 285
= More than 2 L to the terminal CCD per day.

possible explanation is a low open probability for the Na^+ channel, but this basis for the hyperkalemia is unlikely because renin level was low, not high. This constellation suggested that a so-called Cl^- shunt is a good option as a diagnosis.

What additional studies might help clarify this pathophysiology?

A Cl^- shunt seems to respond to bicarbonaturia or a protocol that lowers the $[Cl^-]$ in the CCD. The TTKG rose with bicarbonaturia; it also rose with Cl^--free urine. One would expect to see the excretion of urine with little Na^+ and Cl^- when a deficit of NaCl is present.

Why was metabolic acidosis present?

The urine net charge was positive (more Na^+ + K^+ than Cl^-), which suggests a low rate of excretion of NH_4^+ (confirmed later by direct measurements). The acidosis and low NH_4^+ excretion were no longer evident when normokalemia was present, so the basis for the low NH_4^+ excretion was hyperkalemia (see the discussion of Question 1.24).

DISCUSSION OF CASE 11.5
Treatment Threatens More Than the Protozoa
(Case presented on page 471)

Why has hyperkalemia developed?

Because this development of hyperkalemia is acute, one should begin by considering two initial events: first, there may be a greater input of K^+ from the diet, cell lysis, or a shift of K^+ from the ICF (e.g., lack of insulin); or second, there may be a decreased rate of excretion of K^+. A low flow in the CCD raises the probability of a low osmolar load (e.g., anorexia and/or a very low GFR). The very low TTKG suggests that the low $[K^+]$ in the urine is important.

TTKG
$[K^+]$ in urine (18)
   $\div$ (U/P)$_{osm}$ (577/268)
   $\div$ $[K^+]$ in plasma (5.6)
= 1.5

What is the most likely intrarenal defect?

1. **$[K^+]$ vs flow rate**: The excretion of K^+ is the product of the $[K^+]$ in the urine and the urine flow rate. Translating these events to the CCD reveals a somewhat reduced volume (excretion of 480 mOsm) but a $[K^+]$ that is much lower than expected (TTKG of 1.5 vs the expected value of 10; see margin note). The low flow rate is due to the low protein intake, which leads to low urea formation (catabolism does not result in as much protein oxidation as does oxidation of the usual dietary intake of protein).

2. **Renal vs prerenal cause for low TTKG**: Because hypoaldosteronism may be present (low ECF volume), a physiologic dose of aldosterone was given; 2 hours after receiving 100 μg of $9\alpha F$, the TTKG did not rise in freshly voided urine. Hypoaldosteronism, if present, is therefore not the sole cause of the low TTKG.

3. **Channel analysis in the CCD**: A low TTKG in this setting implies either an abnormally low flux via the Na^+ channel or

Note
Another possible, but unlikely, mechanism is a lower conductance for K^+ in the CCD.

increased permeability to Cl^- in the luminal membrane of the CCD. The low ECF volume with renal Na^+ wasting is more consistent with an Na^+ channel problem than with a Cl^- permeability issue, which would be associated with ECF volume expansion.

4. **Inhibition of Na^+ channels**: Aside from low levels of aldosterone, drugs that are cationic, such as amiloride, inhibit Na^+ channel flux. Pat was taking trimethoprim, an antimicrobial that bears a positively charged amine that can act like amiloride. Later, his renin and aldosterone results were reported, and both were elevated.

There is an emergency measure that one can take to make trimethoprim (TMP) inactive in the urine while maintaining its antimicrobial actions in the body. If the active form of TMP is its cationic form, cationic (TMP^+) can be converted to its electroneutral form (TMP^0) by lowering the $[H^+]$ in the urine (raise the urine pH). This can be achieved by administering $NaHCO_3$ to lower the $[H^+]$ in the urine in the following equation.

$$H^+ + TMP^0 \longleftrightarrow TMP^+$$

The pK for TMP is 7.2, and this is in an appropriate range for this therapeutic intervention. In contrast, raising the urine pH cannot have the same effect on pentamidine because its pK is close to 10 (pentamidine is a drug that has the same complications as TMP^+).

How could one deduce that a nonrenal factor contributed to the degree of his hyperkalemia?

The usual amount of K^+ that must be retained in an adult to achieve a high plasma $[K^+]$ is many hundred millimoles. Because the patient was not consuming large amounts of K^+-rich foods (see Table 10.2), one could deduce that there was a large shift of K^+ from his ICF. Possible contributing factors are the non–anion gap type of metabolic acidosis, necrosis of cells, and a lack of insulin. Perhaps an α-adrenergic effect (due to the low ECF volume) is inhibiting β cells in his pancreas from releasing insulin appropriately.

In what ways will an infusion of saline help correct his hyperkalemia?

There are several ways:
1. **Shift K^+ into cells**: This can help by restoring the ECF volume and thereby removing the stimulus for his α-adrenergic response.
2. **Make TMP a less effective blocker of the ENaC in the CCD**: There are two possibilities here. First, expansion of the ECF volume can depress proximal reabsorption of HCO_3^-, leading to more distal delivery of HCO_3^-, which could help raise the $[K^+]$ in the lumen of the CCD. Second, by having a higher volume traverse the CCD, the $[TMP^+]$ will fall owing to the same amount of this agent dissolved in a larger volume.
3. **Higher flow rate in the CCD**: Having more osmoles when ADH acts will result in a higher flow rate in the CCD and thereby more excretion of K^+.

Summary of Main Points

- Hyperkalemia is an important electrolyte disorder because it predisposes the patient to potentially lethal cardiac arrhythmias.
- Although intake and shift of K^+ from the ICF may contribute to hyperkalemia, reduced excretion of K^+ in the urine is virtually always present in chronic hyperkalemia.
- An unexpectedly low rate of excretion of K^+ implies either a low flow rate in the CCD (low osmole excretion rate) or, more commonly, a low $[K^+]$ in the luminal fluid of the CCD.
- The major causes of a low $[K^+]$ in the luminal fluid of the CCD are an Na^+ channel with a low open probability (e.g., low aldosterone bioactivity or drugs such as amiloride, trimethoprim, or pentamidine) or a Cl^--shunt type of disorder. Evaluating the ECF volume, the ability to excrete an Na^+-free and Cl^--free urine with salt restriction, and the TTKG after mineralocorticoid administration helps in the resolution of the differential diagnosis.
- In an emergency, the adverse cardiac effects of hyperkalemia can be attenuated by infusing Ca^{2+} salts. This infusion can be followed by measures to shift K^+ into cells (insulin, $NaHCO_3$). Longer-term strategies include dietary restriction of K^+, binding of K^+ in the GI tract with resins, and/or promoting the excretion of K^+ by increasing the flow rate (loop diuretics) or $[K^+]$ (aldosterone, bicarbonaturia). The specific choice of these strategies depends on the type of lesion that is present.

Discussion of Questions

11.1 What is the total K^+ content in the platelets of 1 L of blood? (Assume 400,000 cells/mm³, a 150 mmol/L $[K^+]$ in the ICF, and a platelet volume of 1 μ³.)

The platelet count in normal blood is 4×10^5 cells/mm³, which is equivalent to 4×10^{11} cells per liter (1 cm³ = 1 mL).

If the volume of an individual platelet is 1 μ³ (equal to 1×10^{-15} L), the total platelet ICF volume is the product of these two numbers, or 4×10^{-4} L.

The $[K^+]$ in the ICF of a platelet was given as 150 mmol/L, so the total K^+ content of platelets is 150 mmol $\times 4 \times 10^{-4}$ L, or 6×10^{-2} mmol. If lysed, the rise in the $[K^+]$ would be only 0.06 mmol/L.

To get an appreciable rise in the plasma $[K^+]$ from the platelet disruption, the platelets must be increased considerably in volume; a change in the platelet number is much less important.

11.2 What sets the limit on K^+ uptake into cells?

When a K^+ enters a cell, either an anion must enter or a cation (Na^+ or H^+) must exit to maintain electroneutrality. Because there is a limit to the synthesis of new intracellular anions, and because the major anion available to enter is a Cl^- and it primarily has an ECF distribution, an exit of Na^+ or H^+ sets the limit on K^+ entry in an acute setting. The total quantity of Na^+ that can exit is equal to the Na^+ content in the ICF (300 mmol in a 70-kg adult; i.e., 10 mmol/L $\times$ 30 L of ICF). The $[H^+]$ gradient across cells and the content of HCO_3^- in the ECF (375 mmol) set the upper limit on a countermovement of K^+ for H^+.

11.3 How might β-blockers cause a severe degree of hyperkalemia?

There are several settings in which it is important to have the "K^+-shift defense" operating at its greatest efficiency (for example, following heavy physical exercise, when trauma causes cell necrosis, after a large K^+ intake, during renal failure, in insulin plus aldosterone deficiencies, and after surgery); β-blockade at these times may cause severe hyperkalemia.

11.4 What happens to the plasma [K⁺] during exercise?

The plasma $[K^+]$ may rise by several mmol/L following exhausting exercise. Although all the mechanisms are not clearly defined, the most likely cause is depolarization of muscle cells, which yields a high interstitial $[K^+]$ that is washed into the circulation (i.e., K^+ are not restricted to the T tubules). Cell damage (muscle, red blood cells mechanically ruptured by persistent pressure on the soles of the feet) may make a small contribution to this rise. In exercise, the hyperkalemia is particularly well tolerated by the otherwise normal subject, and its duration is short-lived. $β_2$-Adrenergic activity helps in minimizing the degree and the duration of the hyperkalemia.

Note
- A deficiency in carnitine palmitoyltransferase (i.e., a diminished ability to oxidize fatty acids and therefore an increased sensitivity to carbohydrate deprivation) is an example of a disease with a problem regenerating ATP.
- There are important K^+ channels that are regulated by ATP.

11.5 Why do patients with a problem regenerating ATP in muscle cells suffer from weakness but not hyperkalemia?

This is not known, but hyperkalemia is not generally observed. If these patients lack ATP, the $Na^+K^+ATPase$ should stop pumping ions. Because these patients do not become hyperkalemic, they probably have markedly reduced K^+ conductance in their cell membranes.

11.6 How much of a K⁺ load might a patient receive if 1 L of blood is digested in the GI tract in the course of a GI bleed?

One liter of blood has only 0.4 L of red blood cells. The $[K^+]$ in the ICF is as high as 150 mmol/L; therefore, the quantity of K^+ released is only 60 mmol/L of blood ingested. The plasma contains another 2.4 mmol (0.6 L $\times$ 4 mmol/L).

11.7 Does aldosterone act only on the kidney and the ICF-ECF interface to lower the plasma [K⁺]?

No. Aldosterone also acts on the colon to promote fecal K^+ loss, but this loss is only quantitatively important in patients with chronic renal failure, in whom almost half of the daily K^+ load is excreted in this manner.

The mechanisms involved in gastrointestinal K^+ loss are analogous to those in the cortical distal nephron. In addition, glucocorticoids promote K^+ loss via the colon.

Aldosterone also promotes the loss of K^+ in sweat. This loss can become important in athletes who train in hot environments.

11.8 An otherwise healthy patient presents with hyperkalemia associated with mild ECF volume expansion and hypertension, metabolic acidosis with a normal plasma anion gap, and an unexpectedly low urine $[K^+]$. No drugs were taken. What is the lesion in this patient?

Hyperkalemia should lead to aldosterone release and enhanced K^+ excretion. These changes did not occur. Therefore, aldosterone is either absent or not working. The absence of aldosterone as a primary lesion would lead to Na^+ loss and ECF volume contraction. This patient does not have a typical aldosterone deficiency because the ECF volume is expanded.

If aldosterone is present and is preventing Na^+ loss, why does it not lead to K^+ loss? Recall that a major action of aldosterone is to promote Na^+ reabsorption in the CCD (it opens the Na^+ channels). In this case, if the accompanying anions (Cl^-) were reabsorbed in parallel, there would not be a luminal negative voltage, and there would be little secretion of K^+ and H^+; the low secretion of H^+ (together with hyperkalemia-induced inhibition of NH_4^+ excretion) could cause the metabolic acidosis. The lesion is very likely a "Cl^--shunt disorder." It is also possible that there is a very low conductance for K^+ in the CCD; this will cause hyperkalemia, but it should not directly lead to NaCl retention. Perhaps the negative lumen voltage would increase the reabsorption of Cl^- in the CCD.

Note
See page 449 for a flow chart on causes of hyperkalemia with low excretion of K^+.

11.9 A patient has a severe degree of hyperkalemia and ECF volume contraction. A random urine sample has the following values: $[Na^+] = 3$ mmol/L, $[K^+] = 80$ mmol/L, $[Cl^-] = 23$ mmol/L. What should be done to increase the rate of excretion of K^+ promptly?

There is little leverage to raise the $[K^+]$ in the urine further by giving mineralocorticoids (you may be able to raise it twofold if the urine osmolality is now 1200 mOsm/kg H_2O). A better strategy is to raise the urine flow rate with a loop diuretic, which should increase the rate of excretion of K^+ considerably. Of course, NaCl must be infused more rapidly than it is excreted to result in reexpansion of the ECF volume.

Hyperglycemia

OBJECTIVES

☐ To explain why a severe degree of hyperglycemia develops.

☐ To explain how hyperglycemia causes a shift of water across cell membranes and an osmotic diuresis and why hyperglycemia is often associated with catabolism of lean body mass.

☐ To provide the rationale for designing appropriate intravenous therapy for a patient with a severe degree of hyperglycemia.

☐ To demonstrate in a quantitative fashion the factors that determine the fall in the concentration of glucose that occurs during treatment of a patient with a severe degree of hyperglycemia.

Outline of Major Principles

1. Hyperglycemia requires a relative lack of insulin or a resistance to the actions of insulin.

2. When considering a high concentration of any substance in plasma, one should analyze its rate of input and output independently. A severe degree of hyperglycemia usually requires a low output of glucose, including a low glomerular filtration rate (GFR). On occasion, there may be an excessive intake of glucose and little reduction in the GFR.

3. The concentration of glucose in plasma will decline early during therapy, primarily as a result of dilution by administered fluid and by glucosuria. Metabolism of glucose is a minor pathway for the removal of glucose at this time.

4. The actions of insulin become important in lowering the blood glucose level many hours after administration of this hormone.

5. The major short-term complications of hyperglycemia are shifts of water across cell membranes and losses of Na^+ and K^+ via osmotic diuresis.

Note
To describe the actions of low net insulin more completely, the authors include both the low levels of insulin and high levels of glucagon, the normal hormonal responses to fasting with hypoglycemia. For full ketoacid production, a low insulin level and a high glucagon level are required.

INTRODUCTORY CASE
Terry Is Confused
(Case discussed on page 504)

Terry, age 72 years, has had noninsulin-dependent diabetes mellitus

TABLE 12.1 **Terry's Values on Admission**

The urine output was very low on admission.

		Normal	**Terry**
Na^+	mmol/L	140	126
K^+	mmol/L	4.0	4.1
Cl^-	mmol/L	103	82
HCO_3^-	mmol/L	25	25
pH		7.40	7.40
$[H^+]$	nmol/L	40	40
P_aCO_2	mm Hg	40	40
Glucose	mmol/L (mg/dL)	4 (72)	50 (900)
Creatinine	μmol/L (mg/dL)	80 (0.9)	200 (2.3)
Urea	mmol/L (mg/dL)	4 (11)	20 (56)

(NIDDM) for the past 10 years; since she lost weight, her diabetes has been under reasonable control. Two weeks ago, her physician prescribed a thiazide diuretic to treat hypertension (160/95 mm Hg). Since she began taking this medication, Terry has not felt well, her urine output has increased, thirst has become prominent (she has been drinking a large quantity of apple juice) and, more recently, she has become lightheaded when standing. Today, Terry's daughter found her quite confused. In the hospital the two principal new findings are confusion and a marked degree of extracellular fluid (ECF) volume contraction (her blood pressure is now 130/60 mm Hg).

Laboratory results (summarized in Table 12.1) reveal a marked degree of hyperglycemia, hyponatremia, and a high value for creatinine in plasma.

> What is the basis for her severe degree of hyperglycemia?
> Why does Terry have hyponatremia?
> What is the appropriate therapy?
> Why will the concentration of glucose fall during therapy?

PART A

General Approach to a Severe Degree of Hyperglycemia

- A very high concentration of glucose indicates a low GFR and possibly a high input of glucose.
- A large change in the concentration of glucose can occur rapidly because its pool size is small and the rate at which it is consumed can be very rapid.

Background

It is beyond the scope of this text to describe the normal metabolism of glucose in any detail. Nevertheless, the following points should serve as a review.

Fuel oxidation in the brain
Because fatty acids cannot cross the blood-brain barrier at a significant rate, fatty acids are never an important fuel for the brain. The brain can burn only two fuels: the first is ketoacids if they are present, and the second is glucose. When the levels of ketoacids and glucose fall (in response to the actions of insulin), the brain will have insufficient fuel for its needs.

TABLE 12.2 **Degree of Hyperglycemia and Its Clinical Significance**

| Concentration of Glucose | | Clinical Significance |
mmol/L	mg/dL	
3–3.5	55–65	Normal fasted state
4–8	70–140	Normal fed state
10–15	180–270	Relative insulin deficiency
>25	>390	Relative lack of insulin plus a low GFR, and/or possibly a very large intake of glucose

1. In normal metabolism, glucose is very important because it is the principal fuel for the central nervous system (CNS). Only when individuals do not eat might the supply of glucose be inadequate to meet this demand (Table 12.2); in this setting, the brain oxidizes ketoacids.

2. Outside the CNS (see margin note), there is a *hierarchy of fuel oxidation*: fatty acids, if present, are the preferred fuel to oxidize, then ketoacids; if neither fatty acids nor ketoacids are available, glucose can be oxidized. The basis for this hierarchy is that pyruvate dehydrogenase (PDH), the highly regulated enzyme that controls the oxidation of glucose, is inhibited by acetyl-CoA, NADH, and adenosine triphosphate (ATP), the products of the oxidation of fatty acids or ketoacids (Figure 12.1). A lack of insulin or a resistance to its actions makes fatty acids or ketoacids available for oxidation.

3. A mild degree of hyperglycemia is the result of a lack of insulin. A severe degree of hyperglycemia requires either an extraordinarily large intake of glucose or, much more commonly, a low excretion of glucose because the GFR is so low.

Hierarchy of fuel oxidation
The hierarchy depends on which fuel generates acetyl-CoA, the substrate for the TCA cycle. When acetyl-CoA is formed from fat-derived fuels, this intermediate cannot be formed from carbohydrates or proteins.

Quantitative Aspects

The approach to an abnormal concentration of a metabolite (glucose in this case) requires an analysis of two factors, its rate of input and

Note
This figure is an oversimplification. It depicts events in the liver (synthesis of glucose, glycogen, and fatty acids) with events in nonhepatic organs (oxidation of ketoacids).

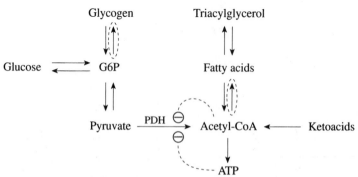

Figure 12.1 Hyperglycemia caused by limited metabolism of glucose. For oxidation, the critical fact is that acetyl-CoA, NADH (not shown), and ATP, the products of fatty acid or ketoacid oxidation, inhibit PDH. The enzyme pathways in the hatched ovals are active only when levels of insulin are high (levels of glucagon are low).

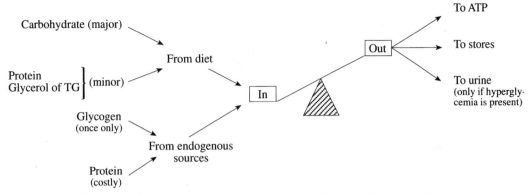

Figure 12.2   Analysis of the input and output of glucose. Balance in any compartment is a function of the rates of input versus output. The sources for glucose are illustrated on the left side of this figure. (TG = triacylglycerol.)

its rate of output (Figure 12.2). The quantity of glucose in the body is very small relative to the amount of glucose consumed and oxidized each day (Figure 12.3).

Pool Size of Glucose

> • Glucose is distributed in 50% of total body water.
> • The pool of glucose is close to 100 mmol, or 18 g.

To calculate the amount of glucose in the body, one must consider the following facts: the volume of distribution of glucose is the ECF plus the intracellular fluid (ICF) of organs that do not require insulin to transport glucose across their cell membranes (most organs other than skeletal muscle; see margin note). In the ECF, the concentration of glucose is normally close to 5 mmol/L, or 100 mg/dL (1 g/L), for easy arithmetic. Therefore, the body contains close to 100 mmol (18 g) of glucose (see margin note).

Quantity of Glucose Oxidized Each Day

A normal adult consumes close to 1500 mmol (270 g) of carbohydrate each day (see Figure 12.3). In addition, glucose is synthesized during the metabolism of proteins (333 mmol, or 60 g) and triglycerides (glycerol of dietary origin can yield close to 100 mmol, or about 18 g, of glucose). In this example, balance is maintained, so a net of 1933 mmol of glucose must be removed directly or indirectly each day.

How Much Glucose Is Stored as Glycogen?

> • The size of the pool of glycogen in the liver is only 600 mmol (100 g).
> • Liver glycogen can provide glucose on a "one time only" basis.
> • The synthesis of glycogen will be slow when insulin is given to a patient with chronic, severe hyperglycemia.
> • For the most part, glycogen in muscle (2500 mmol, 450 g) cannot be converted directly to glucose.

Clinical pearl
Extremely sensitive controls maintain a tiny pool of glucose in the body despite a high flux of glucose through the body. If these controls do not operate properly, hyperglycemia will develop and may do so rapidly.

Volumes in a 70-kg adult
• Total body water: close to 45 L
• ECF: 15 L
• ICF where glucose distributes: 4–5 L
• Concentration of glucose = 5 mmol/L.
• Volume of distribution is the ECF (15 L) plus 5 L of ICF.
• 5 mmol/L × 20 L = 100 mmol.

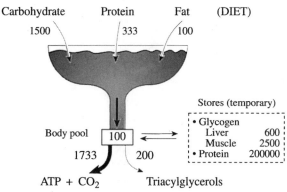

Figure 12.3   Glucose content vs turnover of glucose. The pool of glucose in the body (represented by the solid rectangle) is very small relative to the turnover of glucose each day. Conversion of endogenous protein to glucose is not rapid compared with the production of glucose from dietary sources. All the numbers are in millimoles of glucose; multiply by 0.18 to convert to grams.

Note
The daily input (and output in balance) of glucose exceeds the pool size of glucose by close to 20-fold

Liver

The liver in a 70-kg adult can store about 600 mmol (100 g) of glucose; this store can empty quickly under the catabolic signals of a lack of insulin and high levels of glucagon (called *"low net insulin"*, see margin note).

Conversion of glucose to glycogen is rapid if a person is exposed chronically to high net insulin signals; if, however, the net insulin levels are low and then raised abruptly, as in a patient with diabetes mellitus in poor control, conversion to glycogen will be very slow.

Net insulin
The combined effects of insulin and glucagon. "Low net insulin" refers to low levels of insulin and high levels of glucagon. "High net insulin" indicates high levels of insulin and low levels of glucagon.

Conversion of glucose to glycogen
Two major types of change occur in the presence of insulin: rapid change in the levels of activators and inhibitors of enzymes, and slower change involving the number of enzyme molecules. This latter type of change requires the synthesis of new proteins, a process that may require a period of hours. This delay is the major reason why the administration of insulin to a patient with hyperglycemic hyperosmolar syndrome does not lead to a prompt fall in glycemia.

Muscle

Large amounts of glucose (2500 mmol, or 450 g) are also stored as glycogen in skeletal muscle. Synthesis here requires high net insulin levels and, for rates to be rapid, there must be longer periods of exposure to high net insulin levels. Breakdown of glycogen in muscle does not result in the release of glucose (muscle lacks the enzyme glucose-6-phosphatase); rather, lactic acid will be released. The major stimuli for the breakdown of glycogen in muscle are exercise and adrenaline, not hypoglycemia in a direct way.

QUESTION

(Discussion on page 509)

12.1 *In a patient with hypoglycemia, glycogen in muscle breaks down. Why? How might this pathway be activated in a patient with hyperglycemia?*

Analysis of the Rate of Removal of Glucose

- Metabolic removal of glucose is via oxidation or conversion to storage compounds. During hyperglycemia with insulin

> deficiency, renal excretion is the only major path for re-
> moval of glucose.

Removal by Metabolism

There are two major means of removing glucose from the circulation via metabolism: oxidation to regenerate ATP and conversion of glucose to its storage form, glycogen. In the liver, glucose is also converted to stored fat, but this pathway usually proceeds at a slow rate.

Oxidation of Glucose

> • Oxidation of fat-derived fuels prevents the complete oxida-
> tion of glucose.

For simplicity, the following generalization can be made: oxidation of fat-derived fuels prevents the oxidation of glucose because PDH, the key regulatory enzyme, is inhibited by the products of fatty acid and ketoacid oxidation (see Figure 12.1).

If ketoacids are not present, the brain can oxidize close to 28 mmol (5 g) of glucose per hour. In contrast, if ketoacidosis is present, this oxidation is curtailed markedly, and the only major option for removal of glucose is glucosuria.

QUESTION

(Discussion on page 509)

12.2 *In what organ(s) might glucose be oxidized to CO_2 at an appreciable rate in a patient with chronic hyperglycemia?*

Conversion to Storage Forms

> • There is virtually no conversion of glucose to stores when
> net insulin levels are low.

The pathway for the conversion of glucose to glycogen requires the hormonal setting of high net insulin, which leads to synthesis (induction) of relevant enzymes plus provides the signals required for conversion of glucose to glycogen. Conversely, the hormonal setting of low net insulin, which is typical of fasting with hypoglycemia, requires that the conversion of glucose to glycogen be slow. There is little or no conversion of glucose to fat in this hormonal situation. Thus, because of the effects of a relative lack of insulin, one should expect the level of glucose to decline at a slow rate when insulin is given to a diabetic with poor glycemic control.

Clinical pearl
In a metabolic setting in which glucose cannot be removed by metabolism, any input of glucose is too much glucose.

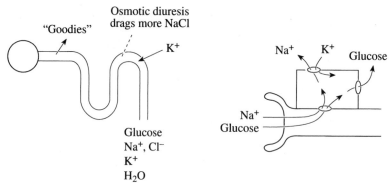

Figure 12.4 Reabsorption of glucose by the kidney. Reabsorption occurs in the proximal convoluted tubule. Limits are usually set by the GFR; stimulation occurs with a low "effective" circulating volume and metabolic acidosis.

Excretion of Glucose in the Urine

- During severe hyperglycemia, the only important means for removal of glucose is excretion.
- Excretion of glucose falls when the GFR falls.
- The usual maximum rate of glucose reabsorption by the kidney is 325 g/day (1800 mmol/day).

Calculation
In a 70-kg adult, 1 kg of lean body mass can supply the brain with glucose for 24 hours:
- The brain needs 120 g of glucose (480 kcal) per day.
- 120 g of glucose is derived from 200 g of protein (60% of protein to glucose).
- 200 g of protein is derived from 1 kg of muscle (80% water).

Quantities
In briefest terms, the plasma glucose in normal individuals after a meal is less than 8 mmol/L (140–150 mg/dL), and the normal kidney can reabsorb 1800 mmol (325 g) of glucose per day. Because the usual GFR in a 70-kg adult is 180 L/day, the filtered load of glucose will not exceed 1800 mmol (325 g) as long as the plasma glucose is less than 10 mmol/L (180 mg/dL).

The only pathways for removal of glucose in a patient with hyperglycemia and low net insulin levels are oxidation of glucose in the brain and urinary excretion of glucose. Valuable water-soluble nutrients such as glucose (referred to as "goodies" in Figure 12.4) must normally not be excreted. Because there are only small stores of glucose in the body, the excretion of glucose will result in the loss of precious fuels for vital organs (brain). Further, a loss of glucose in the urine will "drag" valuable ions (e.g., Na^+, K^+) and water in the urine (osmotic diuresis). In addition, if the body has to rely on high rates of production of glucose from endogenous compounds such as proteins to maintain the pool of glucose, the cost in terms of loss of lean body mass will be great (see margin note).

The general features of reabsorption of glucose in the proximal convoluted tubule reflect the general properties of this nephron segment—a high capacity relative to the normal filtered load (see Figure 12.4). Quantitatively, the maximal reabsorption of glucose is linked to the GFR and exceeds the normal filtered load (Table 12.3). Quantitative considerations appear in the margin.

The main reasons that the concentration of glucose might fall during therapy are reexpansion of the ECF volume (via dilution) and the consequent rise in the GFR, which markedly enhances glucosuria. Table 12.3 indicates just how much glucose will be excreted with a given rise in GFR.

QUESTION

(Discussion on pages 509–510)

12.3 *A patient with NIDDM has hyperglycemia (50 mmol/L, 900* *mg/dL). Assume that the GFR is normal. What are the implications for the intake of glucose and the electrolyte balance during the next 24 hours?*

TABLE 12.3 **Effect of Hyperglycemia and the GFR on the Excretion of Glucose**

Excretion of glucose (g/day) = [GFR (L/day) × plasma glucose (g/L) − 325 g glucose reabsorbed/day]. Note the very high levels of glucosuria when there is both hyperglycemia and a near-normal GFR. A usual diet will supply 270 g of glucose each day, but in a patient with chronic steady-state hyperglycemia, expect an *excretion of 175 g of glucose per day.* Hence, one can predict the GFR required to maintain a given degree of hyperglycemia and the rate at which the concentration of glucose will fall once the GFR rises abruptly.

Glucose (mg/dL)	GFR (L/day)			
	180	100	50	25
	Glucose excreted (g/day)			
200	35	0	0	0
400	395	75	0	0
600	755	275	0	0
1000	1475	675	175	0
1500	2375	1175	425	50

Excretion of 175 g of glucose per day
This rate of excretion reflects the intake of 275 g of glucose and the metabolism of 100 g in organs that do not need insulin to promote the oxidation of glucose (e.g., the brain).

What Permits a Severe Degree of Hyperglycemia to Develop?

A lack of insulin or resistance to its actions is necessary for a modest degree of hyperglycemia to develop. For a modest degree of hyperglycemia to become severe, usually either the renal excretion of glucose will be low or the intake of glucose will be high.

Low Excretion of Glucose

As shown in Table 12.3, the excretion of glucose will be low during severe hyperglycemia only if the GFR is reduced; most commonly, this reduction is secondary to prerenal failure, which, in turn, is due to an osmotic diuresis with a resultant negative Na^+ balance (Table 12.4). The excretion of glucose can also be low in patients with chronic renal disease who cannot produce an osmotic diuresis because of their very low GFR.

Summary
A combination of factors is required to develop a severe degree of hyperglycemia. A relative deficiency of insulin leads to poorly controlled diabetes mellitus. A severe degree of hyperglycemia requires excessive intake of glucose or, more commonly, a low excretion of glucose (a low GFR resulting from ECF volume contraction).

Clinical pearl
If the ECF volume is not low in a patient with a severe degree of hyperglycemia, look for chronic renal disease rather than a prerenal cause for the low GFR.

Osmotic diuresis
During an osmotic diuresis, the $[Na^+]$ in fluid exiting the proximal tubule is two-thirds that of plasma, but more liters exit. The net result is no change in absolute Na^+ reabsorption in the proximal convoluted tubule. A smaller quantity of Na^+ is reabsorbed in the loop of Henle, so delivery to the distal nephron is increased. If all the extra Na^+ delivered are not reabsorbed, a natriuresis occurs.

TABLE 12.4 **Composition of 1 L of Glucose-Induced Osmotic Diuresis**

The values are approximations. Later in time, there will be a marked contraction of the ECF volume and little caloric intake. The volume of urine will then become much smaller (see margin note).

Glucose		Urea	Na^+	K^+
g/L	mmol/L	mmol/L	mmol/L	mmol/L
54	300	100–200	40–50	20–30

K⁺ loss in DKA or HHS

K⁺ loss in DKA or HHS
- Early in the natural history of DKA or HHS, there is a large K⁺ loss in the urine.
- Later, even though there is distal Na⁺ delivery and high aldosterone levels, the [K⁺] in urine is not high (Table 12.5). The authors speculate that chronic glucosuria may lower the open probability of the Na⁺ channel in the luminal membrane of the cortical collecting duct (possibly by glycation) and thereby yield a low transtubular [K⁺] gradient.

Note
See the margin of page 497 for a calculation of the net catabolism of endogenous protein and the yield of glucose and urea.

TABLE 12.5 **Composition of Fluids Containing Glucose**

All examples are based on 1 L volume. Reprinted with permission from Halperin and Rolleston, *Clinical Detective Stories* (London: Portland Press, 1993).

Sample	Glucose g	Glucose mmol	Sodium mmol	Potassium mmol
Plasma (normal)	0.9	5	140	4
Urine (osmotic diuresis)	54	300	50	28
Intake				
D₅W	50	275	0	0
Apple juice	132	732	0	32
Sweetened drinks	110	612	2	0
Normal saline	0	0	152	0

High Intake of Glucose

The second component that may contribute to a severe degree of hyperglycemia is an extraordinary input of glucose, which can overwhelm the normal kidney's ability to excrete it. Most commonly, the source of glucose is excessive quantities of fruit juices or sweetened soft drinks consumed in response to thirst (Table 12.5). Given the very large capacity to excrete glucose, a degree of reduction in GFR is required for these patients to maintain hyperglycemia on a chronic basis. Very rarely, an increased endogenous input of glucose can result transiently from the breakdown of protein (e.g., with increased protein reabsorption from a major gastrointestinal blood loss). This source of glucose is revealed by an evaluation of the urea appearance rate.

PART B

Impact of Hyperglycemia on Fluid and Electrolytes

Hyperglycemia has two major influences on the ECF and ICF volumes. First, as a result of the increased number of osmoles (glucose) restricted to the ECF, severe hyperglycemia will lead to a shift of water from the ICF to the ECF, which will expand the ECF volume and lower the [Na⁺] in the ECF. Second, water and electrolytes will be lost in the urine because hyperglycemia induces an osmotic diuresis.

Shift of Water Across Cell Membranes

- During severe hyperglycemia, myocytes will shrink, and hepatocytes will swell. Of greater importance, brain cell size is probably close to normal.

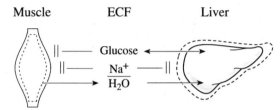

Figure 12.5 Hyperglycemia and the shift of water. Water will move across cell membranes if the concentration of particles restricted to the ECF or ICF changes. The concentration of glucose will always be much higher in the ECF than in the ICF of muscle. Hence, muscle shrinks during hyperglycemia (dashed line); as a result, the concentration of Na^+ in the ECF falls. In contrast, in liver cells, the concentration of glucose is equal to that in the ECF. Hence, hyperglycemia per se has no influence on water shifts in the liver. Hyponatremia, however, will cause water to enter hepatocytes, and they will swell (dashed line). Overall, the volume of the ECF will rise if no excretion of water or electrolytes occurs because the volume of ICF in muscle is at least fourfold larger than that of cells that behave like hepatocytes.

There are two types of particles to consider with respect to shifts of water:

1. Certain particles (urea, ethanol) are "ineffective" in causing a shift of water because they always ultimately achieve an equal concentration in the ECF and ICF.

2. Particles that are restricted to one or other compartment (e.g., Na^+ in the ECF) will cause water to shift into or out of that compartment when their concentrations rise or fall, respectively.

Given these two categories of particles, it remains to be defined whether glucose is a particle with no influence on water shift or one that causes water to exit from the ICF.

Glucose appears to be an "ineffective" osmole in many cells where its transport is independent of insulin (e.g., hepatocytes), because its concentration will be equal in both the ECF and the ICF. In contrast, the concentration of glucose is always much higher outside cells that depend on insulin for the transport of glucose (e.g., myocytes), and the behavior of glucose is similar to Na^+ with respect to water shifts (Figure 12.5).

At any stage of hyperglycemia, it is difficult to be certain of the overall volume of individual brain cells. During severe hyperglycemia, water moves out of myocytes and leads to hyponatremia because there is a gain of water without Na^+ in the ECF. In quantitative terms, muscle contains close to half of the water in the body (25 of 45 L in a 70-kg adult). The volume of distribution of glucose will be 19 L (15 L of ECF and about 4 L of ICF). One can calculate that if the concentration of glucose rises to almost 50 mmol/L, the volume of the ECF should increase by 1.5 L (see margin note). The converse will also be true when the concentration of glucose falls from 50 to 5 mmol/L; 1.5 L of water will shift back from the ECF into the ICF, and a decrease in the volume of the ECF will result.

Change in ECF volume when 1000 mmol of glucose is retained
1. Background:
   - Glucose distributes in ECF (15 L) + 4 L of ICF.
   - ECF contains 2100 mmol of Na^+ (140 mmol/L × 15 L).
   - The body contains 12,600 "effective" mOsm (2 × 140 mmol/L × 45 L).
2. Add 1000 mmol of glucose to its distribution volume (19 L):
   - Total body osmolality = total osmoles (12,600 + 1000)/45 L = 302.2 mOsm/L.
   - Now glucose distribution volume has 6320 "effective" milliosmoles (1000 mmol + (2 × 140 × 19 L)).
3. New ECF volume:
   - Divide osmoles in glucose distribution volume (6320) by new osmolality (302.2 mOsm/L) = 20.9 L.
   - ECF volume = (15/19) × 20.9 L = 16.5 L.
   - Therefore, ECF volume rises by 1.5 L, and the rise in concentration of glucose is 1000 mmol/20.9 L = 47.8 mmol/L.

The Impact of an Osmotic Diuresis on Body Fluid Compartments

> • The major losses of Na^+, K^+, and water during hyperglycemia are the result of the osmotic diuresis induced by glucose.

Total losses of Na^+, K^+, and water have been determined in two types of studies:

1. balance studies in patients who had insulin therapy withheld;
2. retrospective studies involving quantification of the net amounts of Na^+, K^+, and water that were retained during therapy in patients with diabetic ketoacidosis (DKA).

Each of these types of studies has its own limitations. The average losses of electrolytes and water to anticipate during severe hyperglycemia are displayed in a quantitative fashion in Table 12.6.

Sodium

During an osmotic diuresis, the $[Na^+]$ in the urine at presentation is usually close to 50 mmol/L (see Table 12.4). Quantitatively, the net loss of Na^+ at the time of presentation in patients with DKA ranges 3–9 mmol/kg body weight; an average loss of 7 mmol/kg is quite common. This value represents a net loss that is equivalent to 25% of the total body Na^+ (close to 500 of 2000 mmol in a 70-kg subject); it is detected clinically by a markedly contracted ECF volume, which results in an impaired circulating volume and tissue perfusion.

Potassium

Although the net loss of K^+ is close to 5 mmol/kg of body weight, it is difficult to determine the exact impact this loss has on the ECF and ICF volumes. Close to half of the K^+ lost from the ICF is in conjunction with phosphate (typically about 2 mmol/kg). Because the net charge on intracellular phosphodiesters is in effect close to −1, an equal amount of K^+ should leave the cells with phosphate.

The remaining half of K^+ loss will largely represent ECF volume

Replacement of K^+ deficit
• That portion of intracellular K^+ loss associated with a countermovement of Na^+ or H^+ can be replaced with KCl.
• That portion of intracellular K^+ loss associated with a loss of phosphate cannot be replaced with KCl. Phosphate and time for the anabolic effects of insulin (days) are required to restore K^+ stores in the ICF.

K^+ and phosphate vs K^+ and Na^+
• Phosphate in cells is in a macromolecular form. Hence, one needs to lose almost 300 mmol of K^+ with phosphate to lose 1 L of ICF (see Chapter 6).
• For every 150 mmol of Na^+ that enters cells in exchange for K^+ that are excreted with Cl^-, the ECF loses 1 L if there is no change in osmolality. The K^+ loss that occurs in conjunction with entry of Na^+ into cells contracts the ECF volume but does not change the ICF volume (no particle loss in the ICF).

TABLE 12.6 **Typical Deficits in a Patient with DKA**

	Quantity	Comment	Danger of Therapy
Na^+	5–10 mmol/kg	• Restore quickly	• Too rapid a rise in the $[Na^+]$
K^+	5–10 mmol/kg	• Must wait for insulin to shift K^+ into cells if hyperkalemic • Look at the excretion of K^+ when deciding the rate of infusion of K^+	• Hyperkalemia initially • Hypokalemia 2 h later • Half of the K^+ was excreted with phosphate (see margin note)
H_2O	Usually many liters	• Half ICF, half ECF	• Too rapid a repair of water deficit and, thereby, hyponatremia
HCO_3^-	Can be >500 mmol of H^+ retained because of buffering in the ICF	• If plasma anion gap is increased, do not give HCO_3^- unless acidosis is very severe	• A rapid fall in plasma $[K^+]$ (strong opinions held, but not backed up by data)

loss because most of the K^+ will be shifted in exchange for Na^+; this shift equates to at most 1.5 L of ECF fluid. As shown in Figure 10.1, some of this loss of K^+ results from an "exchange" of K^+ for H^+.

Water

The usual electrolyte-free water deficit on presentation is said to be 2–3 L in the adult with severe hyperglycemia. This deficit will be quite variable depending on what the intake of water was during the illness. Because patients do not present with a record of their recent balances, it is possible to calculate only a component of free water deficit from the $[Na^+]$ in plasma, the body weight, and an estimation of the ECF volume.

Metabolic Cost of Glucosuria

If 1 L of osmotic diuresis contains 300 mmol (54 g) of glucose, this value could represent the breakdown of 0.5 kg of lean body mass if the source of glucose was gluconeogenesis from endogenous proteins (see the calculation in the margin note). Hence, there is a large metabolic cost to excrete this urine if its source is endogenous compounds. Further, because this glucose was derived from 90 g of protein, the urine should contain 500–600 mmol of urea. If the cells containing this protein were destroyed, they would release all of their K^+ and phosphate (close to 45 mmol).

Calculation
- 1 lb = 454 g.
- Muscle is 80% water, so each pound of muscle contains close to 90 g of protein.
- 60% of protein can be converted to glucose.
- 0.6×90 g = 54 g.
- Therefore, each liter of osmotic diuresis represents 1 lb (0.5 kg) of muscle in a diabetic in poor control who has not consumed food.
- 90 g of protein will yield 500 mmol of urea.

PART C

Design of Intravenous Therapy for Hyperglycemia

The major issues with regard to intravenous therapy in patients with a severe degree of hyperglycemia are summarized in Table 12.7. They include the following:

1. Replace the majority of the large deficit of ECF particles and volume as rapidly as needed. There should be a further decline in ECF volume because of the expected shift of water from the ECF to the ICF as the level of glycemia declines.

2. Replace ongoing losses of electrolytes and water in urine.

3. Replace the deficit of water and particles in the ICF slowly. Replace the electrolyte-free water deficit associated with resynthesis of glycogen and proteins slowly because these processes take considerable time to occur.

Therapy must be tailored to the individual patient. The time during which each of these issues must be addressed differs from

Clinical pearls
- "Drinker" is our designation for a patient with severe hyperglycemia caused by an excessive intake of fruit juices or sweetened soft drinks. In the "drinker," the deficit in ECF volume may be mild and could be replaced more slowly.
- "Prune" is our designation for a patient with severe hyperglycemia (caused by a low excretion of glucose from a reduced GFR) and clinical evidence of severe ECF volume depletion. In the "prune," replace the ECF volume aggressively.

TABLE 12.7 **Summary of the General Strategy for Intravenous Therapy in a Patient with a Severe Degree of Hyperglycemia**

Compartment	Speed	IV Tonicity	Comments
ECF			
Replace deficit	• Fast	• Isosmotic to ECF	• No shift of water into or out of the ICF
Replace volume of ECF that shifted into ICF	• Slow	• Isotonic (see margin note)	• Depends on decline in glycemia
Ongoing Losses via Urine	• Depends on urine output	• Infuse at [Na$^+$] and [K$^+$] in urine	• Fast in "drinker" • May rise during therapy in "prune"
ICF			
Encourage gain of ICF particles	• Slow, many hours	• Water without Na$^+$	• Replace water when particles are replaced (K$^+$ and H$_2$PO$_4$$^-$)

Note

When glucose disappears from the ECF, water enters the ICF, and the [Na$^+$] in plasma rises. Now the ECF volume is lower, but the [Na$^+$] is close to normal. Hence, the ECF needs reexpansion with fluid restricted to the ECF (isotonic saline). This calculation implies the expected degree of hyponatremia for a given degree of hyperglycemia (often not the case due to loss of electrolyte-free water in the osmotic diuresis).

Calculation
• Assume a blood glucose of 50 mmol/L.
• Glucose was distributed in 15 L on admission.
  Total glucose = 750 mmol.
• After therapy, the concentration of glucose will be 10 mmol/L, and glucose will distribute in 19 L.
  Total = 190 mmol.
• With no other input or output of glucose, 560 mmol of glucose will be excreted, and the osmotic diuresis will be close to 2 L.
• Calculate the rate of appearance of urea to reflect net production of glucose (1.72 mmol of urea for each mmol of glucose).

one patient to another and depends on the cause of the hyperglycemia, the magnitude of the deficits, and the underlying cardiovascular status of the patient. Each of these issues will now be considered in more detail.

Replacing the Deficit of ECF Volume

The deficit of ECF volume and the rate at which this deficit must be replaced must be estimated on clinical grounds. If the patient is hemodynamically unstable, the ECF volume must be reexpanded very quickly with a solution that is isotonic to the patient. Isotonic saline (154 mmol/L NaCl and therefore about 300 mOsm/L) is the best choice because its osmolality approximates the patient's effective osmolality.

In addition to the clinical impression of the deficit of ECF volume on admission, two other factors must be considered. First, the decline of hyperglycemia will cause water to enter cells. The resulting deficit of ECF volume must be replaced with isotonic saline. Second, some of the K$^+$ given will enter cells and lead to a shift of Na$^+$ from the ICF back into the ECF; this shift will expand the ECF volume. Hence, give one less millimole of NaCl for every millimole of KCl infused.

Replacing Ongoing Losses of Electrolytes and Water

Losses of electrolytes and water are easy to estimate from the urine volume and the approximate composition of the urine during an osmotic diuresis (see Table 12.4); these values can be measured, if necessary (urine electrolytes). Solutions used to replace ongoing losses will thus be hypotonic and will reflect the composition of electrolytes in the urine.

During treatment, most of the glucose in the body may be excreted in the urine once the GFR rises appreciably (see Table 12.3). If each liter of osmotic diuresis contains close to 300 mmol of glucose, there is the potential for the additional loss of several liters by osmotic diuresis. These ongoing losses of Na$^+$, K$^+$, and water need to be replaced during therapy. The degree of osmotic diuresis may be even higher in the patient who has consumed a large quantity of glucose because the pool of glucose may be larger (smaller degree of contraction of ECF volume); also, the gastrointestinal tract may contain a hidden pool of glucose when gastric emptying is delayed in response to gastroparesis (commonly seen in these patients).

Restoring the Deficit of Water and Particles in the ICF

The general principle for therapy of the ICF is to replace this deficit slowly. Consider separately the three components of the loss of ICF volume.

Deficit of Electrolyte-Free Water

If the plasma $[Na^+]$ fell more or less than 1.5 mmol/L for every 100 mg/dL (5.5 mmol/L) rise in glycemia (see margin note), there is an additional imbalance in electrolyte-free water that must be adjusted during therapy. It is not clear whether a rapid increase in the concentration of Na^+ in the plasma of patients with severe hyperglycemia poses the same risk for the development of osmotic demyelination as do other settings of hyponatremia. During therapy for severe hyperglycemia, cerebral edema can develop and is a common observation, as judged indirectly from radiologic evidence.

Shift of Water Caused by a Fall in Glycemia

The concentration of glucose will usually decline to the 10–15 mmol/L (180–270 mg/dL) range in 6–8 hours. In a patient with a blood sugar of 50 mmol/L (900 mg/dL), this decline will cause the $[Na^+]$ in the ECF to rise by 7% because the ECF lost 1 of its 14 L (see the calculation on page 495).

Loss of ICF Particles

One need not replace ICF water associated with the loss of K^+ in the acute management of a patient with severe hyperglycemia because considerable time is needed to replace the anions (phosphate) lost with K^+. Obviously, the part of the deficit of K^+ that is due to a shift of cations (largely Na^+) must be replaced acutely to prevent the expected degree of hypokalemia caused by the actions of insulin; this replacement of intracellular Na^+ with K^+ will not change the ICF volume.

Fall in [Na⁺] when plasma concentration of glucose rises
1. Background from page 495:
   - Add 1000 mmol of glucose.
   - Concentration of glucose rose by 47.8 mmol/L.
   - ECF volume = 16.5 vs 15 L.
2. Calculation:
   - Original content of Na^+ in the ECF is 2100 mmol (140 mmol/L × 15 L).
   - $[Na^+]$ in plasma is now 127 mmol/L (2100 mmol/16.5 L).
3. Relationships in plasma:
   - $[Na^+]$ fell 13 mmol/L (140 to 127 mmol/L).
   - Concentration of glucose rose 47.8 mmol/L.
   - $[Na^+]$ fell 1.5 mmol/L/5.5 mmol/L (100 mg/dL) rise in glycemia.

```
  ╭─────────────╮
  │  P A R T  D │
  ╰─────────────╯
```

Clinical Aspects of a Severe Degree of Hyperglycemia

Hyperglycemic hyperosmolar nonketotic coma (HHNC)
This term is commonly used to define a clinical syndrome in which hyperglycemia, but not ketoacidosis, predominates. It is a misnomer because ketoacids are almost always present, and coma is rare.

The hyperglycemic hyperosmolar syndrome (HHS) includes a heterogeneous population of patients who have in common the hallmarks of this diagnosis: a marked degree of hyperglycemia (most often much greater than 27.5 mmol/L, or 500 mg/dL) and hyperosmolality (usually more than 320 mOsm/kg H_2O). The more common name is *hyperglycemic hyperosmolar nonketotic coma*. Because coma is rare and a certain degree of ketoacidosis is present (sufficient to suppress the oxidation of glucose by the brain), this name is misleading and the authors prefer not to use it.

Based on the underlying pathophysiology for the development of hyperglycemia, four subtypes of patients emerge: the "drinker," the patient in a catabolic state, the "prune," and the patient with renal failure. These divisions are somewhat arbitrary because they can represent a continuum, and each patient may have a mixed set of causes for hyperglycemia. It is useful, however, to categorize individual patients because each subtype has unique dangers and requires a different approach to therapy; these principles also apply to patients with diabetic ketoacidosis and a significant degree of hyperglycemia.

The following issues for each subtype are addressed: diagnosis, therapeutic issues, and dangers to anticipate.

Diagnosis

Distinguishing between excessive input and low output of glucose as the major determinants of the severity of hyperglycemia provides the basis for this classification (Figure 12.6). The three questions in the figure should be answered.

Question 1: What is the rate of excretion of glucose?

Patients with a high rate of excretion of glucose will have a rate of urine flow of at least 2–3 mL/min. This category includes those with an exogenous source of glucose (the "drinker") and those with a very high rate of production of glucose from endogenous sources (upper gastrointestinal bleeding and/or a very high rate of catabolism). This latter distinction requires the answer to a second question.

Urea:glucose ratio
When the source of glucose production is protein, urea is made with glucose, and the expected ratio of urea to glucose is 1.7:1. The appearance of glucose without urea implies that glycogen or dietary glucose was the source of this glucose.

Question 2: What is the rate of appearance of urea relative to that of glucose?

Patients with an endogenous protein source for glucose will have a high rate of appearance of urea, and the quantity of glucose formed from protein sources can be quantitated via the *urea:glucose ratio*. Each millimole of glucose is made with 1.7 mmol of urea during the conversion of amino acids to glucose. Therefore, one must

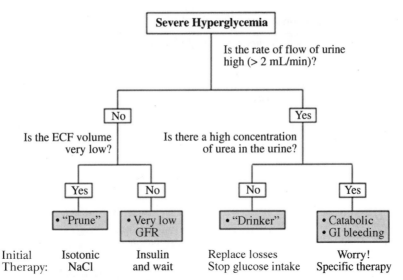

Figure 12.6   Clinical approach to the patient with hyperglycemia. The purpose of this approach is to identify those patients whose primary reason for hyperglycemia is high input of glucose vs those with a low output of glucose. Obviously, most patients will have some degree of excessive intake of glucose and a degree of reduction of the GFR. Nevertheless, if polyuria is present, it should be emphasized because it will help with decision-making concerning intravenous fluid administration.

calculate the appearance of new urea in the body (the concentration of urea in plasma × total body water) plus the quantity of urea excreted in that time interval. The appearance of glucose is its concentration in plasma × one-half total body water plus the quantity of glucose excreted.

In patients with a low rate of excretion of glucose, a renal mechanism is present that permits continued severe hyperglycemia. These patients can be grouped based on ECF volume.

Question 3: In a patient with a low excretion of glucose, is the ECF volume very low?

Patients with chronic renal insufficiency who were unable to mount an osmotic diuresis will have an expanded ECF volume caused by a shift of water from the ICF. Patients with prerenal failure will have very low GFR because of severe contraction of the ECF volume.

Therapeutic Issues

The issues to consider are summarized in Table 12.8. One must replace the deficits of Na^+, K^+, and water as well as the ongoing losses of electrolytes and water. There is some controversy concerning the immediate need for insulin (see margin note). Each of these issues will be considered in the common clinical settings.

There are many interacting phenomena that combine to determine the patient's eventual plasma $[Na^+]$. Probably the rate of correction of chronic hyponatremia is not as critical in the severely hyperglycemic patient. Nevertheless, hypernatremia is a distinct risk, and it must be avoided.

Note
Insulin is needed to:
• Treat severe hyperkalemia
• Prevent severe ketoacidosis
Insulin is not needed acutely to lower blood sugar (dilution and renal excretion will do that).

TABLE 12.8 **Issues During Diagnosis and Therapy of HHS**

Subgroup of HHS	Diagnostic Feature	Unique Threat	Therapeutic Emphasis
Polyuric group The "drinker"	• Urine > 3 mL/min • Ingestion of glucose • Low urea excretion	• Delayed hypernatremia	• Stop glucose intake • Replace ECF volume • Give free water • Match IV solution to urine
The patient in a catabolic state	• Urine > 3 mL/min • High urea in blood and/or urine	• Loss of lean body mass or gastrointestinal blood loss	• Give insulin (stop catabolism) • Defend blood volume if there is GI bleeding • Give free water
Oliguric group The "prune"	• Oliguria • Very low ECF volume	• Shock • More severe hyperkalemia	• Reexpand ECF volume rapidly at first
The patient with chronic renal insufficiency	• Expanded ECF volume	• Congestive heart failure • Hyperkalemia	• With insulin, the fall in glucose may be slow • Hypoglycemia may occur after 6–8 h

Preexisting Status

1. **Degree of ECF volume depletion**: This is important because it determines the degree of hyperglycemia and the rapidity with which an osmotic diuresis will occur.
2. **Water deficit at the time of presentation**: The degree of this deficit is not readily evident even if one corrects the plasma [Na$^+$] for the degree of hyperglycemia because there is also a large and unknown amount of loss of particles (and water) from the ICF (K$^+$ and phosphate in RNA). Renal water loss is a function of the GFR and the degree and duration of hyperglycemia.
3. **The degree of hyperglycemia**: This is important because it determines the amount of water that leaves the ECF and enters the ICF during therapy.
4. **Magnitude of K$^+$ deficit**: There are two types of K$^+$ loss from the ICF that are almost equal in amount. The first occurs along with a deficit of phosphate and is not replaced in acute management. The second involves a cation "exchange." When K$^+$ is given as its Cl$^-$ salt, K$^+$ enters the ICF, and Na$^+$ will return to the ECF.

Intracellular particle loss
If particles are lost from the ICF compartment, one can no longer calculate the change in ICF volume from the plasma [Na$^+$].

Events During Therapy

1. **Rapidity of correction of the ECF volume depletion**: This could influence the magnitude and rapidity of the osmotic diuresis and hence the rate of water loss in the urine.
2. **The choice of replacement fluids**: Initially, fluids isotonic to the patient should be given to reexpand the ECF volume. This fluid will become hypertonic if KCl is added to isotonic saline.
3. **The magnitude of the osmotic diuresis during therapy**: The magnitude of the renal water loss is itself determined by many of the preceding processes such as the degree of hyperglycemia and the rapidity with which it is corrected.

The "Drinker"

The main issue is that patients with high input and output of glucose are not usually in great danger. The priorities in treating these patients include removing the source of glucose and then replacing ongoing losses of electrolytes and water (see margin note). Any initial deficits should be replaced as well (recognize the degree of ECF volume contraction, an inappropriate $[Na^+]$ for the degree of hyperglycemia, and the degree of hyperkalemia). As a result of kaliuresis during the early osmotic diuresis, a large deficit of K^+ is likely at presentation. The usual values to anticipate are a $[K^+]$ in plasma of close to 5.5 mmol/L and a deficit of K^+ of close to 5 mmol/kg of body weight (see Table 12.6).

Therapy should be tailored to measured serum and urinary electrolytes, but, generally, hypotonic saline supplemented with KCl is required. Insulin is not required acutely if there is not an excessive degree of hyperkalemia or catabolism or if there is no imminent threat of severe ketoacidosis.

The Patient in a Catabolic State

Rarely, patients may have excessive breakdown of body proteins. Catabolism of protein yields glucose and urea. If a patient loses 1 kg of lean body mass or digests 1 L of blood, 667 mmol of glucose and close to 1200 mmol of urea will be produced. This production might aggravate the degree of hyperglycemia in a patient with low net insulin. The clinical settings are gastrointestinal bleeding or excessive levels of glucocorticoids (usually given exogenously). In these settings, insulin may be valuable to decrease the rate of oxidation of amino acids.

The "Prune"

The first therapeutic priority for this subgroup of patients is administration of isotonic saline to restore effective circulating volume. Once the ECF volume is reexpanded and/or the urine output rises, switch to hypotonic saline. These patients may have a low GFR and enhanced reabsorption of Na^+ for a prolonged period after the ECF volume is restored so that the extra Na^+ administered will be retained. Replacement of K^+ and the use of insulin are the same as indicated in the "drinker."

The Patient with Chronic Renal Insufficiency

Severe hyperglycemia in this group of patients cannot be treated by dilution or inducing diuresis; insulin is therefore required to lower the plasma glucose concentration. Administration of K^+ should be avoided unless the patient is hypokalemic on presentation. Because insulin may take hours to lower the level of glucose, a delay in resolution of hyperglycemia should be anticipated, and hypoglycemia should be avoided once the concentration of glucose has begun to fall appreciably. Frequent monitoring of the blood glucose is the best way to avoid hypoglycemia.

Dangers to Anticipate

In all patients, there is the threat of the underlying illness and the general problems related to a slower circulation (e.g., thrombotic

Losses in urine
The anticipated losses depend on the quantity of glucose to excrete and the composition of the urine.
- 1 L of urine contains 300 mmol of glucose.
- Glucose distributes in close to half of body water.
- Therefore, for every 15 mmol/L (270 mg/dL) rise in the concentration of glucose in plasma, expect 1 L of urine.

Calculation
- 1 L of blood and 1 kg of lean body mass contain 200 g of protein.
- 60% of protein → glucose, so 200 g of protein → 120 g of glucose.
- Molecular weight of glucose is 180, so 120 g of glucose is 667 mmol.

events). These threats are not discussed. Specific items are the following:

1. **The drinker**: Delayed hypernatremia should be avoided by assuring that electrolyte-free water intake matches its exit from the ECF.

2. **The patient in a catabolic state**: Loss of lean body mass should be reduced by avoiding catabolic hormones (glucocorticoids, catecholamines) and by using insulin. Delayed hypernatremia is a risk, as with the drinker. Gastrointestinal blood loss should also be ruled out as a source of protein for gluconeogenesis. With cell lysis, hyperkalemia is also a potential threat.

3. **The prune**: Hypotension should be treated with normal saline to restore tissue perfusion and gradually improve renal function so that glucose can be excreted.

4. **The patient with chronic renal insufficiency**: Patients with this background may present with pulmonary edema caused by a shift of water from ICF into ECF. Pulmonary edema may be poorly tolerated if underlying cardiac disease is present.

PART E

Review

DISCUSSION OF INTRODUCTORY CASE
Terry Is Confused
(Case presented on page 486)

What is the basis for her severe degree of hyperglycemia?

A severe degree of hyperglycemia has two components. First, there must be "hormonal permission" to have hyperglycemia (i.e., a low level of insulin or a resistance to its actions). Second, there must be a low rate of removal or a large exogenous source of glucose.

Hormonal Permission. Terry had several possible reasons for developing relative insulinopenia (NIDDM, α-adrenergic response to ECF volume contraction, drug actions—thiazides—K^+ deficiency or advanced age). Terry also had reasons for a high level of adrenaline, a hormone that opposes the actions of insulin. The concentration of adrenaline should be high because of ECF volume contraction. Adrenaline will stimulate the release of fatty acids by activating hormone-sensitive lipase and will also inhibit the release of insulin from her β cells.

Reduced Output of Glucose. The major source of output of glucose should be via renal excretion when hyperglycemia is severe (see Table 12.3). Terry's GFR is already low as a result of her age and her longstanding NIDDM. She has a further reduction in her GFR because of the ECF volume contraction.

Terry will not be able to oxidize glucose at an appreciable rate because most of her organs will be oxidizing fatty acids, and her brain will be oxidizing ketoacids in this setting.

Increased Input of Glucose. Terry drank fruit juice, which has a high concentration of glucose (see Table 12.5).

Summary. Although an excessive intake of carbohydrates was probably important 1 week before admission, a reduced degree of glucosuria was the critical factor in sustaining the severe degree of hyperglycemia. This low glucosuria was the expected response to a fall in her GFR as a result of ECF volume contraction.

Why does Terry have hyponatremia?

There are several factors operating. She has a loss of Na^+ in the osmotic and drug-induced diuresis and an increased desire to drink water in the setting of ADH release. Of more importance, Terry is severely hyperglycemic.

The degree of hyponatremia at presentation was as expected for the level of glycemia (i.e., there was no evidence of an additional free water excess or deficit, see margin note).

What is the appropriate therapy?

The major threats to Terry are cardiovascular collapse and possibly acute tubular necrosis from the marked ECF volume contraction. Although Terry is not acidemic, the anion gap in her plasma is increased in magnitude, and she has a component of ketoacidosis. She is not acidemic probably because her plasma $[HCO_3^-]$ was increased due to the metabolic alkalosis associated with diuretic therapy. The other early danger to anticipate is severe hypokalemia once insulin acts because she had an unusually low $[K^+]$ in plasma on admission (4.1 mmol/L vs the expected 5.5 mmol/L). This low $[K^+]$ was probably the result of the excessive kaliuresis (osmotic and pharmacologic diuretics).

Isotonic saline should be infused to restore her ECF volume. Because the clinical estimate of the deficit of ECF volume was 3 L, most of this volume should be replaced rapidly using a tonicity adjusted to Terry. Further intravenous therapy with 150 mmol/L saline should be given to replace the water that shifts into cells as hyperglycemia abates. The volume of urine and electrolytes in urine should also be replaced when the urine flow increases (see margin note). The deficit of intracellular water is not an immediate concern; phosphate need not be administered acutely because it takes time to resynthesize intracellular macromolecules.

The deficit of K^+ is larger than expected, so K^+ should be added to the initial intravenous solutions (at least 10 mmol/L) (see margin note). If insulin becomes part of the treatment (or is released from her β cells), a fall in plasma $[K^+]$ will be likely, especially because she had an unusually low $[K^+]$ on admission. The anticipated fall in the plasma $[K^+]$ might be close to 1 mmol/L when insulin acts.

Why will the concentration of glucose fall during therapy?

The concentration of glucose should fall as a result of dilution (infusion of saline), glucosuria (300 mmol/L of urine), and metabolism (which is slow initially, even if insulin is given). The rate of fall in the concentration of glucose should be 100 mg/dL (5.5 mmol/L) per hour until it approaches 270 mg/dL (15 mmol/L). Because there is no major threat of acidosis and the $[K^+]$ in plasma is lower

Fall in [Na⁺] when plasma concentration of glucose rises
1. Background from page 495:
   • Add 1000 mmol of glucose.
   • Concentration of glucose rose by 47.8 mmol/L.
   • ECF volume = 16.5 vs 15 L.
2. Calculation:
   • Original content of Na^+ in the ECF is 2100 mmol (140 mmol/L × 15 L).
   • $[Na^+]$ in plasma is now 127 mmol/L (2100 mmol/16.5 L).
3. Relationships in plasma:
   • $[Na^+]$ fell 13 mmol/L (140 to 127 mmol/L).
   • Concentration of glucose rose 47.8 mmol/L.
   • $[Na^+]$ fell 1.5/mmol/L/5.5/mmol/L (100 mg/dL) rise in glycemia.

Note
As the urine output increases, her intravenous fluid can be changed to half-isotonic saline with 20 mEq KCl per liter until the urine electrolytes are known.

Note
For tonicity considerations, the KCl infused should be considered equivalent to NaCl in the IV.

than expected, insulin should be withheld during the first several hours of therapy.

Cases for Review

CASE 12.1
An Apple Juice Overdose
(Case discussed on page 506)

A 40-year-old female had a 1-week history of extreme thirst and polyuria. She drank large volumes of fruit juice. She did not have a history of diabetes mellitus but did have acute pancreatitis 1 year ago. The only abnormalities on physical examination were related to a modest degree of contraction of her ECF volume. There was no obvious disturbance in CNS function, and acetone was not detected on her breath. The urine flow was brisk, but the rate of excretion of urea was not high. Laboratory results on admission are summarized in Table 12.9.

Why was the hyperglycemia so severe?
What is the appropriate therapy?

CASE 12.2
A Sudden Shift in Emphasis
(Case discussed on page 508)

A 30-year-old male with long-standing insulin-dependent diabetes mellitus has renal and heart failure. He ingested a carbohydrate-rich meal after stopping his usual administration of insulin because of episodes of hypoglycemia. Laboratory data are provided in Table 12.9.

What do you expect to happen to his degree of congestive heart failure?
What is the appropriate therapy?

Discussion of Cases

DISCUSSION OF CASE 12.1
An Apple Juice Overdose
(Case presented on page 506)

Why was the hyperglycemia so severe?

TABLE 12.9 **Blood Values on Admission in Cases 12.1 and 12.2**

Blood or Plasma		Apple Juice Overdose	Shift in Emphasis
Glucose	mmol/L (mg/dL)	90 (1620)	50 (900)
Na$^+$	mmol/L	116	126
K$^+$	mmol/L	6.9	5.9
Creatinine	μmol/L (mg/dL)	115 (1.0)	1150 (10)
Urea	mmol/L (mg/dL)	4.0 (11)	30 (84)

Hyperglycemia develops primarily as a result of a low net level of insulin. This hormonal change could reflect destruction of β cells in the pancreas (pancreatitis) and an α-adrenergic response to ECF volume contraction.

Her severe degree of hyperglycemia and high rate of excretion of glucose (brisk urine flow rate) imply a high intake of glucose (history). There could also be a high production of glucose from endogenous sources (see margin note). If glycogen breakdown in muscle was the source of glucose, there would be muscular contraction and a high rate of release of L-lactate (not present) or high protein catabolism (urea excretion was not high). Hence, this is a "drinker" type of hyperglycemia. Given the twofold higher concentration of glucose in fruit juice compared with that in urine during an osmotic diuresis (see Table 12.5 and Table 12.4), the excretion of glucose following the intake of 1 L of apple juice will oblige the excretion of 2 L of water plus close to 100 mmol of Na^+ and close to 50 mmol of K^+ (see Table 12.4). With time, the ECF volume will decline somewhat if the intake of Na^+ is inadequate to match these losses. This decline will lead to ECF volume contraction, to a reduction in the GFR, and to a more severe degree of hyperglycemia.

Note
The stimulus to metabolism of muscle glycogen, which eventually becomes glucose in the ECF, is muscle contraction (exercise or seizure).

What is the appropriate therapy?

Avoid a Cardiac Arrhythmia. Because a severe degree of hyperkalemia was present (chance of cardiac arrhythmias) and the ECG displayed a pattern indicating hyperkalemia, Ca^{2+} and insulin should be given. The expected loss of K^+ in the urine in the first hour will be small because the $[K^+]$ in the urine in HHS or DKA is only about 20 mmol/L (see Table 12.4). Given a urine volume of 200 mL in 1 hour (3 mL/min), only 4 mmol of K^+ will be excreted in this hour. Further, one cannot raise this urinary $[K^+]$ by giving aldosterone. Attempts to replace the anticipated deficit of K^+ should not be initiated until the $[K^+]$ in plasma approaches 4 mmol/L (see margin note). The plasma $[K^+]$ may have been this high due to the consumption of apple juice which has a high K^+ content. Other possibilities should be ruled out if the $[K^+]$ does not fall appropriately with therapy.

K^+ deficit
Replace only that portion associated with a gain of Na^+ or H^+ acutely. Replacing the K^+ plus phosphate deficit requires time for anabolic events to occur.

Lower the Concentration of Glucose in Plasma. One aim of therapy is to lower the concentration of glucose in plasma while preventing contraction of the ECF and ICF volumes. Stopping the intake of glucose should lead to a prompt fall in blood sugar as a result of glucosuria; minor factors that cause a decline in glycemia will be the dilution of glucose (ECF volume reexpansion) and the metabolism of glucose. If the patient has a large dilated stomach containing carbohydrate, there may be a much slower fall in glycemia.

Maintain a Normal ECF Volume. Clinically, a deficit of about 1 L of ECF volume was estimated and should be replaced with 150 mmol/L saline, which has almost the same "effective osmolality" as the patient. During the first 6 hours, an additional 1.5 L of isotonic saline will be required to prevent contraction of the ECF volume when hyperglycemia declines and water shifts into myocytes.

Replace Losses in the Urine. The urinary excretion of water and Na^+ should be replaced stoichiometrically. Approximately 3.5 L of osmotic diuresis is likely to be excreted (glucose surplus of 1000 mmol), so a total of almost 200 mmol of Na^+ will need to be replaced. Hypernatremia should be avoided by adjusting the osmolality of intravenous fluids for the ongoing losses of Na^+ and water; also take into consideration the degree of hyperglycemia.

In summary, the main purpose of therapy is to correct the unusual degree of hyperkalemia with an administration of insulin. Restoration of the ECF volume will remove the inhibitory signals to insulin secretion and raise the GFR, which, in turn, will lead to a prompt fall in glycemia. One should anticipate ongoing renal water losses from the osmotic diuresis and replace these losses.

DISCUSSION OF CASE 12.2
A Sudden Shift in Emphasis
(Case presented on page 506)

What do you expect to happen to his degree of congestive heart failure?

In the setting of insulinopenia and a very low GFR, the glucose ingested will lead to a severe hyperglycemia, which, in turn, will lead to a shift of water from the ICF to the ECF volume. Because there is no major osmotic diuresis, an extra liter or so of water will be retained in the ECF and aggravate the degree of congestive heart failure.

What is the appropriate therapy?

The best therapy is the administration of insulin. Because excretion of glucose is not possible, insulin is the only option for lessening the degree of hyperglycemia (and the shift of water out of the ECF). Fat-derived fuels were most likely present in the setting of relative insulinopenia (allowing this degree of hyperglycemia), so one could not expect a maximal rate of oxidation of glucose (25 g/hr) early in therapy.

Hyperkalemia is also a concern in this patient. Its degree will be diminished by the insulin therapy.

If the degree of heart failure becomes critical, the blood volume could be lowered promptly by phlebotomy. Alternatively, hemodialysis could be used to control the volume of the ECF and lessen the degree of hyperglycemia.

Summary of Main Points

When outlining the appropriate therapy for patients with a severe degree of hyperglycemia, identify the subgroup to which the patient belongs (see Figure 12.6) and address the following issues:

> - **Concerning Na^+:** Is the degree of contraction of the ECF volume a major threat? How large is the deficit of Na^+? Will it increase or decrease in the next several hours? How large was the shift of Na^+ into the ICF?
> - **Concerning water:** How large is the deficit of water (compare expected vs observed $[Na^+]$ in plasma)? How much

water was lost from the ICF and the ECF? Is the deficit different in individual organs? How much more water will be lost during the first 5–6 hours of therapy? Will a rapid rise in [Na$^+$] cause osmotic demyelination?

- **Concerning glucose**: How quickly will the concentration of glucose fall during the next 5–6 hours? How much will be excreted, metabolized, and produced? Does it matter what the source of this glucose is? Does it matter how quickly the concentration of glucose will fall?

- **Concerning K$^+$**: There is a large deficit of K$^+$ despite hyperkalemia. Expect a large fall in [K$^+$] (about 1 mmol/l) once insulin acts. This fall will be increased with the administration of HCO$_3$$^-$.

Therapy must reflect the underlying pathophysiology and complications.

Discussion of Questions

12.1 In a patient with hypoglycemia, glycogen in muscle breaks down. Why?

There are two major stimuli for the breakdown of glycogen in muscle. First, with local anaerobiosis (a sprint), the need to regenerate ATP rapidly leads to glycogenolysis. Second, glycogenolysis is augmented when adrenaline levels rise. The adrenergic response to hypoglycemia should lead to the breakdown of glycogen in muscle. The product of this glycogenolysis is L-lactic acid, which may be released from muscle cells.

How might this pathway be activated in a patient with hyperglycemia?

The key to the control of glycogenolysis in muscle is adrenaline. The release of this hormone is augmented by a contracted ECF volume, a feature common to most patients with hyperglycemia. In addition, adrenaline can be released in response to stress or an underlying illness that precipitated the hyperglycemia.

12.2 In what organ(s) might glucose be oxidized to CO$_2$ at an appreciable rate in a patient with chronic hyperglycemia?

In chronic hyperglycemia caused by a relative lack of insulin, more fatty acids are released from adipose tissue. Because fatty acid oxidation inhibits the oxidation of glucose, high levels of fatty acids will limit the oxidation of glucose in all organs that can take them up. The blood-brain barrier prevents fatty acids from entering brain cells at an appreciable rate; therefore, in the absence of ketoacid accumulation, the brain is the only organ that oxidizes glucose to CO$_2$ during hyperglycemia.

12.3 A patient with NIDDM has hyperglycemia (50 mmol/L, 900 mg/dL). Assume that the GFR is normal. What are

the implications for the intake of glucose and the electrolyte balance during the next 24 hours?

It is extremely rare that a very high level of glucose can be maintained in the circulation when the GFR is normal because the kidney has an enormous capacity to excrete glucose in this setting (see Table 12.3). This patient therefore has an enormous intake of glucose or a very unusual renal lesion of hyperreabsorption of glucose. Only in the former setting will there be very large losses of water, Na^+, and K^+. Judging from Table 12.3, one might expect an excretion of close to 1500 g of glucose. At a glucose concentration of 50 g/L of urine, the urine volume could conceivably be 30 L/day, and a loss of 1500 mmol of Na^+ could be anticipated (see Table 12.4). It is obvious from these numbers that one of the assumptions in the question is not valid—i.e., the GFR is much lower than predicted, or the values do not represent a steady state.

Suggested Readings

Acid-Base

The following five sources provide background in the area of acid-base balance.

Halperin, M. L., and R. L. Jungas. 1983. Metabolic production and disposal of hydrogen ions. *Kidney Int.* 24:709–13.

Hochachka, P., and T. Mommsen. 1983. Protons and anaerobiosis. *Science* 219:1391–97.

Oh, M. S., and H. J. Carroll. 1992. Whole body acid-base balance. In *The kidney today: Selected topics in renal science.* Ed. G. M. Berlyne, 89–104. Basel: Karger.

Rahn H. 1979. Acid-base balance and the "milieu interieur." In *Claude Bernard and the internal environment: A memorial symposium.* Ed. E. Robin, 179–90. New York: Marcel Dekker, Inc.

Relman, A., E. Lennon, and J. Lemann, Jr. 1961, vol. 6. Endogenous production of fixed acid and the measurement of the net balance of acid in normal subjects. *J. Clin. Invest.* 1621–30.

The following two articles provide background in the area of intracellular pH.

Aw, T. Y., and D. P. Jones. 1989. Heterogeneity of pH in the aqueous cytoplasm of renal proximal tubule cells. *FASEB J.* 3:52–58.

Boron, W. F. 1992. Control of intracellular pH. In *The kidney: Physiology and pathophysiology.* 2nd ed. Ed. D. W. Seldin and G. Giebisch, 219–64. New York: Raven Press Ltd.

The following four articles provide background in the area of buffering.

Fernandez, P., R. Cohen, and G. Feldman. 1989. The concept of bicarbonate distribution space: The crucial role of body buffers. *Kidney Int.* 36:747–52.

Oh, M. 1991. Irrelevance of bone buffering to acid-base homeostasis in chronic metabolic acidosis. *Nephron* 59:7–10.

Swan, R. C., and R. F. Pitts. 1955. Neutralization of infused acid by nephrectomized dogs. *J. Clin. Invest.* 34:205–12.

Vasuvattakul, S., L. Warner, and M. L. Halperin. 1992. Quantitative role of the intracellular bicarbonate buffer system in response to an acute acid load. *Am. J. Physiol.* 262:R305–R309.

The following eleven articles provide background in the area of renal influences on bicarbonate balance.

Alpern, R. J. 1990. Cell mechanisms of proximal tubule acidification. *Physiol. Rev.* 70:79–114.

Cohen, R. M., G. M. Feldman, and P. C. Fernandez. 1997. The balance of acid, base and charge in health and disease. *Kidney Int* 52:287–93.

Edelman, C. M., et al. 1967. Renal bicarbonate reabsorption and hydrogen ion excretion in normal infants. *J. Clin. Invest.* 46:1309–17.

Halperin, M. L., et al. 1992. Biochemistry and physiology of ammonium excretion. In *The kidney: Physiology and pathophysiology.* 2nd ed. Ed. D. W. Seldin and G. Giebisch, 1471–89. New York: Raven Press Ltd.

Kamel, K., et al. 1990. The removal of an inorganic acid load in subjects with ketoacidosis of chronic fasting: The role of the kidney. *Kidney Int.* 38:507–11.

Knepper, M., R. Packer, and D. Good. 1989. Ammonium transport in the kidney. *Physiol. Rev.* 69:179–249.

Lin, S-H, et al. 1998. Physiological role of the potential alkali load in the diet of the rat for acid-base balance. *Am. J. Physiol.* 274:F1037–F1044.

Packer, R. K., C. A. Curry, and K. M. Brown. 1995. Urinary organic anion excretion in response to dietary acid and base loading. *J. Am. Soc. Nephrol.* 5:1624–629.

Uribarri, J., and M. S. Oh. 1995. Acid-base balance in dialysis patients: A reassessment. *Semin. Dialysis* 8:68–71.

Uribarri, J., et al. 1998. Acid production in chronic hemodialysis. *J. Am. Soc. Nephrol.* 9:1–8.

Zhao, J., et al. 1998. Effect of basolateral HCO_3 or CO_2 on HCO_3 reabsorption by the rabbit superficial S-2 proximal tubule. *FASEB J* 12:A2442.

The following three articles provide background in the area of organic acid production and the GI tract.

Cummings, J. H., and G. T. MacFarlane. 1997. Role of intestinal bacteria in nutrient metabolism. *J. Parent. Ent. Nutr.* 21:357–65.

Halperin, M. L., and K. S. Kamel. 1996. Turning sugar into acids in the gastrointestinal tract. *Kidney Int.* 49:1–8.

Spital, A., and R. H. Sterns. 1994. Metabolic acidosis following jejunoileal bypass. *Am. J. Kidney Dis.* 23:135–37.

The following seven articles provide background in the area of diagnostic tests.

Dyck, R., et al. 1990. A modification of the urine osmolal gap: An improved method for estimating urine ammonium. *Am. J. Nephrol.* 10:359–62.

Goldstein, M., et al. 1986. The urine anion gap: A clinically useful index of ammonium excretion. *Am. J. Med. Sci.* 29:198–202.

Halperin, M. L., et al. 1988. The urine osmolal gap: A clue to estimate urine ammonium in "hybrid" types of metabolic acidosis. *Clin. Invest. Med.* 11:198–202.

Kamel, K. S., et al. 1996. Anion gap: Do the anions restricted to the intravascular space have modifications in their valence? *Nephron* 73:382–89.

Oh, M., and H. Carroll. 1977. The anion gap. *N. Engl. J. Med.* 297:814–17.

Stewart, P. A. 1983. Modern quantitative acid-base chemistry. *Can. J. Physiol. Pharmacol.* 61:1444–61.

Van Leeuwen, A. M. 1964. Net cation equivalency (base-binding power) of the plasma proteins. *Acta Med. Scand.* 176:36–57.

The following seven articles provide background in the area of renal influences on ketoacidosis.

Atchley, D., et al. 1933. On diabetic acidosis: A detailed study of electrolyte balances following withdrawal and reestablishment of insulin therapy. *J. Clin. Invest.* 12:297–325.

Flatt, J. 1972. On the maximal possible rate of ketogenesis. *Diabetes* 21:50–53.

Halperin, M. L., K. S. Kamel, and S. Cheema-Dhadli. 1992. Lactic acidosis, ketoacidosis, and energy turnover: "Figure" you made the correct diagnosis only when you have "counted" on it—Quantitative analysis based on principles of metabolism. *Mt. Sinai J. Med.* 59:1–12.

Halperin, M. L., and F. S. Rolleston. 1993. *Clinical detective stories: A problem-based approach to clinical cases in energy and acid-base metabolism.* London: Portland Press.

Kamel, K. S., et al. 1993. Rate of production of carbon dioxide in patients with a severe degree of metabolic acidosis. *Nephron* 64:514–17.

Schreiber, M., et al. 1994. Ketoacidosis: An integrative view. *Diabetes Rev.* 2:98–114.

Schreiber, M., et al. 1996. Can a severe degree of ketoacidosis develop overnight? *J. Am. Soc. Nephrol.* 7:191–97.

The following three articles provide

background on the ketoacidosis of fasting.

Hannaford, M. C., et al. 1982. Protein wasting due to the acidosis of prolonged fasting. *Am. J. Physiol.* 243:E251–E256.

Kamel, K. S., et al. 1998. Prolonged total fasting: a feast for the integrative physiologist. *Kidney Int.* 53:531–39.

Owen, O. E., S. Caprio, and G. A. Reichard, Jr. 1983. Ketosis of starvation: A revisit and new perspectives. *Clin. Endocrinol. Metab.* 12:359–79.

The following three articles provide background on alcoholic ketoacidosis.

Halperin, M. L., et al. 1983. Metabolic acidosis in the alcoholic: A pathophysiologic approach. *Metabolism* 32:308–15.

Kamel, K. S., et al. 1995. Metabolic acidosis in the alcoholic: An emphasis on intracellular events. *Endocrinologist* 5:278–85.

Wrenn, K. D., et al. 1991. The syndrome of alcoholic ketoacidosis. *Am. J. Med.* 91:119–28.

The following two articles provide quantitative data about the production of L-lactic acid during exercise.

Cheetham, M. E., et al. 1986. Human muscle metabolism during sprint running. *J. Appl. Physiol.* 61:54–60.

Osnes, J. B., and L. Hermansen. 1972. Acid-base balance after maximal exercise of short duration. *J. Appl. Physiol.* 32:59–63.

The following three articles deal with the treatment of L-lactic acidosis.

Cohen, R., and H. Woods. 1983. Lactic acidosis revisited. *Diabetes* 32:181–91.

Halperin, M. L., K. S. Kamel, and S. Cheema-Dhadli. 1992. Lactic acidosis, ketoacidosis, and energy turnover: "Figure" you made the correct diagnosis only when you have "counted" on it—Quantitative analysis based on principles of metabolism. *Mt. Sinai J. Med.* 59:1–12.

Robinson, B. 1989. Lactic acidemia. In *Metabolic basis of inherited disease.* Ed. C. Scriver, A. Beaudet, W. Sly, and D. Valle, 869–88. New York: McGraw-Hill.

The following four articles address therapy of metabolic acidosis with NaHCO3.

Arieff, A. I. 1991. Indications for use of bicarbonate in patients with metabolic acidosis. *Br. J. Anaesth.* 67:165–77.

Halperin, M. L., et al. 1994. Rationale for the use of sodium bicarbonate in a patient with lactic acidosis due to a poor cardiac output. *Nephron* 66:258–61.

Halperin, F. A., et al. 1996. Alkali therapy extends the period of survival during hypoxia: Studies in rats. *Am. J. Physiol.* 271:R381–R387.

Narins, R. G. 1994. Bicarbonate therapy in lactic and ketoacidosis. *Diabetes Rev.* 2.

The following two articles provide background for changing the emphasis of the classification of metabolic acidosis.

Carlisle, E., et al. 1991. Glue-sniffing and distal renal tubular acidosis: Sticking to the facts. *J. Am. Soc. Nephrol.* 1:1019–27.

Halperin, M. L., S. Vasuvattakul, and A. Bayoumi. 1991. A modified classification of metabolic acidosis: A pathophysiologic approach. *Nephron* 60:129–33.

Renal Tubular Acidosis

The following articles are of interest from a historic perspective.

Albright, F., et al. 1946. Osteomalacia and late rickets: Various etiologies met in United States with emphasis on that resulting from specific form of renal acidosis, therapeutic indications for each etiological subgroup, and relationship between osteomalacia and Milkman's syndrome. *Medicine* 25:399–479.

Morris, R. C. J. 1969. Renal tubular acidosis: Mechanisms, classification and implications. *N. Engl. J. Med.* 281:1405–13.

Soriano, J., et al. 1967. Proximal renal tubular acidosis: A defect in bicarbonate reabsorption with normal urinary acidification. *Pediatr. Res.* 1:81–98.

Wrong, O., and H. E. F. Davies. 1959. The excretion of acid in renal disease. *Q. J. Med.* 28:259–313.

The following eight articles provide background on the pathophysiology of RTA.

Bruce, L. J., et al. 1997. Familial distal renal tubular acidosis is associated with mutations in the red cell anion exchanger (Band 3, AE1). *J. Clin. Invest.* 100:1693–707.

Cohen, E. P., et al. 1992. Absence of $H^+ATPase$ in cortical collecting tubules of a patient with Sjögren's syndrome and distal renal tubular acidosis. *J. Am. Soc. Nephrol.* 3:264–71.

Donnelly, S. M., et al. 1992. Might distal renal tubular acidosis be a proximal disorder? *Am. J. Kid. Dis.* 19:272–81.

Halperin, M. L., et al. 1974. Studies on the pathogenesis of type I (distal) renal tubular acidosis as revealed by the urinary P_{CO_2} tensions. *J. Clin. Invest.* 53:669–77.

Halperin, M. L., et al. 1992. In *Clinical disorders of fluid and electrolyte metabolism.* 5th ed. Ed. M. H. Maxwell. C. R. Kleeman, and R. G. Narins, 910–31. New York: McGraw Hill.

Kamel, K. S., et al. 1997. A new classification for renal defects in net acid excretion. *Am. J. Kid. Dis.* 29:126–36.

Vasuvattakul, S., et al. 1992. Should the urine P_{CO_2} or the rate of excretion of NH_4^+ be the gold standard to diagnose distal renal tubular acidosis? *Am. J. Kid. Dis.* 19:72–75.

Vasuvattakul, S., A. Gougoux, and M. L. Halperin. 1993. A method to evaluate renal ammoniagenesis in vivo. *Clin. Invest. Med.* 16:265–73.

The following three articles deal with the pathophysiology of metabolic alkalosis.

Galla, J. H., et al. 1991. Adaptations to chloride-depletion alkalosis. *Am. J. Physiol.* 261:R771–R781.

Galla, J. H., and R. G. Luke. 1987. Pathophysiology of metabolic alkalosis. *Hosp. Pract.* 22:123–46.

Kassirer, J. P., and W. B. Schwartz. 1966. The response of normal man to selective depletion of hydrochloric acid. *Am. J. Med.* 40:10–18.

The following two articles deal with the reabsorption of bicarbonate during metabolic alkalosis.

Maddox, D., and F. Gennari. 1986. Load dependence of proximal tubular bicarbonate reabsorption in chronic metabolic alkalosis in the rat. *J. Clin. Invest.* 77:709–16.

Wesson, D. E. 1994. Combined K^+ and Cl^- repletion corrects augmented H^+ secretion by distal tubules in chronic alkalosis. *Am. J. Physiol.* 35:F592–F603.

The following three articles deal with the treatment of metabolic alkalosis.

Halperin, M. L., A. Scheich. 1994. Should we continue to recommend that a deficit of KCl be treated with NaCl? A fresh look at chloride-depletion metabolic alkalosis. *Nephron* 67:263–69.

Kassirer, J. P., and W. B. Schwartz. 1966. Correction of metabolic alkalosis in man without repair of potassium deficiency. *Am. J. Med.* 40:19–26.

Scheich, A., et al. 1994. Does saline "correct" the abnormal mass balance in meetabolic alkalosis associated with chloride-depletion in the rat. *Clin. Invest. Med.* 17:448–60.

The following seven articles provide information about respiratory acid-base disorders.

Arbus, G. S. 1973. An in vivo acid-base nomogram for clinical use. *Can. Med. Assoc. J.* 109:291–92.

Bercovici, M., et al. 1983. Effect of acute changes in the P_aCO_2 on acid-base parameters in normal dogs and dogs with metabolic acidosis or alkalosis. *Can. J. Physiol. Pharmacol.* 61:166–73.

Brackett, N. C., J. J. Cohen, and W. B. Schwartz. 1965. Carbon dioxide titration curve of normal man. *N. Engl. J. Med.* 272:6–12.

Kamel, K. S., et al. 1993. Rate of production of carbon dioxide in patients with a severe degree of metabolic acidosis. *Nephron* 64:514–17.

Krapf, R., et al. 1991. Chronic respiratory alkalosis: The effect of sustained hyperventilation on renal regulation of acid-base equilibrium. *N. Engl. J. Med.* 324:1394–1401.

Schwartz, W. B., N. C. Brackett, and J. J. Cohen. 1965. The response of extracellular hydrogen ion concentration to graded degrees of chronic hypercapnia: The physiologic limits of the defense of pH. *J. Clin. Invest.* 44:291–301.

Weinberger, S. E., R. M. Schwartzstein, and J. W. Weiss. 1991. Hypercapnia. *N. Engl. J. Med.* 321:1223–31.

The following two articles provide information about mixed acid-base disturbances.

Bear, R., et al. 1977. Effect of metabolic alkalosis on respiratory function in patients with chronic obstructive lung disease. *Can. Med. Assoc. J.* 117:900–03.

Narins, R., and M. Emmett. 1980. Simple and mixed acid-base disorders: A practical approach. *Medicine* 59:161–87.

The following four articles provide a background for the molecular section on acid-base balance.

Alpern, R. J., O. W. Moe, and P. A. Preisig. 1995. Chronic regulation of the proximal tubular Na/H antiporter: From HCO_3 to SRC. *Kidney Int.* 48:1386–96.

Sabolic, I., et al. 1997. Regulation of AE1 anion exchanger and H^+-ATPase in rat cortex by acute metabolic acidosis and alkalosis. *J. Clin. Invest.* 51:125–37.

Soleimani, M., and G. Singh. 1993. Physiologic and molecular aspects of the Na^+/H^+ exchangers in health and disease processes. *J. Investig. Med.* 43:419–30.

Unwin, R., et al. 1996. Unravelling the molecular mechanisms of kidney stones. *Lancet* 348:1561–565.

The following two articles provide a background in the area of integrative aspects of metabolic acidosis.

Asplin, J. R. 1996. Uric acid stones. *Semin. Nephrol.* 16:412–24.

Graham, K. A., et al. 1996. Correction of acidosis in CAPD decreases whole body protein degradation. *Kidney Int.* 49:1396–1400.

Sodium and Water

The following four review articles provide background concerning salt and water balance.

Baylis, P. H., and C. J. Thompson. 1988. Osmoregulation of vasopressin secretion and thirst in health and disease. *Clin. Endocrinol.* 29:549–76.

Feig, P. U., and D. K. McCurdy. 1977. The hypertonic state. *N. Engl. J. Med.* 297:1444–54.

Schrier, R. W. 1992. An odyssey into the milieu interieur: Pondering the enigmas. *J. Am. Soc. Nephrol.* 2:1549–59.

Sonnenberg, H. 1990. Renal regulation of salt balance: A primer for non-purists. *Pediatr. Nephrol.* 4:354–57.

The following two articles provide a reference source on Na^+ and water balance.

Fitzsimons, J. T. 1993. Physiology and pathophysiology of thirst and sodium appetite. In *Clinical disturbances of water metabolism.* Ed. D. W. Seldin and G. Giebisch, 65–97. New York: Raven Press Ltd.

Robertson, G. L. 1993. Regulation of vasopressin secretion. In *Clinical disturbances of water metabolism.* Ed. D. W. Seldin and G. Giebisch, 99–118. New York: Raven Press Ltd.

The following seven articles provide background concerning the physiology of renal water handling.

Gowrishankar, M. 1998. Minimum urine flow rate during water deprivation: Importance of the permeability of urea in the inner medulla. *Kidney Int.* 53:159–66.

Jamison, R. L., D. R. Roy, and H. E. Layton. 1993. Countercurrent mechanisms and its regulation. In *Clinical disturbances of water metabolism.* Ed. D. W. Seldin, and G. H. Giebisch, 119–56. New York: Raven Press.

Macknight, A. D. C., J. Grantham and A. Leaf. 1993. Physiologic responses to changes in extracellular osmolality. In *Clinical disturbances of water metabolism.* Ed. D. W. Seldin and G. Giebisch, 31–49. New York: Raven Press Ltd.

Marples, D., et al. 1996. Hypokalemia-induced down regulation of Aquaporin-2 water channel expression in rat kidney medulla and cortex. *J. Clin. Invest.* 97:1960–968.

Oh, M. S., et al. 1997. Chronic hyponatremia in the absence of ADH: Possible role of decreased delivery of filtrate. *J. Am. Soc. Nephrol.* 8:108A.

Oh, M. S., and M. L. Halperin. 1997. The mechanisms of urine concentration in the inner medulla. *Nephron* 75:384–93.

Soroka, S. D., et al. 1997. Minimum urine flow rate during water deprivation: Importance of the urea and non-urea osmole concentration and excretion rate. *J. Am. Soc. Nephrol.* 8:880–86.

The following five articles provide background concerning the physiology of renal reabsorption of Na$^+$.

Aperia, A. C. 1995. Regulation of sodium transport. *Cur. Opin. Nephrol. Hypertens.* 4:416–20.

Forte, L. R., and F. K. Hamra. 1996. Guanylin and uroguanylin: Intestinal peptide hormones that regulate epithelial transport. *News in Physiol. Sci.* 11:17–24.

Honrath, U., et al. 1997. Effect of sympathetic and angiotensin-aldosterone systems on the renal salt conservation in the rat. *Am. J. Physiol.* 272:F538–F544.

Veress, A. T., et al. 1997. Renal resistance to ANF in salt-depleted rats independent of sympathetic or ANG-aldosterone systems. *Am. J. Physiol.* 272:F545–F550.

Zhang, Y., et al. 1996. Rapid redistribution and inhibition of renal sodium transporters during acute pressure natriuresis. *Am. J. Physiol.* 270:F1004–F1014.

The following two articles deal with the control of cell volume.

Grinstein, S., W. Furuya, and L. Bianchini. 1992. Protein kinases, phosphatases, and the control of cell volume. *News in Physiol. Sci.* 7:232–37.

Gullans, S. R., and J. G. Verbalis. 1993. Control of brain volume during hyperosmolar and hypoosmolar conditions. *Annu. Rev. Med.* 44:289–301.

The following five articles deal with the pathophysiology of hyponatremia.

Gowrishankar, M. G., et al. 1996. What is the impact of potassium excretion on the intracellular fluid volume? Importance of urine anions. *Kidney Int.* 50:1490–495.

Hahn, R. G. 1991. The transurethral resection syndrome. *Acta Anaesth Scand* 35:557–67.

Silver, S. M., R. H. Sterns, and M. L. Halperin. 1996. Brain swelling after dialysis: Old urea or new osmoles. *Am. J. Kid. Dis.* 28:1–13.

Steele, A., et al. 1997. Postoperative hyponatremia despite isotonic saline infusion: A phenomenon of "desalination." *Ann. Intern. Med.* 126:20–25.

Verbalis, J. G. 1991. Hyponatremia: Answered and unanswered questions. *Am. J. Kid. Dis.* 18:546–52.

The following eleven articles focus on the controversy about the rate of treatment of hyponatremia.

Arieff, A. I., and J. C. Ayus. 1991. Treatment of symptomatic hyponatremia: Neither haste nor waste. *Crit. Care Med.* 19:748–51.

Ayus, J. C., and A. I. Arieff. 1996. Brain damage and postoperative hyponatremia: The role of gender. *Neurology* 46:323–28.

Berl, T. 1990. Treating hyponatremia: Damned if we do and damned if we don't. *Kidney Int.* 37:1006–18.

Decaux, G., et al. 1981. Treatment of the syndrome of inappropriate secretion of antidiuretic hormone with furosemide. *N. Engl. J. Med.* 304:329–30.

Laureno, R., and B. I. Karp. 1997. Myelinolysis after correction of hyponatremia. *Ann. Intern. Med.* 126:57–62.

Lohr, J. W. 1994. Osmotic demyelination syndrome following correction of hyponatremia: Association with hypokalemia. *Am. J. Med.* 96:408–13.

Oh, M. S., H. J. Kim, and H. J. Carroll. 1995. Recommendations for treatment of symptomatic hyponatremia. *Nephron* 70:143–50.

Soupart, A., et al. 1994. Prevention of brain demyelination in rats after excessive correction of chronic hyponatremia by serum sodium lowering. *Kidney Int.* 45:193–200.

Soupart, A., and G. Decaux. 1996. Therapeutic recommendations for management of severe hyponatremia: Current concepts on pathogenesis and prevention of neurologic complications. *Clin. Nephrol.* 46:149–69.

Sterns, R. H., E. C. Clark, and S. M. Silver. 1993. Clinical consequences of hyponatremia and its correction. In *Clinical disturbances of water metabolism,* Ed. D. W. Seldin and G. Giebisch, 225–36. New York: Raven Press Ltd.

Wijdicks, E. F., and T. S. Larson. 1994. Absence of postoperative hyponatremia syndrome in young, healthy females. *Ann. Neurol.* 35:626–28.

The following two articles deal with cerebral salt wasting.

Harrigan, M. R. 1996. Cerebral salt wasting: A review. *Neurosurgery* 38:152–60.

Laredo, S., et al. 1996. Coexistence of central diabetes insipidus and salt wasting: The difficulties for diagnosis, changes in natremia, and treatment. *J. Am. Soc. Nephrol.* 7:2527–532.

The following three articles deal with aspects of hypernatremia.

Marsden, P. A., and M. L. Halperin. 1985. Pathophysiologic approach to patients presenting with hypernatremia. *Am. J. Nephrol.* 5:229–35.

Perez, G. O., J. R. Oster, and G. L. Robertson. 1989. Severe hypernatremia with impaired thirst. *Am. J. Nephrol.* 9:421–34.

Star, R. A. 1993. Clinical consequences of hypernatremia and its correction. In *Clinical disturbances of water metabolism.* Ed. D. W. Seldin and G. Giebisch, 237–47. New York: Raven Press Ltd.

The following four articles deal with polyuria.

Magner, P. O., and M. L. Halperin. 1987. Polyuria—a pathophysiological approach. *Med. N. Am.* 15:2971–78.

Narins, R. G., and L. J. Riley. 1991. Polyuria: Simple and mixed disturbances. *Am. J. Kid. Dis.* 17:237–41.

Robertson, G. L. 1988. Differential diagnosis of polyuria. *Annu. Rev. Med.* 39:425–42.

Star, R. A. 1993. Pathogenesis of diabetes insipidus and other polyuric states. In *Clinical disturbances of water metabolism.* Ed. D. W. Seldin and G. Giebisch, 211–24. New York: Raven Press Ltd.

The following three articles deal with the clinical interpretation of urine electrolytes.

Halperin, M. L., and K. L. Skorecki. 1986. Interpretation of the urine electrolytes and osmolality in the regulation of body fluid tonicity. *Am. J. Nephrol.* 6:241–45.

Kamel, K., et al. 1990. Urine electrolytes and osmolality: When and how to use them. *Am. J. Nephrol.* 10:89–102.

Rose, B. D. 1986. New approach to disturbances in the plasma sodium concentration. *Am. J. Med.* 81:1033–40.

The following two review articles deal with hyperglycemia and hyponatremia.

Halperin, M. L., et al. 1993. Clinical consequences of hyperglycemia and its correction. In *Clinical disturbances of water metabolism.* Ed. D. W. Seldin and G. Giebisch, 249–72. New York: Raven Press Ltd.

Roscoe, J., et al. 1975. Hyperglycemia-induced hyponatremia: Metabolic considerations in calculation of serum sodium depression. *Can. Med. Assoc. J.* 112:452–53.

The following two articles deal with diuretics.

Brater, D. C. 1993. Resistance to diuretics: Mechanisms and clinical implications. *Adv. Nephrol.* 22:349–69.

Rose, B. D. 1991. Diuretics (clinical conference). *Kidney Int.* 39:336–52.

The following six articles provide background on some of the molecular aspects of Na$^+$ and water.

Bichet, D. G., A. Oksche, and W. Rosenthal. 1997. Congenital nephrogenic diabetes insipidus. *J. Am. Soc. Nephrol.* 8:1951–958.

Chattopadhyay, N., A. Mithal, and E. M. Brown. 1996. The calcium-sensing receptor: A window into the physiology and pathophysiology of mineral ion metabolism. *Endocr. Rev.* 17:289–307.

Fontaine, B. 1994. Primary periodic paralysis and muscle sodium channel. *Adv. Nephrol.* 23:191–97.

Knepper, M. A. 1997. Molecular physiology of urinary concentrating mechanism: Regulation of aquaporin water channels by vasopressin. *Am. J. Physiol.* 272:F3–F12.

Nielsen, S., et al. 1996. Cellular and subcellular localization of the vasopressin-regulated urea transporter in the kidney. *Proc. Natl. Acad. Sci. USA* 93:5495–500.

Rossier, B. C. 1997. Cum grano salis: The epithelial sodium channel and the control of blood pressure. *J. Am. Soc. Nephrol.* 8:980–92.

Potassium

The following article is of general interest on K$^+$.

Forbes, G. B. 1995. Potassium: The story of an element. *Perspect. Biol. Med.* 38:554–66.

The following eleven articles provide background on the physiology of the excretion of K$^+$.

Carlisle, E. J. F., et al. 1991. Modulation of the secretion on potassium by accompanying anions in humans. *Kidney Int.* 39:1206–12.

Halperin, M. L., et al. 1996. Urea recycling: An aid to the excretion of potassium during antidiuresis. *Nephron* 72:507–11.

Kamel, K. S., et al. 1994. Disorders of potassium homeostasis: An approach based on pathophysiology. *Am. J. Kidney. Dis.* 24:597–613.

Lang, F., and W. Rehwald. 1992. Potassium channels in renal epithelial transport regulation. *Physiol. Rev.* 72:1–32.

Lin, S-H, et al. 1997. Control of the excretion of potassium: Lessons learned from studies during chronic fasting. *Am. J. Physiol.* 273:F796–F800.

Schuster, V., and J. Stokes. 1987. Chloride transport by the cortical and outer medullary collecting duct. *Am. J. Physiol.* 253:F208–F212.

Vasuvattakul, S., et al. 1993. Kaliuretic response to aldosterone: Influence of the content of potassium in the diet. *Am. J. Kid. Dis.* 21:152–60.

Velazquez, H., F. S. Wright, and D. W. Good. 1982. Luminal influences on potassium secretion: Chloride replacement with sulfate. *Am. J. Physiol.* 242:F46–F55.

Wingo, C. S., and F. E. Armitage. 1993. Potassium transport in the kidney: Regulation and physiologic relevance of H$^+$, K$^+$-ATPase. *Semin. Nephrol.* 13:213–24.

Wright, F. S., and G. Giebisch. 1992. Regulation of potassium excretion. In *The kidney: Physiology and pathophysiology.* 2d ed. Ed. D. W. Seldin and G. Giebisch, 2209–47. New York: Raven Press Ltd.

Young, D. B. 1988. Quantitative analysis of aldosterone's role in potassium regulation. *Am. J. Physiol.* 255:F811–F822.

The following nine articles deal with movement of K$^+$ across cell membranes.

Adrogue, H. J., and N. E. Madias. 1981. Changes in plasma potassium concentration during acute acid-base disturbances. *Am. J. Med.* 71:456–67.

Akaike, N. 1988. Regulation of sodium and potassium in muscle of potassium-deficient rats. *News in Physiol. Sci.* 3:25–27.

Brown, A. M. 1992. Ion channels in action potential generation. *Hosp. Pract.* 27:125–32.

Brown, R. S. 1986. External potassium homeostasis. *Kidney Int.* 30:116–27.

Gowrishankar, M. G., et al. 1996. What is the impact of potassium excretion on the intracellular fluid volume: Importance of urine anions. *Kidney Int.* 50:1490–495.

Magner, P. O., et al. 1988. The plasma potassium concentration in metabolic acidosis: A re-evaluation. *Am. J. Kid. Dis.* 11:220–24.

Moore, R. D. 1983. Effects of insulin upon ion transport. *Biochem. Biophys. Acta* 737:1–49.

Rosa, R. M., M. E. Williams, and F. H. Epstein. 1992. Extrarenal potassium metabolism. In *The kidney: Physiology and pathophysiology.* 2d ed. Ed. D. W. Seldin and G. Giebisch, 2165–90. New York: Raven Press Ltd.

Swan, R. C., and R. F. Pitts. 1955. Neutralization of infused acid by nephrectomized dogs. *J. Clin. Invest.* 34:205–12.

The following three articles provide background on diurnal excretion of K$^+$.

Moore-Ede, M. C. 1986. Physiology of the circadian timing system: Predictive versus reactive homeostasis. *Am. J. Physiol.* 250:R735–R752.

Schwartz, W. J. 1996. Internal timekeeping. *Sci. Med.* 3:44–53.

Steele, A., et al. 1994. What is responsible for the diurnal variation in potassium excretion? *Am. J. Physiol.* 258.

The following five articles provide information on drugs and hyperkalemia.

Choi, M. J., et al. 1993. Trimethoprim-induced hyperkalemia in rats. *N. Engl. J. Med.* 328:703–06.

Kamel, K. S., et al. 1992. Studies to determine the basis for hyperkalemia in recipients of a renal transplant who are treated with cyclosporine. *J. Am. Soc. Nephrol.* 2:1279–84.

Ponce, S., et al. 1985. Drug-induced hyperkalemia. *Medicine* 64:357–70.

Schreiber, M. S., et al. 1996. Antikaliuretic action of trimethoprim is minimized by raising urine pH. *Kidney Int.* 49:82–87.

Velazquez, H., et al. 1993. Renal mechanism of trimethoprim-induced hyperkalemia. *Ann. Intern. Med.* 119:295–301.

The following three articles provides background on the renal interactions of magnesium and K+.

Hebert, S. C. 1996. Extracellular calcium-sensing receptor: Implications for calcium and magnesium handling in the kidney. *Kidney Int.* 50:2129–139.

Kamel, K. S., et al. 1998. Studies on the pathogenesis of hypokalemia in Gitelman's syndrome. Role of bicarbonaturia and hypomagnesemia. *Am. J. Nephrol.* 18:42–49.

Quamme, G. A. 1997. Renal magnesium handling: New insights in understanding old problems. *Kidney Int.* 52:1180–195.

The following five articles provide background on the relationship between potassium and hypertension.

Kamel, K. S., and M. L. Halperin. 1994. Hyperkalemia with mild ECF volume contraction: Studies to provide a possible physiologic interpretation. *Clin. Invest. Med.* 17:414–19.

Krishna, G. G., and S. C. Kapoor. 1993. Potassium supplementation ameliorates mineralocorticoid-induced sodium retention. *Kidney Int.* 43:1097–103.

Lathrop, G. M., and F. Soubrier. 1994. Genetic basis of hypertension. In *Curr. Opin. Nephrol. Hypertens.* Ed. B. M. Brenner, 200–06.

Mune, T., et al. 1995. Human hypertension caused by mutations in the kidney isozyme of 11β-hydroxysteroid dehydrogenase. *Nat. Gene.* 10:394–99.

Rossier, B. C.: Cum grano salis. 1997. The epithelial sodium channel and the control of blood pressure. *J. Am. Soc. Nephrol.* 8:980–992.

The following seventeen articles provide background on some of the molecular aspects of K+ homeostasis.

Cannon, S. C., R. H. Brown, Jr., and D. P. Corey. 1991. A sodium channel defect in hyperkalemic periodic paralysis: Potassium-induced failure of inactivation. *Neuron* 6:619–26.

Clore, J., A. Schoolwerth, and C. O. Watlington. 1992. When is cortisol a mineralocorticoid? *Kidney Int.* 42:1297–1308.

George, A. L., Jr. 1995. Molecular genetics of ion channel diseases. *Kidney Int.* 48:1180–190.

Gitelman, H. J. 1994. Unresolved issues in the pathogenesis of Bartter's syndrome and its varients. *Curr. Opin. Nephrol. Hypertens.* 3:471–74.

Gordon, R. D. 1986. Syndrome of hypertension and hyperkalemia with normal glomerular filtration rate. *Hypertension* 8:93–102.

Griggs, R. C., and L. J. Ptacek. 1992. The periodic paralyses. *Hosp. Pract.* 27:123–37.

Guay-Woodford, L. M. 1995. Molecular insights into the pathogenesis of inherited renal tubular disorders. *Curr. Opin. Nephrol. Hypertens.* 4:121–29.

Lehmann-Horn, F., et al. 1991. Altered gating and conductance of Na^+ channels in hyperkalemic periodic paralysis. *Pflugers Arch.* 418:297–99.

Lifton, R. P., et al. 1992. A chimeric 11β-hydroxylase/aldosterone synthetase gene causes glucocorticoid-remediable aldosteronism and human hypertension. *Nature* 355:262–65.

Monder, C. 1991. Corticosteroids, receptors, and the organ-specific functions of 11β-hydroxysteroid dehydrogenase. *FASEB J* 5:3047–54.

Riccardi, D., et al. 1996. Localization of the extracellular Ca^{2+}-sensing receptor and PTH/PTHrP receptor in rat kidney. *Am. J. Physiol.* 271:F951–F956.

Schambelan, M., A. Sebastian, and F. C. Rector, Jr. 1981. Mineralocorticoid-resistant renal hyperkalemia without salt wasting (type II pseudohypoaldosteronism): Role of increased renal chloride reabsorption. *Kidney Int.* 19:716–27.

Schild, L., et al. 1995. A mutation in the epithelial sodium channel causing Liddle disease increases sodium channel activity in *Xenopus Laevis* oocyte expression system. *Proc. Natl. Acad. Sci. USA* 92:5699–703.

Simon, D. B., et al. 1996. Gitelman's variant of Bartter's syndrome, inherited hypokalaemic alkalosis, is caused by mutations in the thiazide-sensitive Na-Cl cotransporter. *Nat. Genet.* 12:24–30.

Simon, D. B., et al. 1996. Bartter's syndrome, hypokalaemic alkalosis with hypercalciuria, is caused by mutations in the Na-K-2Cl cotransporter NKCC2. *Nat. Genet.* 13:183–88.

Simon, D. B., et al. 1997. Mutations in the chloride gene, CLCNKB, cause Bartter's syndrome type III. *Nat. Genet.* 17:171–78.

Warnock, D. G. 1993. Liddle's syndrome: 30 years later. *J. Nephrol.* 6:142–48.

The following two articles provide information about the utility of the TTKG.

Ethier, J. H., et al. 1990. The transtubular potassium concentration in patients with hypokalemia and hyperkalemia. *Am. J. Kid. Dis.* 15:309–15.

West, M. L., P. O. Magner, and R. M. A. Richardson. 1988. A renal mechanism limiting the degree of potassium loss in severely hyperglycemic patients. *Am. J. Nephrol.* 8:373–78.

The following three articles provide information about the treatment of hypokalemia and hyperkalemia.

Donnelly, S. M., et al. 1991. Hypokalemia. In *Current therapy in nephrology and hypertension.* 3rd ed. Ed. J. P. Kassirer, 1015–23. Philadelphia: B. C. Decker, Inc.

Kurtz, I., and L. G. Fine. 1991. Hyperkalemia. In *Current therapy in nephrology and hypertension.* 3rd ed. Ed. J. P. Kassirer, 1023–28. Philadelphia: B. C. Decker, Inc.

Tannen, R. 1985. Diuretic-induced hypokalemia. *Kidney Int.* 28:988–1000.

Hyperglycemia

The following four articles provide background on aspects of carbohydrate metabolism.

Bjorntorp, P., and L. Sjostrom. 1978. Carbohydrate storage in man: Speculations and some quantitative considerations. *Metabolism* 27:1853–85.

Jungas, R. L., M. L. Halperin, and J. T. Brosnan. 1992. Lessons learned from a quantitative analysis of amino acid oxidation and related gluconeogenesis in man. *Physiol. Rev.* 72:419–48.

Martin, B. J. 1990. Gut transit with exercise. *Gastroenterology* 99:290.

Randle, P. 1986. Fuel selection in animals. *Biochem. Soc. Trans.* 14:799–806.

The authors recommend the following textbook.

Halperin, M. L., and F. S. Rolleston. 1993. *Clinical detective stories: A problem-based approach to clinical cases in energy and acid-base metabolism.* London: Portland Press.

The following five articles provide information on the renal handling of glucose.

Deetjen, P., H. V. Baeyer, and H. Drexel. 1992. Renal glucose transport. In *The kidney: Physiology and pathophysiology.* 2nd ed. Ed. D. W. Seldin and G. Giebisch, 249–72. New York: Raven Press Ltd.

Halperin, M. L., et al. 1980. Quantitative aspects of hyperglycemia in the diabetic: A theoretical approach. *Clin. Invest. Med.* 2:127–30.

Kurtzman, N., and V. Pillay. 1973. Renal reabsorption of glucose in health and disease. *Arch. Intern. Med.* 131:901–04.

Magner, P. O., and M. L. Halperin. 1990. Effect of metabolic acidosis on glucose reabsorption in rats with acute hyperglycemia. *Can. J. Physiol. Pharmacol.* 68:79–83.

Mogensen, C. 1971. Maximum tubular reabsorption capacity for glucose and renal hemodynamics during rapid hypertonic glucose infusion in normal and diabetic subjects. *Scand. J. Clin. Lab. Invest.* 28:101–09.

The following two articles help define the deficits of electrolytes in patients with a severe degree of hyperglycemia.

Danowski, T. S., et al. 1949. Studies in diabetic acidosis and coma, with particular emphasis on the retention of administered potassium. *J. Clin. Invest.* 28:1–9.

Nabarro, J., A. Spencer, and J. Stowers. 1952. Metabolic studies in severe diabetic ketosis. *Quart. J. Med.* 82:225–43.

The following three articles deal with clinical aspects of hyperglycemia.

Arieff, A. I., and H. J. Carroll. 1971. Hyperosmolar nonketotic coma with hyperglycemia: Abnormalities of lipid and carbohydrate metabolism. *Metabolism* 20:529.

Gedulin, B. R., and A. A. Young. 1998. Hypoglycemia overrides amylin-mediated regulation of gastric emptying in rats. *Diabetes* 47:93–97.

West, M., et al. 1986. A quantitative analysis of glucose loss during acute therapy for the hyperglycemia hyperosmolar syndrome. *Diabetes Care* 9:465–71.

The following article deals with hyperglycemia and hyponatremia.

Halperin, M. L., et al. 1993. Clinical consequences of hyperglycemia and its correction. In *Clinical disturbances of water metabolism*, ed. D. W. Seldin and G. Giebisch, 249–72. New York: Raven Press Ltd.

Roscoe, J., et al. 1975. Hyperglycemia-induced hyponatremia: Metabolic considerations in calculation of serum sodium depression. *Can. Med. Assoc. J.* 112:452–53.

Index